High Altitude Medicine and Physiology

Fourth edition

John B. West, MD, PhD, DSc, FRCP, FRACP
Professor of Medicine & Physiology, School of Medicine, University of California,
San Diego, USA

Robert B. Schoene, MD
Clinical Professor of Medicine, School of Medicine, University of California,
San Diego, USA

James S. Milledge, MB, ChB, MD, FRCP
Formerly Consultant Respiratory Physician and Scientific Member Medical Research
Council, Northwick Park Hospital, Harrow. Hon Professor, Physiology Dept. University
College London. UK

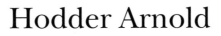

Hodder Arnold

A MEMBER OF THE HODDER HEADLINE GROUP

Dedicated to the memory of Michael Ward (1925–2005) who was lead author of the previous three editions of this book and whose pioneering book, *Mountain Medicine* (published in 1975), was the forerunner to this volume.

First published in Great Britain in 1989 by Chapman and Hall
Second edition 1998
Third edition 2000
This fourth edition published in 2007 by
Hodder Arnold, an imprint of Hodder Education and a member of the Hodder Headline Group,
338 Euston Road, London NW1 3BH

http://www.hoddereducation.com

Whilst the advice and information in this book are believed to be true and accurate at
the date of going to press, neither the author[s] nor the publisher can accept any legal
responsibility or liability for any errors or omissions that may be made. In particular (but
without limiting the generality of the preceding disclaimer) every effort has been made
to check drug dosages; however it is still possible that errors have been missed. Furthermore,
dosage schedules are constantly being revised and new side-effects recognized. For these
reasons the reader is strongly urged to consult the drug companies' printed instructions
before administering any of the drugs recommended in this book.

British Library Cataloguing in Publication Data
A catalogue record for this book is available from the British Library

Library of Congress Cataloging-in-Publication Data
A catalog record for this book is available from the Library of Congress

ISBN   978 0 340 913 444

1 2 3 4 5 6 7 8 9 10

Commissioning Editor: Philip Shaw
Project Editor: Heather Fyfe
Production Controller: Karen Tate
Cover Designer: Laura DeGrasse

Typeset in 10/12 pt Minion by Charon Tec (A Macmillan Company), Chennai, India
www.charontec.com
Printed and bound in Great Britain by CPI Bath

What do you think about this book? Or any other Hodder Arnold title?
Please visit our website: **www.hoddereducation.com**

Contents

Preface

This new edition of *High Altitude Medicine and Physiology* incorporates some major changes. First, Michael Ward has retired after spearheading the first three editions. Indeed it was his previous book, *Mountain Medicine*, which provided the initial impetus for this text which has enjoyed considerable success as a standard work in the area. With Michael's departure, Robert 'Brownie' Schoene has joined us thus adding new young blood. The three of us previously worked extensively together at high altitude during the 1981 American Medical Research Expedition to Everest and this makes a nice comparison with the three original editors who were together on the 1960–61 Silver Hut Expedition.

Brownie Schoene is well known to physicians and physiologists interested in high altitude. He has studied the control of ventilation at high altitude, particularly the importance of the hypoxic ventilatory response for tolerating extreme altitude. In addition, with Peter Hackett, he carried out some remarkable investigations high on Denali where climbers with high altitude pulmonary edema consented to bronchoalveolar lavage. These bold studies showed that the alveolar fluid had a very high protein concentration and contained numerous cells thus proving that it was a high permeability type of edema caused by damage to the pulmonary capillaries. His expertise in high altitude medicine and physiology complements that of the other two editors very well.

In addition to this change in editors, there have been major changes in the scientific content of the book with updates in many areas. Since the last edition, the area of genetics has assumed great importance along with other advances in molecular biology and medicine. There are now numerous allusions to these topics throughout the text, particularly in the areas of mechanisms of oxygen sensing, regulation of the pulmonary circulation particularly hypoxic pulmonary vasoconstriction, adaptation of permanent residents of high altitude, and tolerance to extreme altitude. It was thought preferable to deal with genetic and molecular mechanisms throughout the text rather than have a specific chapter devoted to them. Other areas where extensive updating has occurred include sections on women and children at high altitude, the role of vascular endothelial growth factor, neurological disorders at high altitude, athletic training using high altitude, recent work on high altitude pulmonary edema, and the problems of patients with existing diseases who plan to go to high altitude.

All this new information could substantially increase the size of the book but we have tried to avoid this by prudent pruning. For example, we have reduced the length of the sections on cold injury. Although this topic can be important at high altitude, injuries caused by cold are certainly not limited to this environment. Cold injury was one of the primary interests of Michael Ward, and in this new edition we have attempted to include sufficient information to inform people who go to high altitude about prevention and treatment without going into as much detail as in the previous editions.

In addition to these substantial changes in scientific content, a number of formatting changes have been made to make the book easier to read. We have kept the summaries at the beginning of each chapter but these have been highlighted to make them clearer. Additional tables have also been incorporated; for example, dealing with the features and the treatment of some of the most important high altitude diseases including acute mountain sickness, high altitude pulmonary edema, and high altitude cerebral edema.

Finally, the rapid pace of advances in the area of high altitude medicine and physiology clearly justifies a new edition. In the six years since the last edition appeared there have been several international meetings of the International Society for Mountain Medicine, various international Hypoxia meetings, and a welter of new material appearing in journals. The journal *High Altitude Medicine and Biology* which had just begun publication when the last edition appeared has now become established as the international journal in the field.

Increasingly, lowlanders go to high altitude to trek, ski or climb, and there is also a large increase in the number of people who now work at high altitude, for example in mines or with telescopes. Even more important perhaps is the large population of permanent residents of high altitude who have generally received short shrift in the past partly because many are in poorly developed countries. However, there is presently a great increase in interest in diseases such as chronic mountain sickness and high altitude heart diseases of residents. Our hope, as was the case for previous editions of this book, is that it will continue to improve the health and safety of all people who visit, live or work at high altitude.

John B. West
Robert B. Schoene
James S. Milledge

Acknowledgments

We wish to acknowledge help from many friends and colleagues who have read and commented helpfully on parts of the text, especially John English FRCP, Sukhamay Lahiri Ph.D. and Frank Powell, Ph.D.

We gratefully acknowledge the invaluable help of Jon Preisemberger, administrative assistant to JBW, and Pat Howell who read and corrected the chapters and proofs from JSM. We wish to thank our Project Editor, Heather Fyfe, and the staff at Hodder Arnold and our proofreader, Annette Abel, for seeing the publication through.

We would also like to thank all those who contribued to the original work on which much of this book is based. These include Sherpas, porters, climbers, scientists and other supporters who made the projects possible. We remember too, with gratitude, all those who share the adventure of science with colleagues in the high places of the world.

Conversion tables

Table F.1 Conversion of pressure units mmHg (millimeters of mercury) to kPa (kilopascals)

mm Hg	kPa
1	0.133
10	1.33
20	2.67
30	4.00
40	5.33
50	6.67
60	8.00
80	10.7
100	13.3
200	26.7
300	40.0
500	66.7
700	93.3
760	101.3

1 torr = 1 mmHg

Table F.2 Conversion of height units and barometric pressure according to the ICAO Standard Atmosphere. Note that in the great mountain ranges the actual pressure will usually be higher than given by the table (Chapter 2)

Altitude		Pressure mmHg
m	ft	
0	0	760
1 000	3 281	674
2 000	6 562	596
3 000	9 843	526
4 000	13 123	462
5 000	16 404	405
6 000	19 685	354
7 000	22 966	308
8 000	26 247	267
9 000	29 258	231

Table F.3 Conversion of temperature units, °C (degrees Celsius) to °F (degrees Fahrenheit)

°C	°F
−40	−40
−30	−20
−25	−13
−20	−4
−15	5
−10	14
−5	23
0	32
5	41
10	50
15	59
20	68
25	77
50	86
35	95
40	104

Table F.4 Conversion of energy units, kcal (kilocalories) to kJ (kilojoules)

kcal	kJ
50	209.4
100	418.8
250	1 047
500	2 094
1 000	4 188
2 000	8 375
3 000	12 563
4 000	16 750
5 000	20 938
6 000	25 126

List of abbreviations

A–a	alveolar–arterial	FVC	forced vital capacity
ACE	angiotensin converting enzyme	HACE	high altitude cerebral edema
ADH	antidiuretic hormone	HAGA	high altitude global amnesia
AFC	alveolar fluid clearance	HAPE	high altitude pulmonary edema
AMREE	American Medical Research Expedition to Everest	HCVR	hypercapnic ventilatory response
		HIF-1α	hypoxia-inducing factor 1α
AMS	acute mountain sickness	HVR	hypoxic ventilatory response
ANP	atrial natriuretic peptide	IH	intermittent hypoxia
AVP	arginine vasopressin	IUGR	intrauterine growth retardation
BAL	bronchoalveolar lavage	LH	luteinizing hormone
BCAA	branched-chain amino acid	LHTL	living high, training low
BMR	basal metabolic rate	LVF	left ventricular failure
BP	blood pressure	MRI	magnetic resonance imaging
BTPS	body temperature, ambient pressure, saturated with water vapor	MVV	maximal voluntary ventilation
		NO	nitric oxide
CBF	cerebral blood flow	17-OHCSs	17-hydroxy corticosteroids
CCK	cholecystokinin	OSA	obstructive sleep apnea
CMS	chronic mountain sickness	PA,CO_2	alveolar partial pressure of carbon dioxide
CNS	central nervous system		
COPD	chronic obstructive pulmonary disease	Pa,CO_2	arterial partial pressure of carbon dioxide
CSA	central sleep apnea		
CSF	cerebrospinal fluid	PA,O_2	alveolar partial pressure of oxygen
CT	computerized tomography	Pa,O_2	arterial partial pressure of oxygen
DCO	diffusing capacity of carbon monoxide	PCO_2	partial pressure of carbon dioxide
DLCO	diffusing capacity of the lung for carbon monoxide	PO_2	partial pressure of oxygen
		$P_{ET}CO_2$	end-tidal partial pressure of carbon monoxide
2,3-DPG	2,3-diphosphoglycerate		
ECF	extracellular fluid	PI,H_2O	pressure of inspired water vapor
ECG	electrocardiogram	PI,O_2	ambient to inspired partial pressure of oxygen
EEG	electroencephalogram		
EMG	electromyogram	P_i	intracellular phosphate
eNOS	endothelial nitric oxide synthase	Pv,O_2	mixed venous partial pressure of oxygen
EPO	erythropoietin	PAL	physical activity level
ERPF	effective plasma renal flow	PAP	pulmonary artery pressure
ESQ	Environmental Symptom Questionnaire	PCV	packed cell volume
		PPA	pulmonary artery pressure
ET-1	endothelin-1	PPH	primary pulmonary hypertension
FEV_1	forced expiratory volume in 1 s	PRA	plasma renin activity
FSH	follicle stimulating hormone	PRK	photorefractive keratectomy

PTE	thrombo-embolic disease		SIGA	secretory immunoglobulin A
PV	plasma volume		SL	sea level
RBCs	red blood cells		STPD	standard temperature and pressure, dry gas
RCM	red cell mass			
RDBPC	randomized, double-blind, placebo-controlled trial		SWS	slow wave sleep
			T_3	triiodothyronine
REDST	thiol disulfide redox state		T_4	thyroxine
REM	rapid eye movement		TIA	transient ischemic attack
RK	radial keratotomy		TSH	thyroid stimulating hormone
ROS	reactive oxygen species		UKIRT	United Kingdom Infrared Telescope
RQ	respiratory quotient		$\dot{V}_{O_2,max}$	maximum oxygen consumption kg^{-1}
$Sa,_{O_2}$	arterial oxygen saturation		VDH	ventilatory deacclimatization from hypoxia
SIDS	sudden infant death syndrome			
SiEp	serum immunoreactive erthyropoietin concentration		VEGF	vascular endothelial growth factor
			WBCs	white blood cells

History

SUMMARY

The history of high altitude medicine and physiology is one of the most colorful in the whole of the life sciences. Although there were a few anecdotal references to medical problems at high altitude before 1600, Joseph de Acosta's description of acute mountain sickness, originally published in 1590, is a watershed. Shortly after this the mercury barometer was invented by Evangelista Torricelli in 1644, and very quickly it was recognized that barometric pressure declined with altitude. Robert Boyle and Robert Hooke constructed the first air pump for physiological measurements in 1660 and Boyle then proposed his famous law. During the seventeenth and eighteenth centuries the nature of respiration was elucidated and the respiratory gases were first clearly described by Lavoisier in 1777. Soon the effects of acute ascent to high altitude were dramatically shown by the early balloonists including several fatalities from the severe hypoxia. The French physiologist, Paul Bert, was the first to clearly identify the low partial pressure of oxygen as responsible for high altitude illness with his landmark publication *La Pression Barométrique* in 1878.

When climbing became popular in the European Alps in the mid-nineteenth century many instances of acute mountain sickness were described. The construction of the Observatoire Vallot in France and the Capanna Margherita in Italy facilitated early medical and physiological studies of high altitude. The early twentieth century saw the beginning of special expeditions to high altitude to make medical and physiological measurements including the important Pikes Peak Expedition of 1911. A lively topic at this time was the possibility of oxygen secretion by the lung and this was finally resolved in favor of passive diffusion. Attempts to climb the highest mountain in the world, Mount Everest, comprise a great saga culminating in the first ascent in 1953 when supplemental oxygen was used, and the first ascent without bottled oxygen in 1978.

More recently, there have been several dedicated expeditions to explore the physiology of extreme altitude and generally an enormous increase in high altitude life sciences research. An important area has been the medical and physiological problems of permanent residents of high altitude, and also ways of improving the quality of life for people who are required to work at high altitude.

1.1 INTRODUCTION

This chapter provides an overall view of the history of high altitude medicine and physiology. More information about specific events is given at the beginning of subsequent chapters. Readers who desire more details can find these in West (1998). Table 1.1 shows a chronology of some of the principal events in the development of high altitude medicine and physiology.

1.2 CLASSICAL GREECE AND ROME

It is perhaps surprising that there are so few references to the ill effects of high altitude in the extensive writings of classical Greece and Rome. The Greek epics and myths, in particular, are so rich in the accounts of travels and the foibles of human nature that one might expect there to be a reference to the deleterious effects of high altitude but this is generally not the case. However, seventeenth century writers believed that the ancient Greeks were aware of the thinness of the air at high altitude. For example, Robert Boyle (1627–91) claimed that Aristotle (384–322 BC) held this view when he wrote:

> That which some of those that treat of the height of Mountains, relate out of *Aristotle*, namely, That those that ascend to the top of the Mountain *Olympus*, could not keep themselves alive, without carrying with them wet Spunges, by whose assistance they could respire in that Air, otherwise too thin for Respiration:... (Boyle 1660, p. 357)

However, modern historians have not been able to find this statement in Aristotle's extensive writings. Similar attributions to Aristotle can be found in the writings of Francis Bacon (1561–1626) and St Augustine of Hippo (354–430).

1.3 CHINESE HEADACHE MOUNTAINS

There is a tantalizing reference to what may have been acute mountain sickness in the classical Chinese history the *Ch'ien Han Shu* which dates from about 30 BC. One of the Chinese officials was warning about the dangers of traveling to the western regions, probably part of present day Afghanistan, when he stated that travelers would not only be exposed to attacks from robbers but they would also become ill. One of the translations reads:

> Again, on passing the Great Headache Mountain, the Little Headache Mountain, the Red Land, and the Fever Slope, men's bodies become feverish, they lose colour, and are attacked with headache and vomiting; the asses and cattle being all in like condition. . . .

Several people have tried to identify the site of the Headache Mountains suggesting for instance that it is the Kilik Pass (4827 m) in the Karakoram Range on the route from Kashgar to Gilgit (Gilbert 1983). However, there is not universal agreement on this.

1.4 POSSIBLE EARLY REFERENCE TO HIGH ALTITUDE PULMONARY EDEMA

Fâ-Hien was a Chinese Buddhist monk who made a remarkable journey through China and adjoining countries in about 400 AD. He related that when crossing the 'Little Snowy Mountains' (probably in Afghanistan) his companion became ill, 'a white froth came from his mouth' and he died. It is tempting to identify this as the first description of high altitude pulmonary edema.

1.5 JOSEPH DE ACOSTA'S DESCRIPTION OF MOUNTAIN SICKNESS

Joseph de Acosta (1540–1600) was a Jesuit priest who traveled to Peru in about 1570. While he was there he ascended the Andes and gave a very colorful account of illness associated with high altitude. This was first published in 1590 in Spanish (Acosta 1590) (Fig. 1.1), and an English translation entitled *The Naturall and Morall Historie of the East and*

Table 1.1 Chronology of some principal events in the development of high altitude medicine and physiology

Year	Event
c. 30 BC	Reference to the Great Headache Mountain and Little Headache Mountain in the *Ch'ien Han Shu* (classical Chinese history)
1590	Publication of the first edition (Spanish) of *Historia Natural y Moral de las Indias* by Joseph de Acosta with an account of mountain sickness
1644	First description of the mercury barometer by Torricelli
1648	Demonstration of the fall in barometric pressure at high altitude in an experiment devised by Pascal
1777	Clear description of oxygen and the other respiratory gases by Lavoisier
1783	Montgolfier brothers initiate balloon ascents
1786	First ascent of Mont Blanc (4807 m) by Balmat and Paccard
1878	Publication of *La Pression Barométrique* by Paul Bert
1890	Viault describes high altitude polycythemia
1890	Joseph Vallot builds a high altitude laboratory at 4350 m on Mont Blanc
1891	Christian Bohr publishes *Uber die Lungenathmung*, giving evidence for both oxygen and carbon dioxide secretion by the lung
1893	High altitude station, Capanna Regina Margherita, is built on a summit of Monte Rosa at 4559 m
1906	Publication of *Hohenklima und Bergwanderungen* by Zuntz *et al.*
1909	The Duke of the Abruzzi reaches 7500 m in the Karakoram without supplementary oxygen
1910	Zuntz organizes an international high altitude expedition to Tenerife
1910	August Krogh publishes *On the Mechanism of Gas-Exchange in the Lungs*, disproving the secretion theory of gas exchange
1911	Anglo-American Pikes Peak expedition (4300 m); participants C. G. Douglas, J. S. Haldane, Y. Henderson and E. C. Schneider
1913	T. H. Ravenhill publishes *Some Experiences of Mountain Sickness in the Andes*, describing *puna* of the normal, cardiac and nervous types
1920	Barcroft *et al.* publish the results of the experiment carried out in a glass chamber in which Barcroft lived in a hypoxic atmosphere for 6 days
1921	A. M. Kellas finishes his manuscript on 'A consideration of the possibility of ascending Mt. Everest' which remained unpublished until 2001
1921–22	International High Altitude Expedition to Cerro de Pasco, Peru, led by Joseph Barcroft
1924	E. F. Norton ascends to 8500 m on Mount Everest without supplementary oxygen
1925	Barcroft publishes *Lessons from High Altitude*
1935	International High Altitude Expedition to Chile, scientific leader D. B. Dill
1946	Operation Everest I carried out by C. S. Houston and R. L. Riley
1948	Carlos Monge M. publishes *Acclimatization in the Andes*, about the permanent residents of the Peruvian Andes
1949	H. Rahn and A. B. Otis publish *Man's Respiratory Response During and After Acclimatization to High Altitude*
1952	L. G. C. E. Pugh and colleagues carry out experiments on Cho Oyu near Mount Everest in preparation for the 1953 expedition
1953	First ascent of Mount Everest by Hillary and Tenzing (with supplementary oxygen)
1960–61	Himalayan Scientific and Mountaineering Expedition in the Everest region, scientific leader L. G. C. E. Pugh. Silver Hut laboratory at 5800 m, measurements up to 7440 m
1968–79	High altitude studies on Mount Logan (5334 m), scientific director C. S. Houston
1973	Italian Mount Everest Expedition with laboratory at 5350 m, scientific leader P. Cerretelli

(*continued*)

Table 1.1   (Continued)

Year	Event
1978	First ascent of Everest without supplementary oxygen by Reinhold Messner and Peter Habeler
1981	American Medical Research Expedition to Everest, scientific leader J. B. West
1985	Operation Everest II, scientific leaders C. S. Houston and J. R. Sutton
1983 to present	Research at Capanna Regina Margherita (4559 m) by O. Oelz, P. Bärtsch and co-workers from Zurich, Bern and Heidelberg
1984 to present	Studies at Observatoire Vallot (4350 m) on Mont Blanc by J.-P. Richalet and co-workers
1990 to present	Research at Pyramid Laboratory, Lobuje, Nepal by P. Cerretelli and co-workers
1994	British Mount Everest Medical Research Expedition, leaders S. Currin, A. Pollard, D. Collier
1997	Operation Everest III (COMEX '97), leader J.-P. Richalet
1998	Medical Research Expedition to Kangchenjunga, leaders S. Currin, D. Collier, J. Milledge

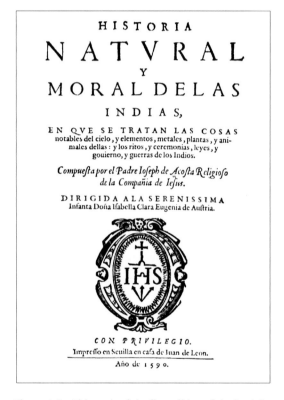

Figure 1.1   Title page of the first edition of the book by Joseph de Acosta published in Seville in 1590.

West Indies appeared in 1604 (Acosta 1604). Here are some passages from his account when the party were near the top of Mount Pariacaca.

> I was suddenly surprized with so mortall and strange a pang, that I was ready to fall from the top to the ground. . . .

He then went on to add:

> I was surprized with such pangs of straining & casting, as I thought to cast up my heart too; for having cast up meate, fleugme & choller, both yellow and greene; in the end I cast up blood, with the straining of my stomacke. To conclude, if this had continued, I should undoubtedly have died. . . .

This is followed by an often-quoted passage:

> I therefore perswade my selfe that the element of the aire is there so subtile and delicate, as it is not proportionable with the breathing of man, which requires a more grosse and temperate aire, and I beleeve it is the cause that doth so much alter the stomacke, & trouble all the disposition.

It should be noted that this not a typical account of acute mountain sickness which usually comes on gradually and is not associated with severe vomiting. The description sounds more like a gastrointestinal upset.

Acosta's book was widely read and, for example, Robert Boyle was familiar with his description of mountain sickness. Various people including Gilbert (1991) have attempted to identify the site of Pariacaca but there is some disagreement over this.

1.6 INVENTION OF THE BAROMETER

A key advance in high altitude science was the recognition that barometric pressure falls with

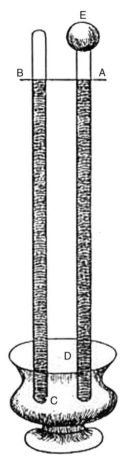

Figure 1.2 Torricelli's drawing of his first mercury barometer, from his letter to Michelangelo Ricci of 1644.

increasing altitude. In 1644 Evangelista Torricelli (1608–47) wrote a letter to his friend Michelangelo Ricci in which he described how he had filled a glass tube with mercury and inverted it so that one end was immersed in a dish of the same liquid (Torricelli 1644) (Fig. 1.2). The mercury descended to form a column about 76 cm high, and Torricelli argued that the mercury was supported by the weight of the atmosphere acting on the dish. His letter included the striking sentence: 'We live submerged at the bottom of an ocean of the element air, which by unquestioned experiments is known to have weight....' This was a conceptual breakthrough. Torricelli also speculated that on the tops of high mountains the pressure might be less because the air is 'distinctly rare.'

However, it was left to Blaise Pascal (1623–62) to prove that barometric pressure falls with increasing altitude. In 1648 he persuaded his brother-in-law, Florin Perier, to carry a mercury barometer up the Puy-de-Dôme in central France. This was an elaborate experiment with careful controls and he was successful in showing that on the summit the pressure had fallen by approximately 12% of its value in the village of Clermont.

1.7 INVENTION OF THE AIR PUMP

The first effective air pump was constructed by Otto von Guericke (1602–86) who was mayor of the city of Magdeburg in central Germany. In a famous experiment he constructed two metal hemispheres that fitted together accurately when the air within them was pumped out. Two teams of horses were then unable to separate the two hemispheres, graphically demonstrating the enormous force that could be developed by the air pressure.

However, Guericke's pump was cumbersome to operate and it was impossible to place objects in the hemispheres to study the effects of the reduced air pressure. This was first done by Robert Boyle (1627–91) and his colleague Robert Hooke (1635–1703). Hooke was a mechanical genius who designed an air pump consisting of a piston inside a brass cylinder. Above this was a large glass receiver into which various objects and small animals could be placed (Fig. 1.3). In his groundbreaking book *New Experiments Physico-Mechanicall, Touching the Spring of the Air, and its Effects...* (Boyle 1660), he demonstrated the effects of a reduced atmospheric pressure in a variety of experiments. In one of these a lark was placed in the receiver and Boyle wrote:

the Lark was very lively, and did, being put into the Receiver, divers times spring up in it to a good height. The Vessel being hastily, but carefully clos'd, the Pump was diligently ply'd, and the Bird for a while appear'd lively enough; but upon a greater Exsuction of the Air, she began manifestly to droop and appear sick, and very soon after was taken with as violent and irregular Convulsions, as are wont to be observ'd in Poultry, when their heads are wrung off. ...

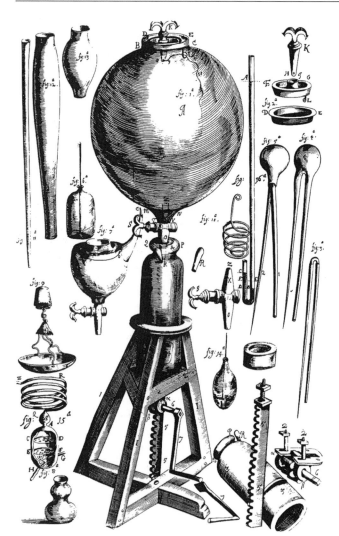

Figure 1.3   Air pump constructed by Robert Boyle and Robert Hooke. This enabled them to carry out the first experiments on hypobaric hypoxia. From Boyle (1660).

Following these experiments Hooke made a chamber large enough for a man to sit in it while it was partially evacuated and he reported to the young Royal Society:

> that himself had been in it, and by the contrivance of bellows and valves blown out of it one tenth part of the air (which he found by a gage suspended within the vessel) and had felt no inconvenience but that of some pain in his ears at the breaking out of the air included in them, and the like pain upon the readmission of the air pressing the ear inwards.

1.8 DISCOVERY OF OXYGEN

Progress in the remainder of the seventeenth century and most of the eighteenth century was largely stymied until the nature of the respiratory gases was characterized. There is not space to follow the interesting story here of the work of Boyle, Hooke, Lower and Mayow in the seventeenth century and the discovery of oxygen by Joseph Priestley (1733–1804), Carl Scheele (1742–86) and Antoine Lavoisier (1743–94). John Mayow (1641–79) was aware in 1674 of what he called 'nitro-aerial spirit' which we now recognize as oxygen but his work was largely ignored for almost

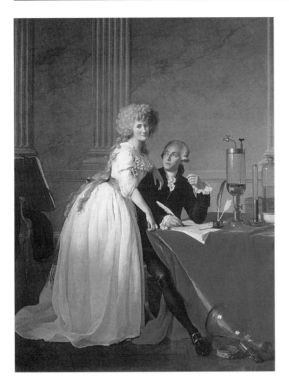

Figure 1.4   Antoine Lavoisier (1747–1794) with his wife Marie-Anne (1759–1836), who was his laboratory assistant. From the painting by David, 1780.

a century. Both Priestley and Scheele independently isolated oxygen but Priestley was confused about its nature, believing that it was 'unphlogisticated air,' and Scheele's report was delayed because of publication problems. It was left to the brilliant French chemist Lavoisier (Fig. 1.4) to clearly describe the three respiratory gases. In 1777 he stated:

> Eminently respirable air [he later called it *oxygine*] that enters the lung, leaves it in the form of chalky aeriform acids [carbon dioxide] . . . in almost equal volume. . . . Respiration acts only on the portion of pure air that is eminently respirable . . . the excess, that is its mephitic portion [nitrogen], is a purely passive medium which enters and leaves the lung . . . without change or alteration. The respirable portion of air has the property to combine with blood and its combination results in its red color.

Carbon dioxide had been discovered earlier by Joseph Black (1728–99) while he was a medical student although he used the term 'fixed air.'

1.9 FIRST BALLOON ASCENTS AND THE RECOGNITION OF SEVERE ACUTE HYPOXIA

The Montgolfier brothers, Joseph (1740–1810) and Jacques (1745–99), invented the man-carrying balloon, first using heated air, and later hydrogen. The first free ascent of a manned balloon took place in Paris in 1783. It was not long before these adventurous balloonists became aware of the deleterious effects of high altitude on the body. For example, Alexandre Charles (1746–1823) (of Charles' Law) ascended in a hydrogen-filled balloon in December 1783 and reported 'In the midst of the inexpressible rapture of this contemplative ecstasy, I was recalled to myself by a very extraordinary pain in the interior of my right ear. . . .' He correctly attributed this to the effects of air pressure.

However, more ominous effects were soon noted. Jean Blanchard (1753–1809) claimed to have ascended to an altitude of over 10 000 m in 1785 (although the altitude was contested) and reported that 'Nature grew languid, I felt a numbness, prelude of a dangerous sleep. . . .' However, much more dramatic were the events in 1862 when James Glaisher (1809–1903) and Henry Coxwell (1819–1900) rose to an altitude which was estimated to exceed 10 000 m. Glaisher became partly paralyzed and then unconscious, and Coxwell lost the use of his hands, and could only open the valve of the balloon by seizing the cord with his teeth. Glaisher also reported losing his sight before his partial paralysis.

The most famous and tragic balloon ascent was by three French aeronauts Gaston Tissandier (1843–99), Joseph Crocé-Spinelli (1843–75) and Theodore Sivel (1834–75) in their balloon *Zénith* in 1875. Paul Bert (see below) had recommended that they take oxygen but they had too little and there were difficulties in inhaling it. Tissandier's report (1875) is dramatic.

> Towards 7500 meters, the numbness one experiences is extraordinary. . . . One does not suffer at all; on the contrary. One experiences

inner joy, as if it were an effect of the inundating flood of light. One becomes indifferent. . . . Soon I wanted to seize the oxygen tube, but could not raise my arm. . . . Suddenly I closed my eyes and fell inert, entirely losing consciousness.

When the balloon ultimately reached the ground, Sivel and Crocé-Spinelli were dead, having perished as a result of the severe hypoxia. The disaster caused a sensation in France.

1.10 MOUNTAIN SICKNESS IN MOUNTAINEERS

During the nineteenth century mountaineering became popular particularly in the European Alps. The result was many descriptions of acute mountain sickness, some of which seem to us today to be greatly exaggerated. One of the first was from the great German naturalist Alexander von Humboldt (1769–1859) when he reached very high altitudes on two volcanoes in South America in 1799. On Chimborazo at an altitude of about 5540 m he stated that the whole party felt 'a discomfort, a weakness, a desire to vomit, which certainly arises as much from the lack of oxygen in these regions as from the rarity of the air.' Another early account was by Horace-Bénédict de Saussure (1740–99) on Mont Blanc (4807 m) in 1787. When he was near the summit he stated:

I therefore hoped to reach the crest in less than three quarters of an hour; but the rarity of the air gave me more trouble than I could have believed. At last I was obliged to stop for breath every fifteen or sixteen steps. . . . This need of rest was absolutely unconquerable; if I tried to overcome it, my legs refused to move. . .

Numerous other reports of the deleterious effects of high altitude while climbing mountains are given in the first chapter of Paul Bert's book *La Pression Barométrique* (1878).

1.11 PAUL BERT AND THE PUBLICATION OF *LA PRESSION BAROMÉTRIQUE*

The French environmental physiologist Paul Bert (1833–86) is often cited as the father of modern high

altitude physiology and medicine. The publication of his great book *La Pression Barométrique* in 1878 was certainly an important landmark. One of his principal findings was that the deleterious effects of exposure to low pressure could be attributed to the low P_{O_2}. He did this by exposing experimental animals to a low pressure of air on the one hand (hypobaric hypoxia), and to gas mixtures at normal pressure but with a low oxygen concentration (normobaric hypoxia) on the other. In this way he showed that the critical variable was the P_{O_2}. *La Pression Barométrique* is essential reading for anybody with a serious interest in the history of high altitude medicine and physiology. For one thing, there is a long introductory section on the history as Bert saw it, and this makes fascinating reading today. Bert wrote with a charming style and urbane wit. The book not only deals with the medical and physiological effects of low pressure but high pressure as well.

Many of Bert's studies were carried out at the Sorbonne in Paris which was equipped with both low pressure and high pressure chambers (Fig. 1.5). At one stage he tested the three French balloonists Tissandier, Crocé-Spinelli and Sivel who were referred to above and he actually warned them that they had insufficient oxygen but the warning letter arrived too late.

La Pression Barométrique includes many interesting passages. For example, it contains the first graphs of the oxygen and carbon dioxide dissociation curves in blood. Bert also speculated that polycythemia might occur at high altitude and this was shown a short time later by compatriots including Viault (1890). At one point Bert speculated on the possible reduction of metabolism in frequent visitors to high altitude and people who live permanently there. This short section will be cited partly because it gives a good feel for the style of Bert and his pungent wit.

We see that very probably, in the habitual conditions of our life, we commit excesses of oxygenation as well as of nourishment, two kinds of excess, which are correlative. And just as peasants, who eat much less than we do, but utilizing all that they absorb, produce in heat and work a useful result equal, if not superior, to that of city dwellers; just as a Basque mountaineer furnished with a piece of bread and a few onions makes expeditions which require of the member of the *Alpine Club* who accompanies him the absorption of

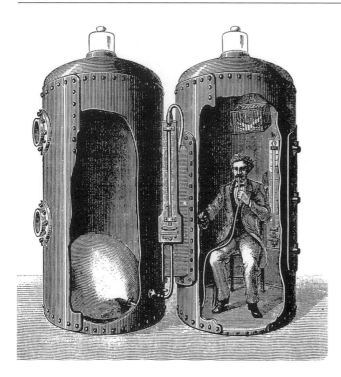

Figure 1.5 Low pressure chambers used by Paul Bert at the Sorbonne. From Bert (1878).

a pound of meat, so it may be that the dwellers in high places finally lessen the consumption of oxygen in their organism, while keeping at their disposal the same quantity of vital force, either for the equilibrium of temperature, or the production of work. Thus we could explain the acclimatization of individuals, of generations, of races. (Bert 1878, p. 1004 in the English translation)

1.12 HIGH ALTITUDE LABORATORIES

1.12.1 Observatoire Vallot

Towards the end of the nineteenth century the pace of discoveries in high altitude medicine and physiology accelerated rapidly partly as the result of the publication of *La Pression Barométrique*. This was a period when two high altitude laboratories were established. The first was the Observatoire Vallot on Mont Blanc which was installed in 1890. Joseph Vallot (1854–1925) conceived the idea of placing a small building at an altitude of about 4350 m, which is about 460 m below the summit of Mont Blanc. With typical French panache he was not satisfied with a simple hut, but in addition there were a comprehensive laboratory, a well-appointed

kitchen, and attractive interior decorations including a French tapestry of courtly ladies in the eighteenth century style. The laboratory was used for research in several of the physical sciences including astronomy and glaciology, but physiological studies were also carried out including some of the first observations of periodic breathing at high altitude (Egli-Sinclair 1893). The Observatoire Vallot is still in use today although it has been considerably modified. Access is challenging because usually a night has to be spent at the Grands Mulets (3050 m) followed by a climb over the snow and ice the following day. Alternatively, a helicopter ascent is possible.

In 1891 a young physician, Dr Jacottet, died in the Observatoire Vallot from what was almost certainly high altitude pulmonary edema. A description of the illness including the post mortem findings is in Mosso's book *Life of Man on the High Alps* (Mosso 1898) referred to in the next section.

1.12.2 Capanna Margherita

Shortly after the construction of the Observatoire Vallot, an even higher structure was placed on one of the peaks of Monte Rosa in Italy at an altitude of

4559 m. The original hut was completed in 1893 and 10 years later it was enlarged by the influential Italian scientist, Angelo Mosso (1846–1910) to include a laboratory for physiological and medical studies. The structure owes its name to Queen Margherita of Savoy who was a lover of alpinism and a generous patron of science. In fact she visited the Capanna in 1893 and spent the night there.

Mosso was a physiologist with very broad interests particularly in the area of exercise and environmental physiology. Some of the early studies in the Capanna Margherita were reported in his book *Fisiologia dell'uomo sulle Alpi: studii fatti sul Monte Rosa* (Mosso 1897), and this was translated into English as *Life of Man on the High Alps* (Mosso 1898). Among the projects carried out at the Capanna were some on periodic breathing, and also total ventilation at high altitude. In fact, Mosso believed that the deleterious effects of high altitude were related to the low carbon dioxide levels in the blood rather than the reduced P_{O_2} as previously proposed by Paul Bert. Mosso coined the term 'acapnia' to describe this condition which he thought was important in the development of acute mountain sickness. An interesting event at the Capanna was the illness of an Italian soldier, Pietro Ramella, who developed what was thought to be a respiratory infection and from which he recovered. In retrospect this may have been high altitude pulmonary edema as was the case with Jacottet at the Observatoire Vallot. The Capanna Margherita has been enlarged over the years and is the site of a very active research program at the present time (Fig. 1.6).

1.13 EARLY SCIENTIFIC EXPEDITIONS TO HIGH ALTITUDE

In the early 1900s the tradition began of organizing expeditions to high altitude locations to carry out medical and physiological research. One of the first was organized by Nathan Zuntz (1847–1920), Professor of Animal Physiology in Berlin, who was the first author of an influential book on high altitude physiology published in 1906 (Zuntz *et al.* 1906). The expedition was to Tenerife in the Canary Islands and experiments were carried out at the Alta Vista hut at an altitude of 3350 m. Among the members of the expedition were Joseph Barcroft

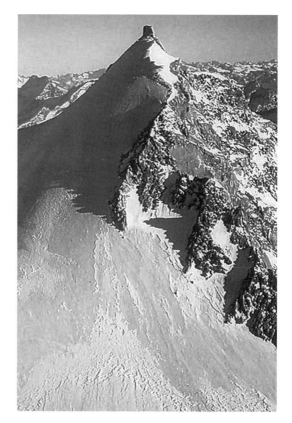

Figure 1.6 Contemporary photograph of the Capanna Margherita on one of the peaks of Monte Rosa. It is the site of an active research program on high altitude medicine and physiology.

(1872–1947) and C.G. Douglas (1882–1963) and they made an interesting observation on the alveolar gases and acclimatization. Barcroft was the only member of the party who showed no significant fall in alveolar P_{CO_2} at the Alta Vista hut; that is, he was the only person who did not exhibit an increase in ventilation, and he was also the only person who was incapacitated by acute mountain sickness. By contrast, the alveolar P_{CO_2} of Douglas fell from 41 to 32, and that of Zuntz fell from 35 to 27 mmHg and both of these members had no mountain sickness. This was corroborative evidence that mountain sickness was caused by the low P_{O_2} as suggested by Paul Bert, rather than the low P_{CO_2} as proposed by Angelo Mosso.

A very important expedition took place in 1911 when an Anglo-American group led by J.S. Haldane (1860–1936) went to Pikes Peak just outside Colorado Springs where there was a hotel on the

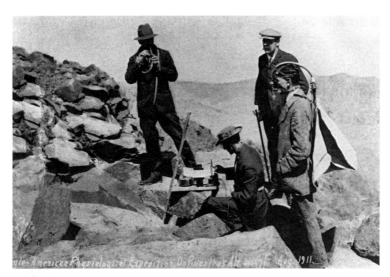

Figure 1.7 Members of the Anglo-American Pikes Peak Expedition of 1911. Left to right: Henderson taking samples of alveolar gas, Schneider sitting and recording his respiration, Haldane standing, and Douglas wearing a 'Douglas bag' to collect expired gas during exercise. From Henderson (1939).

summit at an altitude of 4300 m (Fig. 1.7). One of the advantages of Pikes Peak was a cog railway all the way to the summit. The expedition was carefully planned so that there were measurements at a lower altitude prior to the ascent. Then a rapid ascent was made and the party stayed on the summit where extensive data were collected. Finally, measurements were made again when the participants returned to low altitude. Many important observations were made. The hyperventilation that accompanies ascent to high altitude was documented with the alveolar P_{CO_2} falling to about 2/3 of its sea level value over 2 weeks on the summit. Periodic breathing was confirmed. The polycythemia was studied with the percentage of hemoglobin in the blood increasing over several weeks on the summit to values between 115 and 154% of normal as measured by color changes in the blood. All the measurements were reported in a long paper (Douglas *et al.* 1913).

The members of the expedition also believed that they had obtained evidence for oxygen secretion at high altitude. In fact, the report stated that the arterial P_{O_2} at rest was as much as 35 mmHg above the alveolar value on the summit, whereas at or near sea level the two values were the same. The investigators proposed that oxygen secretion was the most important factor in acclimatization. To this day it is not clear where this large error was made in the measurements.

Oxygen secretion was an important controversy around this time and Haldane actually believed in it until his death in 1936. In fact the second edition of

his book on respiration (Haldane and Priestley 1935) has a whole chapter devoted to the evidence for oxygen secretion. Haldane had originally developed the notion after visiting Christian Bohr (1855–1911) in Copenhagen who was a great champion of oxygen secretion. However, the error was exposed in the view of most physiologists by August Krogh (1874–1949) and his wife Marie (1874–1943) in a series of papers published in 1910.

Mabel FitzGerald (1872–1973) was invited to join the Pikes Peak expedition but did not spend any time in the laboratory for reasons that are not entirely clear. Instead she visited various mining camps in Colorado at altitudes between 1500 and 4300 m where she measured the alveolar P_{CO_2} in acclimatized miners and produced data on acclimatization to moderate altitudes that are still extensively cited (FitzGerald 1913, 1914). Although she studied at Oxford University for a number of years it was not the custom then to give degrees to women. However, the university relented in 1972 when she was 100 years old and awarded her an honorary M.A. degree.

Another classical expedition to high altitude was the International High Altitude Expedition to Cerro de Pasco, Peru which took place in 1921–22 under the leadership of Joseph Barcroft (1872–1947). An attractive feature of this location at an altitude of about 4330 m was that it could be reached by railway from Lima, and the expedition fitted out a railway baggage van as an efficient laboratory (Fig. 1.8). Again there was a very extensive scientific program and the report occupied 129 pages (Barcroft *et al.*

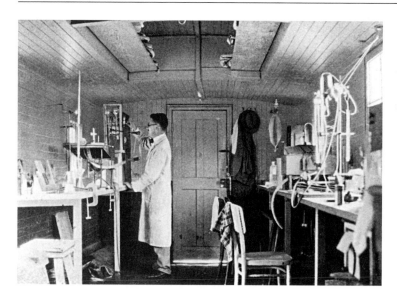

Figure 1.8 Laboratory of the International High Altitude Expedition to Cerro de Pasco, Peru, 1921–22. This was set up in a railroad car. From Barcroft *et al.* (1923).

1923). The topic of oxygen secretion was investigated but no support for it was found. In fact, the P_{O_2} in arterial blood measured by a bubble equilibration method was about 3 mmHg lower than that in alveolar gas. There was an increase in red blood cell concentration by about 20–30% over the sea level value. The arterial oxygen saturation fell during exercise at high altitude and this fall was correctly attributed to the failure of the P_{O_2} to equilibrate between alveolar gas and pulmonary capillary blood because of diffusion limitation. Extensive measurements of neuropsychological function showed that this was impaired at high altitude. In fact, Barcroft made the famous statement 'All dwellers at high altitude are persons of impaired physical and mental powers.'

One of the novel features of this expedition was its studies of permanent residents of high altitude. Cerro de Pasco was a substantial mining town with a large permanent population. It was shown that the red cell concentrations in the permanent residents had values of 40–50% above what would be expected at sea level, that is substantially higher than the newcomers to high altitude. It was also found that the permanent residents of Cerro tended to have lower arterial oxygen saturations of 80–85%, one of the first intimations that highlanders have lower ventilations than newcomers to high altitude.

In 1935 the International High Altitude Expedition to Chile took place under the scientific leadership of D.B. Dill (1891–1986). A number of measurements were made at a mining camp, altitude 5334 m, and these resulted in a classical paper entitled 'Blood as a physicochemical system. XII. Man at high altitudes' (Dill *et al.* 1937). Extensive measurements of exercise were carried out showing, for example, that in one of the members the maximal oxygen consumption fell from 3.72 to 1.80 L min^{-1} at the altitude of the high camp (compared with sea level) while the maximal heart rate fell from 190 to 132 beats min^{-1}. A particularly interesting finding made by Edwards (1936) was that in well-acclimatized subjects the maximal levels of blood lactate were remarkably low, certainly much lower than in acute hypoxia or in subjects without acclimatization. This so-called 'lactate paradox' has been observed on many occasions since and is still not fully understood.

1.14 PERMANENT RESIDENTS OF HIGH ALTITUDE

A large number of people live permanently at high altitude. For example, about 140 million people live at altitudes above 2500 m (WHO 1996) and it has been estimated that each year some 40 million travel to similar altitudes for work or recreation. The high altitude populations are mainly in underdeveloped regions of the world including the South American Andes, the Tibetan plateau and, to a lesser extent,

Ethiopia. Partly as a result of this, these large populations have not received the attention they deserve.

Just as many people regard Paul Bert as the father of modern high altitude physiology, Carlos Monge Medrano (1884–1970) merits the title of father of the study of permanent high altitude residents. He started the influential Peruvian school in Lima and this was subsequently continued by Alberto Hurtado Abadilla (1901–83) and Monge's son, Carlos Monge Cassinelli (1921–2006). The Peruvian school remains very active today with high altitude scientists such as Fabiola León-Velarde, and there are also groups in Argentina, Bolivia, Chile, China and Tibet who are now doing extensive work on high altitude residents.

Mention was made earlier of Barcroft's unguarded statement that 'All dwellers at high altitude are persons of impaired physical and mental powers' (Barcroft 1925). Monge took great exception to this and in his influential book *Acclimatization in the Andes* (Monge M. 1948) he referred to 'the incredible statement of Professor Barcroft, the Cambridge physiologist, who after staying 3 months at Cerro de Pasco. . . .' Monge made the point that because of the 'climatic aggression' of high altitudes as he referred to it, Andean man should not be assessed using the same criteria as people who live near sea level. In fact, at one stage, Monge attributed Barcroft's statement to the fact that the latter had mountain sickness at the time!

Monge made extensive studies of the ability of permanent residents of the Andes to withstand the hypoxia and cold of the environment. Nevertheless he is best known for his work on chronic mountain sickness, also known as Monge's disease, which he set out in his book *La Enfermedad de los Andes* (Monge M. 1928). In this he describes the condition associated with severe polycythemia, cyanosis and vague neuropsychological complaints including headache, dizziness, somnolence and fatigue. Initially the condition was thought to be polycythemia vera but was later shown to be distinct.

Alberto Hurtado (1901–83) was a physiologist who trained under Monge and who made extensive studies of the high altitude residents of Morococha at an altitude of 4550 m. Typically, the arterial P_{O_2} was only 45 mmHg with a corresponding arterial oxygen saturation of 81%. However, interestingly, because of the polycythemia which raised the hemoglobin concentration to nearly 20 g dL^{-1}, the arterial oxygen concentration was actually above the normal sea level value. The son of Carlos Monge Medrano, Carlos Monge Cassinelli was a biologist with broad interests in high altitude including comparative physiology. However, he was very interested in the relationships between high altitude, polycythemia and chronic mountain sickness and many of his studies are reported in a classical book (Winslow and Monge C. 1987).

1.15 HIGH ALTITUDE STUDIES FROM THE LAST 50 YEARS

There have been such a wealth of high altitude studies during this period that it is impossible to do them justice, and furthermore many of them will be alluded to in subsequent chapters of this book and so only a brief summary is given here. Many of the studies have concentrated on the effects of extreme altitude.

In 1944 Charles Houston (1913–) and Richard Riley (1911–2001) carried out a remarkable study known as Operation Everest I at the US Naval School of Aviation Medicine in Pensacola, Florida. Four volunteers lived continuously in a low pressure chamber for 35 days and were gradually decompressed to the equivalent of the altitude of Mount Everest. The project was justified to the Navy on the grounds that it was relevant to improving the tolerance of aviators to high altitudes. Alveolar gas and arterial blood studies were carried out and the most striking finding was that it was possible for resting, partly acclimatized subjects to survive for 20 min or so at a simulated altitude that actually exceeded the summit of Mount Everest. This came about because they were using the Standard Atmosphere which predicts a substantially lower pressure on the summit than actually exists.

A major high altitude physiologist at this time was L.C.G.E. Pugh (1909–94) who was closely associated with the first successful ascent of Everest in 1953. During 1952 Pugh and others conducted physiological studies on the nearby mountain Cho Oyu to clarify some of the logistics of tolerating extreme altitude including ventilation rates, maximal oxygen consumptions, effects of oxygen breathing, hydration, food and clothing. Pugh's contributions were a major factor in the ultimate success of the expedition when Edmund Hillary (1919–) and Tenzing Norgay

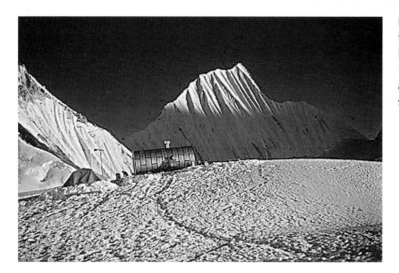

Figure 1.9 Main laboratory of the Himalayan Scientific and Mountaineering Expedition, 1960–61. The Silver Hut was at an altitude of 5800 m about 16 km south of Mount Everest.

(1914–86) became the first people to reach the highest point in the world.

In 1960–61 Pugh was the scientific leader of the Himalayan Scientific and Mountaineering Expedition now universally known as the Silver Hut Expedition. The reason for the name is that the scientists wintered for several months at an altitude of 5800 m in a wooden structure painted silver (Fig. 1.9). The extensive scientific program was largely devoted to studies of exercise, pulmonary gas exchange, the control of ventilation, polycythemia, the electrocardiogram and neuropsychological function (Pugh 1962a). Many of the studies are referred to in later chapters of this book.

In 1981 the American Medical Research Expedition to Everest set out to obtain the first data from the Everest summit itself and made measurements that so far have not been repeated. Among the remarkable findings were alveolar P_{O_2} and P_{CO_2} values of 35 and 7–8 mmHg and an arterial pH (based on the measured alveolar P_{CO_2} and blood base excess) of over 7.7. The barometric pressure on the summit was 253 mmHg., and the maximal oxygen consumption measured using the summit inspired P_{O_2} was just over $1\,\mathrm{L\,min^{-1}}$.

Four years later Houston and John Sutton (1941–96) carried out Operation Everest II at a US Army facility in Natick, Massachusetts which was basically similar to Operation Everest I in design but much more sophisticated in the measurements that could be made. Again the volunteers were gradually decompressed to the barometric pressure on the Everest summit and a large series of measurements that could not be made in the field were completed. These included cardiac catherization which showed substantial increases in pulmonary artery pressures with ascent, particularly on exercise. An interesting aspect was that after a few days the pulmonary hypertension could not be reversed by giving oxygen, suggesting that some remodeling of the pulmonary circulation had taken place. Other important information was obtained on pulmonary gas exchange, changes in skeletal muscle by biopsy, and neuropsychological changes. Another simulated ascent of Mount Everest using a low pressure chamber was carried out in 1997 (called Operation Everest III (COMEX '97)) and, again, important new information was obtained in a number of areas.

The atmosphere

SUMMARY

Most of the medical problems that occur at high altitude are caused by the low partial pressure of oxygen in the atmosphere which in turn is due to the decrease in barometric pressure as altitude increases. The relationship between barometric pressure and altitude is therefore important, especially in regions of the world such as the Andes and Himalayas where large numbers of people reside at high altitude. Recent work has clarified the pressure–altitude relationship with much better accuracy than previously. Considerable confusion occurred in the past by assuming that the relationship follows the standard atmosphere. In fact, the pressures are usually substantially higher at a given altitude because the relationship between barometric pressure and altitude is latitude-dependent, and most of the high mountains of the world are relatively near the equator. At extreme altitudes, the variation of barometric pressure with season is sufficient to affect human performance. This is particularly true of the summit of Mount Everest where climbers are near the limit of tolerance to hypoxia. Other atmospheric factors such as temperature, humidity and solar radiation are also important.

2.1 INTRODUCTION

It has been known since the time of Paul Bert and the publication of *La Pression Barométrique* (Bert 1878) that most of the deleterious effects of high altitude on humans are caused by hypoxia. This, in turn, is a direct result of the reduction in atmospheric pressure. Yet in spite of the fact that Bert's book appeared almost 130 years ago, there is still confusion in the minds of some physicians and physiologists about the relationship between barometric pressure and altitude, particularly at extreme heights. For example, some environmental physiologists are still surprised to learn that the barometric pressure at the summit of Mount Everest is considerably higher than that predicted by the standard pressure–altitude tables used by the aviation industry, and that humans can reach the summit without supplementary oxygen only because the tables are inapplicable.

Although most of the undesirable effects of high altitude are due to hypoxia, under some circumstances additional deterioration results from cold, dehydration, solar radiation, and even ionizing radiation. However, most of these hazards of the environment can be avoided by proper clothing or shelter. Only hypoxia is unavoidable unless, of course, supplementary oxygen is available. The low barometric pressure in itself has no physiological sequelae unless the decompression is rapid, for example in the case of the explosive decompression that occurs when a window fails in a pressurized aircraft. Rapid decompression causes so-called barotrauma as a result of the very rapid enlargement of airspaces within the body including the lungs and middle ear cavity. Such accidents can also occur in ascent from deep diving, but are not considered here.

That low pressure per se is innocuous was not always realized. Indeed, early theories of mountain sickness included a number of exotic explanations based on the reduced pressure itself (Bert 1878, pp. 342–7 in the 1943 translation). One was weakening of the coxofemoral articulation; it was thought that barometric pressure was an important factor in pressing the head of the femur into its socket and that, at high altitudes, the necessary increase in action of the neighboring muscles resulted in fatigue. Another hypothesis was that superficial blood vessels would dilate and rupture if the barometric pressure which normally supported them was reduced. Indeed, modern day medical students occasionally raise issues of this kind when they are first introduced to high altitude physiology. A further theory was that distension of intestinal gas would interfere with the action of the diaphragm and also impede venous return to the heart. All these theories neglect the fact that, when humans ascend to high altitude, all the hydrostatic pressures in the body fall together. In other words, although the pressure outside the superficial blood vessels falls, the pressure inside the vessels falls to the same extent and therefore the pressure differences across the vessels are unchanged.

2.2 BAROMETRIC PRESSURE AND ALTITUDE

2.2.1 Historical

A general historical introduction can be found in Chapter 1, but some additional background material related to the atmosphere is included here. The notion that air has weight and therefore exerts a pressure at the surface of the earth eluded the ancient Greeks and had to wait until the Renaissance. Galileo (1638) was well aware of the force associated with a vacuum and therefore the effort required to 'break' it, but he thought of this in the context of a force required to break a copper wire by stretching it, that is, the cohesive forces within the substance of the wire. It was left to Galileo's pupil Torricelli to realize that the force of a vacuum is due to the weight of the atmosphere. In addition he wondered whether the air

pressure became less on the tops of high mountains where the air 'begins to be distinctly rare …' as he put it. Torricelli made the first mercury barometer, though barometers filled with other liquids had apparently been constructed previously, for example by Gaspar Berti. These were unsatisfactory because of the effect of the vapor pressure of the liquid.

A landmark experiment took place in 1648 when the French philosopher and mathematician Blaise Pascal suggested that his brother-in-law, F. Périer, take a barometer to the top of the Puy-de-Dôme (1463 m) in central France to see whether the pressure fell (Pascal 1648). The results were communicated to Pascal in a delightful letter by Périer in which he described how the level of the mercury barometer fell some three pouces (about 75 mm) during the ascent of '500 fathoms' of altitude (probably about 900 m). The experiment had elaborate controls. For example, the Reverend Father Chastin, 'a man as pious as he is capable', stood guard over one barometer in the town of Clermont while Périer and a number of observers (including clerics, counselors, and a doctor of medicine) took another to the top of the mountain. On returning, it was found that the first barometer had not changed, and Périer even checked it again by filling it with the same mercury that he had taken up the mountain. Another observation was made the next day on the top of a high church tower in Clermont, and this also showed a fall in pressure, though of much smaller extent.

A few years later, Robert Boyle carried out experiments with the newly invented air pump and wrote his influential book *New Experiments Physico-Mechanicall Touching the Spring of the Air, and its Effects*. In the second edition of this book published in 1662 he formulated his famous law, which states that gas volume and pressure are inversely related (at constant temperature) (Boyle 1662). Recent commentaries on both the original book and Boyle's law are available (West 1999b and 2005).

An influential analysis of the relationships between altitude and barometric pressure was made by Zuntz *et al.* in 1906. They pointed out the important effect of temperature on the pressure–altitude relationship noting that, on a fine warm day, the upcurrents carry air to high altitudes and thus increase the sea level barometric pressure. Indeed, this is the basis for weather prediction based on barometric pressure.

Zuntz *et al.* (1906, pp. 37–9) gave the following logarithmic relationship for determining barometric pressure at any altitude:

$$\log b = \log B - \frac{h}{72\,(256.4 + t)}$$

where h is the altitude difference in meters, t is the mean temperature (°C) of the air column of height h, B is the barometric pressure (mmHg) at the lower altitude, and b is the barometric pressure at the higher altitude. Note that this expression implies that the higher the mean temperature, the less rapidly does barometric pressure decrease with altitude. In addition, if temperature were constant, $\log b$ would be proportional to negative altitude, that is, the pressure would decrease exponentially as altitude increased. Zuntz *et al.* cite Hann's *Lehrbuch der Meteorologie* where the pressure–altitude relationship is given in a slightly different form (Hann 1901).

The expression by Zuntz *et al.* was used by FitzGerald (1913) in her study of alveolar P_{CO_2} and hemoglobin concentration in residents of various altitudes in the Colorado mountains during the Anglo-American Pikes Peak expedition of 1911. She showed that barometric pressures calculated from the Zuntz formula agreed closely with pressures observed in the mountains when a sea level pressure of 760 mmHg and a mean temperature of the air column of +15°C were assumed. Kellas (2001) used the same expression to predict barometric pressures in the Himalayan ranges, obtaining a value of 251 mmHg for the summit of Mount Everest, assuming a mean temperature of 0°C. This was almost the same as the pressure of 248 mmHg given by Bert (Bert 1878, Appendix 1) in contrast to the erroneously low values used 70 years after Bert because of the inappropriate application of the standard atmosphere (section 2.2.3). However, a major difficulty with the use of the Zuntz formula is the sensitivity of the calculated pressure to temperature and the fact that the mean temperature of the air column is not accurately known. For example, the barometric pressure on the summit of Mount Everest was calculated by Kellas to be 267 mmHg for a mean temperature of +15°C, but only 251 mmHg for a mean temperature of 0°C.

2.2.2 Physical principles

Barometric pressure decreases with altitude because the higher we go, the less atmosphere there is above us pressing down by virtue of its weight. If the atmosphere were incompressible, as is very nearly the case in a liquid, barometric pressure would decrease linearly with altitude, just as it does in a liquid. However, because the weight of the upper atmosphere compresses the lower gas, barometric pressure decreases more rapidly with height near the earth's surface. If temperature were constant, the decrease in pressure would be exponential with respect to altitude, but because the temperature decreases as we go higher (at least, in the troposphere), the pressure falls more rapidly than the exponential law predicts.

The relationships between pressure, volume and temperature in a gas are governed by simple laws. These derive from the kinetic theory of gases which states that the molecules of a gas are in continuous random motion, and are only deflected from their course by collision with other molecules, or with the walls of a container. When they strike the walls and rebound, the resulting bombardment results in a pressure. The magnitude of the pressure depends on the number of molecules present, their mass and their speed:

- **Boyle's law** states that, at constant temperature, the pressure (P) of a given mass of gas is inversely proportional to its volume (V), or PV = constant (at constant temperature). This can be explained by the fact that as the molecules are brought closer together (smaller volume), the rate of bombardment on a unit surface increases (greater pressure).
- **Charles' law** states that at constant pressure, the volume of a gas is proportional to its absolute temperature (T), or V/T = constant (at constant pressure). The explanation is that a rise in temperature increases the speed and therefore the momentum of the molecules, thus increasing their force of bombardment on the container. Another form of Charles' law states that at constant volume, the pressure is proportional to absolute temperature. (Note that absolute temperature is obtained by adding 273 to the Celsius temperature. Thus 37°C = 310 K.)

- The **ideal gas law** combines the above laws thus: $PV = nRT$, where n is the number of gram molecules of the gas and R is the 'gas constant'. When the units employed are mmHg, liters and kelvin, then $R = 62.4$. Real gases deviate from ideal gas behavior to some extent at high pressures because of intermolecular forces, which are neglected in the derivation of the real gas law.
- **Dalton's law** states that each gas in a mixture exerts a pressure according to its own concentration, independently of the other gases present. That is, each component behaves as though it were present alone. The pressure of each gas is referred to as its partial pressure or tension (now obsolete). The total pressure is the sum of the partial pressures of all gases present. In symbols: $P_x = PF_x$, where P_x is the partial pressure of gas x, P is the total pressure and F_x is the fractional concentration of gas x. For example, if half the gas is oxygen, $FO_2 = 0.5$. The fractional concentration always refers to dry gas.
- The **kinetic theory of gases** explains their diffusion in the gas phase. Because of their random motion, gas molecules tend to distribute themselves uniformly throughout any available space until the partial pressure is the same everywhere. Light gases diffuse faster than heavy gases because the mean velocity of the molecules is higher. The kinetic theory of gases states that the kinetic energy ($0.5\,mv^2$) of all gases is the same at a given temperature and pressure. From this it follows that the rate of diffusion of a gas is inversely proportional to the square root of its density (**Graham's law**).

On the basis of different rates of diffusion, one might expect that very light gases such as helium would separate and be lost from the upper atmosphere. This does happen to some extent at extreme altitudes. However, at the altitudes of interest to us, say up to 10 km, convective mixing maintains a constant composition of the atmosphere.

Vertically, the atmosphere can be divided on the basis of temperature variations into the troposphere, the stratosphere and regions above that. The troposphere is the region where all the weather phenomena take place and is the only region of interest to high altitude medicine. Here, the temperature decreases approximately linearly with altitude until a low of about −60°C is reached. The troposphere extends to an altitude of about 19 km at the equator but only to about 9 km at the poles. The average upper limit is about 10 km.

Above the troposphere is the stratosphere where the temperature remains nearly constant at about −60°C for some 10–12 km of altitude. The interface between the troposphere and stratosphere is known as the tropopause.

Beyond the stratosphere, temperatures again vary with altitude. One of the important components of this region is the ionosphere where the degree of ionization of the molecules makes short-wave radio propagation possible.

2.2.3 Standard atmosphere

With the development of the aviation industry in the 1920s it became necessary to develop a barometric pressure–altitude relationship that could be universally accepted for calibrating altimeters, low pressure chambers and other devices. Although it had been recognized for many years that the relationship between pressure and altitude was temperature dependent and, as a result, latitude dependent, there were clear advantages in having a model atmosphere that applied approximately to mean conditions over the surface of the earth. This is often referred to as the ICAO standard atmosphere (1964) or the US standard atmosphere (NOAA 1976). These two are identical up to altitudes of interest to us.

The assumptions of the standard atmosphere are a sea level pressure of 760 mmHg, sea level temperature of +15°C and a linear decrease in temperature with altitude (lapse rate) of 6.5°C km^{-1} up to an altitude of 11 km (Table 2.1). Haldane and Priestley (1935, p. 323) gave the following expression for the pressure–altitude relationship of the standard atmosphere in the second edition of their textbook *Respiration*:

$$\frac{P_0}{P} = \left(\frac{288}{288 - 1.98H} \right)^{5.256}$$

where P_0 and P are the pressures in mmHg at sea level and high altitude respectively, and H is

Table 2.1   Barometric pressures (in mmHg) from the standard atmosphere (ICAO 1964) and a model atmosphere (West 1996a): the latter is a better fit for most sites where high altitude physiology and medicine are studied

Altitude		Standard pressure		Model atmosphere	
kilometers	feet	Barometric pressure	Inspired P_{O_2}[a]	Barometric pressure	Inspired P_{O_2}
0	0	760	149	760	149
1	3 281	674	131	679	132
2	6 562	596	115	604	117
3	9 843	526	100	537	103
4	13 123	462	87	475	90
5	16 404	405	75	420	78
6	19 685	354	64	369	67
7	22 966	308	54	324	58
8	26 247	267	46	284	50
9	29 528	231	38	247	42
10	32 810	199	31	215	35

[a] The P_{O_2} of moist inspired gas is 0.2094 $(P_B - 47)$.

the height in thousands of feet. A more rigorous description is given in the *Manual of the ICAO Standard Atmosphere* (ICAO 1964).

It should be emphasized that this model atmosphere was never meant to be used to predict the actual barometric pressure at a particular location. Rather it was developed as a model of more or less average conditions within the troposphere with full recognition that there would be local variations caused by latitude and other factors. Nevertheless, the standard atmosphere has assumed some importance in respiratory physiology because it is universally used as the standard for altimeter calibrations, and it has frequently been inappropriately used to predict the pressure at various specific points of the earth's surface, particularly on high mountains.

Haldane and Priestley (1935) clearly understood that the standard atmosphere predicted barometric pressures considerably lower than those given by the expression of Zuntz *et al.* (1906), which had been shown by FitzGerald to predict accurately pressures in the Colorado mountains when a mean air column temperature of +15°C was assumed.

Nevertheless, some physiologists have used the standard atmosphere for predicting the pressure at great altitudes, for example on Mount Everest (Houston and Riley 1947, Riley and Houston 1951, Rahn and Fenn 1955, Houston *et al.* 1987). The barometric pressure calculated in this way for the Everest summit (altitude 8848 m) is 236 mmHg, which is far too low. In retrospect, one of the reasons for the indiscriminate use of the standard atmosphere was undoubtedly its very frequent employment in low pressure chambers during the very fertile period of research on respiratory physiology during World War II.

Climbers using altimeters from sports shops, including those on some wristwatches, should be aware that these use the standard atmosphere to convert barometric pressure to altitude. The difference between the readings given by these altimeters and the true altitude up to about 3000 m is unimportant for navigation in the mountains. From 4000 to 5000 m a climber should add 3% to the altimeter reading to get a truer altitude. From 5000 to 6000 m the change is 4%, from 6000 to 8000 m the change is about 5%, and above 8000 m it is 6–7%. Of course, if the altimeter also reads pressure, the best solution is to relate this to altitude using the model atmosphere equation.

2.2.4 Variation of barometric pressure with latitude

The limited applicability of the standard atmosphere is further clarified when we look at the relationship between barometric pressure and altitude for different latitudes (Fig. 2.1). This shows that the barometric pressure at the earth's surface and at an altitude of 24 km is essentially independent of latitude. However, in the altitude range of about 6–16 km, there is a pronounced bulge in the barometric pressure near the equator both in winter and summer. Since the latitude of Mount Everest is 28°N, the pressure at its summit (8848 m) is considerably higher than would be the case for a hypothetical mountain of the same altitude near one of the poles.

The cause of the bulge in barometric pressure near the equator is a very large mass of very cold air in the stratosphere above the equator (Brunt 1952, p. 379). In fact, paradoxically, the coldest air in the atmosphere is above the equator. This is brought about by a combination of complex radiation and convective phenomena which result in a large up-welling of air near the equator. Another corollary of the same phenomenon is that the height of the tropopause is much greater near the equator than near the poles. These latitude-dependent variations of pressure are of great physiological significance for anyone attempting to climb Mount Everest without supplementary oxygen, because they result in a barometric pressure on the Everest summit which is considerably higher than that predicted from the model atmosphere. By the same token, a climber at a high latitude such as Mount McKinley (Denali) is at a considerable disadvantage because of the low barometric pressure, especially in the winter months.

2.2.5 Variation of barometric pressure with season

Not only does barometric pressure alter with latitude, but there are marked variations according to the month of the year. For example, Fig. 2.2 shows the mean monthly pressures for an altitude of 8848 m as obtained from radiosonde balloons released from

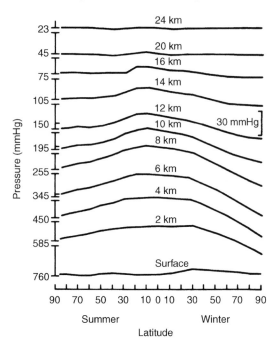

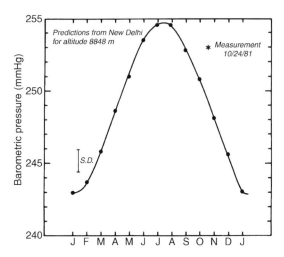

Figure 2.1 Increase of barometric pressure near the equator at various altitudes in both summer and winter. Vertical axis shows the pressure increasing upwards according to the scale on the right. The numbers on the left show the barometric pressures at the poles for various altitudes; the altitude of Mount Everest is 8848 m. (From Brunt 1952.)

Figure 2.2 Mean monthly pressures for 8848 m altitude as obtained from weather balloons released from New Delhi, India. Note the increase during the summer months. The mean monthly standard deviation (SD) is also shown. The barometric pressure measured on the Everest summit on 24 October 1981 (*) was unusually high for that month. (From West *et al.* 1983a.)

New Delhi, India, over a period of 15 years. Delhi has about the same latitude as Everest. Note that the mean pressures were lowest in the winter months of January and February (243.0 and 243.7 mmHg, respectively) and highest in the summer months of July and August (254.5 mmHg for both months). The monthly standard deviation showed a range of 0.65 mmHg (July) to 1.66 mmHg (December). The daily standard deviation was as low as 1.54 in the summer and as high as 2.92 in the winter. The standard deviation shown on Fig. 2.2 is the mean of the monthly standard deviation for the 12 months of the year.

The single measurement of barometric pressure (253.0 mmHg) made by Pizzo on the summit of Mount Everest on 24 October 1981 (West *et al.* 1983a) is also shown on Fig. 2.2. This was 4.3 mmHg higher than that predicted from the data shown in Fig. 2.1, which is twice the daily standard deviation of barometric pressure for the month of October. It should be added that Pizzo had an exceptionally fine day for his summit climb, the temperature on the summit being measured as −9°C, much higher than expected for that altitude (section 2.3.1).

Figure 2.3 combines the effects of latitude and month of the year on the barometric pressure at an altitude of 8848 m. The data are for the northern hemisphere, and the pressures for the months of January (midwinter), July (midsummer) and October (preferred month for climbing in the post-monsoon period) are compared. The profile for the month of May, which is the usual month for reaching the summit in the pre-monsoon season, is almost the same as that for October. The data are the means from all longitudes (Oort and Rasmusson 1971). The data clearly show the marked effects of both latitude and season on barometric pressure. It is interesting that in midsummer the pressure reaches a maximum near the latitude of Mount Everest (28°35′N). Figure 2.3 shows that if Mount Everest was at the latitude of Mount McKinley (63°N), the pressure on the summit would be very much lower.

Radiosonde balloons are released from meteorological stations all over the world twice a day, and the resulting data on the relationship between barometric pressure and altitude are available from constant pressure charts. Details on how to obtain these are given in West (1993a). Using these data it can be shown that the barometric pressure on the Everest summit was 251 mmHg when Messner and

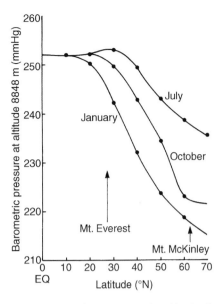

Figure 2.3   Barometric pressure at the altitude of Mount Everest plotted against latitude in the northern hemisphere for midsummer, midwinter, and the preferred month for climbing in the post-monsoon period (October). Note the considerably lower pressures in the winter. The arrows show the latitudes of Mount Everest and Mount McKinley. (From West *et al.* 1983a.)

Habeler made their first ascent without supplementary oxygen in 1978. In August 1980, Messner made the first solo ascent without supplementary oxygen and he was fortunate that the barometric pressure was unusually high at 256 mmHg. When Sherpa Ang Rita made the first winter ascent on 22 December 1987, the barometric pressure was only 247 mmHg.

2.2.6 Barometric pressure–altitude relationship for locations of importance in high altitude medicine and physiology

We have seen that the standard atmosphere generally underestimates the pressures on the high mountains which are of interest to people concerned with high altitude medicine and physiology. Recently, it has been possible to define the barometric pressure–altitude relationship in the Himalayan and Andean ranges with some accuracy, and it transpires that the relationship holds for many other locations where high altitude medicine and physiology are studied.

As already stated, the first direct measurement of barometric pressure on the Everest summit was obtained by Pizzo in 1981 during the course of the American Medical Research Expedition to Everest (West *et al.* 1983a). The value was 253 mmHg, as shown on Fig. 2.2. During the same expedition, careful measurements of barometric pressure were made at two other locations on Mount Everest where the altitudes were accurately known. These were the Base Camp (altitude 5400 m) and Camp 5, just above the South Col (altitude 8050 m). These points lay very close to a straight line on a log pressure–altitude plot and therefore allowed the barometric pressure–altitude relationship at very high altitudes on Mount Everest to be accurately described for the first time (Fig. 2 in West *et al.* 1983a). This relationship is of great physiological interest because, as discussed in Chapter 12, the pressure near the summit is so low that the P_{O_2} is very near the limit for human survival.

More recently, additional measurements have been made at very high altitudes on Mount Everest (West 1999a). Another direct measurement was made on the summit in May 1997 and this agreed within 1 mmHg of Pizzo's measurement of 253 mmHg. In addition, a large number of measurements were reported from a barometer that telemetered information from the South Col (altitude 7986 m). When these points were added to those obtained during the 1981 expedition (Fig. 2.4), they greatly increase our confidence in the barometric pressure–altitude relationship.

Two other pieces of data have more recently come to light: Charles Corfield made a single measurement of the barometric pressure on the Everest summit at 10 a.m. on 5 May 1999. He used a Kollsman aneroid barometer and the value was 253 mmHg (personal communication). The air temperature was −18°C, and this had been shown not to affect the calibration of the barometer. The other data point comes from measurements made on the South Col by the Italian Ev-K2-CNR program. They reported 52 measurements of barometric pressure on 29 and 30 September and 1 October 1992 (personal communication). The mean value was 383.0 mbar (287 mmHg). This is the same pressure as that found by the MIT group in August 1997 (West 1999a). These two additional pieces of data fit very well with the other measurements listed above.

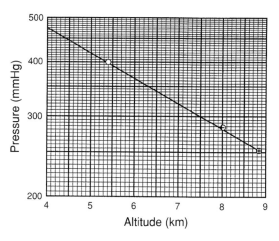

Figure 2.4 Barometric pressure–altitude relationship for Mount Everest. The circles show data from the 1981 American Medical Research Expedition to Everest. The cross at the summit altitude (8848 m) is from the 1997 NOVA expedition. The cross at an altitude of 7986 m is from measurements made by the Massachusetts Institute of Technology in 1998. The standard deviations are too small to show on the graph. The line corresponds to the model atmosphere equation: $P_B = \exp(6.63268 - 0.1112h - 0.00149h^2)$ where h is in kilometers. (From West 1999a.)

2.2.7 Model atmosphere equation

It is now possible to provide a barometric pressure–altitude relationship that accurately predicts the pressure at most locations of interest to high altitude medicine and physiology (West 1996a). The data are shown in Fig. 2.5. The prediction is particularly good if the locations lie within 30° of the equator, and especially if the pressure is measured in the summer months. Since many studies of high altitude medicine and physiology are carried out in locations and times that fulfill these criteria, the relationship is very useful in practice. The equation of the line is

$$P_B = \exp(6.63268 - 0.1112h - 0.00149h^2)$$

where P_B is the barometric pressure (in mmHg) and h is the altitude in kilometers. This has been called the **model atmosphere equation**, and is useful for theoretical calculations in high altitude physiology such as predicting the effects of oxygen enrichment at different altitudes. The algorithms for both the standard and model atmospheres are

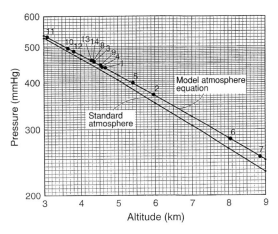

Figure 2.5 Barometric pressure–altitude relationship corresponding to the model atmosphere equation. Note that it predicts the altitudes of many locations of interest in high altitude medicine and physiology very well. The lower line shows the standard atmosphere which predicts pressures that are too low. The locations and measured pressures are as follows: 1) Collahuasi mine, Chile, 438 mmHg; 2) Aucanquilcha mine, Chile, 372 mmHg; 3) Vallot observatory, France, 452 mmHg; 4) Capanna Margherita, Italy, 440 mmHg; 5) Mount Everest Base Camp, Nepal, 400 mmHg; 6) Mount Everest South Col, 284 mmHg; 7) Mount Everest summit, 253 mmHg; 8) Cerro de Pasco, Peru, 458 mmHg; 9) Morococha, Peru, 446 mmHg; 10) Lhasa, Tibet, 493 mmHg; 11) Crooked Creek, California, 530 mmHg; 12) Barcroft laboratory, California, 483 mmHg; 13) Pikes Peak, Colorado, 462 mmHg; 14) White Mountain summit, California, 455 mmHg. (From West 1996a.)

available on the web at <http://medicine.ucsd.edu/phys/convert.html>.

2.2.8 Barometric pressure and inspired P_{O_2}

As we have seen, the composition of the atmosphere is constant up to altitudes well above those of medical interest so it is safe to assume that the concentration of oxygen in dry air is approximately 20.94%. However, the effects of water vapor on the inspired P_{O_2} become increasingly important at higher altitudes.

When air is inhaled into the upper bronchial tree, it is warmed and moistened and becomes saturated with vapor at the prevailing temperature.

The water vapor pressure at 37°C is 47 mmHg and this, of course, is independent of altitude. Thus the P_{O_2} of moist inspired gas is given by the expression

$$PI_{,O_2} = 0.2094 \, (P_B - 47)$$

where P_B is barometric pressure. This equation shows how much more important water vapor pressure becomes at very high altitudes. For example, at sea level, the water vapor pressure at 37°C is only 6% of the total barometric pressure. However, on the summit of Mount Everest, where the barometric pressure is about 250 mmHg, the water vapor pressure is nearly 19% of the total pressure, and the inspired P_{O_2} is correspondingly further reduced (see Table 2.1).

It has been pointed out from time to time that a relatively small reduction in body temperature at extreme altitude would confer a substantial increase in inspired P_{O_2}. For example, if the body temperature fell to 35°C where the water vapor is 42 mmHg, the P_{O_2} of moist inspired gas would be increased from 42.5 to 43.5 mmHg. This increase of 1 mmHg would be beneficial because the arterial P_{O_2} would increase by approximately the same extent, and since the oxygen dissociation curve is very steep at this point, there would be an appreciable gain in arterial oxygen concentration. However, there is no evidence that body temperature falls at extreme altitude. Nor is it reasonable to assume that the temperature in the alveoli where gas exchange takes place would be significantly less than the body core temperature.

2.2.9 Physiological significance of barometric pressure at high altitude

Since the barometric pressure directly determines the inspired P_{O_2}, it is clear that the variations of barometric pressure with latitude and season, as described in sections 2.2.4 and 2.2.5, will affect the degree of hypoxemia in the body. For example, a climber on Mount McKinley in Alaska, which is situated at a latitude of 63°N, will be exposed to a considerably lower barometric pressure on the summit than would be the case for a mountain of the same height located in the tropics (see Fig. 2.3).

The reduction in inspired P_{O_2} resulting from the lower barometric pressure will not only reduce exercise performance but may also increase the risk of altitude illness. In fact there is evidence that this may be the case at the comparatively modest altitudes of Summit County, Colorado (2650–2950 m) as reported by Reeves *et al.* (1994). They found that barometric pressure and environmental temperature averaged 8 mmHg and 23°C lower in winter compared with summer months. While the number of visits to the Summit Medical Center (2773 m) was nearly the same in the two periods, the proportion of patients with high altitude pulmonary edema was higher in winter, though interestingly there was no difference in the incidence of acute mountain sickness. Cold seemed to be more important than barometric pressure.

The variations of barometric pressure with latitude and season become particularly significant from a physiological point of view at extreme altitudes such as near the summit of Mount Everest. For example, it has been shown that if the pressure on the Everest summit conformed to the standard atmosphere, it would be impossible to climb the mountain without supplementary oxygen (West 1983). In addition, the variation of barometric pressure with month of the year shown in Fig. 2.2 indicates that it would be considerably more difficult to reach the summit without supplementary oxygen in the winter as a result of the reduced inspired P_{O_2}, quite apart from the obvious difficulties of lower temperatures and high winds. Although there have now been many ascents of Everest without supplementary oxygen in the pre- and post-monsoon seasons, only one person has made a winter ascent without supplementary oxygen. This was Sherpa Ang Rita on 22 December 1987 when the barometric pressure was 247 mmHg based on radiosonde balloon data for that date. Therefore the pressure was much higher than it typically becomes in midwinter, for example in late January (see Fig. 2.2). This topic is considered in more detail in Chapter 12.

2.3 FACTORS OTHER THAN BAROMETRIC PRESSURE AT HIGH ALTITUDE

2.3.1 Temperature

Temperature falls with increasing altitude at the rate of about 1°C for every 150 m. This lapse rate is essentially independent of latitude. The consequence is that on a very high mountain, such as Mount Everest, the average temperature near the summit is predicted to be about −40°C. Most climbers choose the warmer months of the year. In May, a temperature of −27°C was measured at an altitude of 8500 m on Everest (Pugh 1957), although Pizzo obtained a temperature of −9°C on the summit in October (West *et al.* 1983a). In the winter the temperatures are much lower. However, even then they do not approach the extremely low temperatures seen in northern Canada or Siberia during midwinter.

More important than temperature per se is the wind chill factor. Wind velocities on Himalayan peaks have often been estimated to be in excess of 150 km h^{-1}, though few measurements have been made. Such high winds result in extremely severe chill factors at low temperatures and can make climbing impossible. Cold injury is common in the mountains and is discussed in Chapter 23.

2.3.2 Humidity

Absolute humidity is the amount of water vapor per unit volume of gas at the prevailing temperature. This value is extremely low at high altitude because the water vapor pressure is so depressed at the reduced temperature. Thus even if the air is fully saturated with water vapor, the actual amount will be very small. For example, the water vapor pressure at +20°C is 17 mmHg but only 1 mmHg at −20°C.

Relative humidity is a measure of the amount of water vapor in the air as a percentage of the amount that could be contained at the prevailing temperature. This value may be low, normal or high at altitude. The disparity between absolute and relative humidities is explained by the fact that even saturated air is unable to contain much water vapor because of the very low temperature. If this air is warmed without allowing additional water vapor to form, its relative humidity falls.

The very low absolute humidity at high altitude frequently causes dehydration. First, the insensible water loss caused by ventilation is great because of the dryness of the inspired air. In addition, the levels of ventilation may be extremely high, especially on exercise (Chapter 11), and this increases water loss. For example, near the summit of Mount Everest, the total ventilation is increased some five-fold compared with sea level for the same level of activity. Pugh (1964b) calculated that during exercise at 5500 m altitude, the rate of fluid loss from the lungs alone was about 2.9 g water per 100 L of ventilation (body temperature and pressure, saturated with water vapor, or BTPS). This is equivalent to about 200 mL of water per hour for moderate exercise.

However, it is likely that Pugh's calculation gives erroneously high values because the temperature of expired gas is below body temperature, and the gas is probably not fully saturated with water even at this lower temperature (Loewy and Gerhartz 1914, Burch 1945, Webb 1951, Ferrus et al. 1980). Using an equation given by Ferrus et al. (1984), Milledge (1992) calculated that the water loss is only about 30–40% of that calculated assuming that the expired gas is fully saturated at body temperature in a climber at extreme altitude. Actual measurements during climbing at extreme altitude would be valuable.

There is evidence that the dehydration resulting from these rapid fluid losses does not produce as strong a sensation of thirst as at sea level. As a result, it is necessary for climbers to drink large quantities of fluids at high altitude to remain hydrated even though they have little desire to do so. For people climbing 7 h a day at altitudes over 6000 m, 3–4 L of fluid are required in order to maintain a urine output of 1.5 L day^{-1} (Pugh 1964b). Even so, it appears that people living at very high altitude are in a state of chronic volume depletion (Blume et al. 1984). In a group of subjects living at an altitude of 6300 m during the American Medical Research Expedition to Everest, serum osmolality was significantly increased compared with sea level despite the fact that ample fluids were available and the lifestyle in terms of exercise and diet was not exceptional (Blume et al. 1984).

2.3.3 Solar radiation

The intensity of solar radiation increases markedly at high altitude for two reasons. First, the much thinner atmosphere absorbs fewer of the sun's rays, especially those of short wavelength in the near ultraviolet region of the spectrum. Second, reflection of the sun from snow greatly increases radiation exposure.

The reduced density of the air causes an increase in incident solar radiation of up to 100% at an altitude of 4000 m compared with sea level (Elterman 1964). The fact that mountain air is so dry is another important factor because water vapor in the atmosphere absorbs substantial amounts of solar radiation.

The efficiency with which the ground reflects solar radiation is known as its albedo. This varies from less than 20% at sea level to up to 90% in the presence of snow at great altitudes (Buettner 1969). Mountaineers are familiar with the extreme intensity of solar radiation, especially on a glacier in a valley between two mountains. Here the sunlight is reflected from both sides as well as from the snow or ice on the glacier and the heat can be very oppressive despite the great altitude. A consequence of this is the extreme variation in temperature which has been noted in camps under these conditions.

2.3.4 Ionizing radiation

The intensity of cosmic radiation increases at high altitude because there is less of the earth's atmosphere to absorb the rays as they enter from space. This is the reason why cosmic radiation laboratories are often located on high mountains. It has been shown that, at an altitude of 3000 m, the increased cosmic radiation results in an increased radiation dose to a human being of approximately 0.0007 Gy year^{-1} (70 mrad year^{-1}). This should be considered in relation to the normal background radiation dose from all sources of 0.0005–0.004 Gy year^{-1} (50–400 mrad year^{-1}). The increased ionizing radiation of high altitude has been cited as one of the factors causing acute mountain sickness (Bert 1878), but there is no scientific basis for this assertion.

3

Geography and the human response to altitude

SUMMARY

The highland areas of the world support considerable populations. The climate is harsh and methods of cultivation have to be adapted to the terrain. Terracing has been brought to a fine art in the mountain regions, although the South American altiplano and the Tibetan plateau allow normal methods of cultivation. Animal husbandry and mining are important, and tourism is becoming increasingly popular and can contribute significantly to the economy of mountainous regions.

Mountains often form boundaries between cultures. Highland peoples have developed a physique that enables them to survive under severe conditions of cold and hypoxia. Commerce in high valleys without roads depends on porters and without their remarkable capacity to carry loads the economy would remain static. Acclimatization to hypoxia is complex and far reaching and depends on the severity and rate at which oxygen lack is imposed (Chapter 4). Local cold tolerance but not general cold acclimatization occurs, and protection is mainly by cultural methods, clothing and shelter.

3.1 INTRODUCTION

Although the expression 'high altitude' has no precise definition, the majority of individuals have certain clinical, physiological, anatomical and biochemical changes which occur at levels above 3000 m. Individual variation is, however, considerable and some people are affected at levels as low as 2000 m. For sea level visitors, an altitude of 4600–4900 m represents the highest acceptable level for permanent habitation; for high altitude residents 5800–6000 m is the highest so far recorded (West 1986a). Indeed, the highest permanent human habitation is probably the town of La Rinconada, a town of about 7000 inhabitants in southern Peru, at an altitude of 5100 m (West 2002a). Although even altitude residents are affected by the altitude, the limit of permanent habitation is probably dictated by economic, rather than physiological, factors. Above 5000 m, even in the tropics, crops cannot be grown and animals cannot be pastured all year round. Nomadic and semi-nomadic peoples regularly take their flocks to pastures higher than 5000 m but these are not permanent dwellings. In South America, archaeological sites have been found at 6271 m on Llullaillaco, but there is no evidence that these were permanent dwellings.

The main areas of the world above 3000 m are:

- The Tibetan plateau
- The Himalayan range and its valleys
- The Tien Shan and Pamir
- The mountain ranges of east Turkey, Iran, Afghanistan and Pakistan
- The Rocky Mountains and Sierra Nevada of the USA and Canada
- The Sierra Madre of Mexico
- The Andes of South America
- The European Alps
- The Pyrenees between Spain and France
- The Atlas Mountains of North Africa
- The Ethiopian highlands
- The mountains of East and South Africa
- The plateau and mountains of Antarctica
- Parts of New Guinea and other small regions such as Hawaii, Tenerife and New Zealand

The European Alps do not support a large high altitude population, but the region is vitally important because of its position at the crossroads of Europe and because modern investigation into all aspects of mountain science originated there.

The three main regions that support large populations are the Tibetan plateau and Himalayan valleys, the Andes of South America and the Ethiopian Highlands. Although the plateau and peaks of Antarctica are a large area of high altitude there is no indigenous population.

3.1.1 European Alps

The early development of all branches of mountain science resulted from the increasing ability to travel in these inhospitable regions, due to developments in mountaineering and skiing. The word 'alp' is based originally on a Celtic word meaning 'high mountain': the modern use of this word meaning 'high pasture' dates from the Middle Ages.

The history of the European Alps is the story of how this region, constrained by its geographical position and topography, became a vital and indispensable link in the communications of the whole of Europe. The discovery of 'Similaun Man', some

5000 years old, at a height of 3210 m shows that considerable altitudes were reached by local people when crossing from one valley to another. The deposition of gold bracelets to propitiate the mountain gods was common from prehistory to the Middle Ages and many offerings have been found in the neighborhood of the Great St Bernard Pass. Here the Roman deity Poeninus presided over the crossing and he is commemorated in the present day name, Pennine Alps.

The century between 50 BCE and 50 CE was the first period in which the whole of the European Alps came into the orbit of one political system, the Roman Empire, with communications linking Rome via the Alpine passes with the periphery of that empire. Many of the names used for subregions, such as Alps Maritimae and Alps Cottiae, are still in use today.

The native population was neither static nor homogenous, but it was the Romans who established the main framework of communication in this region. However, their roads had little impact on the essential pasturalism of the Alpine economy and the mountains themselves were feared by the Romans as the abode of dragons and evil forces. The people, with their susceptibility to goiter, were not much admired either.

It was not until the nineteenth century that gradual easing of communications opened up the whole region to the outside world and ignorance turned to knowledge and understanding (Snodgrass 1993).

3.1.2 Himalayas and Tibetan plateau

The Himalayas form a topographically extremely complex region, extending 1500 miles from Nanga Parbat (8125 m) in the west to Namcha Barwa (7756 m) in the east. At their western extremity they are part of a confused mass of peaks, passes and glaciers where the western Kun Lun, Karakoram, Pir Panjal and Pamirs form an area the size of France. The Himalayas contain the world's highest mountain, Mount Everest (8848 m), and many other peaks over 7500 m. The main range forms the watershed between Central Asia and India, and there are middle ranges at intermediate altitudes. The outer Himalayas (up to 1500 m) form foothills rising from the plains of India.

The Tibetan plateau is an area occupied by Tibetans, who have a well-defined culture. It extends in the south to the Himalayas and high Himalayan valleys. To the west the plateau is demarcated by the northward curve of the Himalayas which continues into Kashmir, Baltistan and then to Gilgit and the Karakoram. To the north the peaks (up to 7700 m) of the Kun Lun range, 1500 miles long, mark off the plateau of Tibet from Xinjiang (Chinese Turkestan). To the east it extends to the Koko Nor or Qinghai Lake and, further south, the valleys of Qinghai and Sikiang and the gorge country of south-east Tibet.

The area covers about 1.5 million square miles and is the largest and highest plateau in the world, much of it at an altitude of 4600–4900 m. It presents an enormous range of climate and topography. 'Every 10 li (3 miles) heaven is different.' The major climatic contrast is between the southern side of the Himalayas and the high valleys exposed to the summer Indian monsoon with very high rainfall, particularly in the east, and the aridity and low rainfall of the Tibetan plateau. The change is so abrupt that in some passes in the eastern Himalayas, vegetation may change from tropical to subarctic within a few yards.

The Tibetans believe that in the prehistoric era their land was a large sea, Tethys, which, according to the theory of plate tectonics, is correct. The Royal Society/Chinese Academy of Sciences Tibet Geotraverse in 1985–86 established that the thickness of the Tibetan plateau crust, which at 70 km is about twice as much as normal, is due mainly to folding and thrusting that has occurred as a result of India colliding with Asia, rather than India moving under Asia and elevating to a plateau (Chang et al. 1986). In mythology, Tibetans are descended from the union of a forest monkey and a female demon of the rocks, with the site of the first cultivated field being at Sothang in south-east Tibet, but other legends place their origin further east.

The Tibetans have always regarded themselves as living in the northern part of the world; the Indians, however, considered the Himalayas to be the abode of the gods and inhabited by a race of supermen gifted with special knowledge, particularly of magic, and this probably accounts for the popular European belief of Tibet as a place where the immortal sages dwell, guarding the ultimate secrets. Far from being isolated, however, Tibetans have been subject to influences from China, India, Central Asia and the Middle East for many centuries

(Stein 1972). Permanent buildings are found up to 3500 m with nomadic populations at higher levels. Neolithic human remains have been found near Lhasa (Ward 1990, 1991).

With increasing numbers of Han Chinese immigrants there are more than 3.0 million people living over 3000 m, and it is estimated that the amount of this land available for agriculture is only 5% of the total. In the valleys, fields are terraced; on the plateau, larger fields are found in sheltered areas on valley floors, but all are threatened by snow, hail, wind and erosion. The opening of the Golmud to Lhasa rail link in July 2006 means that it is possible now to travel from all parts of China to Lhasa by rail. This has been a prodigious enterprise. The link is 1100 km; three-quarters of it at altitudes over 4000 m (West 2004a). The numbers of Han Chinese at altitude in Tibet, as visitors or immigrants, are bound to increase as a result. This immigrant population are at higher risk of altitude illness than Tibetans (Chapter 17).

3.1.3 Andes of South America

The highland zone extends from Colombia in the north to central Chile in the south, and is flanked by an arid desert on its west, with a deeply eroded escarpment to the east, which adjoins the Amazon basin.

The central Andean region has three broadly defined areas running parallel with the Pacific Ocean: the cordillera occidentale, the altiplano, a broad undulating plain at 4000 m in the middle, and the cordillera orientale in the east.

The earliest archeological evidence for human occupation dates back 20 000 years (MacNeish 1971) and has been found at Ayacucho, Peru at 2900 m; other early finds are recorded in central Chile, Venezuela and Argentina. The skeleton of a man who lived 9500 years ago has been found at Lauricocha (4200 m) in Peru (Hurtado 1971). The pre-Inca civilizations were situated mainly along the Pacific Coast and the population subsisted mainly on seafood. Little is known of the highland population during this period.

The Inca civilization only achieved a position of major importance in the 100 years preceding the Spanish invasion of 1532. Spanish settlement of highland areas was hindered by ecological restraints imposed by altitude and the nature of the terrain, and, after consolidation of Spanish rule, Peru remained under colonial domination for 300 years, achieving independence in 1824.

Both agriculture and stock raising dominate the subsistence economy, with the upper limit of agriculture at 4000 m and the upper limit of vegetation at 4600 m. Mining is carried out at even greater altitudes and tourism is increasingly popular.

3.1.4 Ethiopian highlands

No well-circumscribed highland zone exists. The country is intersected by a number of rift valley systems, establishing a connection between the African rift valley in the south and the Red Sea. The valley systems divide the country into three reasonably well-defined regions: the western highlands, the eastern highlands and the rift valley itself with the lowland area.

The northern part of the western highlands, the Amhara highlands, attains the greatest altitude (2400–3700 m). The highest peak of Ethiopia, Ras Dashau (4620 m), is a volcanic outcrop and Lake Tana, the origin of the Blue Nile, lies at the center of the region. Much of Ethiopian history centers on this area, which has been settled for many centuries. It is inhabited by the largest of Ethiopia's many population groups, the Amharas and Tigraeans, who are the descendants of people who came from southern Arabia prior to 1000 BCE (Sellassie 1972).

Gondar (3000 m), in the Amhara highlands, with a population of 100 000, became the second largest city in Africa, and it remained the capital of Ethiopia until the middle of the first century, when Addis Ababa was founded.

Much of the population of Ethiopia lives above 2000 m and in the highland area two types of cultivation, by plough and by hoe, predominate. Teff, a type of grass which produces a small seed, is grown up to 3000 m and is the mainstay of the agricultural economy.

3.2 POPULATION

Most of the high altitude areas of the world are in the economically least developed regions and for this reason population numbers in relation to altitude

are difficult to obtain. Although the total population living in mountainous regions is estimated at 400 million, the majority live at low altitude in the valleys. De Jong (1968) 'guessed' that between 13 and 14 million people lived at altitudes above 3000 m. The United Nations Food and Agricultural organization (FAO) recently published data indicating that 45.6 million people lived at altitudes above 2500 m, 13.2 million above 3500 m and 4.1 million of these at altitudes above 4500 m (Huddleston *et al.* 2003).

In South America large populations have lived at high altitude since prehistory and the Andean population at the time of the Spanish conquest was estimated at between 4.5 and 7.5 million. In 1980 it was considered that between 10 and 17 million were living at over 2500 m and in Peru 30–40% of the population of 4 million lived at or above this height, with 1.5% living at over 4000 m.

In Asia and Africa the estimates are less accurate. On the Tibetan plateau, which consists of the autonomous region of Tibet (Xizang) and Qinghai province, the population is estimated as between 4 and 5 million. Lhasa (3658 m), in 1986, had about 130 000 inhabitants, mainly Tibetan, but recent immigration of Han Chinese has increased this number. Relatively small groups, nomads (at up to 5450 m) and miners (at up to 6000 m), live at higher levels. Fairly large numbers live at altitudes exceeding 3000 m in the upper valleys of eastern Tibet, and in Nepal about 60 000 live above this level, with a number of villages in Dolpo being at 5000 m (Snellgrove 1961). In Ethiopia about 50% of the total population of 26 million live above 2000 m. Small populations in Mexico, the USA and the former USSR live above 3000 m, for instance in Kyrgyzstan.

In tropical latitudes permanent settlements are usually placed where both pasture and timber can be used and the upper limit of habitation may fall between the two. Further from the equator the upper limit falls below the timber line and variation in temperature becomes seasonal; the upper pasturelands are thus used for a semi-nomadic economy. Permanently inhabited villages are found at lower levels, with isolated groups of buildings or shelters on the pastures occupied for the grazing season and evacuated during the winter. Considerable migration may occur and part of the population may always be on the move. One mine, now closed, was worked at 5950 m in South America; although the miners lived at rather lower altitudes, the caretakers lived there permanently (West 1986a).

Those who spend periods at greater altitude are mountaineers, who have evolved specialized techniques of movement above the snow line. In winter, movement across snow is essential for the feeding of livestock quartered in isolated shelters. Since prehistoric times boards have been placed on the feet to facilitate movement. The earliest references to primitive skis are found in the Nordic sagas of 3000 BCE and, in northern Norway, rock engravings of skiers are dated at around 2500 BCE. In the UK skis were used in Cumberland at the start of the eighteenth century. The modern sport dates from 1870. No historical evidence of the use of skis has been found in South American or Tibetan populations.

Highland populations, being strategically placed between prosperous lowland centers, play a vital role in trade. Because they are physiologically well adapted they are capable of crossing high mountain passes with heavy loads and use their animals to carry produce. Major mountain passes have for centuries been arteries for trade, the movement of people and ideas, and the dissemination of disease. The closing of passes such as the Nangpa La between the two different economies of Tibet and Nepal caused a fall in living standards until readjustments had been made.

3.3 TERRAIN

Although mountain country varies widely, there are two distinct types: the high, flat, plateaux (Tibet and the altiplano of South America) and deep valleys (Himalayas and Andes) (Fig. 3.1).

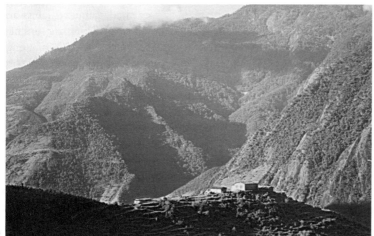

Figure 3.1 Contrasting terrain and climate at altitude. (a) Typical mountainous country on southern slopes of the Himalaya. (b) The north Tibetan plateau with the Kun Lun range in the background.

(a)

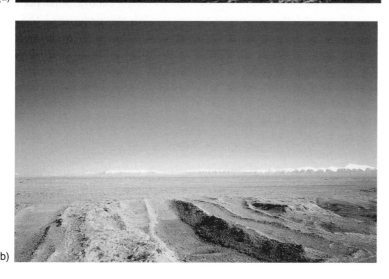

(b)

Plateaux can support large populations and large towns but they may be isolated by virtue of distance from lowland cities, which are usually the center of government, commerce and industry.

In mountain valleys, because flat ground is at a premium, populations tend to be smaller, with groups perched on slopes and ridges far from one another. The placing of houses in sunny positions is more difficult and isolation within the community is common. Communications are easily severed by land slips, avalanches and other natural disasters. The funneling effect of valleys on wind may increase its velocity with an ensuing stunting effect on vegetation and trees. This also restricts the placing of houses, as does the availability of water and the possibility of natural disasters.

3.4 CLIMATE

The climate near the ground at high altitude has several basic features. At any given latitude, seasonal variation of monthly temperature is less at high altitude than at sea level and, as the equator is reached, seasonal variation virtually disappears. Diurnal variations are considerable, and can show a range of 30°C. This is because of high levels of long-wave radiation that occur in cloudless skies during the day and escape to clear skies at night. In overcast conditions the diurnal variation decreases.

With increasing altitude the temperature falls. There is no uniform value for decline, or lapse rate, although the figure 1°C for every 150 m is usually given.

Solar radiation is an important factor in maintaining thermal balance in humans at extreme altitude. High winds are also a feature of mountains. A gust of 231 mph has been recorded on Mount Washington (1917 m) in the eastern USA.

3.4.1 Rainfall

In Asia, the monsoon flows from east to west across India, cooling as it is forced to ascend by the Himalayas. Water vapor condenses and falls as rain, and as it passes to the west the monsoon becomes depleted of water; the eastern Himalayas are thus very wet, the western dry. In Darjeeling the annual

rainfall is 2000–3000 mm a year; in the central Himalayas at Simla it is 1500 mm, but in the west at Ladakh it is only 75 mm. The Karakoram is arid whereas the eastern Himalayan region is tropical.

There is also considerable north–south variation with subarctic species on the Tibetan plateau and tropical species often only a few hundred yards away to the south. This is particularly marked on some passes in the eastern Himalayas. On the plateau, although 'monsoon' clouds are seen on the Tangulla range, about 700 km north of Lhasa, precipitation is small. In the deserts of the Tarim basin and Tsaidam to the north of the Tibetan plateau, annual rainfall may be less than 100 mm.

In the Andes the Pacific coastal strip is desert – 'It never rains in Lima.' Along the whole length of the coast the cold Humboldt current cools the air above the sea, reducing its capacity to retain moisture which normally falls as rain. Once air passes over the land, it is warmed again and increases its capacity to retain moisture, making rain unlikely.

The western slopes of the Andes are dry; cacti and eucalyptus trees flourish and only a few high mountains are snow covered. The eastern slopes which descend to the Amazon basin become progressively more humid and tree covered.

The rainfall in the UK and Europe is influenced by the Gulf Stream. Records kept between 1884 and 1901 by the observatory on the summit of Ben Nevis, Scotland (1300 mm), the highest peak in the UK, show that the average daily sunshine was only 2 h and the annual rainfall was 3500 mm, as much or more than Darjeeling (MacPhee 1936).

3.4.2 Temperature

The fall in temperature globally with altitude has been discussed in Chapter 2. However, the temperature of mountain regions is very variable and records of the observatory on the summit of Ben Nevis (1300 m) between 1884 and 1901 show that the mean temperature over these 17 years was −0.1°C; the lowest temperature was −17°C and the highest +19°C. On the plateau of the Cairngorms in Scotland, which has an average height of around 1000 m, similar temperatures have been recorded with winds gusting to over 160 km h^{-1} (100 mph).

In North America, Alaska and the Yukon a number of peaks of 6000 m lie within the Arctic Circle.

Temperatures of −30°C at 5500–6000 m have been recorded, with gale force winds, in the winter (Mills 1973b).

In the European Alps, the average temperature was −13°C during a winter expedition up to 4000 m, carried out over several days, in the Bernese Oberland in Switzerland (Leuthold *et al.* 1975); gale force winds were not uncommon. Temperatures on the summit of Everest (8848 m) in winter are probably of the order of −60°C; in summer the average temperature would be about −30°C. Hillary recorded a temperature of −27°C at 8500 m on Everest at 3 a.m. on 29 May 1953, the day the first ascent was made (Ward 1993b). On the Changthang (the northern part of the Tibetan plateau), which has an average height of 4900 m, there are few days when the temperature reaches as high as 10°C, and −25°C has been recorded.

In Lhasa (3658 m) there are about 100 days a year when the temperature is around 10°C; in summer it may rise as high as 27°C but in the winter it falls to −15°C.

In Antarctica, the lowest recorded temperature is −88.2°C and the highest 15.2°C. The dangers of cold injury, therefore, are likely to complicate accidents or illness in mountain regions.

3.4.3 Humidity

Ambient humidity influences heat loss from the body by evaporation and, in regions where the humidity is high, heat regulation is more difficult. In arid areas with a low humidity, heat regulation is easier.

3.4.4 Solar radiation

Although temperature falls with altitude there is increased exposure to solar radiation (Chapter 2). The amount of radiation absorbed by the body depends on clothing and posture. The clear mountain air permits an increased degree of direct radiation which is enhanced by indirect radiation reflected from the snow. The altitude of the sun is also important (Chrenko and Pugh 1961). The solar heat absorbed depends on the type of clothing; dark clothing absorbs more radiation than light-colored clothing.

3.4.5 Ultraviolet radiation

There appears to be some increase in the level of ultraviolet radiation at high altitude. Snow reflects up to 90% of ultraviolet radiation, compared with 9–17% reflected from ground covered by grass (Buettner 1969), so in snow-covered terrain the combination of direct (incident) and reflected ultraviolet radiation is considerable.

3.5 ECONOMICS

Most mountain communities depend on animal husbandry and agriculture; mining is important in some regions but more recently tourism has assumed a greater significance.

Animal husbandry predominates in regions above the limit of agriculture. On the Tibetan plateau, or Changthang, which covers two-thirds of Tibet, there are immense herds of yak, sheep and goats herded by nomads. Similar nomadic culture was traditional in mountainous regions of central Asian countries such as Kyrgyzstan, though now most herdsmen are semi-nomadic, living in town or village houses in the winter and in their traditional felt covered tents (yurts) in the summer. In the bitter climate nomadic pastoralism is the only viable and economic way of life and this may have started between 9000 and 10 000 years ago. The survival of the animals depends exclusively on natural fodder, which creates problems as the sedges and grasses have only a short growing season between May and September. Because there are no areas on the plateau where grass will grow in the winter they cannot escape the climate and, as extensive migration would weaken the stock, only short distances, up to 40 miles, are traversed. Each family has a 'home base', which is sometimes a house, and migrates to set areas whose boundaries, though not fenced, are all well known. On the Tibetan plateau tents made of yak and sheep's wool are used as dwellings. Further north camels are common (Goldstein and Beall 1989). In the upper Himalayan valleys the pattern is similar, with flocks spending the summer on pastures up to 5000 m, but below the snow line; in the winter they return to more permanent and protected locations at 4000 m.

The llama *(Lama glama)* and yak *(Bos grunniens)* are extremely important to the economy of the

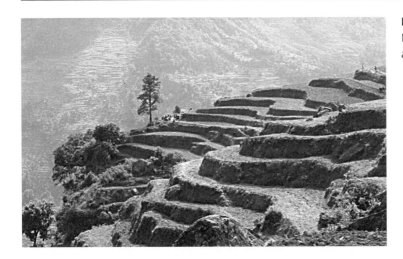

Figure 3.2   Typical terraces in Nepal after harvesting, late autumn.

populations of the South American altiplano, and of Tibet and the Himalayan valleys. Both these species show genetic adaptation to high altitude (Chapter 17).

The limiting factor in agriculture is the number of months that the soil remains frozen; only a single period of the year may be available for cultivation. The type of crop may influence the size of population. Potatoes introduced into the high Himalayan valleys of Nepal between 1850 and 1860 increased the population of Sola Khumbu in the Everest region from 169 households in 1836 to 596 in 1957 (Fuhrer-Haimendorf 1964, p. 10). Immigrants came from Tibet over the Nangpa La, a glacier pass of 5800 m, and, because food was more abundant, were able to adopt the religious life and built many new monasteries. Increasing the productivity of the land, as well as the area under cultivation in Tibet, may change the pattern of life near the centers of population under the present Chinese-organized regime.

Level land may have to be manufactured in the form of terraces. This technique to produce land for agriculture from even steeply sloping hillsides is found in almost all mountainous areas but especially in the Himalayas and Andes. The terraces range in size from a few square feet to a relatively large area, but which is usually too small for pasture (Fig. 3.2). Irrigation may involve ingenious construction of water conduits from surrounding streams. The task of building and maintaining terraces is considerable, especially as manure has to be carried up and placed manually. Despite this, terracing is a marked feature of populated mountain valleys and, as it involves ownership and

maintenance by groups rather than individuals, the social implications are important. High grazing pasture (alps) is also communal pasture land and this too has social overtones.

Mining, which is often carried out above the pasture level or in rocky terrain, may involve the building of special towns and roads. In Tibet gold mining has been carried on for centuries, often at 5000 m. However, shallow trenches were used and no deep mines were worked. Recently, a gold mine has been established at 4500 m in northern Chile, and other mines are being opened at comparable altitudes. In recently opened mines at high altitude in Chile there are no resident high altitude populations. The miners live at low altitude with their families and commute to the mine for a period of a week or 10 days followed by the same period off duty at low altitude. Thus they never fully acclimatize nor are they unacclimatized. This intermittent exposure to altitude has been of interest to physiologists (Richalet *et al.* 2002) and is further discussed in Chapter 27.

Tourism, particularly skiing, may involve developing an area which has no natural amenities except good snow fields and glaciers. In 2001 about 20 000 tourists visited the Everest region out of about 100 000 trekkers and almost 300 000 tourists to Nepal.

3.6 LOAD CARRYING

Loads are carried by all who visit mountainous regions. In the valleys of the Himalayas professional

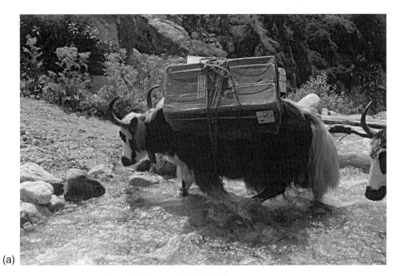

(a)

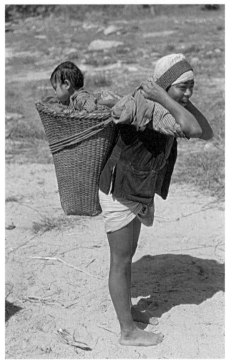

(b)

Figure 3.3 Load carrying in the Himalayas. (a) A yak carrying expedition equipment. (b) A young Nepalese porter with typical basket and head strap carrying his young sister and a load.

porters carry much of the merchandise and the economy depends on them, together with yak and mule transport (Fig. 3.3a).

Observations by Pugh in 1952 and 1953 on the march in to Everest (Pugh 1955) suggest that loads of 40–50 kg, with an addition of 10 kg personal baggage, are carried routinely by porters for 10–12 h over 10–12 miles each day. Often ascents and descents of 1000–1200 m are made, with loads of tea or paper weighing over 60 kg occasionally being carried.

As the body weight of porters is usually 45–60 kg, and the average height just over 150 cm, each porter carries his own weight in merchandise.

Where possible, loads are carried in a conical, light but strong, wicker basket, 22 by 30 cm at the base and 50 by 70 cm at the top, with a height of 60 cm (Fig. 3.3b). Larger sizes are available for carrying bulky loads such as leaf mold. Loads are supported by a strap passing over the forehead and under the lower end of the basket. When in position the upper end of the basket is level with the top of the porter's head. The center of gravity therefore is as close as possible to a vertical line passing through the center of the pelvis, thus reducing the torque on the spine. The advantage of the head band is that it allows direct transmission of the load to the vertebral column, with muscles being used for balancing rather than support, as when shoulder straps are used. This method of carrying has to be learnt as a child, and the neck muscles in all such Himalayan porters are extremely well developed. In East Africa heavy loads are carried in this way or just balanced on the head. It has been suggested that this method of load carrying, if practiced from childhood, is more economic, in terms of oxygen consumption, than the Western method in a rucksack (Maloiy et al. 1986). Minetti et al. (2006) found Nepalese porters to have greatly increased performance in load carrying compared with Caucasian mountaineers. This was especially true of uphill walking (+60% in speed and +39% in mechanical power) but they showed greater efficiency also in downhill walking when carrying a load. The authors thought the porters' superior performance could be partly explained by better balance control; they had less oscillations of the trunk than the mountaineers, due presumably to skill acquired over a lifetime of load carrying. Thus they did not waste energy in the unproductive muscle contraction needed by the mountaineers to keep their balance.

Marching technique depends on the weight of the load. With loads of 50 kg, stops are made every 2–3 min, with rests lasting 0.5–1.0 min after a distance of 70–250 m has been covered, depending on the gradient. With lighter loads, rests for 2–3 min every 10 min are normal. Longer pauses are made every hour.

During rests, the loads are supported on a T-stick about 1 m long, and the porter does not sit down. When longer rests are taken, loads are placed on the top of stone walls conveniently placed beside the track, usually in the shade of a large tree.

Heart rate in porters walking up steep paths varies between 150 and 170 beats min^{-1}; on the level between 100 and 124 beats min^{-1} and downhill between 80 and 104 beats min^{-1}.

At about 3700 m, porter loads are reduced to 25 kg (gross weight 35 kg) which are carried to 5700 m. Exhaustion, when it occurs, is due to overwork; that is, not enough rest days. Few porters have any interest in climbing mountains and so tend to give up when the effects of hypoxia appear.

With high altitude Sherpas, load-carrying ability is considerable. Without supplementary oxygen on Everest in 1933 eight porters carried loads weighing 10–15 kg to an altitude of 8300 m, as they did on the Swiss Everest Expedition in 1952.

Low altitude porters carry their own food, eating tsampa (pre-cooked barley) or ata (wheat flour), which is made into a paste or dough, three times a day. Four seers (4 kg) of tsampa is the standard ration for each man for 3.5 days, equivalent to 14.6 kJ (3500 kcal) man^{-1} day^{-1}.

Mountaineers also carry considerable loads to high altitude but use shoulder straps, climb more slowly and stop less frequently.

3.7 HOUSES AND SHELTER

Cultural mechanisms that provide a comfortable microclimate and reduce heat loss have been developed in all high altitude communities. The ideal house should be draught-free with a low ratio of surface area to volume and well constructed of material which diminishes the daily extremes of temperature. The roof should be well insulated.

In the Andes the adobe (dried mud) building has the first meter or so of the walls made of stone, the roof is of tile, grass or tin and walls are plastered with mud to provide an airtight structure; the roof is tightly fitted and the floor may be wood or dirt. Because of the method of construction the diurnal change is reduced (Baker 1966). In the Himalayas the thermal protection of stone structures built for semi-nomadic occupation appears to be less. Traditional Sherpa houses often have only one floor, with stone walls and wooden roofs held on with stones. The ground floor is without windows and provides quarters for animals; the first floor is for human habitation. Windows usually have no glass, but have wooden shutters, and an open fire is placed in the center of one side, but this provides only a transient increase in temperature. Nowadays, in places like Namche Bazaar, where the benefits of greatly increased tourism have increased wealth, better housing with glass in the windows is to be found. However, in areas less popular with trekkers, such as the Rolwaling Valley, traditional Sherpa houses are still common.

In north Bhutan houses are similarly constructed but animals are kept in a yard. Cracks between stones in both Bhutanese and Sherpa houses are filled with earth. Tibetan houses may be of more than one floor and are often in terraces. Glass is rare and the houses are heated by an open fire or stove. Nomads have tents with a loose wide weave which enables warm air to be entrapped but allows egress of smoke from open fires and is waterproof. However, some semi-nomadic families have a stove with a chimney.

In Central Asia the nomads traditionally live in yurts. These tent-like structures have a wooden frame, the tunduk, covered with felt. The floor and walls are covered with rugs. Yurts are circular with an opening in the center of the conical roof allowing smoke to escape. This opening can be covered or 'cowled' against the prevailing wind. The yurt can be quickly dismantled and transported on pack animals, yaks, camels or horses.

3.8 CLOTHING

Because of the generally low temperature and loss of heat, particularly due to radiation and convection, clothing with good insulation is necessary to provide a warm microclimate. Trapped, still air is the best insulation and wool is the best naturally available insulating material; it resists compacting and loses only 40% of its insulating value when wet. Garments that are loosely woven entrap more air than those that are tightly woven.

A multiple layered system for garments is preferable to one thick layer because insulation can be varied at will, thus minimizing perspiration. The outer layer should be as impermeable to wind as possible. A sheepskin coat is the best naturally available garment that has many of these characteristics, and is usually worn with cotton or wool undergarments.

In general, Andean clothing conforms to the above model and natural clothing is adequate for the conditions encountered. Measurements of insulation of normal clothing without hats, shawls and ponchos showed values for men slightly less than those for women (Little and Hanna 1978). The greatest increase in surface temperature occurred in the hands and feet. At night, Andean highlanders, who use a bedding of skins, can maintain their metabolic rate by light shivering that does not disturb sleep.

In the high Himalayan valleys and Tibet, clothing assemblies are similar. The main garment is a thick sheepskin 'chupa' with long, wide sleeves which, when extended, keep the hands warm; gloves are never used. Normally the garment is gathered around the waist by a belt and hitched up to the knees so that there is a pocket for loose objects in front of the chest. When the belt is loosened the garment extends to the ground and thus can be used as a sleeping robe; often in warm conditions one or both shoulders are left bare. Under this is a woolen shirt and often long woolen, cotton or sheepskin trousers. Soft leather boots with decorative wool leggings extending to the knees are packed with grass, straw or leaves but a Tibetan often may walk in bare feet in the snow or through streams. Some wear a felt hat or balaclava and, to prevent snow blindness, yak hair is put in front of the eyes if goggles are not available (Desideri 1712–27, Moorcroft and Trebeck 1841, Vol. 1 p. 399). Other methods used by Tibetans include blackening the eyelids and wearing masks with tiny eye holes, the rims of which are blackened (MacDonald 1929, p. 182). Cotton clothing is favored at high temperatures and low altitudes, but nomads wear wool or sheepskin. Many now wear wool sweaters and leather boots. Tibetan nomads sleep resting on their elbows and knees with all their clothes piled on their backs (Holditch 1907, Duff 1999b). This 'fetal position' diminishes surface area and therefore heat loss: contact with the ground is also minimal.

Some Tibetan lamas have developed the ability to 'warm without fire'. The central core temperature is kept raised under cold conditions, both by increasing the metabolic rate, probably by continuous light shivering, and also by the practice of g-tum-mo yoga (an advanced form of Tibetan yoga), which appears to involve peripheral vasodilatation (Pugh 1963, Benson et al. 1982).

Children have oil rubbed over their bodies and adults seldom wash, the natural skin oils forming a protective layer. Very few Tibetans living on the plateau are obese (Bell 1928).

3.9 HUMAN RESPONSE TO COLD AND ALTITUDE

The main environmental stresses of living in mountain regions are cold and the hypoxia of altitude.

3.9.1 Cold

Temperature is a more important factor than altitude in colonizing high mountainous regions; high altitude residents seem to withstand cold better than sea level visitors to altitude.

Most of the process of adaptation to cold consists of the adoption of clothing and housing which reduce cold stress by maintaining a microclimate as close as possible to the preferred temperature. However, some studies have demonstrated different physiological responses in high altitude residents to experimental cold stress compared with low altitude controls. These have been summarized by Little and Hanna (1978) in drawing from work on Andean and Tibetan high altitude residents.

In response to abrupt exposure to cold, high altitude residents, when contrasted with sea level Caucasian control subjects, show the following responses:

- No dramatic fall of core temperature
- A slightly elevated basal metabolic rate
- Consistently high surface temperatures in extremities
- A slightly greater loss of body heat

These changes are probably the result of lifelong intermittent exposure to modest cold stress rather than cold plus altitude. Pugh (1963) found a number of these responses in a Nepalese pilgrim studied at 4500 m, who came from a village at only 1800 m. Benson *et al.* (1982) found similar changes in Tibetans practicing g-tum-mo yoga. The elevation of basal metabolic rate may be the effect of hypoxia and cold acting together (Little and Hanna 1978). Further aspects of cold adaptation are considered in Chapter 23.

3.9.2 Hypoxia

In order to colonize the mountainous regions above about 3000 m, acclimatization to the chronic hypoxia of altitude is important. This response to hypoxia is discussed in detail in Chapter 4. People born and brought up at altitude have certain advantages over lowlanders and this is discussed in Chapters 4 and 17. However, long-term residence also carries the risk of chronic mountain sickness and high altitude pulmonary hypertension (Chapter 21). The question of whether altitude populations have undergone adaptation in the biological sense of genetic selection for that environment is hotly debated. There is some evidence that this has happened to a degree in the case of Tibetans (see Chapter 17).

Altitude acclimatization and deterioration

SUMMARY

Altitude acclimatization is the physiological process which takes place in the body on exposure to hypoxia at altitude (or in a chamber). It comprises a number of responses by different systems in the body, which mitigate, to a degree, the effects of the fall in oxygen partial pressure so that the tissues of the body are defended against this fall to a remarkable degree. Advantageous though this process is, it does not restore performance to that at sea level. Probably the most important change is the increase in breathing (minute ventilation) due to stimulation of the peripheral chemoreceptor (carotid bodies) by hypoxia and changes in the chemical control of breathing. Another is the well-known increase in haemoglobin concentration in the blood. The time courses of these responses vary but most of the changes take place over a period of days up to a few weeks. Individuals vary in the speed and extent to which they can acclimatize. Apart from past history of acclimatization there are no good predictors of future performance. A recent interest is in the effect of intermittent hypoxia. Intermittent hypoxia, in sufficient dose, can produce some of the changes of acclimatization.

Adaptation is a term used to describe the changes which take place over generations by natural selection enabling animals and humans to function better at altitude.

Deterioration is a condition that is evident after some time spent at extreme altitude. It develops over weeks above about 5500 m, and over days above 8000 m. It is characterized by loss of appetite, weight loss, lethargy, fatigue, slowness of thought and poor judgement.

4.1 THE PHYSIOLOGICAL RESPONSE TO HYPOXIA

4.1.1 Introduction

The response of the body to hypoxia depends crucially on the rate as well as the degree of hypoxia. For instance the effect on a pilot of sudden loss of oxygen supply in an unpressurized aircraft at the height of the summit of Mount Everest is quite different from the effect of similar altitude on a climber who has spent some weeks at altitude. The pilot would probably lose consciousness in a few minutes (Fig. 4.1) whereas the climber, though very breathless, will not only remain conscious but also be able to work out his route and climb slowly upward.

The symptoms of acute hypoxia are few and subtle (Fig. 4.1). The effect of acute, often severe, hypoxia has been studied intensively since Paul Bert first pointed out the danger of ascent to high altitude to early balloonists (Chapter 1). Figure 4.1 shows the effect of sudden exposure to various increasing

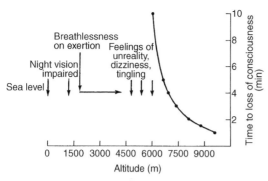

Figure 4.1 The effect of sudden exposure to various altitudes. At extreme altitude consciousness will be lost after an average time indicated by the curve on the right. There is considerable variability in this time. (Data from Sharp 1978.)

altitudes. At modest altitude breathlessness may be felt on exertion and some rise in heart rate noticed but the main effect is on the central nervous system. At levels as low as 1500 m night vision is impaired (Pretorius, 1970). At 4000–5000 m some tingling of the fingers and mouth may be noticed but, although the subject would now definitely be hypoxic, there would be very little subjective sensation to indicate this fact. Above about 5000 m some subjects may become unconscious and above 7000 m most will do so (Sharp, 1978). There is considerable individual variation in response to acute hypoxia. Figure 4.1 shows the average time to loss of consciousness after sudden exposure to given altitudes. It will be seen that, on acute exposure to the altitude equivalent to the summit of Everest, the unacclimatized subject remains conscious for only about 2 min.

By contrast the effect of hypoxia on an acclimatized person is much less. The main symptom is shortness of breath on exertion. The preferred rate of climbing amongst mountaineers is at about 50% $V_{O_2,max}$. This typically requires a ventilation of about 50 L min^{-1} at sea level, whereas at 6300 m the ventilation for this work rate will be about 160 L min^{-1}, close to the maximum voluntary ventilation at sea level. The difference between the pilot and the climber is due to a series of adaptive changes in the body known as acclimatization.

As oxygen is such a vital substrate for mammalian life it is not surprising that hypoxia causes many deleterious effects on many systems in the body. Some of these changes are addressed in later chapters; the term acclimatization is reserved for

those changes resulting from hypoxia which are beneficial.

4.1.2 Definition of altitude acclimatization

To mountaineers, acclimatization is the process by which they become more comfortable at altitude and find they can perform better than when they first arrived at a particular altitude. Subjectively, there is both relief of symptoms of acute mountain sickness and a return of some of their climbing performance lost on arrival at altitude. For physiologists, altitude acclimatization is, strictly, the sum of all the beneficial changes in response to altitude hypoxia, but it is often defined by the increase in ventilation and the consequent reduction in P_{CO_2} (and increase in P_{O_2}).

4.1.3 Rate of acclimatization

The changes involved in acclimatization occur in various systems and with varying time courses. These are illustrated in Fig. 4.2, which shows the futility of the frequently asked question, 'How long does it take to become acclimatized?' However, the most important changes are in the cardio-respiratory system and the blood with time courses of days or a few weeks.

Early changes in acclimatization were recently studied in six lowlanders (Lundby *et al.* 2004a). Subjects were studied at sea level (normoxic and acute hypoxia) and after 2 and 8 weeks acclimatization at 4100 m in Bolivia. Local high altitude (HA) residents were also studied at altitude. Some results from this study are shown in Fig. 4.3 for rest (a) and maximum exercise (b). It can be seen that the hematocrit rises during the first 2 weeks to close to the HA residents' value and is no higher at 8 weeks (see below). The P_{a,O_2} continues to rise for 8 weeks and is still below that of the HA residents. Changes in P_{a,CO_2} appear to be complete at 2 weeks while the alveolar to arterial P_{O_2} difference ((A–a) P_{O_2}) rises with acute hypoxia, is greater at 2 weeks and falls slightly at 8 weeks. The HA residents have very low values for this parameter. The situation at maximum work rate is similar except that the P_{a,CO_2} continues to fall due to increased exercise ventilation.

HYPOXIA

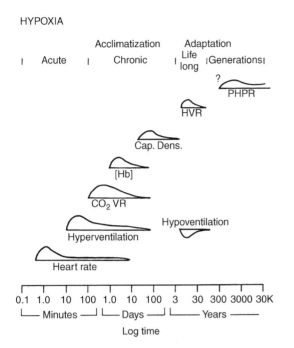

Figure 4.2   Time courses of a number of acclimatization and adaptive changes plotted on a log time scale, the curve of each response denoting the rate of change, which is fast at first then tails off. Included are: heart rate, hyperventilation and hypoventilation, the carbon dioxide ventilatory response (HCVR), hemoglobin concentration ([Hb]), changes in capillary density (Cap. Dens.), hypoxic ventilatory response (HVR) and pulmonary hypoxic pressor response (PHPR).

The improvement in Pa,O_2 is impressive and no doubt contributes to the improved performance so frequently noted by mountaineers during the course of an expedition.

In some cases the changes of acclimatization involve a biphasic response; for instance, the heart rate response to hypoxia shows a rise within a few minutes, followed by a fall over weeks at altitude (Chapter 7). The change measured can include two responses with different time courses. For instance minute ventilation involves the rapid hypoxic ventilatory response within a few minutes, followed by slow changes in both central and peripheral chemoreceptor response over 1–20 days (Chapter 5). Similarly, the well-known increase in hemoglobin concentration is due to a rapid decrease in plasma volume, followed by a slow increase in red cell mass (Chapter 8).

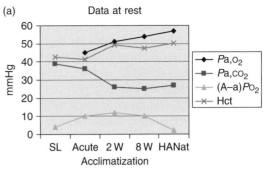

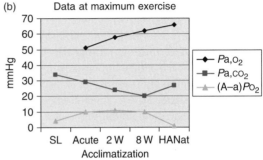

Figure 4.3   Changes in Pa,O_2, Pa,CO_2, (A–a)PO_2 and hematocrit (Hct) at sea level (SL) under normoxia and acute hypoxia, at altitude (4100 m) after 2 weeks (2W) and 8 weeks (8W) acclimatization, mean results in six lowlanders and eight Amarya high altitude natives (HA Nat); at rest (a) and maximum exercise (b). (Drawn using data from Lundby et al. 2004a.)

4.1.4 Hypoxia: is there a difference between hypobaric and normobaric hypoxia?

Since the studies of Paul Bert (1878) it has been accepted that the effects of hypoxia are due to the reduced partial pressure of oxygen (PO_2) and are the same however this reduction is achieved. Hypoxia can be produced either by lowering the barometric pressure, hypobaric hypoxia, as happens when we ascend to high altitude, or by reducing the percentage of oxygen (O_2%) in the inhaled gas mixture, normobaric hypoxia. Apart from the effects of hypoxia, hypobaria has some physiological effects, especially if imposed suddenly upon the subject. These relate to possible bubble formation in the blood and tissues as in decompression sickness experienced by divers coming to the surface too fast and also in aircrew subject to explosive decompression at great altitudes. However, in the case of travelers taking some hours or mountaineers taking days to reach altitude this is not a problem though it cannot be ruled out in chamber studies where rates of ascent may be fast enough to cause micro-bubble formation.

A number of studies have addressed this question and have reported some differences in the effect of these two types of hypoxia. Roach *et al.* (1996) studied nine subjects exposed to 9 h of either normobaric or hypobaric hypoxia equivalent to 4564 m, or to normoxic hypobaria (increased O_2% at lowered pressure). They found that acute mountain sickness symptom (AMS) scores were significantly higher in hypobaric hypoxia than in normobaric hypoxia. Normoxic hypobaria resulted in virtually no symptoms. In a recent study (Loeppky *et al.* 2005b) the same authors extended these results, confirming the effect on AMS scores and finding differences in fluid balance and in some endocrine responses. They found no differences in Sa,O_2. Savourey *et al.* (2003) looked for differences in cardio-respiratory variables between the two forms of hypoxia (altitude equivalent 4500 m) given for 40 min in 18 subjects. They found that hypobaric hypoxia resulted in lower ventilation, lower Pa,O_2, Sa,O_2, Pa,CO_2, and higher pH, suggesting, if true, that there is a problem in gas exchange under hypobaric hypoxia not present in normobaric hypoxia. The significance of these studies remains to be established.

4.2 ACCLIMATIZATION AND ADAPTATION

4.2.1 Acclimatization

The term 'altitude acclimatization' refers to the process whereby lowland humans and animals respond to the reduced partial pressure of oxygen (PO_2) in the inspired air. It refers only to the changes in response to hypoxia seen as beneficial as opposed to changes which result in illness such as acute mountain sickness. Acclimatization is then a series of physiological processes. Other changes, resulting in illness, are pathological.

The processes of acclimatization all tend to reduce the fall in PO_2 as oxygen is transported through the body from the outside air to the tissues. However, even in the best acclimatized individual the tissue PO_2 is not restored to the sea level

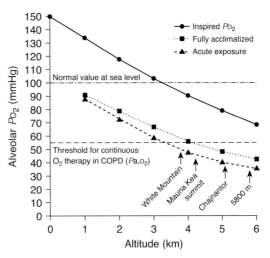

Figure 4.4 PA,O_2 of unacclimatized (acute exposure) and acclimatized subjects at altitudes from 1000 to 6000 m. Also plotted, as dashed lines, are the normal sea level PA,O_2 of 100 Torr, and the value at which patients with chronic obstructive pulmonary disease (COPD) are entitled to continuous oxygen therapy, 55 Torr. Note that even acclimatized subjects are below this latter value when above altitudes of about 4000 m. (From West 2004b, with permission.)

value and performance remains impaired. This is illustrated in Fig. 4.4 which shows the inspired PO_2 and arterial PO_2 (Pa,O_2) of a subject exposed to acute hypoxia and after acclimatization. Also shown are the normal Pa,O_2 at sea level and the Pa,O_2 at which continuous O_2 therapy is advised for patients with chronic obstructive lung disease. It can be seen that even acclimatized subjects are below this level at altitudes above 4000 m.

4.2.2 Adaptation

People born and bred at altitude have certain characteristics which distinguish them from even well-acclimatized lowlanders. There is debate about whether these are due to environmental, operating during early growth, or genetic causes. The term adaptation is used for characteristics thought to be due to natural selection, working on the gene pool. Adaptation, in this sense, has certainly taken place in animals such as the yak and llama. In the case of the yak one example is the loss of the hypoxic pulmonary pressor response which seems to be due to a single dominant gene (Harris, 1986). There is some evidence of a similar adaptation in Tibetans resident at high altitude for generations. This is, at present, only suggestive though recent studies tend to support this notion (see Chapter 17).

4.3 THE OXYGEN TRANSPORT SYSTEM

4.3.1 Introduction

Figure 4.5 shows the oxygen transport system at sea level and at high altitude. This diagram can be used as a 'table of contents' of changes due to acclimatization, which will be followed in succeeding chapters. P_{O_2} falls at each stage as oxygen is transported from outside air, ambient P_{O_2} to inspired, to alveolar, to arterial, to mixed venous which approximates to the mean tissue P_{O_2}. This forms a staircase or cascade of P_{O_2}. The process of acclimatization can

be thought of as reducing each step in this cascade as far as possible.

4.3.2 Ambient to inspired P_{O_2} ($PI_{,O_2}$)

The ambient P_{O_2} of dry air at sea level is about 160 mmHg (20.9% of 760 mmHg the barometric pressure). At an altitude of 5800 m in the example shown in Fig. 4.5, the barometric pressure is just half that at sea level (Chapter 2) so the ambient P_{O_2} is also half the sea level value, 80 mmHg. The drop seen in the figure from ambient to inspired P_{O_2} of about 10 mmHg is due to the addition of water vapour to the inspired air as it is wetted and warmed to body temperature in the nose, mouth, larynx and trachea. The water vapor pressure at body temperature is 47 mmHg, and this displaces almost 10 mmHg P_{O_2}. This physical cause of P_{O_2} reduction is beyond the control of the body and so applies equally at altitude, though its effect is proportionately more important there.

4.3.3 Inspired to alveolar P_{O_2} ($PA_{,O_2}$)

At sea level there is a drop of about 50 mmHg at this point in the oxygen transport system. This drop can be thought of as being due to the addition of carbon dioxide and the uptake of oxygen and so depends, in part, on the metabolic rate. However, it also depends on alveolar ventilation and for a given O_2 uptake and CO_2 output the size of this reduction is entirely due to ventilation. A doubling of ventilation results in a halving of this drop. If ventilation were infinite there would be no reduction and alveolar gas would be fresh air. After acclimatization at 5800 m resting alveolar ventilation is approximately doubled and this step in the system, as shown in Fig. 4.5, is halved.

This increase in ventilation is one of the most important aspects of acclimatization and the mechanisms underlying it, the changes in control of breathing, are dealt with in Chapter 5.

Figure 4.5 shows also the effect of exercise on the oxygen transport system (the dashed lines). At sea level the $PA_{,O_2}$ is little changed by exercise but at altitude the increase of ventilation is far greater in response to exercise than at sea level, so that with exercise the $PA_{,O_2}$ is increased and $PA_{,CO_2}$ decreased (Chapter 11).

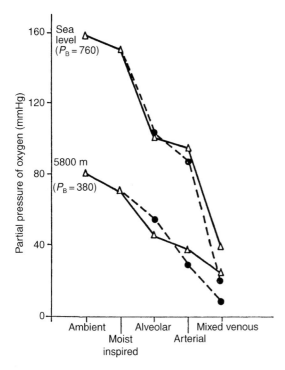

Figure 4.5   The oxygen transport system from outside air through the body at sea level and at an altitude of 5800 m. P_B, barometric pressure; $\triangle$ rest; $\bullet$ maximum exercise. Ref Pugh 1964a (Pugh, L.C.G.E. Man at high altitude, *Scientific Basis of Medicine, Annual Review*, pp. 32–54, 1964)

4.3.4 Alveolar to arterial P_{O_2} (Pa,$_{O_2}$)

Oxygen passes across the alveolar–capillary membrane by diffusion resulting in a small pressure drop but in the normal lung this accounts for less than 1 mmHg. The total alveolar–arterial (A–a)P_{O_2} gradient at sea level is about 6–10 mmHg. The major part of this gradient is due to ventilation/perfusion ratio (V/Q) inequalities. Even in the healthy lung the matching of ventilation to blood flow is not perfect. In lung disease such as emphysema or pulmonary embolism this mismatching results in much greater (A–a)P_{O_2} gradients and in significant hypoxemia. For a full discussion of this important topic see West (1986c).

At altitude, at rest there is little change in the (A–a)P_{O_2} gradient from its value at sea level. The V/Q ratio inequality is modestly reduced, because of the increase in pulmonary artery pressure due to hypoxia (Chapter 7), reducing the gravitational effect on the distribution of blood flow in the lung. However, this is not enough to cause any measurable increase in the diffusing capacity of the lung during acclimatization (West 1962a).

On exercise at high altitude, however, the (A–a)P_{O_2} gradient increases significantly and becomes important in limiting exercise performance. This is shown as the dashed line in Fig. 4.5. This diffusion limitation, shown by West $et\ al.$ (1962), is explored more fully in Chapters 6, 11 and 12.

4.3.5 Arterial to mixed venous P_{O_2} (PvO_2)

The last drop in P_{O_2} shown in Fig. 4.3 from arterial to mixed venous is due to the uptake of oxygen in the systemic capillaries. Its magnitude is influenced by the metabolic rate, the cardiac output and the oxygen-carrying capacity of the blood, i.e. the hemoglobin concentration ([Hb]). Probably the best known aspect of acclimatization is the increase in [Hb].

A modest increase in [Hb] is probably beneficial in that it increases the oxygen-carrying capacity of the blood and at altitudes up to about 4000 m this is sufficient to balance the reduction in oxygen saturation due to reduced Pa,$_{O_2}$ and restore the oxygen content of arterial blood to sea level values (though now at a lower P_{O_2}). However, the increase in viscosity of the blood is the price paid and this increases

vascular resistance and contributes to raised pulmonary arterial pressure. This certainly happens in patients with chronic mountain sickness where hematocrits of over 80% are seen. If the rise in vascular resistance is too great, the cardiac output falls and so oxygen delivery is reduced. It has been shown that reducing the hematocrit in these patients never reduces exercise performance and usually increases it (Winslow and Monge 1987a). There is also the increased risk of vascular disorders. A recent report on the effect of hemodilution in lowlanders at 5260 m also showed that lowering the [Hb] by 24% had no effect on $V_{O_2,max}$ (Calbet $et\ al.$ 2002). With moderate, physiological, increases in [Hb] there seems to be a close reciprocal relationship between [Hb] and blood flow so that oxygen delivery to particular organs, e.g. working muscles or brain, remains constant over a range of [Hb] and V_{O_2}. The question of optimum hemoglobin value is further considered in section 8.5.4.

The $in\ vitro$ oxygen dissociation curve is shifted slightly to the right at moderate altitudes due to an increase in 2,3-diphosphoglycerate (DPG). However, the position of the $in\ vivo$ curve is uncertain because of uncertainties about the $in\ vivo$ pH (Winslow and Monge 1987b). There is probably some degree of respiratory alkalosis which offsets the effect of the 2,3-DPG. At extreme altitude, above about 7000 m there is quite severe respiratory alkalosis and therefore a definite leftward shift in the dissociation curve which is beneficial to the climber at least as far as oxygen delivery to working muscles is concerned. This is because more oxygen is loaded into the blood in the lungs while the unloading of oxygen in the muscles is only slightly reduced, because the difference in position of the curves for normal and higher pH, at very low P_{O_2}, is so small (see Chapter 9, Fig. 9.1).

Cardiac output increases with acute hypoxia but decreases as [Hb] increases with continued stay at altitude over the first 1 to 2 weeks. These changes as well as other effects on the vascular system are discussed in Chapter 7. At the tissue level there is an increase in the density of capillaries due to a reduction in diameter of muscle fibers (Chapter 10).

Taking the body as a whole the mixed venous P_{O_2} can be thought of as reflecting the mean tissue P_{O_2}. It will be seen in Fig. 4.5 that the effect of these processes of acclimatization is to maintain this critical P_{O_2} as near as possible to the sea level value.

Beyond this there is the possibility of adaptation at the tissue level involving the microcirculation and then intracellular mechanisms. These form the subject of Chapter 10.

4.4 PRACTICAL CONSIDERATIONS AND ADVICE

A very real problem in the study of acclimatization is that there is no single measure of the process. Respiratory acclimatization is very important and can be followed by measuring minute ventilation or the alveolar or end-tidal P_{CO_2}. The ventilation rises with acclimatization and the P_{CO_2} falls exponentially over the first few days at altitude. However, climbers find that their performance continues to improve over a longer period; presumably changes in other systems underlie this further acclimatization. This problem of how to measure the degree of acclimatization coupled with the very great individual variation in the rate and final degree of acclimatization means that we still do not have answers to apparently simple questions such as, 'Does exercise speed acclimatization?' There is also the problem that the time of early and rapid acclimatization is also the risk time for AMS. It is hard and perhaps futile to try and separate the effect of any given strategy on preventing AMS and on speeding acclimatization since the two are inextricably commingled. Thus the advice given here is as much about preventing AMS as with acclimatization itself. Also, in the absence of hard data, anecdotal evidence has to be relied on.

4.4.1 Rate of ascent

A rate of ascent which is slow enough to avoid AMS should be chosen. This will inevitably be dictated, in part, by the terrain, availability of camp sites etc. A rule of thumb often given is that above 3000 m each night's camp should be about 300 m above the previous one and that every 2–3 days a rest day be added when the party remains based at the same site for two nights. This is an unnecessarily slow ascent rate for many individuals but will prove too fast for a substantial minority (see Chapter 18 for more discussion and references). Where a greater height gain has to be made, then a rest day should be taken.

During the 'rest' day trips to higher altitude and back are considered beneficial by experienced climbers, probably because the greater altitude and exercise stimulates acclimatization. However, it should be noted that there is some evidence that exercise is a risk factor for AMS (Roach et al. 1999).

4.4.2 Individual variability and acclimatization

As mentioned, there is great individual variation in the rate and degree of acclimatisation. Some may acclimatize rapidly to moderate altitude but then find that they simply cannot tolerate an altitude above say 7000 m. Others may take time to acclimatize but then go well to extreme altitude. Usually, as with susceptibility to AMS, past experience is a good guide to future performance but apart from this there are no reliable predictors for good acclimatization.

4.4.3 Age, gender and experience

There is not much data to answer the oft-asked question about the effects of age or gender on acclimatization. If anything, older people are less susceptible to AMS than the young and seem to acclimatize just as well as do the young. There does not seem to be any important difference between men and women in this respect. There is a strong impression that experienced mountaineers acclimatize better than novices. (See Chapters 25 and 26 for further discussion of acclimatization in women, children and the elderly.)

4.4.4 Pre-acclimatization by continuous or intermittent hypoxia

There is increasing interest in methods by which people can achieve some degree of acclimatization before going to the mountains. There is no doubt that living in a chamber for a number of days at simulated altitude will achieve acclimatization. There is an impression that the degree of acclimatization is not as great as that achieved in the mountains, perhaps because of the lack of exercise. West (1998) argues the case for this being true for the long-term studies of Operation Everest I and II. However, incarceration in a chamber for days or weeks is not practicable or acceptable for most climbers.

Intermittent hypoxia (IH) has been used to see if this stimulus could result in some degree of acclimatization. IH can be achieved by spending a few hours a day in a chamber, sometimes with exercise, i.e. training under hypoxia. Alternatively, sleeping in a hypoxic environment, e.g. at altitude but coming down to train at low altitude, that is, 'living high, training low', a pattern popularized by Levine and Stray-Gunderson (1997). Their proposals were to improve performance of athletes for sea level races but the effect of such a pattern of hypoxic exposure can also give some of the changes of acclimatization (see below). Instead of actually commuting up and down athletes and researchers can achieve the same effect by breathing a low oxygen percentage in a normobaric chamber, or by using a machine to provide low oxygen percentage in the inspired gas via a mask. The machine can be programmed to give any pattern of bursts of hypoxia or normoxia. End points of these studies are usually changes in cardio-respiratory or blood measurements or athletic performance. Whether these indirect measures of acclimatization translate into improvement in performance at altitude is not clear. Savourey et al. (1998) studied the effect of 8 h daily for 5 days at 4500 m equivalent altitude on various hormones and biochemical measures but found very little effect with this dose of pre-acclimatization. Garcia et al. (2000) had their subjects breathe 13% oxygen (equivalent to 3800 m) for 2 h daily for 12 days. They found the hypoxic ventilatory response (HVR) increased significantly reaching a peak at 5 days but there was no change in ventilation, P_{CO_2} or S_{a,O_2}. Katayama et al. (2001) using only 1 h day^{-1} of simulated altitude equivalent to 4500 m a day, for 7 days in six subjects, also found an increase in HVR, resting ventilation and S_{a,O_2} but no effect on the ventilatory response to CO_2 (HCVR). They found that on exercise, the ventilatory equivalent (V_E/V_{O_2}) was increased after this intermittent hypoxia as was the exercise S_{a,O_2} as a result of the increase in ventilation due to increased HVR. Townsend et al. (2002) studied three groups of trained endurance athletes under three conditions:

1. Simulated 'living high, training low' (LHTL), i.e. sleeping in a normobaric chamber in low O_2% equivalent to 2650 m.

2. A group that had four blocks of five nights of hypoxia interspersed with two nights at normoxia.
3. A control group sleeping at normal P_{O_2}.

The study lasted 20 days. Results showed that HVR was increased by LHTL, more so in the continuous than in the group with two nights of normoxia. Resting ventilation, tested in normoxia, was not significantly changed by the exposure, but end-tidal P_{CO_2} ($P_{ET}CO_2$) was decreased in both hypoxic groups, though only by about 2.5 Torr.

The effect of IH on the erythropoietic system has been studied by a number of workers. Garcia et al. (2000) found a reticulocytosis but no change in [Hb] or hematocrit. Schmidt (2002) reviewed this topic and concluded that the effect of IH depended upon the intensity and duration of the hypoxia, both with respect to the length of each burst and the total duration of exposure. Short hypoxic episodes like sleep apnea seem to result in only small increases in Hb concentration due mainly to reduction in plasma volume. There seems to be a critical threshold of about 90 min cumulative hypoxia. Athletes, using longer periods of hypoxia, such as sleeping in hypoxia, show increases in plasma erythropoietin (EPO) concentration, transferin receptor and reticulocyte count, e.g. Koistinen et al. (2000), but an increase in red cell mass has not been found.

It seems that intermittent hypoxia does effect some of the changes seen in acclimatization, depending upon the 'dose' of hypoxia, but not all. However, an extra few days at altitude would probably be as good and much more pleasant.

4.4.5 Carry-over acclimatization

If pre-acclimatization is attempted, how quickly should a climber get out to the mountains? In other words, how long does acclimatization last? There is little hard data to guide us, though one study by Lyons et al. (1995) showed that a group of subjects who had been at 4300 m for 3 weeks retained some beneficial effect after 8 days at low altitude compared with a group who had had no altitude exposure. A later study by the same group (Beidleman et al. 1997) with a similar protocol put some quantification on this carry-over effect. After 8 days at sea level they calculated that, on average, 92% of the effect on Sa,O_2 was retained, 74% of plasma volume and 58% of the lactic acid concentration at 75% $VO_{2,max}$ exercise. For intermittent hypoxia in the study of Townsend *et al.* (2002) quoted above, the HVR increased by 50% over pre-hypoxia values and declined 30% by 2 days after cessation of IH. However, Katayama *et al.* (2001) found most of the effect of IH on HVR, the ventilatory equivalent, and Sa,O_2 to be still present 1 week after stopping IH.

These studies support anecdotal experience. The effect of acclimatization probably falls off exponentially with time over perhaps 2 or 3 weeks, though some feel there is some residual benefit even after months at sea level. It is likely that the time course of the 'off' transients are different for different systems involved in the acclimatization process.

4.5 ALTITUDE DETERIORATION

4.5.1 Introduction

The term 'high altitude deterioration' was first used by members of early Everest expeditions to denote deterioration in mental and physical condition as a result of prolonged stay at altitude. De Filippi (1912) noted the condition during an expedition to the Karakoram. He writes:

> The atmosphere of the expedition did work some evil effect revealing itself only gradually after several weeks of life above 17500 feet in a slow decrease of appetite and consequent lack of nourishment without, however, any disturbance of digestive function.

In this way he distinguished the condition from acute mountain sickness, though the mechanisms, at least of anorexia, may be common to both conditions.

It is well known amongst climbers that staying at extreme altitudes for long is deleterious. Altitudes above 8000 m have been called 'The Death Zone' and summit bids on peaks over this height are wisely planned so as to spend as short a time as possible in this zone. Deterioration can frequently be attributed to factors such as dehydration, starvation, physical exhaustion and cold. However, in the absence of such factors it seems that hypoxia per se can cause deterioration if sufficiently severe (Pugh

Table 4.1 Maximum period spent at varying altitudes without supplementary oxygen (lowlanders)

Height (m)	Period (days)	Expedition
5791	90–100	Silver Hut, 1960–61
6760–7315	11	Everest 1953
7010	11	Everest 1924
7467	8	Makalu 1961
7850	5	Everest 1953
7925	4	Everest 1953
8380	3	Everest 1953
8450	1	Everest 1953
8848	1 (night)	Everest 1953

Modified from Ward 1975.

1962a). Many of the symptoms and signs are seen in prolonged chamber experiments such as Operation Everest II (Houston *et al.* 1987, Rose *et al.* 1988). The altitude at which this becomes manifest is about 5000–6000 m, with considerable individual variation. Highlanders can probably tolerate prolonged periods at a higher altitude better than can most lowlanders (West 1986a). The highest elevation for permanent habitation seems to be about 5334 m (caretakers at a mine in Chile) though economic considerations may mean that there is no reason to live higher than this. For lowlanders, there is probably a maximum altitude for prolonged residence at about this altitude. The experience of spending the winter at 5800 m (the Silver Hut 1960) suggested this was above the critical altitude. Above this altitude deterioration limits the time that can be spent. The higher the altitude, the more rapid is the deterioration. Table 4.1 shows times for sojourns at various altitudes.

4.5.2 Symptoms and signs

High altitude deterioration (in the absence of dehydration, starvation etc.) is characterized by weight loss, poor appetite, slow recovery from fatigue, lethargy, irritability and an increasing lack of willpower to start new tasks (Ward 1954). There is slowing of mental processes, dulling of affect and impaired cognitive function. There may be low systemic blood pressure.

ANOREXIA AND WEIGHT LOSS

Loss of appetite soon after arrival at altitude is part of the symptomatology of acute mountain sickness but after acclimatization, appetite is regained at altitudes below about 5500 m. Above this altitude there is usually further loss of appetite which tends to increase the longer is the time spent at these extreme altitudes. The anorexia tends to be worse in the mornings and for certain types of food, with considerable individual variation. This anorexia results in reduced calorie intake, a negative calorie balance and weight loss. There may also be a degree of malabsorption. Weight loss is the most well attested, objective sign of deterioration. The mechanisms underlying this weight loss are considered further in Chapter 14.

FATIGUE AND SLOW RECOVERY FROM EXERTION

Other symptoms of deterioration, fatigue and slow recovery from exertion, are more subjective and difficult to measure. In the 1970s we made an attempt to find a biochemical basis for the reported symptoms of slow recovery from exhausting exercise at altitude. We followed the resynthesis of muscle glycogen after depletion by exercise at sea level under normoxia (air breathing) and hypoxia (breathing 12% O_2). We found that, although the rate of resynthesis was not significantly slowed by hypoxia in the muscle overall, there was an enhancement of the difference between the type I and type II fibers. This suggested that hypoxia depresses glycogen synthesis in type I though not type II fibers (Milledge *et al.* 1977). This might contribute to the slowness of recovery from severe exercise at high altitude. However, fatigue and lassitude are felt even in the absence of exercise, so there is probably a central effect as well.

SLOWING OF MENTAL PROCESS, DULLING OF EFFECT AND IMPAIRED COGNITIVE FUNCTION

There have been numerous studies of cognitive function at altitude though not many at extreme altitude. They have mostly shown some impairment of some tests involving memory (reviewed by Raichle and Hornbein 2001 and in Chapter 16),

and also speech deterioration with increasing altitude (Leiberman *et al.* 1995). An effect of severe hypoxia, often not appreciated by the subject, is to cause a slowing of mental and physical function. For instance, well-learned acts such as strapping on crampons take much longer at extreme altitude. Similarly, mental tasks such as calculating the remaining supply time of an oxygen cylinder, though still possible, take longer than at low altitude. A recurring theme in accounts of life at extreme altitude is the lethargy, which gets worse with time. There is a great disinclination to get started on a task. The climber, normally a very active person, just wishes to lie dozing in a tent. The emotions, too, seem to be dulled and the capacity to initiate a new plan in the face of the unexpected is reduced. Ward reported after the 1953 Everest Expedition that at Camp 7 on the Lhotsi face, the sight of the exhausted Tom Bourdilon provoked nothing more than the comment, 'Poor old Tom, he's had it!' Ward himself had no doubt that at lower altitude, attempts would have been made to help the exhausted climber (Pugh and Ward 1956). Insight and judgement are impaired and no doubt contribute to fatalities at extreme altitude.

SLEEP

Sleep is disrupted at altitude by more frequent arousals than at sea level and the architecture of sleep is changed with less time spent in REM sleep (Weil and White 2001). Periodic breathing may contribute to this and becomes more frequent the higher the altitude. Climbers are conscious that they have not slept well and feel unrefreshed in the morning. This sleep deprivation may contribute to the psychological element of deterioration. A more detailed description of sleep at altitude is given in Chapter 13.

LOW SYSTEMIC BLOOD PRESSURE

The blood pressure (BP) response to altitude is either no change or a slight rise initially, falling back to sea level values with acclimatization. However, there have been a few reports that at, or returning from, extreme altitude, the BP was low. Pugh and Ward (1956) reported from the 1953 Everest Expedition on a number of climbers returning to their camp from higher on the mountain. One had a BP of 86/66, a second 80/60 and a third 115/90. In Operation Everest II, Reeves noted in his diary about one subject at the simulated altitude of the summit,

> Roger Gough's study today underscored an observation that we have noted repeatedly at these very hypoxic levels. Namely, that when the subjects were not exercising, their arterial blood pressure falls (there was an arterial line in place). In Roger's case, systolic pressure would fall to 80 or less. (Quoted by Houston *et al.* 1991)

The mechanism is unknown. Pugh (personal communication) suggested it might be due to adrenal insufficiency but there is no evidence for this. These observations are only anecdotes and we clearly need more research. If extreme altitude does cause hypotension this could also contribute to the fatigue characteristic of altitude deterioration.

5

Ventilatory response to hypoxia and carbon dioxide

SUMMARY

Of all the changes that take place in the physiology of a person acclimatizing to altitude, those resulting in an increase in ventilation are probably the most important. There are changes in both the hypoxic ventilatory response (HVR) and the hypercapnic ventilatory responses (HCVRs). The changes in HVR are more difficult to measure but it is now accepted that HVR increases with time at altitude over a period of days to a few weeks. The changes in HCVR were characterized over 40 years ago and include a shift to the left and a steepening of the carbon dioxide response line. That is, a person when acclimatized responds to a lower P_{CO_2} and is more sensitive to carbon dioxide than when unacclimatized. The time course of the changes in HCVR is exponential, with almost half taking place in the first 24 h and most of the change being complete in about 2 weeks. These changes in the chemical control of breathing underlie the well-known

increase in ventilation and result in a lower P_{CO_2} and higher P_{O_2} characteristic of acclimatization. The mechanism underlying the increased carbon dioxide sensitivity may be due to the documented reduction in bicarbonate concentration in cerebrospinal fluid (CSF), blood and, presumably, brain extracellular fluid (ECF) but may be due to other mechanisms which make the ventilatory drive appear as if the set point for CO_2 has been reset to a lower value. The mechanisms of the increase in HVR are debatable but probably include changes in both the peripheral chemoreceptors and central processing of the signal in the brain.

HVR does not predict susceptibility to acute mountain sickness (AMS), though subjects susceptible to high altitude pulmonary edema (HAPE) do have low HVRs. High altitude residents have similar HCVR but generally have blunted HVR compared to acclimatized lowlanders. Some studies have found a correlation between HVR and performance at extreme altitude but some elite climbers have HVR in the normal range, and high altitude residents (Sherpas and Andean peoples) who tend to have low HVR perform very well at extreme altitude.

5.1 INTRODUCTION

The increase in ventilation that takes place in the first few days at altitude is one of the most important aspects of the acclimatization process. It results in higher alveolar and arterial Po_2 and lower Pco_2 levels than would have obtained if the ventilation were unchanged. The cause of this increased ventilation is a change in the chemical control of breathing. Interest in the mechanisms underlying these changes goes back to the early years of the twentieth century. Haldane, who had shown that the level of carbon dioxide in the body was stable at sea level, soon realized that altitude resulted in depression of Pco_2 due to increased ventilation. Whilst Haldane and companions were on the Pikes Peak Expedition of 1911, he suggested that his colleague Mabel FitzGerald measure the alveolar Pco_2 in residents at mining camps at various altitudes in Colorado. She found that the Pco_2 fell linearly with altitude (FitzGerald 1913). Since then physiologists have continued to investigate these mechanisms and their work is reviewed in this chapter.

There are two sensing systems for the chemical control of breathing: the peripheral chemoreceptors (the carotid and aortic bodies), and central chemoreceptors situated in the medulla. There are three chemical drives to ventilation: hypoxia, pH and carbon dioxide. The peripheral chemoreceptors principally sense hypoxia, though they also respond to carbon dioxide and pH, whereas the central chemoreceptors respond principally to changes in Pco_2 sensed by the change in pH induced.

5.2 HYPOXIC VENTILATORY RESPONSE (HVR)

5.2.1 Introduction

The HVR is the increase in ventilation brought about by acute hypoxia. This is not a simple linear response and is complicated by the effect of ventilation on Pco_2. As ventilation rises in response to hypoxia, Pco_2 falls and pH rises. Thus the carbon

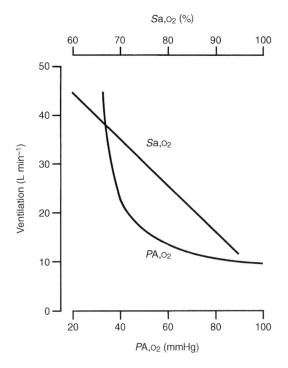

Figure 5.1   Hypoxic ventilatory response (HVR) to decreasing PA,o_2 and to decreasing arterial oxygen saturation (Sa,o_2).

dioxide drive to breathing is reduced and the hypoxic response is masked unless measures are taken to prevent this fall in Pco_2.

If the inspired Po_2 is reduced acutely, i.e. over a period of a few minutes, either by breathing a low oxygen mixture or by decompression in a hypobaric chamber, the minute ventilation is increased. However, this increase in ventilation varies greatly from individual to individual and does not usually begin until the inspired Po_2 is reduced to approximately 100 mmHg (equivalent to about 3000 m altitude) (Rahn and Otis 1949). This corresponds to an alveolar Po_2 of about 50 mmHg. Thereafter, as inspired Po_2 is further reduced ventilation increases more rapidly.

The relationship of ventilation to Po_2 is hyperbolic, as shown in Fig. 5.1. However, if arterial saturation is measured by an oximeter the relationship between it and ventilation is found to be approximately linear (Fig. 5.1). The Pa,o_2 at which ventilation starts to increase corresponds to the Po_2 at which the oxygen dissociation curve begins to steepen, thus HVR protects arterial oxygen content increasing ventilation as saturation begins to fall.

The actual effect of acute hypoxia on ventilation will depend upon whether P_{CO_2} is allowed to fall or not. Unless the experimental arrangement allows control of $PA,_{CO_2}$, a rise in ventilation will result in a fall of P_{CO_2}. This is the normal situation as a person ascends to altitude and HVR measured in this way is termed poikilocapnic. As P_{CO_2} is reduced some drive to breathing will be lost so that the full hypoxic response is not seen. In order to see the full HVR, P_{CO_2} is usually held constant and the response measured is termed the isocapnic HVR.

5.2.2 Time course of ventilatory response to hypoxia: minutes to days

There are three phases to this response, as shown in Fig. 5.2, where P_{CO_2} is used as a (reciprocal) measure of ventilation:

- In the first few seconds to about 10 min there is an increase in ventilation (and fall in P_{CO_2}) if the hypoxia is sufficiently severe.
- From about 20 to 30 min there is a reduction of ventilation back towards the control value (a rise in P_{CO_2}). This is called the hypoxic ventilatory decline (HVD) or 'roll off'. For a fuller discussion of this phenomenon see Smith *et al.* (2001). Bascom *et al.* (1990) showed that HVR declined during this period reaching a nadir at about 5 min. Recently, Vovk *et al.* (2004) have shown that HVR recovers after this 5 min decline, over the next 36 min to pre-hypoxia control values. However, Garcia *et al.* 2000 found this decrease in ventilation in the absence of a change in HVR. They found that the slope of the ventilation/$Sa,_{O_2}$ line was unchanged but its intercept decreased. Clearly the mechanism of HVD is unclear.
- There is further increase in ventilation (reduction in P_{CO_2}) from about 30 min to some days and continuing at a decreasing rate up to about 2 weeks at a given altitude. This is termed respiratory acclimatization and is due to an increase in HVR and the HCVR as discussed in further sections of this chapter.

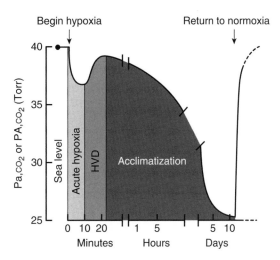

Figure 5.2 Idealized time course of ventilatory acclimatization, using P_{CO_2} as an index of ventilation. (From Smith *et al.* 2001, with permission.)

5.3 CAROTID BODY

Before considering HVR further, the transduction of the hypoxic response will be briefly considered. A transducer effects the conversion of one mode of signal to another, in this case from $Pa,_{O_2}$ to a neural signal by the carotid body.

5.3.1 Historical

The stimulating effect of oxygen lack on respiration had been known for many years before it became apparent in the early years of the twentieth century that, under normal sea level conditions, carbon dioxide was the main chemical stimulus to ventilation.

In the late 1920s, the father and son team of Heymans and Heymans in Belgium, using complex cross-circulation experiments in dogs, localized the main sensing organ for hypoxia to the carotid body (Heymans and Heymans 1927). Not long afterwards Comroe (1938) showed that the aortic bodies have a similar function. These bodies are known collectively as the peripheral chemoreceptors. However, in most animals, including humans, the main organ for transduction of the hypoxic signal is the carotid body and if this is removed or denervated, acute hypoxia actually results in depression of ventilation.

5.3.2 Anatomy and physiology of the carotid body

The human carotid body weighs about 10 mg and is situated just above the bifurcation of the common carotid artery. It has an extremely rich blood flow for its mass and oxygen consumption, and thus it extracts only a very small percentage of the oxygen in the blood presented to it. This explains how it is able to respond to arterial P_{O_2} (or saturation) and not to oxygen content. Thus it responds to hypoxemia but not anemia or reduced flow. This is appropriate since an increase in ventilation would not help the organism overcome the tissue hypoxia caused by anemia or low cardiac output, but does help in a hypoxic environment.

MECHANISM OF RESPONSE TO ACUTE HYPOXIA

An enormous amount of research has been carried out on the carotid body, and it is now generally accepted that the glomus cells (type I), the characteristic cells of the carotid body, are the site of chemoreception and that modulation of neurotransmitter release from the glomus cells by physiological and chemical stimuli affects the discharge rate of the carotid body afferent fibers. Undoubtedly, the signal is modified, enhanced or suppressed by parts of the system not involved with the primary sensing process. The information on the arterial P_{O_2} is sent via the carotid sinus nerve to the respiratory centers in the brain which then affect their output and thus breathing rate, minute ventilation.

There have been, recently, a number of good reviews of the mechanisms by which hypoxemia is sensed by the carotid body and transmitted as increased neural discharge (Lahiri and Cherniack 2001, Prabhakar and Peng 2004, Prabhakar and Jacono 2005, Wilson et al. 2005). Hypoxia may slow down mitochondrial electron transport owing to the presence of a reduced affinity cytochrome in the oxygen transport chain. This could stimulate neurotransmitter release from glomus cells by progressive breakdown of the mitochondrial electrochemical gradient and release of mitochondrial calcium into the cytoplasm. The elevated intracellular calcium would then cause release of the neurotransmitter. Metabolic blockers which interfere with electron transport and oxidative phosphorylation would

have a similar effect (Mulligan et al. 1981, Biscoe and Duchen 1990).

Two hypotheses have been proposed:

- Glomus cells have potassium channels in their cell membranes that are modulated by the partial pressure of oxygen. The probability that the channel is open decreases with hypoxia and acidosis and the result is a reduction in overall potassium conductance which causes membrane depolarization. This could explain chemo-transduction as follows. The membrane depolarizes, voltage sensitive calcium channels open, and these allow extracellular calcium to enter the cell. The elevated intracellular calcium then promotes neurotransmitter release.
- A heme protein (either in the cytosol or mitochondria) is an oxygen sensor and a biochemical event associated with the redox state of the protein triggers transmitter release.

These hypotheses are not mutually exclusive and perhaps the sensors work together as a 'chemosome' over a wide range of P_{O_2} values (Prabhakar and Peng 2004).

The potassium channel has been demonstrated in submicron-sized membrane patches which continue to be modulated by oxygen when removed from the cell. It has been suggested that the channel itself contains a heme group which may interact with oxygen directly, thus modifying channel confirmation and the probability of its being open (Ganfornina and Lopez-Barneo 1991).

Also, there is evidence that non-mitochondrial enzymes such as NADPH oxidases, NO synthase and heme oxygenases may be involved in the hypoxia sensing process. These proteins could contribute to transduction via generation of reactive oxygen species, nitric oxide and/or carbon monoxide (Prabhakar and Overholt 2000).

Dopamine is the most abundant transmitter found in the carotid body. Hypoxia increases the rate of release of dopamine from glomus cells. Norepinephrine (noradrenalin) and 5-hydroxytryptamine are next in abundance. There are also small quantities of acetylcholine and enkephalin-like peptides in some glomus cells. Substance P, endothelin-1, adenosine and purinergic receptors are also present and may be involved with modulating the hypoxic response (Wilson *et al.* 2005).

It should be noted that, although the most important function of the peripheral chemoreceptors (carotid and aortic bodies) is to respond to hypoxia, they do also respond to an increase in Pa,CO_2 and decrease in arterial pH. The greatest response to PCO_2 is via the central chemoreceptors in the brain stem (see section 5.13.1); a recent study (Fatemian *et al.* 2003) suggested that subjects who had had both carotid bodies removed had about 36% lower HCVR than normal subjects.

CHRONIC HYPOXIA

Anatomically, chronic hypoxia results in hypertrophy of the carotid body in animals and man probably due to upregulation of growth factors, e.g. vascular endothelial growth factor (VEGF) (Prabhakar and Jacono 2005). Physiologically, there is an increase in sensitivity over a period of about 30 min to some weeks. The mechanism of this involves a number of systems including those mentioned above and no doubt others. It is likely that during this period gene induction is involved (see section 5.5.1).

5.4 HVR AT SEA LEVEL

5.4.1 Methods for measuring HVR

A number of different methods have been used to measure HVR, each having its advantages and disadvantages. Probably the most popular method for studies involving large numbers of subjects is the rebreathing method using an oximeter to measure oxygen saturation continuously while the PCO_2 is held constant (Rebuck and Campbell 1974). More recently, Robbins and his group in Oxford have used a series of square wave pulses of hypoxia keeping the carbon dioxide constant and then fitting a single compartment model which yields a parameter G_p, the hypoxic sensitivity (Ren and Robbins 1999).

Previously steady state methods have been used, e.g. Cunningham *et al.* (1957), Severinghaus *et al.* (1966a), in which the subject breathed a hypoxic mixture until ventilation was steady, typically 10–20 min. All these methods measure the isocapnic

HVR. Single breath methods have also been used, e.g. Dejours *et al.* (1959), in which a single breath of altered PO_2 was given and the change in tidal volume in the following few breaths observed. Single breath methods were thought to reflect the activity of peripheral and not central chemoreceptors and would not be influenced by HVD. There would also be no time for a significant change in PCO_2. The steady state methods would reflect the activity of both central and peripheral chemoreceptors and the effect of HVD depending upon how long the 'steady state' was held. They are also influenced by changes in cerebral blood flow (CBF) which alter the arterial–venous blood gas difference so that the central chemoreceptors may see a change in PCO_2 even if end-tidal PCO_2 is held constant. The simple and popular progressive hypoxia test is likely to be influenced by both sets of chemoreceptors, HDV and CBF.

It should also be borne in mind that posture influences the HVR (but not HCVR). Usually the subject is seated. The supine position results in a 52% reduction in HVR and microgravity a reduction of 46%, presumably by the same mechanism, that of an increase in the blood pressure in the carotid baroreceptors (Prisk *et al.* 2000).

5.4.2 Variability of HVR: effect of age, specific groups, and drugs

The range of HVR found in healthy sea level residents is wide. The coefficient of variation varies between 23 and 72% in different studies (Cunningham *et al.* 1964, Weil *et al.* 1970, Rebuck and Campbell 1974).

Various groups of subjects at sea level have been shown to have lower HVRs than controls, for instance endurance athletes (Byrne-Quinn *et al.* 1971) and swimmers (Bjurstrom and Schoene 1986). With increasing age HVR becomes lower (Kronenberg and Drage 1973, Chapman and Cherniak 1986, Poulin *et al.* 1993). Alcohol (Sahn *et al.* 1974), respiratory depressant drugs and anesthetics inhibit HVR (Davis *et al.* 1982).

The thiol disulfide redox state (REDST) has an effect on HVR (and erythropoietin production) as shown by treatment with *N*-acetyl-cysteine. Hildebrandt *et al.* (2002) showed that HVR was more than doubled after 6 days treatment with the drug compared with placebo. This treatment greatly increased the REDST and the increase in HVR showed a significant correlation with the increase in REDST state. They suggest that the reduction in HVR with age may be due to the effect of age on REDST.

5.5 HVR AT HIGH ALTITUDE AND INTERMITTENT HYPOXIA

5.5.1 HVR and acclimatization

During the first few days at altitude, respiratory acclimatization takes place. This is shown by an increase in ventilation and a decrease in PA,CO_2. PA,O_2 falls immediately on exposure to acute altitude and then rises (as PA,CO_2 falls) over the next few days. The rise in ventilation on acute exposure to hypoxia is mediated by the HVR (by definition) but further increase in ventilation is due to changes in HCVR (see section 5.12) and HVR with more time at altitude (see below).

The peripheral chemoreceptors are essential for normal respiratory acclimatization, and animals which have had their carotid bodies denervated fail to acclimatize normally (Forster *et al.* 1981, Lahiri *et al.* 1981, Smith *et al.* 1986). After denervation these animals have raised Pa,CO_2, which rises further with acute hypoxia. With chronic hypoxia, at least in some cases, there is a small fall in Pa,CO_2 which has been taken by some workers as evidence of acclimatization (Sorensen and Mines 1970). This and other evidence suggests that chronic hypoxia produces some effect on ventilation via mechanisms other than the carotid body, possibly via cerebral metabolism. All agree, however, that denervated animals appeared ill at altitude and a proportion die.

It might be expected that exposure to hypoxia of some days or months would result in attenuation or sensitization of the HVR. Michel and Milledge (1963) found an increase in the hypoxic parameter A in three out of four subjects after 1–3 months at 5800 m. Parameter A is the 'shape' parameter of the hyperbola relating PA,O_2 to ventilation (Fig. 5.3). The larger the value the greater is the response. There was no change in the other hypoxic parameter, C (the PO_2 at which theoretically ventilation becomes infinite, the PO_2 asymptote of the hyperbola). Cruz *et al.* (1980) also found an increase in parameter A after 74 h of altitude exposure; this was

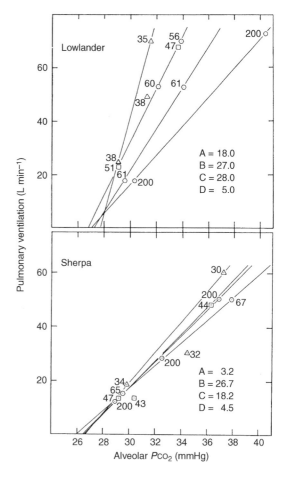

Figure 5.3 Two steady-state inhalation experiments typical of a lowlander (upper panel) and a Sherpa highlander (lower panel). The numbers refer to the PO_2 of each point. There is no significant difference in hypercapnic ventilatory response (HCVR) but the 'closed fan' of the Sherpa indicates very little HVR. Letters A–D refer to the parameters relating HVR (A and C) and HCVR (B and D). (From Milledge and Lahiri 1967.)

not seen in subjects whose PA,CO_2 was not allowed to fall.

The question of a change in chemoreceptor responsiveness during acclimatization was reviewed by Weil (1986), who points out that a number of studies have not found any change in HVR with acclimatization, although the presence of hypocapnic alkalosis, which has a depressant effect on HVR at sea level, may have obscured a real change. However, more recent studies have found an increase in responsiveness. Barnard *et al.* (1987) found neurophysiological evidence of increased sensitivity of the carotid body for hypoxia in cats after chronic hypoxia of 28 days but not after only 2–3 h. Vizek *et al.* (1987) also presented evidence from work in cats of an increase in HVR (parameter *A*) after 48 h hypoxia. Nielsen *et al.* (1988) showed, in goats, an increase in discharge in recordings from a single carotid body afferent during hypoxia over a 6 h period. There was no change for the first hour but a progressive increase thereafter. Note that the goat acclimatizes much faster than humans. From the same laboratory Engwall and Bisgard (1990) found an increase in HVR after 4 h of hypoxia in awake goats.

Apart from an increased response of the carotid body it is possible that acclimatization might result in changes in the CNS leading to an increase in response by the respiratory center to signals from the carotid body. This possibility was tested in a study by Dwinell and Powell (1999) in anaesthetized rats. They found an increase in phrenic nerve discharge in response to supra-maximal stimulation of the carotid sinus nerve in acclimatized rats as compared with control animals suggesting this might be a further mechanism in the increase in HVR with acclimatization.

In humans, Yamaguchi *et al.* (1991), Sato *et al.* (1992, 1994) and Goldberg *et al.* (1992) found a significant increase in HVR in lowland subjects after acclimatization at 3730–4860 m compared with pre-exposure values. Masuda *et al.* (1992) measured HVR serially in seven lowland subjects after arrival at Lhasa (3658 m) as they acclimatized over 27 days. They found a small decrease in HVR over the first 3–5 days then a considerable increase from day 5 to 27. It seems that there are significant differences in response in different subjects especially in the first few days at altitude, and that this may be associated with their susceptibility or resistance to AMS (see section 5.6 and Bartsch *et al.* 2002). These differences may account for some of the variability in results from different studies.

Robbins's group in Oxford has carried out a series of chamber studies in which the inspired gases can be controlled so as to keep the subject's end-tidal P_{CO_2} constant. Thus they are able to study the changes in HVR with hypoxia over the first 8 h and later 48 h with or without the confounding effect of respiratory alkalosis mentioned above. They found that HVR did increase even under isocapnia

(Howard and Robbins 1995). They also showed that acclimatization had taken place even with isocapnia in that ventilation was raised under acute hyperoxia (Tansley *et al.* 1998). Using a 48 h chamber exposure, under either isocapnic or poikilocapnic hypoxia, the increase in hypoxic sensitivity started within 12 h and reached peak at about 36 h. That there was no difference between isocapnic and poikilocapnic results suggests that the respiratory alkalosis (due to reduced P_{CO_2}), normal in early acclimatization, is not an important part of the mechanism for the increase of HVR.

This increase in HVR over the period of a few days to a few weeks could explain the further increase in ventilation over this period of altitude exposure. The mechanism for this increase in HVR is not clear. A recent study in awake goats using selective inhibitors indicates that 5-HT is not essential for this aspect of ventilatory acclimatization (Herman *et al.* 2001). The possibility that HVD might change during acclimatization was considered by Sato *et al.* over a 3 day and a 2 week exposure (1992, 1994) and they found no change. Hupperets *et al.* (2004) extended this period to 8 weeks at a similar altitude (3900 m) and also found that HVD did not change.

A recent study has demonstrated the importance of the hypoxia inducible factor 1α (HIF-1α) in the changes in HVR with acclimatization (Kline *et al.* 2002). In this study transgenic mice, with one chromosome for HIF-1α knocked out, heterozygous (homozygous knock out mice die *in utero*), were compared with wild-type mice. Whereas there was no difference in response to acute hypoxia, the effect of chronic hypoxia (3 days at 0.4 atm) was different. The wild-type mice showed the expected increase in HVR, the knock out mice showed reduced HVR. They showed this result both in terms of ventilation, especially respiratory rate, and in sinus nerve activity, indicating it was an effect in the carotid body as opposed to a purely central effect. HIF-1α induces transcription of many genes that are influenced by hypoxia, including those mentioned above. It may also be the mechanism by which hypoxia effects the potassium channel activity in glomus cells leading to depolarization and increases in calcium concentration and neurotransmitter release (Prabhakar 2000). HIF-1αclearly has a global role as the master regulator of oxygen homeostasis (see section 8.4.1 for further discussion of HIF-1α).

Malik *et al.* (2005) found a clue as to a gene which might be responsible for this aspect of acclimatization, the immediate early gene, *fos B*. This is a member of a family of transcription factor genes active in the brain which are inducible by a variety of stimuli including drugs, hormones and, interestingly, repetitive behavior, as well as hypoxia. They found that mice lacking this gene had the same HVR as wild-type mice but while the latter increased their ventilation and HVR with chronic hypoxia (3 days at 0.4 atm), the mutant mice failed to increase their ventilation or their HVR.

The question of the role of HVR in effecting the change in carbon dioxide response and brain extracellular bicarbonate concentration is considered in section 5.13.

5.5.2 HVR and intermittent hypoxia

With the increase in the use of intermittent hypoxia (IH) in athletic training and also interest in clinical conditions such as obstructive sleep apnea, there have been a number of studies in which the effect of various forms of IH have been used and the effect on HVR observed.

Serebrovskaya and colleagues (1999) gave their subjects three, 5-to-6-min rebreathing sessions per day, separated by two 5-min breaks, for 14 days. During the procedure the end-tidal P_{O_2} progressively decreased from 105–100 mmHg to 50–40 mmHg during the first week and to 40–35 mmHg during the second week as subjective tolerance to hypoxia increased. End-tidal P_{CO_2} (PET_{CO2}) was kept constant. They found that the HVR increased by 43% after the training compared with pre-training control values.

Garcia *et al.* (2000) using 2 h a day of hypoxia (3800 m equivalent) for 12 days found HVR increased to 193% above control by day 5 but then declined to 70% above control by day 12. Katayama *et al.* (2001) showed that as little as 1 h of hypoxia (4500 m equivalent) per day for 7 days significantly increased HVR whilst Townsend *et al.* (2002) in their study of trained athletes 'living high, training low' also found an increase in HVR that was dose dependent. That is, the groups having most hypoxia had greatest increase in HVR and this continued to increase with the number of nights spent in hypoxia. They were also able to show a decrease in

PET_{CO2} of about 3 Torr in normoxia, though no measured change in ventilation.

It seems that IH definitely results in an increase in HVR though whether the change is more, less or about the same as an equivalent dose of hypoxia given continuously is not clear. The effects of IH on other aspects of the physiology of hypoxia are addressed in other chapters.

5.5.3 HVR and altitude residents

Chiodi (1957) reported that altitude residents in the Andes had higher $PA_{,CO_2}$ than acclimatized lowlanders. Severinghaus *et al.* (1966a) showed that Andean Indians born and living at altitude had a blunted HVR and similar findings were reported in Sherpas, natives to high altitude in the Himalayas (Lahiri and Milledge 1967, Milledge and Lahiri 1967). Steady-state inhalation experiments typical of a lowlander and a Sherpa are shown in Fig. 5.3. The 'opened-out fan' of CO_2 response lines of the lowlander indicates a brisk HVR whereas the 'closed fan' of the Sherpa shows that changing $PA_{,O_2}$ between 200 and 30 mmHg has very little effect on ventilation. These early reports have been confirmed and Lahiri (1977) has reviewed the data from these studies. There is considerable variability amongst these people, the HVR varying from almost zero response to values within the lowlander range. One study (Hackett *et al.* 1980) claimed that Sherpas did not show this blunted HVR. However, even this study showed that HVR was lower in Sherpas with the longest altitude exposure. More recently, Zhuang *et al.* (1993) found HVR in Tibetan subjects at 3658 m to be less than in acclimatized Han Chinese at the same altitude.

One large study compared Tibetan with Andean high altitude residents directly. Beall *et al.* (1997a) studied 320 Tibetans and 552 Andean subjects. They found resting ventilation to be higher in Tibetans by a factor of about 1.5, and their HVR to be roughly double that of the Andean subjects. Comparison of these two populations is discussed further in Chapter 17.

Weil *et al.* (1971) showed blunting of HVR in North Americans born and living at Leadville, Colorado (3100 m), HVR being only 10% of that found in the sea level controls. In residents, the blunting of HVR was dependent on the time of residence at altitude. Roughly 50% reduction in HVR was found at about 10 years.

5.5.3 Lowlanders resident at high altitude

Early studies of lowland subjects resident for a few years at high altitude suggested that HVR remained unchanged indefinitely (Sorensen and Severinghaus 1968, Lahiri *et al.* 1969). However, in a study of low-landers resident at altitude for decades (Weil *et al.* 1971) it was shown that blunting did take place slowly.

5.5.4 Highlanders resident at sea level

The HVR was found not to change in high altitude natives who came down to live at low altitude for 10 months (Lahiri *et al.* 1969), but Vargas *et al.* (1998), also in South America, in two studies found no difference in HVR between high and low altitude natives measured at low altitude. In one study the HA natives had been at altitude (>3000 m) for an average of 14 years and had resided at sea level for at least 20 years. In the other study they had lived above 3500 m for at least 20 years and at sea level for no more than 5 years. This study was followed up recently by a group from Lima and Oxford. Gamboa *et al.* (2003) considered the possibility that HVR might differ according to whether the test used a sufficiently short hypoxic exposure to avoid HVD (see section 5.2.2) or not. They found that high altitude natives, from altitudes above 3500 m, resident at low altitude for more than 5 years, when compared with low altitude natives had blunted HVR using a 10 min hypoxic exposure; but using a more acute hypoxic exposure (50 s for each step change of oxygen) most of the difference disappeared. These findings may explain some of the differences in results of previous studies of this topic. Why high altitude natives appear to have greater HVD than sea level natives is not clear.

5.5.5 The development of blunted HVR

Lahiri *et al.* (1976) found evidence in Andean Indians that HVR was normal in children and became blunted only as they grew into adulthood at altitude. They suggested the rate of blunting was more rapid the higher the place of residence. Weil *et al.* (1971) showed that in North American subjects in Leadville, Colorado, blunted HVR also developed but only after decades of high altitude residence.

In cats this blunting is seen after 3–5 weeks if the hypoxia is sufficiently severe. Tatsumi *et al.* (1991) showed blunting of HVR after this time at a simulated altitude of 5500 m. They also found that HVR, measured by recording from the carotid sinus nerve, was blunted. They considered that both central and peripheral parts of the system contributed to the reduction in overall HVR.

These findings prove that the blunting of the HVR takes many years to develop in humans and is due to environmental rather than genetic factors.

5.6 HVR AND ACUTE MOUNTAIN SICKNESS

AMS is a condition affecting otherwise fit people on ascending rapidly to altitude. For details of symptomatology, etiology and treatment see Chapter 18. It would seem axiomatic that a brisk HVR by increasing ventilation reduces the degree of hypoxia and must be protective against AMS. There is some evidence that this may be the case, but it is by no means overwhelming.

Hu *et al.* (1982) showed that six good acclimatizers (no history of AMS) had brisk HVR while four poor acclimatizers (subjects who had AMS on going to altitude) had blunted responses. Richalet *et al.* (1988) found that, in 128 climbers going to altitude on various expeditions, a measure of HVR carried out before departure indicated that a low response was a risk factor for AMS. However, high altitude residents and peoples native to high altitude have blunted HVR (see section 5.5.2) and yet tended to be less subject to AMS than lowlanders. In climbers resident at low altitude, of varying altitude experience, Milledge *et al.* (1988, 1991a) found no correlation between HVR, measured before expeditions to Everest, Mount Kenya and Bolivia, and the symptom score for AMS in the first few days after arrival at altitude.

Masuda *et al.* (1992) found an initial decrease in HVR 1–5 days after arrival at Lhasa (3700 m)

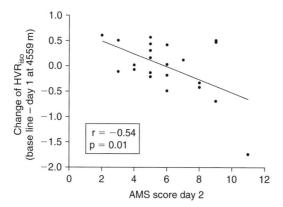

Figure 5.4   Changes in isocapnic HVR between baseline and day 1 at altitude (4559 m) versus Lake Louise acute mountain sickness (AMS) scores on day 2. (From Bartsch *et al.* 2002, with permission.)

followed by an increase and suggested that this might explain why these first few days are the time of risk for AMS. More recently Bartsch *et al.* (2002) examined the correlation of HVR (both iso- and poikilocapnic) measured at sea level, with subsequent development of AMS at 4559 m. They found none. However, they also measured HVR on the first few days after arrival at 4559 m and showed that there was a significant correlation between the change in HVR from the sea level value, to that measured on the first day at altitude, and the AMS symptom score on the next day. That is, subjects who increased their HVR tended to be resistant to AMS, whilst those who, on the second day, had AMS had shown a decrease in HVR on the first day at altitude; see Fig. 5.4.

These studies all considered a correlation, or lack of it, between HVR and simple or benign AMS. The relationship of HVR and HAPE seems clearer. Hackett *et al.* (1988b) studied seven male patients with HAPE and found HVR was low, especially in those with most severe hypoxemia. Bandopadhyay and Selvamurthy (2003) also reported that HVR was lower in a group of soldiers who had suffered from HAPE.

Hohenhaus *et al.* (1995) measured HVR in 30 subjects proved to be HAPE susceptible compared with a control group. They concluded that a low HVR is associated with an increased risk of HAPE but not with simple AMS. HAPE susceptible subjects have a greater hypoxic pulmonary vascular response (HPVR) than HAPE resistant subjects (see

Chapter 20). A low HVR means that their PA,O_2 is likely to be lower than others at a given altitude, especially on exercise (see section 5.7), thus raising their pulmonary artery pressure even higher.

5.7 HVR AND ALTITUDE: PERFORMANCE

Apart from AMS, some people 'go well' at altitude whereas others, just as athletically fit, seem much more adversely affected. In general, there is a good correlation between freedom from AMS and good altitude performance. Again, it would seem advantageous for a mountaineer to have a brisk HVR in order to maintain a better oxygen supply to the working muscles. However, the evidence for this is conflicting.

Climbers with a brisk HVR were found to suffer greater impairment of mental performance at altitude (Hornbein *et al.* 1989), presumably as a result of reduced brain blood flow due to lower Pa,CO_2 (see Chapter 16 for details of this work).

Schoene (1982) showed that 14 high altitude climbers had significantly higher HVR than 10 controls. During the 1981 American Medical Research Expedition to Everest, Schoene *et al.* (1984) extended this work, showing again that the HVR measured before and on the expedition correlated well with performance high on the mountain (Fig. 5.5). They also showed that, at altitude (6300 m), the fall in oxygen saturation on exercise is greater in subjects with a low HVR and least in those with a brisk response. This effect is most obvious at extreme altitude when the Pa,O_2 is well onto the steep part of the O_2 dissociation curve. In part of this study subjects breathed a low oxygen mixture which brought out this effect even more clearly. Thus, subjects with a blunted HVR are not only more hypoxic at rest but have even greater hypoxia on exercise than brisk responders. This is because there is a correlation between HVR and exercise ventilatory response (Martin *et al.* 1978).

Matsuyama *et al.* (1986) found that five climbers who reached an altitude of 8000 m on Kangchenjunga (8486 m) had a higher HVR than five climbers who did not.

However, the blunted HVR in peoples native to high altitude who perform at least as well as lowlanders argues against the necessity for a brisk HVR. They have probably adapted in other ways such as

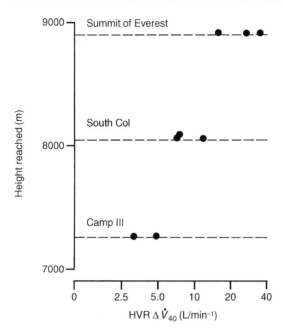

Figure 5.5   HVR and height reached on Mount Everest by eight mountaineers on the American Medical Research Expedition to Everest 1981. (Redrawn from data of Schoene *et al.* 1984.)

having larger lungs with higher diffusing capacities and may have developed differences in metabolism (Chapter 17). There is also evidence of not so brisk HVR in top level climbers. On the British Mount Kongur Expedition four elite climbers were found to have lower HVR than four scientists on the same expedition (Milledge *et al.* 1983c). Schoene *et al.* (1987) studied one of the two climbers to first reach the summit of Mount Everest without supplementary oxygen and found him to have a low HVR. Oelz *et al.* (1986) also showed that six elite climbers who had all reached at least 8400 m without supplementary oxygen had HVRs no different from controls. In a prospective study of 128 climbers going on expeditions to the great ranges, Richalet *et al.* (1988) found that a measure of HVR did not correlate with the height reached, whereas maximal oxygen consumption ($\dot{V}_{O_2,max}$) measured at sea level did.

Serebrovskaya and Ivashkevich (1992) found that subjects with the highest HVR had higher physical capacity at moderate altitude but tolerated extreme hypoxia less well, in that the P_{O_2} at which they had a disturbance of consciousness was higher than subjects with less brisk HVR. This may be explained by the fact that because of their hyperventilation, their P_{CO_2} would be lower and therefore their cerebral blood flow would be lower leading to more severe brain hypoxia.

5.8 HVR AND SLEEP

A feature of sleep at high altitude is periodic breathing. This not only disturbs sleep, the subject often waking with a distressing sensation of suffocation, but also results in quite profound hypoxia for short but repeated periods following the apneic phase of the periodic breathing (see Chapter 13). It may be that these short but repeated periods of profound hypoxia are more detrimental than a steady moderate hypoxia, although the peak and average S_{a,O_2} tend to be higher during periodic breathing (Salvaggio *et al.* 1998). Lahiri *et al.* (1984) have shown that to produce periodic breathing a brisk HVR is needed, so in this respect a brisk HVR may be a disadvantage (see Chapter 13).

5.9 HVR AT ALTITUDE: CONCLUSIONS

Animals that have had their carotid bodies denervated appear sick on being taken to altitude and have a high mortality, so an HVR sufficient to at least counter the central depressant effect of hypoxia is clearly beneficial. Whether a very brisk HVR is more advantageous than a more modest response is questionable. Relative hypoventilation at altitude is possibly a risk factor for AMS (see Chapter 18) but the HVR measured at sea level is only one factor in determining the ventilation after a day or two at altitude. The speed of respiratory acclimatization (rate of change in both HVR and HCVR) may be more important than the sea level HVR (Fig. 5.4).

In subjects with a brisk HVR it seems likely that periodic breathing will begin at lower altitudes and be present for more of the night than in subjects with a more blunted HVR. Mental performance at altitude and even after return to sea level may be more impaired in subjects with a brisk HVR (see Chapter 16).

Lowlanders with little or no altitude experience may possibly acclimatize faster and be freer of AMS if they are endowed with a brisk HVR. Highlanders, with decades of altitude living, probably develop adaptations at the tissue level which allow them to dispense with this 'emergency' response to hypoxia and avoid the need for hyperventilation. They therefore avoid the extra energy cost. Highly experienced climbers may also have made some progress towards this adaptation and so may not require a brisk HVR to avoid mountain sickness and perform well at altitude.

5.10 ALVEOLAR GASES AND ACCLIMATIZATION

It has been pointed out that if PI,O_2 is progressively reduced over a few minutes there is very little effect on ventilation until PI,O_2 has fallen to about 100 mmHg (equivalent to about 3000 m). However, in residents at altitudes lower than this, ventilation is increased. This effect of chronic hypoxia in increasing ventilation (over and above that due to acute hypoxia) is an important aspect of respiratory acclimatization.

Minute ventilation at rest is not easy to measure accurately because the placing of a mouthpiece or a mask on a subject itself tends to increase ventilation. Therefore it is usual to use PA,CO_2 as an index of ventilation, since during steady state there is a close (inverse) relationship between PA,CO_2 and ventilation.

The classical description of the effect of altitude on alveolar gases is by Rahn and Otis (1949) on the oxygen/carbon dioxide diagram (Fig. 5.6). Alveolar gases in subjects acutely exposed to varying PI,O_2 in a decompression chamber are compared with results from residents at various altitudes culled from the literature.

It will be seen that in chronic hypoxia PCO_2 falls in a linear fashion from sea level up to altitudes of about 5400 m, above which PCO_2 falls more rapidly so that the line dips down, that is with increasing altitude, PCO_2 falls but PO_2 falls very little. These are altitudes above the highest permanent habitation and points are from climbers who have been there for some days or weeks. At this altitude complete acclimatization is probably not possible; the physiology is further discussed in Chapter 12.

Figure 5.6 also shows that at about 5000 m the difference in alveolar gases between the two lines, i.e. acclimatized and unacclimatized subjects, is greatest. The PA,CO_2 is 10–12 mmHg lower in acclimatized

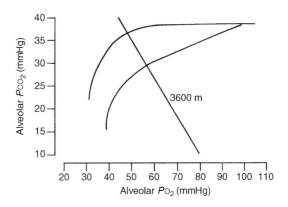

Figure 5.6 Alveolar gas concentrations and altitude. The upper line represents the PO_2 and PCO_2 found in subjects actually exposed to increasing hypoxia in a chamber. The lower line is from residents at various altitudes and from acclimatized mountaineers. (After Rahn and Otis 1949.)

subjects, indicating an increase in ventilation of over 40% compared with unacclimatized subjects.

5.11 ACUTE NORMOXIA IN ACCLIMATIZED SUBJECTS

If acclimatized subjects are returned to normal (sea level) PO_2 either by rapid return to sea level or by breathing a gas mixture appropriately enriched with oxygen their ventilation is reduced and the PA,CO_2 rises but does not return to sea level values. The remaining elevation of ventilation and depression of PA,CO_2 has been termed 'ventilatory deacclimatization from hypoxia' (VDH). The increase in PI,O_2 turns off most of the hypoxic drive and the residual hyperventilation indicates the changes in CO_2 response induced by acclimatization. This VDH is most accurately measured when ventilation is recorded during exercise.

Figure 5.7 shows results from two typical experiments (Milledge 1968). It will be seen that by breathing sea level PI,O_2 the increase in ventilation at altitude compared with sea level is reduced by only 40–50% at any given sub-maximal work rate. This suggests that about half the increase in ventilation is due to the hypoxic stimulus (HVR being increased by acclimatization) and half due to the changes in control of breathing, principally in the response to CO_2, due to acclimatization.

If subjects are returned abruptly to sea level, as after a long chamber experiment, this continued hyperventilation persists for some days. The time course of this VDH is similar to that of acclimatization and has been assumed to be due to similar mechanisms being turned on and off. However, the view that there may be different mechanisms involved is gaining ground (Smith *et al.* 2001) and a chamber study in humans found that VDH was similar in subjects whose P_{CO_2} was allowed to drop (poikilocapnic) compared with those maintained isocapnic during a 48 h exposure to hypoxia (Tansley *et al.* 1998).

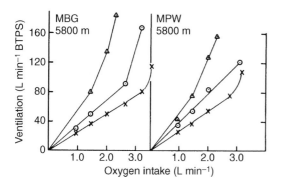

Figure 5.7 Effect of breathing sea level P_{I,O_2} on exercise minute ventilation in two acclimatized subjects (O) compared with their ventilation during air breathing at altitude (Δ) and at sea level (X). (Milledge 1968.)

5.12 CARBON DIOXIDE VENTILATORY RESPONSE AND ACCLIMATIZATION

An important aspect of respiratory acclimatization is the change in carbon dioxide ventilatory response (HCVR) measured either by the steady state (Lloyd *et al.* 1958) or by a rebreathing method (Reed 1967).

The effect of time at altitude on the HCVR is shown in Fig. 5.8, which is from the work of Kellogg (1963). The steady-state method was used in three subjects to measure the HCVR before ascent to White Mountain. The measurement was repeated a few hours after arrival by road at 4350 m and thereafter at intervals as indicated on the figure. It will be seen that the HCVR line shifts progressively leftwards and steepens. Voluntary hyperventilation of only 6 h duration breathing air has a significant effect in shifting the carbon dioxide response curve to the left (Ren and Robbins 1999).

5.13 MECHANISM FOR RESETTING HCVR

5.13.1 Central chemoreceptors

Although the peripheral chemoreceptors are sensitive to changes in P_{CO_2} and hydrogen ion concentration, the main sensor for changes in P_{CO_2} is the central medullary chemoreceptor. This is a paired region of the CNS situated just beneath the surface of the fourth ventricle in the medulla. Work by Mitchell (1963) showed that this area is sensitive to changes in hydrogen ion concentration in the

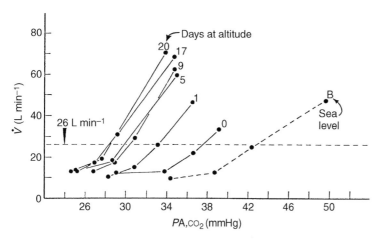

Figure 5.8 Effect of acclimatization on HCVR at an altitude of 4340 m. $\dot{V}$, ventilation. (Reproduced with permission from Kellogg 1963.)

brain ECF. Such changes are brought about primarily by changes in arterial P_{CO_2}. More recent work indicates that in addition there are other sites in the brain stem which are also chemo-sensitive and respond to changes in [H] (Nattie 2002).

The blood–brain barrier is readily permeable to dissolved carbon dioxide, less permeable to hydrogen ions and even less to bicarbonate. Thus, a rise in Pa,CO_2 is rapidly reflected in CSF P_{CO_2} and causes a rapid increase in CSF hydrogen ion concentration. Increases in hydrogen ion concentration sensed by the chemoreceptors result in increased stimulation of the respiratory center and an increase in ventilation.

5.13.2 The importance of CSF bicarbonate

The chemoreceptors sense the hydrogen ion concentration in the brain ECF (or possibly some other extracellular or intracellular compartment) but since this cannot be sampled, the following discussion centers on the CSF acid–base changes which can be measured. See section 5.15.1 for further discussion of the differences between these two compartments.

The Henderson–Hasselbalch equation, which defines the relationship between P_{CO_2}, bicarbonate and pH (hydrogen ion concentration), is shown in Fig. 5.9. This indicates that for hydrogen ion concentration to be held constant, a change of bicarbonate concentration must be followed by a change of P_{CO_2} in the same direction. Assuming the sensitivity of the central chemoreceptors to hydrogen ion concentration remains constant, a reduction in bicarbonate concentration will result in an increase in hydrogen ion concentration which will stimulate the central chemoreceptor and cause a rise in ventilation. This, in turn, will lower the P_{CO_2} and restore the hydrogen ion concentration to normal, but now with a lower P_{CO_2}. Thus a reduction in CSF bicarbonate concentration has the effect of resetting the chemoreceptor to start responding at a lower P_{CO_2} (a shift to the left of the HCVR line). A rise in CSF bicarbonate concentration has the opposite effect and is seen in patients with chronic bronchitis and hypercapnia. If the chemoreceptor responds to log hydrogen ion concentration (i.e. pH), then changes in P_{CO_2} at low values, e.g. 20–21 mmHg, will have

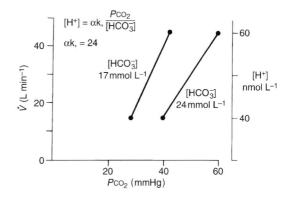

Figure 5.9 Calculated effect of reducing CSF [HCO$_3^-$] on the HCVR using the Henderson–Hasselbalch equation and assuming CSF pH is held constant by ventilatory induced changes in P_{CO_2}. $\dot{V}$, ventilation.

twice the effect of that at normal values, i.e. 40–41 mmHg. This would then explain the steepening of the HCVR seen in acclimatized subjects.

These effects are shown in Fig. 5.10. This is a theoretical representation of the effect on HCVR of a reduction in CSF bicarbonate concentration. A typical HCVR line at sea level is shown on the right. The CSF bicarbonate concentration is 24 mmol L^{-1}. If the CSF bicarbonate concentration is reduced to 17 mmol L^{-1} the chemoreceptor now 'sees' an increased hydrogen ion concentration and ventilation is stimulated until hydrogen ion concentration is reduced to the previous value. The resulting P_{CO_2} values are plotted and joined by a line giving the new HCVR on the left. This looks very similar to the actual effect of acclimatization on HCVR.

It is suggested that the mechanism of the change in HCVR is a reduction in CSF bicarbonate concentration. Evidence for this is provided by the experiments of Pappenheimer et al. (1964) in which they perfused the cerebral ventricles of awake goats with artificial CSF, varying the pH and bicarbonate concentration. They showed that by simply reducing the bicarbonate concentration in the CSF, the HCVR was shifted to the left.

Bisgard et al. (1986) found evidence of the importance of CSF bicarbonate concentration in maintaining the residual ventilation of acclimatization on giving normoxia. These workers perfused the carotid body in awake goats with hypoxemic blood while the rest of the animal, including the brain, was normoxic. Carbon dioxide was added to

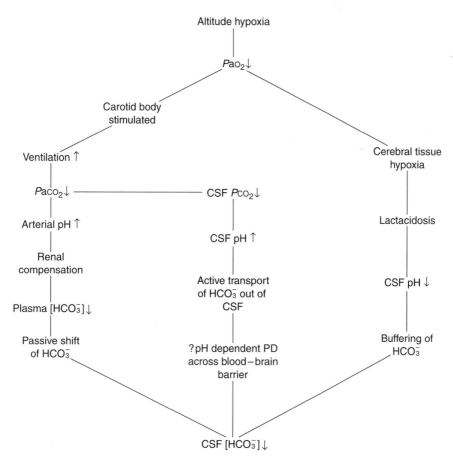

Figure 5.10 Possible mechanisms by which altitude hypoxia could cause a reduction in CSF [HCO$_3^-$]. PD, potential difference.

the inspired gas to maintain normocapnia despite hyperventilation. There was a time-dependent increase in ventilation over the 4h of the experiment, due presumably to increases in HVR. But since brain and body were normocapnic and normoxic there would have been no change in CSF bicarbonate concentration. Full respiratory acclimatization did not take place since, on switching the carotid perfusion to normoxia, ventilation promptly fell to normal.

5.13.3 Reduction in CSF bicarbonate concentration at altitude

In lowlanders going to an altitude of 3800 m the CSF bicarbonate concentration is reduced from a mean sea level value of 24.7 mmol L^{-1} to 20.4 mmol L^{-1} on the second day at altitude and 20.1 mmol L^{-1} on day 8 (Severinghaus *et al.* 1963). Similar results (mean 20.1 mmol L^{-1}) were found at 4880 m (Lahiri and Milledge 1967). Residents at high altitude had similar values, 19.1–21.3 mmol L^{-1} (Severinghaus and Carcelan 1964, Lahiri and Milledge 1967, Sorensen and Milledge 1971). Thus the reduction in CSF bicarbonate concentration of 4.5 mmol L^{-1} measured at altitude might explain the shift of the HCVR line to the left, though respiratory acclimatization probably also involves contributions from other mechanisms such as changes in HVR (see section 5.5.1). The mechanism for the reduction in bicarbonate and the importance of CNS pH was discussed at length in previous editions of this textbook. However, the consensus of opinion now seems to emphasize the changes in HVR rather than in CO$_2$ response as the more important element in the hyperventilation of altitude acclimatization. To quote Smith *et al.* (2001):

> Regulation of CNS [H⁺] as a mechanism of ventilatory acclimatization to hypoxia is an elegant hypothesis with considerable logical appeal. However, it has been difficult to establish any major role for CNS [H⁺] in the control of ventilatory acclimatization, when the entire time course of the process is considered.

5.13.4 Brain intracellular pH

Using magnetic resonance spectroscopy on unacclimatized lowland subjects in a hypobaric chamber, Goldberg *et al.* (1992) found that, after a week at 4267 m simulated altitude, there was no significant change in intracellular pH although on return to normobaria there was a significant intracellular acidosis compared with pre-altitude exposure.

5.14 DYNAMIC CARBON DIOXIDE RESPONSE

Carbon dioxide is eliminated only during expiration; during inspiration it is retained. Therefore the level of carbon dioxide in the blood leaving the lungs must oscillate in time with breathing. During exercise these oscillations will be increased. Yamamoto and Edwards (1960) suggested that these oscillations might be a signal to which the peripheral chemoreceptors could respond over and above the mean level of carbon dioxide in the arterial blood. The response to this putative signal of change in carbon dioxide with time is called the dynamic carbon dioxide ventilatory response. Datta and Nickol (1995) showed that this response could be demonstrated in exercising humans (it had been shown previously in anesthetized cats) by measuring the ventilation during the injection of a small bolus of carbon dioxide either early or late in inspiration. Ventilation was found to be greater with early pulses. Collier *et al.* (1995) showed that this response is absent in acute hypoxia and weak or absent on first arrival at altitude. It is enhanced with acclimatization and is greatest in subjects who have

climbed to over 7000 m. This provides evidence that the ventilatory response of the peripheral chemoreceptor is increased for carbon dioxide as it is for hypoxia (section 5.5.1).

5.15 LONGER TERM ACCLIMATIZATION

5.15.1 Highlanders

People native to high altitude have slightly lower ventilation and higher $Pa,_{CO_2}$ than acclimatized newcomers (Chiodi 1957). This is probably due to their blunted HVR (see section 5.5.2). The HCVR of Andean natives (Severinghaus *et al.* 1966a), Sherpas (Milledge and Lahiri 1967) and Tibetans (Shi *et al.* 1979) has the same slope as that of lowlanders at the same altitude. The position of the carbon dioxide ventilatory response line may be to the right (Severinghaus *et al.* 1966a) or not significantly different from lowlanders (Milledge and Lahiri 1967). That is, there is little difference between highlanders and lowlanders in their carbon dioxide ventilatory response.

5.15.2 Lowlanders

Although most of the respiratory acclimatization takes place within the first few hours and days at altitude, there may be further changes over the following weeks. In humans, there is a further increase in ventilation and $Pa,_{O_2}$ with a further decrease in $Pa,_{CO_2}$ (Forster *et al.* 1974), though in other animals, e.g. pony and goat, the $Pa,_{CO_2}$ reaches the lowest point at 8–12 h and then rises. The rat responds like humans with continued fall in $Pa,_{CO_2}$ up to 14 days (Dempsey and Forster 1982). There is no significant change in acid–base balance over this period to account for this further ventilatory adaptation. This further increase in ventilation is probably due to an increase in HVR, due to changes in both sensitivity of the carotid body over this period (see section 5.5.1) and in changes in control of ventilation from higher centers, such as has been demonstrated in cats by Tenney and Ou (1977). This might be due to activation of genes such as *fos B* (Malik *et al.* 2005) (section 5.5.1).

Pulmonary gas exchange

SUMMARY

Important changes in pulmonary gas exchange occur at high altitude. The most obvious feature is the hyperventilation resulting from hypoxic stimulation of the peripheral chemoreceptors. The hyperventilation reduces the alveolar P_{CO_2} and helps to maintain the alveolar P_{O_2} in spite of the inevitable fall associated with the reduced P_{O_2} of inspired gas. As an example of the extent of the hyperventilation that can occur, climbers on the summit of Mount Everest increase their alveolar ventilation some five-fold and drive the alveolar P_{CO_2} down to less than 10 mmHg. The degree of hyperventilation is very different depending on whether subjects are exposed to acute hypoxia, or whether they have the advantages of acclimatization. With acute hypoxia there may be no increase in ventilation up to altitudes of about 3500 m. However, in acclimatized subjects, essentially any increase in altitude above sea level results in a rise in alveolar ventilation and a fall in alveolar P_{CO_2}. Diffusion of oxygen across the blood-gas barrier is a critical link in the oxygen cascade from the atmosphere to the mitochondria. Diffusion limitation of oxygen transfer across the blood-gas barrier occurs during exercise at even moderate altitudes and at rest at extreme altitude. This is one of the few situations when diffusion limitation for oxygen is seen in the normal lung. Diffusion across the blood-gas barrier is enhanced if the oxygen affinity of hemoglobin is increased, and it is of interest that this occurs at extreme altitude because of the severe respiratory alkalosis. Lowlanders who go to high altitude have a small increase in diffusing capacity caused partly by the polycythemia. Highlanders generally have higher diffusing capacities than lowlanders possibly because of the accelerated growth of the lung in a hypoxic environment. Ventilation–perfusion inequality is a major cause of impaired gas exchange at sea level but is a minor factor at high altitude. However, very high altitudes, particularly associated with exercise, cause ventilation–perfusion inequality possibly because of the development of subclinical pulmonary edema. There is some evidence that gas exchange in the placenta is enhanced at high altitude.

6.1 HISTORICAL

Some aspects of the effects of high altitude on pulmonary gas exchange, particularly the hyperventilation and the cyanosis, have been recognized ever since the early days of the balloonists. For example, in 1804 the eminent French scientist Louis Joseph Gay-Lussac ascended to an altitude of what was thought to be 7020 m in a balloon and reported that his breathing was difficult, and his pulse and respiration were high. There were also reports of discoloration of the hands and face presumably the result of cyanosis. In fact during the ill-fated flight of the *Zénith* referred to in Chapter 1, Tissandier reported that Sivel's face was black. On the other hand, the early balloonists did not complain as much about difficulties with breathing including breathlessness as did high altitude climbers, and this is consistent with the fact that acute hypoxia does not result in as large a ventilatory response as prolonged hypoxia, as we shall see below.

Early mountain climbers were well aware of the shortness of breath at high altitudes. During an early ascent of Mont Blanc by the Swiss physicist Horace-Bénédict de Saussure in 1787, he complained that 'the rarity of the air gave me more trouble than I could have believed. At last I was obliged to stop for breath every 15 or 16 steps. . . .' In fact on the summit he complained that he was 'constantly forced to interrupt my work and devote myself entirely to breathing.' The eminent climber Edward Whymper, during the first ascent of Chimborazo (6420 m) in 1880, gave a colorful description of shortness of breath stating that

we were unable to satisfy our desire for air, except by breathing with open mouths. . . . Besides having our normal rate of breathing largely accelerated, we found it impossible to sustain life every now and then giving spasmodic gulps, just like fishes when taken out of water.

Some of the most striking accounts of breathlessness at high altitude came from the early expeditions to Mount Everest. For example in 1924 at an altitude of about 8380 m, E.F. Norton stated that

our pace was wretched. My ambition was to do twenty consecutive paces uphill without a pause to rest and pant elbow on bent knee; yet I never remember achieving it – thirteen was nearer the mark.

His companion T. Howard Somervell was even more breathless stating 'From taking three or four breaths to a step we were reduced to having to take ten or more.' Finally, Reinhold Messner, who with Peter Habeler made the first ascent of Everest without supplementary oxygen in 1978, stated when he was on the summit 'I have nothing more to do than breathe. . . . I am nothing more than a single, narrow, gasping lung.'

It is remarkable that in spite of so many anecdotal accounts of hyperventilation at high altitude, some of the most eminent physiologists claimed that it did not occur. For example, Paul Bert stated that hyperventilation does not occur at high altitude and wrote

what is really certain is that . . . a dweller in lofty altitudes, does not even try to struggle against the decrease of oxygen in his arterial blood by speeding up his respiration successively, as was first supposed. The observations of Dr. Jourdanet are conclusive. (Bert 1878)

Possibly this error can be traced to the fact that Bert worked exclusively with low pressure chambers that only allowed short-term observations of the effects of acute hypoxia. However, even Angelo Mosso, who had the advantage of studying long-term residents at the Capanna Margherita, reported that although respiratory frequency was increased at high altitude, total ventilation was decreased. He reached this erroneous conclusion because he converted the volumes to standard conditions (0°C and 1000 mmHg in his case) rather than to body temperature and pressure, saturated with water vapor (BTPS).

Turning now to the role of diffusion in pulmonary gas exchange, the controversy over oxygen secretion constitutes one of the most colorful episodes in the history of high altitude medicine. The debate was briefly alluded to in Chapter 1. An early proponent of the secretion hypothesis was the Danish physiologist Christian Bohr. In a paper published in 1891 he compared the P_{O_2} and P_{CO_2} of alveolar gas with that of gas in a tonometer equilibrated with arterial blood taken at the same time (Bohr 1891). In some instances the alveolar P_{O_2} was found to be as much as 30 mmHg below, and the P_{CO_2} as much as 20 mmHg above, the arterial blood values. Bohr's conclusion was: 'In general, my experiments have shown definitely that the lung tissue plays an active part in gas exchange; therefore the function of the lung can be regarded as analogous to that of the glands.' Bohr referred to the secretion ability of the lung as its 'specific function,' and claimed that the active secretion of oxygen and carbon dioxide by the lung could use large amounts of oxygen, up to 60% of the total requirements of the body.

August Krogh was one of Bohr's students and assisted him in his experiments on gas secretion from 1899 to 1908. However, Krogh gradually became persuaded that passive diffusion rather than active secretion could account for the experimental data and in 1910 published a landmark paper on this topic. Since Bohr was his major professor and very jealous of the secretion theory, the introductory section of Krogh's paper required an unusually delicate touch. Part of it reads:

> I shall be obliged in the following pages to combat the views of my teacher Prof. Bohr on certain essential points. . . . I wish here not only to acknowledge the debt of gratitude which I, personally, owe to him, but also to emphasize the fact . . . that the real progress, made during the last twenty years in the knowledge of the processes in the lungs, is mainly due to his labours. . . .

The British physiologist J.S. Haldane visited Bohr in Copenhagen and also became convinced of the secretion theory, at least as far as oxygen was concerned. For example, in 1897 Haldane and Lorraine Smith wrote: 'The absorption of oxygen by the lungs thus cannot be explained by diffusion alone.' Haldane argued that oxygen secretion would be particularly beneficial at high altitudes, and in order to test the hypothesis the Anglo-American expedition to Pikes Peak was organized in 1911. Arterial P_{O_2} was calculated by an indirect method following the inhalation of carbon monoxide, and the results appeared to strongly support the secretion hypothesis. However, the theory was also attacked by Marie Krogh (wife of August) when she developed a method for measuring the diffusing capacity of the lung using small concentrations of carbon monoxide. Her results indicated that the normal lung was capable of transferring very large amounts of oxygen by passive diffusion even when the inspired P_{O_2} was greatly reduced.

Another physiologist who did not accept the secretion story was Joseph Barcroft. He conducted a heroic experiment on himself by living in a sealed glass chamber filled with hypoxic gas for 6 days (Barcroft *et al.* 1920). His left radial artery was exposed 'for an inch-and-a-half' and blood was taken for measurements of oxygen saturation. There was a 'somewhat dramatic moment' when the first blood sample was drawn because it 'looked dark', an observation which was believed to be inconsistent with oxygen secretion. The conclusion was that diffusion was the only mechanism necessary for oxygen transfer across the blood-gas barrier during hypoxia.

Barcroft and his colleagues subsequently tested the secretion hypothesis further on their expedition to Cerro de Pasco (4330 m) in the Peruvian Andes in 1921–22. The diffusing capacity of the lung for carbon monoxide was measured on five members of the expedition both at sea level and at Cerro de Pasco, and only a small increase was found. Barcroft therefore argued that the tendency for the arterial oxygen saturation to fall during exercise at high altitude could be explained by the failure of equilibration of P_{O_2} between alveolar gas and pulmonary capillary blood (Barcroft *et al.* 1923). This was one of the first direct demonstrations of diffusion limitation of oxygen at high altitude, a finding that has been confirmed many times since.

It is remarkable that J. S. Haldane remained a staunch supporter of oxygen secretion all his life. In the second edition of his book *Respiration*, written with J.G. Priestley and published in 1935, a year before Haldane's death, a whole chapter was devoted to evidence for oxygen secretion (Haldane and Priestley 1935). Haldane gradually shifted his position as evidence mounted against the secretion hypothesis. He initially thought that oxygen secretion occurred under all conditions, but later argued that it only became significant at high altitude, and later still that it only occurred after a period of acclimatization. His obsession with this theory long after seemingly overwhelming evidence had been provided against it was remarkable in this great physiologist.

6.2 EFFECTS OF HYPERVENTILATION ON GAS EXCHANGE

The most important feature of pulmonary gas exchange at high altitude is the increase in alveolar ventilation and its consequences. The importance of hyperventilation is emphasized if we look at its role at extreme altitude, for example on the summit of Mount Everest. First we need to refer to two simple equations governing pulmonary gas exchange. The first is the alveolar ventilation equation:

$$\dot{V}_A = \frac{\dot{V}_{CO_2}}{PA,CO_2} \times K$$

where $\dot{V}_A$ is alveolar ventilation, $\dot{V}_{CO_2}$ is the CO_2 production, and PA,CO_2 is the alveolar partial pressure of carbon dioxide. This equation states that if the rate of CO_2 production is constant, the alveolar ventilation and alveolar PCO_2 are inversely related. For example, if the alveolar ventilation is doubled, the PCO_2 is halved.

The second equation is the alveolar gas equation:

$$PA,O_2 = PI,O_2 - \frac{PA,CO_2}{R} + F$$

where PA,O_2 and PA,CO_2 are the alveolar partial pressures of oxygen and carbon dioxide, respectively; PI,O_2 is the inspired partial pressure of oxygen; R is the respiratory exchange ratio; and F is a correction factor that is generally small and can be neglected.

At sea level the normal alveolar ventilation equation results in an alveolar PCO_2 of about 40 mmHg. If we insert this value into the alveolar gas equation, assuming an inspired PO_2 of 150 and a normal respiratory exchange ratio at rest of 0.8, the alveolar PO_2 is given by

$$150 - \frac{40}{0.8} = 100 \text{ mmHg}$$

Now suppose we apply this equation to a climber on the summit of Mount Everest where the barometric pressure is, say, 250 mmHg (see Fig. 2.2). The PO_2 of moist inspired gas is given by:

$$PI,O_2 = 0.2904(P_B - 47)$$

where 0.2094 is the fractional concentration of oxygen, P_B is the barometric pressure, and 47 mmHg is the water vapor partial pressure. This gives an inspired PO_2 of about 43 mmHg. If we now assume

that both the alveolar ventilation and the CO_2 production of the climber at rest are unchanged compared with sea level, his alveolar PCO_2 is 40 mmHg. The alveolar gas equation then gives an alveolar PO_2 of

$$43 - \frac{40}{0.8} = -7 \text{ mmHg}$$

which of course is absurd. However, if the climber now increases his alveolar ventilation fivefold thus reducing his alveolar PCO_2 to 8 mmHg, the alveolar gas equation gives

$$PA,O_2 = 43 - \frac{8}{0.8} = 33 \text{ mmHg}$$

While this value is very low, it is just sufficient to maintain life. This simple calculation shows the crucial importance of hyperventilation at high altitude. The mechanism of the hyperventilation is hypoxic stimulation of the peripheral chemoreceptors as discussed in Chapter 5.

6.3 ACUTE HYPOXIA COMPARED WITH ACCLIMATIZATION

There is a striking difference between the degree of hyperventilation that occurs when subjects are exposed acutely to hypoxia on the one hand, and when they are acclimatized to high altitude on the other. One of the classical studies was performed by Rahn and Otis (1949) and their original results are shown in Fig. 6.1. The data on subjects exposed acutely to high altitude (upper line) were obtained using low pressure chambers. The data for the acclimatized line come from a number of sources including lowlanders who spent various periods at a given altitude, and in some cases permanent residents at high altitudes.

It can be seen that with acute exposure to high altitude there is typically no change in alveolar PCO_2, which implies no change in alveolar ventilation, up to an altitude of about 12 000 ft or about 3600 m. By contrast, acclimatized subjects show a fall in alveolar PCO_2 indicating an increase in alveolar ventilation for any increase in altitude. Note that altitude itself

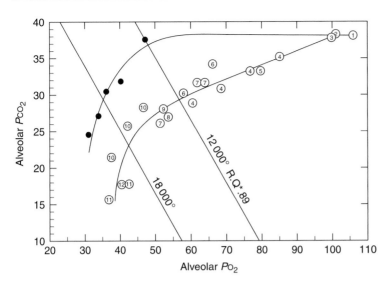

Figure 6.1 Oxygen–carbon dioxide diagram showing the alveolar gas composition in subjects acutely exposed to high altitude (upper line) and after acclimatization (lower line). The two diagonal lines are for a respiratory exchange ratio (RQ) of 0.85 for altitudes of 12 000 ft (3660 m) and 18 000 ft (5490 m). The numbers in the circles show the sources of the data (see original article). (From Rahn and Otis 1949.)

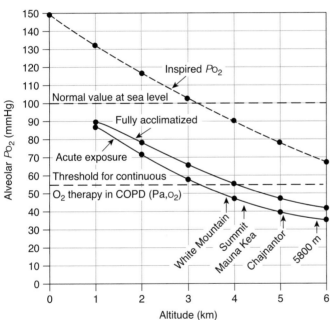

Figure 6.2 Alveolar P_{O_2} at high altitudes following acute exposure (lower line) and full acclimatization (upper line). The values come from the measurements shown in Fig. 6.1 and there is considerable individual variation. The altitudes of several observatories where astronomers work are also shown. Note that fully acclimatized astronomers on the summit of Mauna Kea (4200 m) have an alveolar P_{O_2}, and therefore an arterial P_{O_2}, lower than the threshold for continuous oxygen therapy in patients with chronic obstructive pulmonary disease (COPD) at sea level.

is not shown explicitly on the graph but the intersection of the diagonal RQ lines with the lower horizontal axis indicates the inspired P_{O_2} which falls as altitude increases.

In Fig. 6.2 the P_{O_2} data are redrawn so that they are now plotted against altitude. This plot shows more clearly the relentless fall in alveolar P_{O_2} with increasing altitude for both acute exposure and full acclimatization. However, acclimatization results in an increase in ventilation which lowers the alveolar P_{CO_2} and thus increases the alveolar P_{O_2} at any given altitude according to the alveolar gas equation

shown earlier. The altitudes can be read off the horizontal axis and some important high altitude sites are identified. The summit of Mauna Kea in Hawaii at an altitude of 4200 m is the site of several large telescopes and many astronomers are exposed to this altitude. Additional telescopes are located on the Chajnantor plateau in north Chile at an altitude of 5050 m, and this will shortly be the site of an extremely large radio telescope (Atacama Large Millimeter Array). Other high altitude sites near Chajnantor up to an altitude of 5800 m are being considered for astronomy.

Figure 6.2 emphasizes that in spite of the hyperventilation that occurs at high altitude, severe alveolar hypoxia and therefore arterial hypoxemia may occur. As an example, astronomers on Mauna Kea, even if they are fully acclimatized, have an alveolar P_{O_2} on the average less than 55 mmHg. Their arterial P_{O_2} will therefore be a little lower. Forster (1986) reported that the mean arterial P_{O_2} on the first day at 4200 m was 42 mmHg rising to 44 mmHg on day 5. The severity of the hypoxemia is further indicated by the fact that an arterial P_{O_2} of 55 or less is the criterion for continuous oxygen administration at sea level if that degree of arterial hypoxemia is caused by chronic obstructive pulmonary disease. This emphasizes the severe hypoxemia that occurs even in fully acclimatized subjects at these altitudes. In fact astronomers at Mauna Kea never become fully acclimatized because of the limited time they spend there.

Figures 6.1 and 6.2 emphasize the advantages of acclimatization in raising the alveolar P_{O_2} at high altitude. However, it is interesting that permanent residents of high altitude often have lower alveolar P_{O_2} values and higher alveolar P_{CO_2} values than fully acclimatized lowlanders. This is discussed in section 5.15.1.

6.4 PHYSIOLOGY OF DIFFUSION IN THE LUNG

6.4.1 Fick's law of diffusion

Fick's law of diffusion states that the rate of transfer of a gas through a sheet of tissue is proportional to the area of the tissue and to the difference in gas partial pressure between the two sides, and inversely proportional to the tissue thickness. The area of the blood-gas barrier in the human lung is some 50–100 m^2, and the thickness is less than 0.3 mm in many places, so the dimensions of the barrier are well suited to diffusion.

In addition, the rate of gas transfer is proportional to a diffusion constant which depends on the properties of the tissue and the particular gas. The constant is proportional to the solubility of the gas and inversely proportional to the square root of its molecular weight. This means that carbon dioxide diffuses about 20 times more rapidly than oxygen through tissue sheets since its solubility is about

24 times greater at 37°C and the molecular weights of carbon dioxide and oxygen are in the ratio of 1.375 to 1.

Fick's law can be written as

$$\dot{V}_{gas} = \frac{A}{T} D \left(P_1 - P_2 \right)$$

where $\dot{V}$ is volume of gas per unit time, A is area, T is thickness, D is the diffusion constant, and P_1 and P_2 denote the two partial pressures.

For a complex structure such as the blood-gas barrier of the human lung, it is not possible to measure the area and thickness during life. Instead, we combine A, T and D and rewrite the equation as

$$\dot{V}_{gas} = D_L \left(P_1 - P_2 \right)$$

where D_L is the diffusing capacity of the lung.

The gas of choice for measuring the diffusing capacity of the lung is carbon monoxide (at very low concentrations) because the avidity of hemoglobin for this gas is so great that the partial pressure in the capillary blood is extremely small (except in smokers) and thus the uptake of the gas is solely limited by the diffusion properties of the blood-gas barrier. (The complication caused by finite reaction rates is considered below.) Thus if we rewrite the above equation as

$$D_L = \frac{\dot{V}_{CO}}{P_1 - P_2}$$

where P_1 and P_2 are the partial pressures of alveolar gas and capillary blood respectively, we can set P_2 to zero. This leads to the equation for measuring the diffusing capacity of the lung for carbon monoxide:

$$D_L = \frac{\dot{V}_{CO}}{P_{A,CO}}$$

In words, the diffusing capacity of the lung for carbon monoxide is the volume of carbon monoxide transferred in mL min^{-1} $mmHg^{-1}$ of alveolar partial pressure.

6.4.2 Reaction rates with hemoglobin

Early workers assumed that all of the resistance to the transfer of oxygen from the alveolar gas into the capillary blood could be attributed to the diffusion process within the blood-gas barrier. However, when the rates of reaction of oxygen with hemoglobin were measured using a rapid reaction apparatus, it became clear that the rate of combination with hemoglobin might also be a limiting factor. If oxygen is added to deoxygenated blood, the formation of oxyhemoglobin is quite fast, being well on the way to completion in 0.2 s. However, oxygenation occurs so rapidly in the pulmonary capillary that even this rapid reaction significantly delays the loading of oxygen by the red cells. Thus the uptake of oxygen can be regarded as occurring in two stages:

- Diffusion of oxygen through the blood-gas barrier (including the plasma and red cell interior)
- Reaction of the oxygen with hemoglobin (Fig. 6.3)

In fact it is possible to sum the two resulting resistances to produce an overall resistance (Roughton and Forster 1957).

We saw above that the diffusing capacity of the lung is defined as

$$D_{\mathrm{L}} = \frac{\dot{V}_{\mathrm{gas}}}{P_1 - P_2}$$

that is, the flow of gas divided by the pressure difference. It follows that the inverse of D_{L} is pressure difference divided by flow and is therefore analogous to electrical resistance. Consequently the resistance of the blood-gas barrier in Fig. 6.3 is shown as $1/D_{\mathrm{M}}$ where M denotes membrane. The rate of reaction of oxygen with hemoglobin can be described by θ, which gives the rate in mL min^{-1} of oxygen which combine with 1 mL blood mmHg^{-1} Po_2. This is analogous to the 'diffusing capacity' of 1 mL of blood and, when multiplied by the volume of capillary blood (V_c), gives the effective 'diffusing capacity' of the rate of reaction of oxygen with hemoglobin. Again its inverse, $1/(\theta V_c)$, describes the resistance of this reaction.

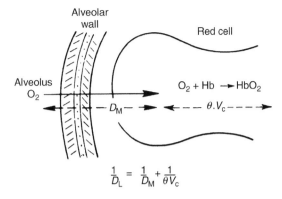

Figure 6.3   The measured diffusing capacity of the lung (D_{L}) is made up of two components, one due to the diffusion process itself (D_{M}), and one attributable to the time taken for oxygen to react with hemoglobin (θV_c).

It is possible to add the resistances offered by the membrane and the blood to obtain the total resistance. Thus the complete equation is

$$\frac{1}{D_{\mathrm{L}}} = \frac{1}{D_{\mathrm{M}}} + \frac{1}{\theta V_{\mathrm{c}}}$$

In practice the resistances offered by the membrane and blood components are approximately equal in the normal lung.

6.4.3 Rate of oxygen uptake along the pulmonary capillary

By using Fick's law of diffusion, and data on reaction rates of oxygen with hemoglobin, it is possible to calculate the time course of Po_2 along the pulmonary capillary as the oxygen is loaded by the blood. The application of Fick's law to this situation is not trivial because of the chemical bond which forms between oxygen and hemoglobin. This means that the relationship between Po_2 and oxygen concentration in the blood is nonlinear, as shown by the oxygen dissociation curve. This problem was first solved by Bohr (1909) and the numerical integration procedure which he developed is known as the Bohr integration. A further complication occurs because, as oxygen is being taken up, carbon dioxide is given off, and this alters the position of the oxygen dissociation curve. A full treatment of this latter process should take into account not only the rate of diffusion of carbon

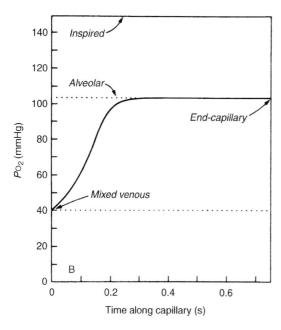

Figure 6.4 Calculated time course for P_{O_2} in the resting human pulmonary capillary at sea level. Note that there is ample time for equilibration of the P_{O_2} between alveolar gas and end-capillary blood. $\dot{V}_{O_2}$ 300 mL min^{-1}; D_{M,O_2} 40 mL min^{-1} mmHg^{-1}. (From West and Wagner 1980.)

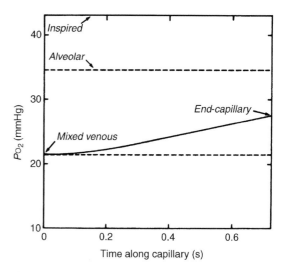

Figure 6.5 Calculated time course of the P_{O_2} along the pulmonary capillary for a climber at rest on the summit of Mount Everest. Note that there is considerable diffusion limitation of oxygen uptake with a large alveolar end-capillary P_{O_2} difference. P_B 253 mmHg; $\dot{V}_{O_2}$ 350 mL min^{-1} (From West *et al.* 1983b.)

dioxide through the blood-gas barrier, but also the rates of reaction of carbon dioxide in blood. Since not all the rate constants are known under all the required conditions, some assumptions and simplifications are necessary.

Figure 6.4 shows a typical time course calculated for the lung of a resting subject at sea level (Wagner and West 1972, West and Wagner 1980). The diffusing capacity of the blood-gas barrier itself (D_M) was assumed to be 40 mL min^{-1} mmHg^{-1}, and the time spent by the blood in the pulmonary capillary was taken as 0.75 s (Roughton 1945). Other assumptions include a resting cardiac output of 6 L min^{-1} and oxygen uptake of 300 mL min^{-1}.

Note that the blood comes into the lung with a P_{O_2} of 40 mmHg and the P_{O_2} rapidly rises to almost the alveolar P_{O_2} level by the time the blood has spent only about one-third of its available time in the capillary. The rate of rise of P_{O_2} in the latter two-thirds of the capillary is extremely slow, and there is a negligible P_{O_2} difference between alveolar gas and end-capillary blood.

This time course can be contrasted with that calculated for a resting climber breathing air on the summit of Mount Everest (Fig. 6.5). Again, the membrane diffusing capacity of the blood-gas barrier was assumed to be 40 mL min^{-1} mmHg^{-1} based on measurements made on acclimatized lowlanders at an altitude of 5800 m (West 1962a). The oxygen uptake was taken to be 350 mL min^{-1}, and other blood and alveolar gas variables were taken from measurements made on the American Medical Research Expedition to Everest (West *et al.* 1983b). The time spent by the blood in the pulmonary capillary was assumed to be unchanged at 0.75 s because this is determined by the ratio of capillary blood volume to cardiac output (Roughton 1945). The capillary blood volume was shown to be unchanged at 5800 m (West 1962a), and the cardiac output is also the same as at sea level according to the measurements of Pugh (1964c) (section 7.3).

It can be seen that the oxygen profile is very different at this extreme altitude. The blood comes into the lung with a P_{O_2} of only about 21 mmHg, and the P_{O_2} rises very slowly along the pulmonary capillary, reaching a value of only about 28 mmHg at the end. Thus there is a large P_{O_2} difference of some 7 mmHg between alveolar gas and capillary blood. This indicates marked diffusion limitation of oxygen transfer. It can be shown that this diffusion limitation becomes more striking as the oxygen consumption is increased by exercise.

The very different time courses for P_{O_2} shown in Figs 6.4 and 6.5 represent the extremes between sea level and the highest point on Earth for resting humans. At intermediate altitudes, the difference between alveolar and end-capillary P_{O_2} will be considerably reduced at rest and may be negligibly small. However, exercise at high altitude will always tend to cause diffusion limitation of oxygen transfer as originally demonstrated by Barcroft and colleagues (1923).

Whether carbon dioxide elimination is ever limited by diffusion is still unknown. This is partly because some of the reaction rates of carbon dioxide in blood remain uncertain. Many physiologists believe that some diffusion limitation of carbon dioxide output may occur during heavy exercise.

6.4.4 Diffusion and perfusion limitation of oxygen transfer

It is clear from Fig. 6.4 that a resting subject at sea level has no diffusion limitation of oxygen transfer because there is no P_{O_2} difference between alveolar gas and end-capillary blood. Under these conditions, the amount of oxygen which is taken up by the blood is determined by the pulmonary blood flow. This means that oxygen uptake is perfusion limited.

By contrast, Fig. 6.5 shows a situation where oxygen uptake is, in part, diffusion limited. This is indicated by the large P_{O_2} difference between alveolar gas and end-capillary blood. However, under these conditions, oxygen uptake is also partly perfusion limited because increasing pulmonary blood flow will increase oxygen uptake.

At first sight the substantial diffusion limitation of oxygen transfer shown in Fig. 6.4 might be attributed to the low alveolar P_{O_2}, and therefore the smaller driving gradient for oxygen diffusion. However, this is not correct. The conditions under which diffusion and perfusion limitation occur have been clarified by Piiper and Scheid (1980). They used a simplified model with several assumptions including linearity of the oxygen dissociation curve in the working range. This situation is approached during conditions of severe hypoxia when the lung is operating very low on the oxygen dissociation curve.

Using this simplified model, Piiper and Scheid showed that the total transfer rate $\dot{M}$ of a gas is given by the expression

$$\dot{M} = \left(P_A - P_V\right)\dot{Q}\beta\left[1 - \exp\left(\frac{-D}{\dot{Q}\beta}\right)\right]$$

where P_A and P_V are the partial pressures of oxygen in the alveolar gas and venous blood respectively, $\dot{Q}$ is cardiac output, D is the diffusing capacity, and β is the slope of the oxygen dissociation curve (assumed to be linear). The total conductance, G, for gas exchange between alveolar gas and capillary blood may be defined as the transfer rate divided by the total effective partial pressure difference $(P_A - P_V)$, or

$$G = \dot{Q}\beta\left[1 - \exp\left(\frac{-D}{\dot{Q}\beta}\right)\right]$$

This expression clarifies the factors responsible for diffusion and perfusion limitation. The equation shows that if D is very much larger than $\dot{Q}\beta$, the expression inside the large brackets tends to 1, and gas transfer is limited by perfusion only. In this case, the (perfusive) conductance is given by $G = \dot{Q}\beta$. The relative difference between the conductance without diffusion limitation and the actual conductance is an index of diffusion limitation, L_{diff}, as shown in Fig. 6.6.

By contrast, diffusion limitation occurs if $\dot{Q}\beta$ is so large that it greatly exceeds D, or to put it in another way, D becomes relatively very small. In this case the (diffusive) conductance is given by $G = D$. The relative difference between the conductance without perfusion limitation and the actual conductance is an index of perfusion limitation. Zero on the vertical axis of Fig. 6.6 indicates complete perfusion limitation.

Figure 6.6 shows that oxygen uptake is entirely perfusion limited in hyperoxia (extreme right of diagram) and that this is also true for the uptake of the inert gases (those that do not combine with hemoglobin) nitrogen and sulfur hexafluoride. However, oxygen transfer during hypoxia becomes diffusion limited to some extent (middle of diagram) and this is particularly the case during exercise when oxygen

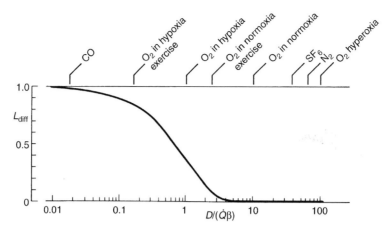

Figure 6.6 Conditions under which diffusion limitation of gas transfer in the lung occurs. L_{diff} is a measure of diffusion limitation; when its value is 1.0, gas transfer is entirely diffusion limited. It can be seen that L_{diff} is greatest for carbon monoxide, and least for oxygen under hyperoxic conditions. D, diffusing capacity; $\dot{Q}$, pulmonary blood flow; β, solubility of the gas in blood, or slope of its dissociation curve. See text for details. (Modified from Piiper and Scheid 1980.)

consumption is greatly increased. For carbon monoxide, gas transfer is essentially diffusion limited under all conditions (left of diagram).

The above analysis emphasizes that an important factor leading to diffusion limitation is an increase in β; that is, the slope of the blood-gas dissociation curve. This is the reason why the uptake of carbon monoxide is entirely diffusion limited; the slope of its dissociation curve is extremely large. An increased slope of the oxygen dissociation curve tending to diffusion limitation occurs for three reasons at high altitude:

- The lung is working on a low part of the oxygen dissociation curve which is very steep.
- The polycythemia of high altitude increases the change in blood oxygen concentration per unit change in P_{O_2}.
- The left shift of the curve caused by the respiratory alkalosis increases its slope. In fact, at extreme altitude, oxygen begins to resemble carbon monoxide to some extent.

For readers who prefer an intuitive explanation to the more formal analysis given above, the essential conclusion can be stated as follows. Diffusion limitation is likely when the 'effective solubility' of the gas in pulmonary capillary blood (that is, the slope of the dissociation curve) greatly exceeds the solubility of the gas in the tissues of the blood-gas barrier. This condition is met for carbon monoxide for which blood has an enormous avidity, and is approached for oxygen at high altitude because of the steepness of its dissociation curve at low P_{O_2} values, and the increased blood hemoglobin concentration.

An analogy is the rate at which sheep can enter a field through a gate. If the gate is narrow but the field is large, the number of sheep that can enter in a given time is limited by the size of the gate. However, if both the gate and the field are small (or both are big) the number of sheep is limited by the size of the field.

6.4.5 Oxygen affinity of hemoglobin and diffusion limitation

It can be shown that increasing the affinity of hemoglobin for oxygen expedites the loading of oxygen in the pulmonary capillary under conditions of diffusion limitation at high altitude. The oxygen affinity of hemoglobin is conveniently expressed by the P_{50}, that is the P_{O_2} for 50% saturation of the hemoglobin. The normal value is about 27 mmHg.

Numerical analysis shows that increasing the affinity (leftward shift of the oxygen dissociation curve) results in more rapid equilibration between the P_{O_2} of alveolar gas and pulmonary capillary blood. A simplified way of looking at this is that the

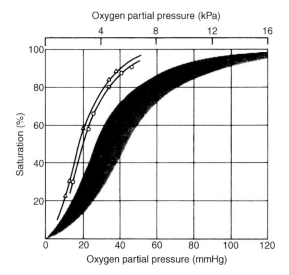

Oxygen partial pressure (kPa)

Oxygen partial pressure (mmHg)

Saturation (%)

Figure 6.7 Oxygen dissociation curves for blood of llama (circle) and vicuna (triangle) compared with other mammals. The left-shifted curve for these high altitude native animals indicates an increased affinity of the hemoglobin for oxygen which assists in oxygen loading along the pulmonary capillaries. (From Hall *et al.* 1936.)

Table 6.1 Strategies for increasing oxygen affinity in chronic hypoxia

Strategy	Subject
Different sequence in globin chain	Human fetus, bar-headed goose, toadfish
Decrease in red cell 2,3-DPG	Fetus of dog, horse, pig
Decrease in ATP	Trout, eel
Different hemoglobin, small Bohr effect	Tadpole
Mutant hemoglobin (Andrew-Minneapolis)	Family in Minnesota
Respiratory alkalosis	Climber at extreme altitude

left-shifted curve keeps the blood P_{O_2} low in the initial stages of oxygen loading and thus maintains a large P_{O_2} difference between alveolar gas and capillary blood during much of the oxygenation time. This increased P_{O_2} difference therefore maintains the driving pressure and accelerates loading.

However, a left-shifted oxygen dissociation curve interferes with the unloading of oxygen in peripheral capillaries because, for a given P_{O_2} in venous blood (required to maintain the diffusion head of pressure to the tissues), the blood unloads less oxygen. It is therefore not intuitively obvious whether the advantages of a left-shifted curve in assisting the loading of oxygen in the pulmonary capillaries outweigh the disadvantages of unloading the oxygen in the peripheral capillaries.

Several pieces of evidence suggest that a high oxygen affinity of hemoglobin is beneficial under hypoxic conditions. For example, the llama and vicuna, animals native to the Peruvian highlands, have left-shifted oxygen dissociation curves (Fig. 6.7), as do some burrowing animals whose environment becomes oxygen depleted (Hall *et al.* 1936). The human fetus, which is believed to have arterial P_{O_2} in the descending aorta of less than

25 mmHg, has a greatly increased oxygen affinity by virtue of its fetal hemoglobin which has a P_{50} at pH 7.4 of about 17 mmHg. Experimental studies have shown that rats with artificially left-shifted oxygen dissociation curves tolerate severe acute hypoxia better than rats with normal dissociation curves (Eaton *et al.* 1974). Again, Hebbel and his colleagues (1978) described a family in which two of the four children had an abnormal hemoglobin (Andrew-Minneapolis) with a P_{50} of 17 mmHg. These two siblings had a higher $\dot{V}_{O_2,max}$ at an altitude of 3100 m than the two with normal hemoglobin.

Numerical modeling gives some basis for these findings by showing that the increased oxygen affinity of the hemoglobin improves oxygenation in the pulmonary capillaries under conditions of diffusion limitation more than it interferes with the release of oxygen by peripheral capillaries (Bencowitz *et al.* 1982). Table 6.1 lists some of the strategies used by animals (including humans) to increase the oxygen affinity of their hemoglobin under hypoxic conditions.

Climbers at very high altitude tend to have an increased arterial blood pH, which causes a leftward shift of the oxygen dissociation curve. This is caused by a respiratory alkalosis which is only partially compensated and was the case for members of the 1981 American Medical Research Expedition to Everest who spent several weeks at an altitude of 6300 m. The mean arterial pH of three subjects was 7.47 (Winslow *et al.* 1984), which is well above the normal range.

At extreme altitudes, there is evidence of extraordinary degrees of respiratory alkalosis. For example, when Pizzo took alveolar gas samples on the summit of Mount Everest, there is good evidence that his arterial pH exceeded 7.7. This value is based on a measured alveolar P_{CO_2} of 7.5 mmHg, and a base excess measured in venous blood taken on the following morning of -5.9 mmol L^{-1}. This extreme respiratory alkalosis caused a marked leftward shift of the oxygen dissociation curve with a calculated *in vivo* P_{50} of about 19 mmHg. Thus a climber on the summit of Mount Everest develops conditions rather similar to those in the human fetus where the arterial P_{O_2} is less than 30 mmHg and the P_{50} is less than 20 mmHg.

6.5 PULMONARY DIFFUSING CAPACITY AT HIGH ALTITUDE

6.5.1 Acclimatized lowlanders

Barcroft and his colleagues measured the diffusing capacity for carbon monoxide in five members of the expedition to Cerro de Pasco in the Peruvian Andes in 1921–2. They used the single breath method which had recently been described by Krogh (1915) and the measurements were made at rest. There was no consistent change from the sea level values though the investigators believed that there was a slight tendency for the diffusing capacity to rise. They pointed out, however, that this change would not be an important element in acclimatization (Barcroft *et al.* 1923). Subsequent investigators have confirmed the absence of change or found only a very small (less than 10%) increase in diffusing capacity for carbon monoxide in resting subjects after periods of up to several months at altitudes of up to 4560 m (Kreuzer and van Lookeren Campagne 1965, DeGraff *et al.* 1970, Guleria *et al.* 1971, Dempsey *et al.* 1978).

Measurements on exercising subjects at altitudes up to 5800 m showed that after 7–10 weeks of acclimatization, there was an increase in pulmonary diffusing capacity of 15–20% (Fig. 6.8). However, this small change could be wholly accounted for by the increased rate of reaction of carbon monoxide with hemoglobin due to hypoxia and by the increased blood hemoglobin concentration (West 1962a).

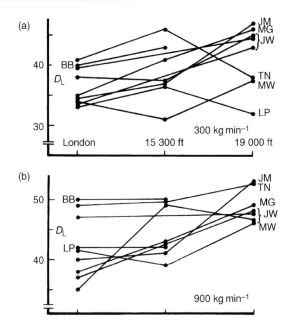

Figure 6.8 Diffusing capacities (D_L) in mL min^{-1} mmHg^{-1} measured at sea level (London), 15 300 ft (4700 m) and 19 000 ft (5800 m) in acclimatized lowlanders exercising at: (a) 300 kg min^{-1} and (b) 900 kg min^{-1}. Note the moderate increase in diffusing capacity of carbon monoxide with altitude. (From West 1962.)

The mechanism of this increase can be explained by reference to Fig. 6.3. The 'resistance' attributable to the rate of combination of oxygen with hemoglobin is given by $1/(\theta V_c)$. It has been found experimentally that the value of θ varies depending on the ambient P_{O_2}. At low P_{O_2} values, θ is increased and therefore the resistance to oxygen transfer is decreased. An additional factor is the increased blood hemoglobin concentration which, for a given value of V_c (capillary blood volume), increases the amount of hemoglobin present. Thus these factors completely accounted for the small observed increase in diffusing capacity for carbon monoxide at high altitude and indicated that there was no change in the diffusion properties of the lung itself after 7–10 weeks of acclimatization at an altitude of 5800 m.

Acute mountain sickness (AMS) has been shown to reduce the diffusing capacity for carbon monoxide at high altitude (Ge *et al.* 1997). The measurements were made 2 days after arrival at 4700 m. The subjects with AMS also showed a lower vital capacity

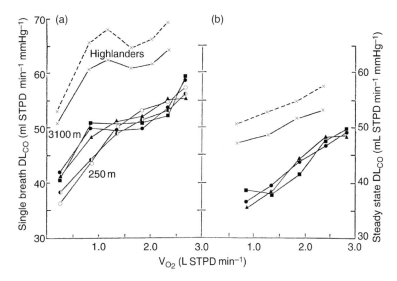

Figure 6.9 Diffusing capacities for carbon monoxide as obtained by the single breath method (a) and steady-state method (b) in three groups of subjects; lowlanders at 250 m (open circle and half-filled circle), lowlanders sojourning at 3100 m (closed circle, triangle and square indicate different periods at this altitude), and native highlanders at 3100 m. The broken line indicates the measured data for highlanders; the continuous line shows the results after correction for $1/\theta$. All the measurements are on white people, the 3100 m data being from Leadville, Colorado. Note the higher diffusing capacities of the highlanders both at rest and on exercise. (From Dempsey *et al.* 1971.)

and arterial P_{O_2}, and an increased alveolar–arterial P_{O_2} gradient (based on arterialized capillary blood) than subjects without AMS. The mechanism was thought to be subclinical pulmonary edema. In another study subjects with a history of high altitude pulmonary edema (HAPE) were found to have a lower diffusing capacity for carbon monoxide during hypoxia and exercise than a HAPE-resistant group (Steinacker *et al.* 1998). The HAPE-susceptible group also had smaller increases in stroke volume, cardiac output and ventilation during exercise. Enhanced pulmonary vasoconstriction was suggested as the mechanism of the lower diffusing capacity.

Interestingly, the diffusing capacity measured during submaximal exercise was reduced following a Himalayan expedition to 4900 m and above compared with measurements made prior to the expedition (Steinacker *et al.* 1996). The fall in diffusing capacity was about 14% and this was accompanied by a reduction in cardiac index of about 16% and $\dot{V}_{O_2,max}$ of about 5%. A possible explanation was the wasting of skeletal muscle which resulted in a reduced cardiac output and therefore diffusing capacity on exercise.

6.5.2 Highlanders

Several studies have shown that people who live permanently at high altitude (high altitude natives or highlanders) have pulmonary diffusing capacities that are about 20–50% higher than the predicted values, or than in lowlander controls (Fig. 6.9). One of the first studies was by Velásquez (1956) who studied 12 native residents of Morococha (altitude 4550 m) and showed that the diffusing capacity for oxygen was consistently higher than in similar subjects at sea level. Remmers and Mithoefer (1969) found that Andean Indians at an altitude of 3700 m had a diffusing capacity for carbon monoxide which was some 50% higher than predicted. High diffusing capacities have also been reported in Caucasians living at an altitude of 3100 m (DeGraff *et al.* 1970, Dempsey *et al.* 1978). The increased diffusing capacities were demonstrated both during rest and exercise.

A potential problem in such studies is the appropriateness of the predicted values for diffusing capacity. For example, in the study by Remmers and Mithoefer (1969), predicted values were obtained from Caucasian North Americans and

(a)

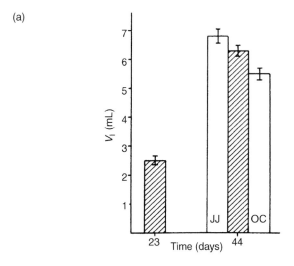

Figure 6.10 (a) Increase in lung volume V_I from day 23 to day 44 of life in three groups of rats exposed to an altitude of 3450 m (JJ), sea level (cross-hatched), and 40% oxygen at sea level (OC). Note that lung volume increased most in the hypoxic and least in the hyperoxic animals. (b) Pulmonary diffusing capacity estimated morphometrically in the same three groups of animals at the 44th day. Note that the diffusing capacities reflected the changes in lung volume. C shows a control group. (From Burri and Weibel 1971.)

(b)

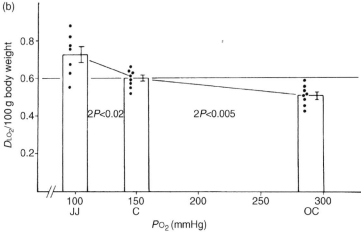

were applied to the South American high altitude Indian population. This may introduce errors because of ethnic differences in body build. However, in other studies such as that by Dempsey *et al.* (1971), diffusing capacities were compared between lowlanders and highlanders in similar ethnic groups (Fig. 6.9).

The increased diffusing capacities can presumably be explained by the larger lungs which result in an increased alveolar surface area and capillary blood volume. Barcroft *et al.* (1923) commented on the remarkable chest development of the Peruvian natives in Cerro de Pasco and these early investigators made chest radiographs to confirm this. The radiographs showed that the ratio of chest width to height was greater in the high altitude natives than in the Anglo-Saxon lowlanders (expedition members). Children who are raised

at altitudes of 3000 m have been shown to have increased lung volumes and diffusing capacities (de Meer *et al.* 1995). It has been shown experimentally that animals exposed to low oxygen partial pressures during their active growth phase develop larger lungs and bigger diffusing capacities than animals reared in a normoxic environment (Fig. 6.10) (Bartlett and Remmers 1971, Burri and Weibel 1971). Beagles raised at an altitude of 3100 m had higher diffusing capacities and lung tissue volume than a control group at sea level (Johnson *et al.* 1985). In a subsequent study on foxhounds it was shown that exposure of pups to 3800 m for only 5 months resulted in higher diffusing capacities in the adults (McDonough *et al.* 2006). These studies provide an adequate explanation for the observed high diffusing capacities, and would also account for the persistence of an increased diffusing capacity for carbon monoxide in highlanders after a pro-longed period spent at sea level as observed by Guleria and his co-workers (1971). However, Lechner *et al.* (1982) presented evidence that the lungs only grow faster in a hypoxic environment and the end result is the same lung volume as in normoxic animals. This discrepancy is unresolved.

The impact of pregnancy on diffusing capacity for carbon monoxide was measured in pregnant and nonpregnant Peruvian women by McAuliffe *et al.* (2003). One group lived at sea level and the other at 4300 m. The diffusing capacities were corrected for the hemoglobin concentration. At sea level, the diffusing capacities of pregnant and non-pregnant women were similar though smaller than those of the women at high altitude consistent with the results discussed earlier.

6.6 DIFFUSION LIMITATION OF OXYGEN TRANSFER AT HIGH ALTITUDE

The main reason for the importance of pulmonary diffusion at high altitude is that it may be a limiting factor in oxygen uptake. A considerable amount of evidence now supports this.

One of the first groups to suggest diffusion limitation of oxygen uptake at altitude was Barcroft and his colleagues (1923). They concluded from their measurements of pulmonary diffusing capacity for carbon monoxide at an altitude of 4300 m that P_{O_2} equilibration between alveolar gas and the blood at the end of the capillary would not be achieved, especially on exercise. Subsequently, Houston and Riley (1947) measured alveolar–arterial P_{O_2} differences in four subjects who spent 32 days in a low pressure chamber in which the pressure was gradually reduced from 760 to 320 mmHg (Operation Everest I). Measurements were made during rest and during relatively low levels of exercise (oxygen uptakes less than 1200 mLmin^{-1} at simulated high altitude). During exercise, the alveolar–arterial P_{O_2} difference was increased to about 10 mmHg, which they correctly ascribed to diffusion limitation.

During the Silver Hut Expedition of 1960–61, measurements of arterial oxygen saturation by ear oximetry were made on five subjects who lived for 4 months at an altitude of 5800 m ($P_B = 380$ mmHg) in a prefabricated hut. The average arterial oxygen saturation at rest was 67% and

this fell at work levels of 300 and 900 kg m min^{-1} to 63% and 56%, respectively (West *et al.* 1962). The progressive fall in arterial oxygen saturation as the work level was raised occurred in the face of an increasing alveolar P_{O_2} and was strong evidence for diffusion limitation of oxygen transfer. Alveolar–arterial differences were calculated and nine measurements at the maximal exercise level gave a mean P_{O_2} difference of 26 mmHg with a standard deviation of 4 mmHg. Calculations based on the Bohr integration procedure showed that the results were consistent with a maximum pulmonary diffusing capacity for oxygen of about 60 mL min^{-1} mmHg^{-1}.

Further evidence for diffusion limitation of oxygen transfer during exercise at very high altitudes was obtained on the 1981 American Medical Research Expedition to Everest. Fifteen subjects spent up to 4 weeks at an altitude of 6300 m ($P_B = 350$ mmHg) and arterial oxygen saturation was measured by oximeter at rest and during increasing levels of work (Fig. 6.11). Again there was a progressive fall in arterial oxygen saturation as the work level was increased from rest to 1200 kg min^{-1}, equivalent to an oxygen consumption of about 2.3 L min^{-1}. The calculated alveolar–arterial P_{O_2} difference at this highest work level was 21 mmHg (West *et al.* 1983c).

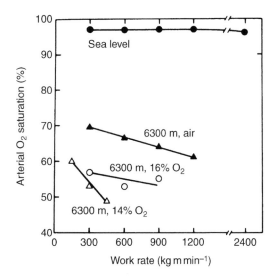

Figure 6.11 Arterial oxygen saturation as measured by ear oximetry plotted against work rate at sea level and 6300 m altitude. The two lower lines were obtained with subjects breathing 16% and 14% oxygen at 6300 m. (From West *et al.* 1983c.)

Figure 6.11 also shows that additional measurements were made with subjects breathing 16% and 14% oxygen at this very high altitude. The latter gave an inspired PO_2 of 42 mmHg, equivalent to that encountered by a climber breathing air on the summit of Mount Everest. Note the very abrupt fall in arterial oxygen saturation as work rate was increased at this highest altitude on Earth. Two subjects performed maximum exercise while breathing 14% oxygen and in one of them the oximeter reading fell to less than 10% oxygen saturation at one point during the experiment! Although the calibration of the oximeter at such values is unreliable, the actual saturation must have been extremely low.

6.7 VENTILATION/PERFUSION INEQUALITY

Ventilation/perfusion inequality is a major cause of impaired gas exchange in lung diseases at sea level such as chronic obstructive pulmonary disease, interstitial lung disease and acute respiratory failure. At high altitude, ventilation/perfusion inequality also becomes important in the presence of lung disease caused, for example, by high altitude pulmonary edema or pulmonary thromboembolism.

In the absence of obvious lung disease ventilation/perfusion inequality generally plays a minor role at high altitude. In fact there is some evidence that the topographical inequality of ventilation/perfusion ratios is actually improved by ascent. The reason is that the increase in pulmonary artery pressure caused by hypoxic pulmonary vasoconstriction causes a more uniform distribution of blood flow in the lung (Dawson 1972) and, other things being equal, this will improve the relationships between ventilation and blood flow. However, the degree of ventilation/perfusion inequality in the normal lung caused by the topographical differences of ventilation and blood flow is so small that this must be a minor effect.

There is evidence that ventilation/perfusion inequality can develop at extreme altitude especially on exercise. These measurements were made by Wagner and his colleagues in the simulated ascent of Mount Everest (Operation Everest II). The measurements of ventilation/perfusion inequality were made using the multiple inert gas elimination technique (Wagner et al. 1974). Inert gas

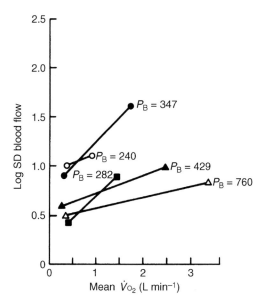

Figure 6.12 Relationship between the degree of ventilation/perfusion inequality in the lung and oxygen uptake in subjects during a simulated ascent of Mount Everest in a low pressure chamber (Operation Everest II). The ordinate shows the log SD of blood flow which is a measure of ventilation/perfusion inequality. Note that both a reduction of barometric pressure (P_B, measured in mmHg) and increase in work rate tended to increase the degree of ventilation/perfusion inequality. (From Wagner et al. 1987.)

exchange is not diffusion-limited, even during maximal exercise.

Figure 6.12 shows the increase in ventilation/perfusion inequality caused both by increasing altitude and increasing work level in the 40-day low pressure chamber experiment (Wagner et al. 1987). The vertical scale shows the mean log standard deviation of the blood flow distribution which is one measure of ventilation/perfusion inequality. It can be seen that this index was about 0.5 during rest at sea level but increased slightly when the oxygen consumption was raised to over 3 L min^{-1} during exercise at sea level. At very high altitude, where the barometric pressure was 347 mmHg, the resting standard deviation rose to approximately 0.9 and it increased further to over 1.5 with exercise. The explanation of these intriguing data is uncertain but may be subclinical pulmonary edema. There was also evidence that rapid ascent was more likely to result in ventilation/perfusion inequality than slow ascent, suggesting that inadequate acclimatization may have been an important factor.

Using these independent measurements of the amount of ventilation/perfusion inequality present, it was possible to separate the contribution of diffusion limitation and ventilation/perfusion inequality to the observed increase of the alveolar–arterial P_{O_2} difference at high altitude. The results are shown in Fig. 6.13. The arterial P_{O_2} was directly measured on arterial blood samples. It can be seen that the measured alveolar–arterial P_{O_2} difference increased to a mean of about 13 mmHg during maximal exercise at a barometric pressure of 347 mmHg where the oxygen consumption was a little over 2 L min^{-1}. At higher simulated altitudes, the maximum alveolar–arterial P_{O_2} differences were smaller. This can be explained by the smaller maximum oxygen uptakes, and the fact that the subjects were operating on the lower, steeper region of the oxygen dissociation curve.

Also shown in Fig. 6.13 are the predicted alveolar–arterial P_{O_2} differences for the degree of ventilation/perfusion inequality measured at the same time by means of the multiple inert gas elimination technique. These predicted P_{O_2} differences decreased as the altitude increased despite the broadening of the distributions of ventilation/perfusion ratios as shown in Fig. 6.11. Again, the reason is that the P_{O_2} values are lower on the curvilinear oxygen dissociation curve. The data allow the total alveolar–arterial P_{O_2} difference to be divided into two components, one caused by ventilation/perfusion inequality, and the rest presumably attributable to diffusion limitation. The results show that, at sea level, essentially all of the alveolar–arterial P_{O_2} difference was attributable to ventilation/perfusion inequality up to an oxygen consumption of nearly 3 L min^{-1}. Above that high exercise level, some diffusion limitation apparently occurred. By contrast, at a barometric pressure of 429 mmHg, the measured alveolar–arterial P_{O_2} difference exceeded that predicted from the amount of ventilation/perfusion inequality when the oxygen uptake was above about 1 L min^{-1}. This was also true at a barometric pressure of 347 mmHg. At the higher simulated altitudes, with barometric pressures of 282 and 240 mmHg, almost all of the observed alveolar–arterial P_{O_2} difference during exercise could be ascribed to diffusion limitation. These elegant studies go a long way towards elucidating the role

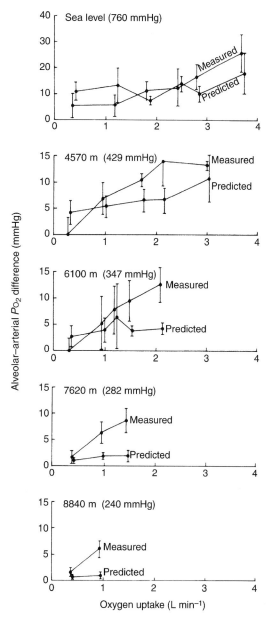

Figure 6.13 Relationship between alveolar–arterial P_{O_2} difference and the oxygen uptake in Operation Everest II (compare Fig. 6.12). The predicted difference refers to that calculated from the measured amount of ventilation/perfusion inequality. Note that, at the highest altitudes, the measured differences considerably exceeded the predicted values, indicating diffusion limitation of oxygen uptake. For the measurements at 240 mmHg, the subjects breathed an oxygen mixture to give an inspired P_{O_2} of 43 mmHg. (From Wagner *et al.* 1987.)

of diffusion in the hypoxemia of high altitude during exercise.

6.8 DIFFUSION IN THE PLACENTA AT HIGH ALTITUDE

The fetus derives its oxygen via the placenta rather than the lung. Gas exchange in the placenta is much less efficient than in the lung and, for example, the P_{O_2} in the descending aorta of the human fetus at sea level is less than 25 mmHg. The fetus must be even more hypoxic at high altitude and it is known that birth weight is reduced at high altitude, and that smaller birth weights at high altitude are associated with increased infant morbidity and mortality (Lichty *et al.* 1957, Moore *et al.* 1998a).

An interesting question is whether the diffusion properties of the placenta are improved at high altitude, just as the diffusing capacity in high altitude natives is apparently raised. There is some evidence for this. Reshetnikova *et al.* (1994) examined 10 normal term placentas from women in Kyrghyzstan up to altitudes of 2800 m and found that there was an increase in capillary volume, and that the harmonic mean thickness of the maternal–fetal barrier fell from 6.9 μm in controls to 4.8 μm at high altitude. They calculated that the morphometric diffusing capacity of the villous membrane for oxygen was significantly increased, by about 80%. Zhang *et al.* (2002) reported that in human placentas at high altitude, the small blood vessels were dilated and were less frequently associated with perivascular cells than in an ethnically matched lowland population. Other evidence of structural differences at high altitude was obtained by Tissot van Patot and colleagues (2003) who showed that fetal capillary density increased at 3100 m compared with 1600 m. However, Mayhew (1991) found somewhat different results in placentas from populations living at 3600 m compared with 400 m altitude in Bolivia. Although there was some improvement in diffusion properties on the maternal side of the placenta, these did not extend to the fetal side. In another study no differences were found in capillary surface area or length, and it was concluded that high altitude pregnancy is not accompanied by increased angiogenesis (Mayhew 2003).

7

Cardiovascular system

SUMMARY

Important changes in the cardiovascular system occur at high altitude. Cardiac output increases following acute exposure to high altitude, but in acclimatized lowlanders and high altitude natives, most measurements show the cardiac output for a given work rate is the same as at sea level. Nevertheless, because of the polycythemia, hemoglobin flow is increased. Heart rate for a given work rate is higher than at sea level, with the result that stroke volume is reduced at high altitude. However, this is not caused by a reduced myocardial contractility; on the contrary, this is preserved up to very high altitudes in normal subjects. Abnormal heart rhythms, such as premature ventricular or atrial contractions, are unusual despite the severe hypoxemia. However, sinus arrhythmia accompanying periodic breathing is very common at high altitude. Changes in systemic blood pressure are variable; several studies report an increase when lowlanders move to high altitude. However, in some instances patients with hypertension at sea level have developed a reduction in pressure on ascent to altitude. Pulmonary hypertension is striking at high altitude, in both newcomers and high altitude natives, particularly on exercise. Tibetans have smaller degrees of pulmonary hypertension than other highlanders. This is also the case in some animals native to high altitude. The hypertension is relieved by oxygen breathing when the exposure to high altitude is acute, but after a few days the response to oxygen is less because of vascular remodeling. Right ventricular hypertrophy and corresponding electrocardiographic changes are seen. Newborn infants sometimes develop right heart failure at high altitude and this also occurs in young soldiers stationed at extreme altitudes.

7.1 INTRODUCTION

The cardiovascular system is an essential link in the transport of oxygen from the air to the mitochondria, and it therefore has an important role in acclimatization and adaptation to the oxygen-depleted environment of high altitude. However, some aspects of the cardiovascular system at high altitude have not been as extensively studied as their importance may suggest. One reason for this is the difficulties of measurement, especially the invasive investigations necessary to reliably measure cardiac output and pulmonary artery pressure. However, echocardiographic assessment of tricuspid regurgitation is increasingly used to estimate systolic pulmonary artery pressure.

In this chapter we look at available data on many aspects of the cardiovascular system, although, as will be seen, there are still many areas of ignorance.

This chapter is closely related to some others. The cerebral circulation is discussed in Chapter 16, and changes in the capillary circulation in high altitude acclimatization and adaptation are considered in Chapter 10. High altitude cerebral edema and high altitude pulmonary edema are discussed in Chapters 19 and 20 respectively.

7.2 HISTORICAL

Early travelers to high altitudes frequently complained of symptoms related to the cardiovascular system. Many of these accounts were collected by Paul Bert and set out in the first chapter of his classical book *La Pression Barométrique* (Bert 1878, p. 29 in the 1943 translation). For example, he quotes the great explorer Alexander von Humboldt at an altitude of 2773 'fathoms' (about 5070 m) on Chimborazo in the South American Andes complaining that 'blood issued from our lips and eyes'. Many other travelers gave accounts of bleeding from the mouth, eyes and nostrils, and they often attributed this to the low barometric pressure which, they argued, did not balance the pressures within the blood vessels. This is fallacious reasoning because all vascular pressures fall along with the ambient atmospheric pressure (section 2.1). These early reports of bleeding are intriguing because this is not a typical feature of mountain sickness as we see it today.

Another common complaint of these early mountain travelers was cardiac palpitations, especially on exercise. Typical is the passage quoted by Bert (Bert 1878, p. 37 in 1943 translation) from the explorer D'Orbigny who stated when he was on the crest of the Cordilleras that 'at the least movement, I felt violent palpitations'. The most observant travelers measured their pulse rate and noted that mild exercise such as horse riding caused it to increase dramatically although it was normal at rest. Cloves of garlic were frequently eaten to relieve these symptoms, which often seem exaggerated to the modern reader.

An interesting historical vignette was the occurrence of peripheral edema in cattle while grazing at high altitude in Utah and Colorado early in the twentieth century (Hecht *et al.* 1962). The condition is known as brisket disease because the edema is most prominent in that part of the animal between the forelegs and neck (brisket). The condition is caused by right heart failure as a result of severe pulmonary hypertension caused by hypoxic pulmonary vasoconstriction. Right heart failure also occurs in some newborn infants at high altitude, especially in Han children born in Tibet (Sui *et al.* 1988). A somewhat similar condition has been described in Indian soldiers stationed at very high altitudes near the border with Pakistan (Anand *et al.* 1990). These conditions are further discussed in Chapter 21.

Early climbers on Mount Everest who became fatigued were sometimes diagnosed as having 'dilatation' of the heart. This was thought to be one of the signs of failure to acclimatize. As late as 1934, Leonard Hill stated that 'degeneration of the heart and other organs due to low oxygen pressure in the tissues, is a chief danger which the Everest climbers have to face' (Hill 1934).

7.3 CARDIAC FUNCTION

7.3.1 Cardiac output

It is generally accepted that acute hypoxia causes an increase in cardiac output both at rest and for a given level of exercise compared with normoxia. These responses are seen at sea level following inhalation of low oxygen mixtures, and on acute exposure to high altitude (Asmussen and Consolazio 1941, Keys *et al.* 1943, Honig and Tenney 1957, Kontos *et al.* 1967, Vogel and Harris 1967). There is also evidence that, in well-acclimatized lowlanders at high altitude, the relationship between cardiac output and work rate returns to the sea level value (Pugh 1964d, Reeves *et al.* 1987). On the other hand, there is some uncertainty about the changes following short periods of acclimatization.

Perhaps the first systematic studies of cardiac output at high altitude were made by Douglas, Haldane and their colleagues (1913) on the Anglo-American Pikes Peak Expedition where they made measurements on themselves by means of ballistocardiography. No consistent changes in stroke volume of the heart were noted. They therefore concluded that cardiac output at rest was proportional to heart rate, which they showed increased over the first 11 days at 4300 m and subsequently decreased towards normal. Barcroft and his colleagues (1923) used an indirect

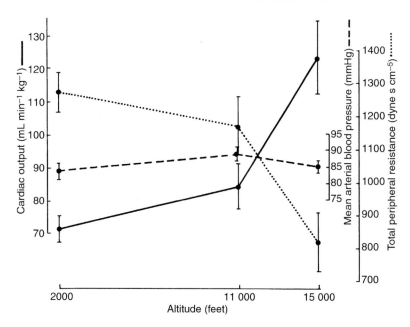

Figure 7.1 Cardiac output (solid line), mean systemic arterial pressure (dashed line), and calculated peripheral resistance (dotted line) during acute exposure to a simulated altitude of 2000 ft (610 m), 11 000 ft (3353 m) and 15 000 ft (4572 m). Measurements were made on 16 subjects after 10, 20, 30 and 40 h at each altitude. The results from the different altitude exposures were pooled. Mean $\pm$ SE indicated by vertical bars (1 dyne = 10^{-5} N). (From Vogel and Harris 1967.)

Fick technique to measure cardiac output in their study of themselves at Cerro de Pasco in the Peruvian Andes at an altitude of 4330 m. They reported essentially no difference in acclimatized subjects compared with sea level.

Grollman (1930) made an impressive series of measurements on Pikes Peak in 1929 using the acetylene rebreathing method. He reported that resting cardiac output increased soon after reaching high altitude, with a maximum value approximately 5 days later. However, by day 12 it had returned to its sea level value. Similar changes were found by Christensen and Forbes (1937) during the International High Altitude Expedition to Chile.

More recent investigators have reported similar findings. Figure 7.1 shows the increase in resting cardiac output during the first 40 h of acute exposure to simulated high altitude (Vogel and Harris 1967). Klausen (1966) found an increase in cardiac output following ascent to an altitude of 3800 m but after 3–4 weeks it had returned to its sea level value. Similar findings were reported by Vogel and his colleagues (1967) on Pikes Peak at an altitude of 4300 m. However, Alexander *et al.* (1967) reported a decrease in cardiac output during exercise after 10 days at 3100 m compared with sea level. The decrease was caused by a fall in stroke volume. Reductions in cardiac output (compared with sea level) after

several days at high altitude were also reported by Wolfel *et al.* (1994) and Sime *et al.* (1974).

In well-acclimatized lowlanders at high altitude, and in high altitude natives, cardiac output in relation to work level is the same as at sea level. This was shown by Pugh (1964d) during the Silver Hut Expedition at an altitude of 5800 m where the measurements were made by the acetylene rebreathing technique (Fig. 7.2). Further measurements were made by Cerretelli (1976a) at the Everest Base Camp where the subjects had acclimatized for 2–3 months. Reeves *et al.* (1987) reported the same finding on subjects during Operation Everest II where a remarkable series of measurements was made down to an inspired P_{O_2} of 43 mmHg, equivalent to that of the Everest summit (Fig. 7.3). Similar results were found in Operation Everest III (COMEX '97) (Boussuges *et al.* 2002). Since the maximal work level is greatly reduced at high altitude it follows that maximal cardiac output is also lower. Bogaard *et al.* (2002) showed that this is not explained by alterations in the function of the autonomic nervous system.

High altitude natives also show the same relationship between cardiac output and oxygen consumption during exercise as at sea level. Vogel *et al.* (1974) studied eight natives of Cerro de Pasco, Peru, at an altitude of 4350 m and again after 8–13

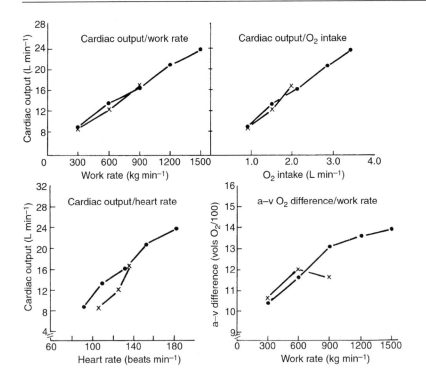

Figure 7.2 Cardiac output in relation to work rate and related variables as obtained from four well-acclimatized subjects during the Silver Hut Expedition. Note that the cardiac output/work rate relationship is the same at an altitude of 5800 m (×, barometric pressure 380 mmHg) as at sea level (●). (From Pugh 1964a.)

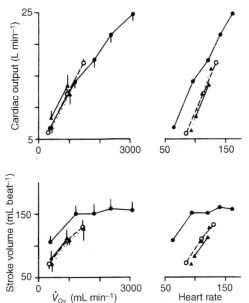

Figure 7.3 Cardiac output (by thermodilution) and stroke volume plotted against oxygen uptake ($\dot{V}_{O_2}$) and heart rate at barometric pressures of 760 (●, $n = 8$), 347 (○, $n = 6$), 282 (▲, $n = 4$) and 240 (▲, $n = 2$) mmHg during Operation Everest II. For the measurements at 240 mmHg, the subjects breathed an oxygen mixture to give an inspired P_{O_2} of 43 mmHg. (From Reeves *et al.* 1987.)

days at Lima (sea level) and showed that the results were almost superimposable (Fig. 7.4).

It is perhaps surprising that cardiac output in well-acclimatized lowlanders and high altitude natives bears the same relationship to work rate (or power) as it does at sea level. After all, there is plenty of evidence of severe tissue hypoxia during exercise at high altitude, and at first sight it seems that one way of increasing the tissue P_{O_2} would be to raise cardiac output and thus peripheral oxygen delivery. However, in a theoretical study, Wagner (1996) argued that although increasing cardiac output improves calculated maximal oxygen consumption at sea level, the improvement becomes progressively less as altitude increases. In fact, calculations done for a subject on the summit of Mount Everest show that maximal oxygen consumption ($\dot{V}_{O_2,max}$) was essentially unchanged as cardiac output was increased from 50 to 150% of its expected value (Fig. 7.5).

A similar picture emerged when hemoglobin concentration was varied between 50 and 150% of its expected value. Note that in the case of both cardiac output and hemoglobin concentration, calculated oxygen delivery to the tissues was greatly increased. The reason for the lack of improvement

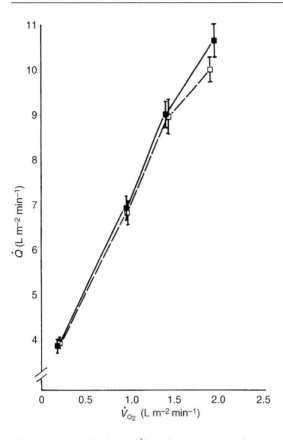

Figure 7.4 Cardiac index ($\dot{Q}$) against oxygen uptake ($\dot{V}O_2$) (both related to body surface area) in high altitude natives at 4350 m (□) and again after 8–13 days at sea level (■). (From Vogel *et al.* 1974.)

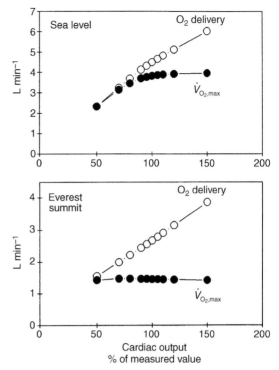

Figure 7.5 Theoretical study of the effects of changing cardiac output on maximal oxygen consumption ($\dot{V}O_{2,max}$) at sea level and at extreme altitude. Note that although $\dot{V}O_{2,max}$ improves at sea level, there is essentially no change at extreme altitude. This is explained by diffusion limitation in the lung and tissues. (From Wagner 1996.)

in $\dot{V}O_{2,max}$ with increases in cardiac output and hemoglobin concentration (and therefore oxygen delivery) is that diffusion impairment of oxygen, both in the lungs and in the muscles, reduces its availability. At medium altitudes, the calculated improvement in $\dot{V}O_{2,max}$ that accompanies an increase in cardiac output or hemoglobin concentration is intermediate between the values at sea level and extreme altitude. Reeves (2004) has also discussed the limited value of increasing cardiac output and hemoglobin concentration at high altitude. Calbert *et al.* (2002) reported that the increase in hemoglobin concentration accompanying acclimatization to 5260 m did not increase $\dot{V}O_{2,max}$ or peak cardiac output.

Although cardiac output in relation to work level is unchanged in acclimatized subjects at high altitude, and in high altitude natives, hemoglobin flow is appreciably increased because of the polycythemia. As long ago as 1930, Grollman suggested that the return of cardiac output to its sea level value was related in some way to the increase in hemoglobin concentration of the blood (Grollman 1930).

7.3.2 Heart rate

Acute hypoxia causes an increase in heart rate both at rest and for a given level of exercise, just as is the case for cardiac output. The higher the altitude, the greater the increase in heart rate. At simulated altitudes of 4000–4600 m where acute exposure depresses the arterial P_{O_2} to 40–45 mmHg, resting heart rates increase by 40–50% above the sea level values (Kontos *et al.* 1967, Vogel and Harris 1967). Benoit *et al.* (2003) showed that when normal subjects are exposed to acute hypoxia, the lowest peak

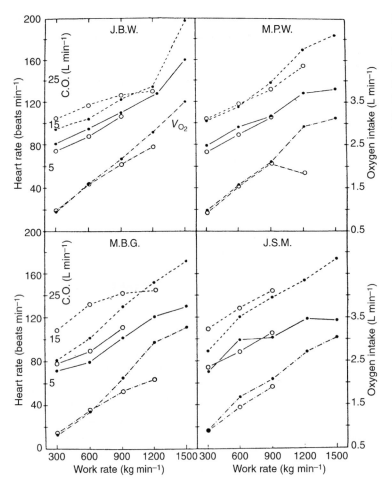

Figure 7.6 Heart rate (HR, – – –), cardiac output (CO, -), and oxygen uptake ($\dot{V}_{O_2}$, -.-.) against work rate in four well-acclimatized subjects at an altitude of 5800 m. Measurements taken at sea level (●) and 5800 m (○, P_B 380 mmHg). (From Pugh 1964d.)

heart rates are seen in those people who have the lowest arterial oxygen saturations.

In acclimatized subjects at high altitude, resting heart rates return to approximately the sea level value up to an altitude of about 4500 m, although there is some individual variation (Rotta *et al.* 1956, Peñaloza *et al.* 1963). On exercise, heart rate for a given work rate or oxygen consumption exceeds the sea level value. Figure 7.6 shows comparisons of heart rate at sea level and at an altitude of 5800 m in four subjects from the Himalayan Scientific and Mountaineering Expedition who had spent several months at that altitude (Pugh 1964d). It can be seen that the sea level values were generally lower than the high altitude measurements. However, in three of the four subjects the data points crossed at the highest work level that was tolerated at the high altitude. In other words, at the highest work level the heart rate was actually less than at sea

level for the same power output. However, in every instance, this crossover was associated with a reduction in measured oxygen consumption, suggesting that at the high work rate, an increasing amount of work was being accomplished anaerobically.

Maximal heart rate, that is the heart rate at maximal exercise, is reduced in acclimatized subjects at high altitude. This is clearly seen from Fig. 7.6. In Operation Everest II, maximal heart rates decreased from 160 ± 7 at sea level to 137 ± 4 at a simulated altitude of 6100 m, 123 ± 6 at 7620 m and 118 ± 3 at 8848 m (Reeves *et al.* 1987). For a given work level, heart rates were greater at high altitude compared with sea level, though, interestingly, there seemed to be little difference between the measurements made at barometric pressures of 347, 282 and 240 mmHg, as shown in Fig. 7.7. This is possibly a reflection of the limited degree of acclimatization of the subjects at

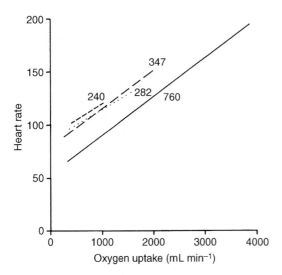

Figure 7.7 Regression lines for heart rate on oxygen uptake at barometric pressures of 760, 347, 282, and 240 mmHg during Operation Everest II. For the measurements at 240 mmHg, the subjects breathed an oxygen mixture to give an inspired Po_2 of 43 mmHg. (From Reeves *et al.* 1987.)

the highest altitudes (West 1988a). The difference between field and chamber studies was emphasized by Lundby and van Hall (2001), who showed that although peak heart rate was reduced at an altitude of 8750 m on Mount Everest, the heart rates were considerably higher than found in chamber experiments. In Operation Everest III (Comex '97) maximal heart rates were also reduced compared with sea level values (Richalet *et al.* 1999). Lundby *et al.* (2001) confirmed that the peak heart rate fell as the altitude is increased.

Richalet (1990) has argued that the reduction of maximal heart rate in acclimatized subjects at high altitude represents a physiological adaptation which reduces cardiac work under conditions of limited oxygen availability. There is good evidence that hypoxia induces downregulation of β-adrenergic receptors in animal hearts (Voelkel *et al.* 1981, Kacimi *et al.* 1992) and the role of the autonomic nervous system in controlling heart rate and cardiac output is well established. Short periods of exposure to hypoxia increase the plasma concentration of epinephrine and norepinephrine (Richalet 1990) and the increase in heart rate caused by hypoxia is abolished by beta-blockers (Kontos and Lower 1963). Mazzeo *et al.* (2003) emphasized the

various roles of α-adrenergic stimulation in response to exercise at 4300 m. Lundby *et al.* (2001b) reported that dopamine D_2 receptors are not involved in the hypoxia-induced decrease in maximal heart rate.

However, the reduction of maximal heart rate in acclimatized subjects at high altitude can be interpreted differently. Since heart rate is actually increased both at rest and at a given work level compared with sea level (except perhaps at the highest work level; Fig. 7.6), it seems reasonable to regard the reduced maximal heart rate simply as a reflection of the reduced maximal work level. For example, it hardly makes sense that a climber on the summit of Mount Everest where the $\dot{V}o_{2,max}$ is only about 1 L min^{-1} should have a maximal heart rate as high as the same person at sea level when the $\dot{V}o_{2,max}$ is 4–5 L min^{-1}.

Oxygen breathing in acclimatized subjects at high altitude reduces the heart rate for a given work level (Pugh *et al.* 1964d). This is shown in Fig. 11.4 where it can be seen that the heart rate for a given work level was actually lower than the corresponding measurements at sea level. A possible explanation for the reduction below the sea level value is the fact that the arterial Po_2 at this altitude of 5800 m with 100% oxygen breathing is higher than at sea level, and also that these subjects had much higher hemoglobin levels than at sea level because of the high altitude polycythemia. It is known that heart rate for a given work rate at sea level is inversely related to hemoglobin concentration (Richardson and Guyton 1959).

7.3.3 Stroke volume

Since stroke volume is determined by cardiac output divided by heart rate, its changes at high altitude can be deduced from those variables described in the last two sections.

Acute hypoxia causes approximately the same increase in cardiac output as in heart rate. The result is no consistent change in stroke volume. This is true for both rest and exercise (Vogel and Harris 1967).

After a few weeks' exposure to high altitude, the cardiac output response to work rate is the same as at sea level (Figs 7.2 and 7.3) but heart rate remains high (Figs 7.6 and 7.7). This means that stroke volume is reduced. The fall in stroke volume has been attributed to depression of myocardial function as a result of myocardial hypoxia (Alexander *et al.* 1967) but, as the next section shows, myocardial contractility is apparently well maintained up to extremely high altitudes in young healthy subjects. The reduction of stroke volume was also confirmed in Operation Everest II where it was shown that oxygen breathing did not increase stroke volume for a given pulmonary wedge or filling pressure. This suggested that the decline in stroke volume was not caused by severe hypoxic depression of contractility (Reeves *et al.* 1987). A possible contributing factor is a fall in plasma volume. A reduction in stroke volume during ascent was also well documented in Operation Everest III (Comex '97) (Boussuges *et al.* 2000). However, Calbert *et al.* (2004) found that plasma volume expansion did not increase maximal cardiac output or oxygen consumption in lowlanders acclimatized to an altitude of 5260 m.

Studies of high altitude natives at an altitude of 4350 m gave results similar to those found in acclimatized lowlanders. Cardiac output against oxygen consumption at high altitude was almost identical to the sea level measurements (Fig. 7.4), whereas heart rate was higher at high altitude and stroke volume was up to 13% less (Vogel *et al.* 1974).

7.3.4 Myocardial contractility

As indicated above, stroke volume is reduced at high altitude both in acclimatized lowlanders and in high altitude natives compared with sea level. The reduced stroke volume could be caused by either reduced cardiac filling or impaired myocardial contractility. A fall in filling pressures could result from either an increased heart rate or a reduction of circulating blood volume, or both.

During Operation Everest II, it was possible to measure both right atrial mean pressure (filling pressure for the right ventricle) and pulmonary wedge pressure (as an index of the filling pressure of the left ventricle). Both these measurements tended to fall as simulated altitude increased (Reeves *et al.* 1987). It was interesting that the right atrial pressures tended to be low despite pulmonary hypertension (section 7.5). In general the relationship between stroke volume and right atrial pressure was maintained. This finding suggests maintenance of contractile function. In addition, as indicated above, oxygen breathing did not increase stroke

volume for a given filling pressure, suggesting that the reduced stroke volume was not caused by hypoxic depression of contractility.

Additional evidence to support the finding of normal myocardial contractility came from a two-dimensional echocardiography study during Operation Everest II (Suarez *et al.* 1987). It was found that the ventricular ejection fraction, the ratio of peak systolic pressure to end-systolic volume, and mean normalized systolic volume at rest were all sustained at a barometric pressure of 282 mmHg, corresponding to an altitude of about 8000 m. Indeed the surprising observation was made that during exercise at the level of 60 W, the ejection fraction was actually slightly higher (79% ± 2% compared with 69% ± 8%) at a barometric pressure of 282 mmHg compared with sea level. The conclusion was that, despite the decreased cardiac volumes, the severe hypoxemia and the pulmonary hypertension, cardiac contractile function appeared to be well maintained. Preservation of left ventricular contractility in spite of the severe hypoxia at simulated high altitude was also well documented in Operation Everest III (COMEX '97) using echocardiographic and Doppler techniques (Boussuges *et al.* 2000).

7.3.5 Abnormal rhythm

Abnormal rhythms (apart from sinus arrhythmia during periodic breathing) are uncommon at high altitude and perhaps this is surprising in view of the very severe arterial hypoxemia. A resting climber on the summit of Mount Everest has an arterial P_{O_2} of around 30 mmHg (West *et al.* 1983b, Sutton *et al.* 1988). During exercise, the arterial P_{O_2} falls even farther, principally because of diffusion limitation across the blood-gas barrier in the lung (West *et al.* 1983b, Sutton *et al.* 1988) (see Chapter 6). Thus the myocardium is exposed to extremely low oxygen levels and it is known that the hypoxic myocardium is prone to rhythm abnormalities (Josephson and Wellens 1984).

In an electrocardiographic study of 19 subjects during the 1981 American Medical Research Expedition to Everest, only one subject had premature ventricular contractions and these were recorded at an altitude of 5300 m. Another climber showed premature atrial contractions at 6300 m (Karliner *et al.* 1985). One subject on the 1960–61 Silver Hut

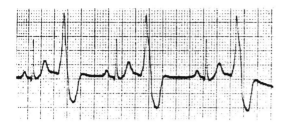

Figure 7.8 Electrocardiogram showing premature ventricular contractions occurring after exercise at 5800 m. (From Milledge 1963.)

expedition showed premature ventricular contractions after exercise at an altitude of 5800 m (Fig. 7.8). However, no other member of the expedition showed any dysrhythmia (Milledge 1963). Occasional premature ventricular contractions and premature atrial contractions have been observed by others (Cummings and Lysgaard 1981). One report suggests that cardiac arrhythmias may become more frequent with aging (Alexander 1999). Thus it appears that extreme hypoxia of the otherwise normal myocardium causes little abnormal rhythm, even at the most extreme altitudes. This conclusion is consistent with the maintenance of normal myocardial contractility even during the extreme hypoxia of very great altitudes (Reeves *et al.* 1987), as discussed in section 7.3.4.

There is a report that permanent inhabitants of mountainous regions (altitude 2800–4000 m) have a higher prevalence of cardiac arrhythmias than low altitude dwellers at rest. However, the rhythm disturbances were less on exercise (Mirrakhimov and Meimanaliev 1981). There are also studies in animals claiming that intermittent hypoxia protects the myocardium against ischemic arrhythmias (Meerson *et al.* 1987, Asemu *et al.* 1999).

Sinus arrhythmia accompanying the periodic breathing of sleep is very common at high altitude (Chapter 13). Indeed, the periodic slowing of the heart can be reliably used to identify the presence of periodic breathing at sea level (Guilleminault *et al.* 1984) and was used in this way with a Holter monitor to detect periodic breathing in climbers at an altitude of 8050 m during the American Medical Research Expedition to Everest (West *et al.* 1986). It is likely that the most extreme arterial hypoxemia for a given altitude occurs during the periodic breathing of sleep following the periods of apnea. It is not surprising that occasional premature ventricular

and premature atrial contractions are then sometimes seen. For example, during the four sleep studies at 8050 m, one individual had occasional premature ventricular contractions, another had atrial bigeminy and a third had occasional premature atrial beats (Karliner *et al.* 1985).

7.3.6 Coronary circulation

The myocardium normally extracts a large proportion of the oxygen from the coronary arterial blood, with the result that the venous Po_2 has one of the lowest values of all organs in the body. Acute hypoxia has been shown to increase coronary blood flow in proportion to the fall in arterial oxygen concentration (Hellems *et al.* 1963). It is perhaps surprising therefore that coronary blood flow has been shown to be reduced in permanent residents of high altitude compared with people at sea level. Moret (1971) measured coronary flow in two groups of people at La Paz (3700 m) and Cerro de Pasco (4375 m) and compared them with a group at sea level. The flow per 100 g of left ventricle was some 30% less in the high altitude natives. A reduction of coronary blood flow of about the same magnitude in lowlanders 10 days after ascent to high altitude (3000 m) was found by Grover *et al.* (1970).

Despite this, there appears to be little evidence of myocardial ischemia in people living at high altitude (Arias-Stella and Topilsky 1971). These authors showed that casts of the coronary vessels had a greater density of peripheral ramifications than those of sea level controls. This might be part of the explanation for the apparent low incidence of angina and other features of myocardial ischemia.

7.4 SYSTEMIC BLOOD PRESSURE

Acute hypoxia causes essentially no change in the mean systemic arterial blood pressure in humans, at least up to altitudes of 4600 m (Kontos *et al.* 1967, Vogel and Harris 1967). This is in contrast to the dog, in which acute hypoxia results in a rise of mean arterial pressure (Kontos *et al.* 1967). However, when lowlanders move to high altitude there is frequently an increase in blood pressure for the first few weeks. In one study of 32 subjects who moved to an altitude between 3500 and 4000 m, 31 of them had an increase in resting blood pressure, and this persisted for some 3 weeks at altitude but returned to normal after descent (Kamat and Banerji 1972). In another study of four sea level residents who moved to an altitude of 4350 m, the mean arterial blood pressure rose from about 100 to about 128 mmHg after arrival and this persisted for 10 days (Vogel *et al.* 1974). In a further report there was a rise in systemic blood pressure in 11 subjects who ascended to 4300 m and it was shown that propanalol given to some of the subjects reduced the rise in pressure suggesting that increased sympathetic activity was a causative factor (Wolfel *et al.* 1994). Another study reported only in an abstract looked at a large number of high school students living at altitudes of about 1200, 1800 and over 2000 m. The mean systolic pressure was slightly elevated at the highest altitude compared with the lowest (Appleton 1967).

In contrast to these increases in systemic blood pressure shortly after moving to high altitude, people who reside there for several years apparently have a decrease in both systolic and diastolic pressure (Marticorena *et al.* 1969, Hultgren 1970). These studies included 100 lowlanders who moved to altitudes of about 3800 to 4300 m for between 2 and 15 years. There is also a report that a stay of 1 year at an altitude of 4500 m resulted in a decrease of systemic systolic and diastolic pressures (Rotta *et al.* 1956).

There is some evidence that patients with systemic hypertension who move to high altitude are improved. Penaloza (1971) found that some patients with systemic hypertension who moved to an altitude of 3750 m had a reduction in their level of systemic blood pressure. This finding is consistent with a study of the prevalence of systemic hypertension at altitudes of 4100 to 4360 m in Peru, compared with two communities at sea level. This showed a prevalence of hypertension in men at least 12 times greater at sea level than at high altitude (Ruiz and Penaloza 1977). The difference was even more marked in women.

In high altitude natives living at 4350 m, Vogel *et al.* (1974) found that the mean brachial arterial blood pressure was consistently higher during exercise than in the same subjects at sea level. By contrast the increase in mean systemic arterial pressure which occurs during the course of heavy exercise is apparently the same in acclimatized lowlanders as it is in sea level residents.

Syncope occasionally occurs at high altitude in otherwise healthy individuals (Nicholas *et al.* 1992, Perrill 1993, Freitas *et al.* 1996, Westendorp *et al.* 1997). This has been seen mainly in young adults, often within 24 h of arrival at altitude, and commonly after a meal including alcohol. Imbalance of the sympathetic–parasympathetic systems is the probable cause.

7.5 PULMONARY CIRCULATION

7.5.1 Pulmonary hypertension

One of the most striking cardiovascular changes at high altitude is the occurrence of pulmonary hypertension caused by an increase in pulmonary vascular resistance. This is seen in subjects exposed to acute hypoxia, in acclimatized lowlanders at high altitude, and in most high altitude natives. The pulmonary hypertension of acute hypoxia is reversed by oxygen breathing, but this is not the case in acclimatized lowlanders or high altitude natives.

In normal subjects at sea level who are given low oxygen mixtures to breathe, mean pulmonary artery pressure almost always increases. In early studies, Motley *et al.* (1947) reported an increase of 13–23 mmHg as a result of breathing 10% oxygen in nitrogen for 10 min. This study followed the initial demonstration by von Euler and Liljestrand (1946) that the pulmonary arterial pressure in the cat increased when the animals breathed 10% oxygen in nitrogen. The increase in pulmonary vascular resistance is caused by vasoconstriction, mainly or solely as a result of contraction of smooth muscle in small pulmonary arteries.

Extensive studies of the effects of acute hypoxia on the pulmonary circulation have been made in humans and in a variety of animals. Figure 7.9 shows a typical study by Barer *et al.* (1970) in anesthetized cats in which the left lower lobe of the lung was made hypoxic and its blood flow was plotted against the alveolar P_{O_2}. Note the typical nonlinear stimulus–response curve. When the alveolar P_{O_2} was altered in the region above 100 mmHg, little change in blood flow and therefore vascular resistance was seen. However, when the alveolar P_{O_2} was reduced to approximately 70 mmHg, a marked increase in vascular resistance occurred, and at very low P_{O_2}

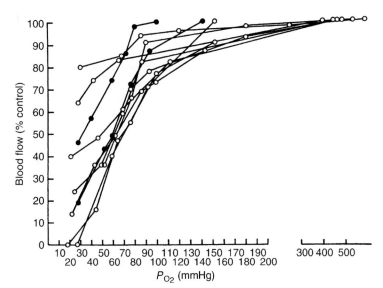

Figure 7.9 Blood flow from left lower lobe of open-chest anesthetized cats plotted against the P_{O_2} of the pulmonary venous blood from the lobe. The lobe was ventilated with different inspired gas mixtures while the rest of the lung was breathing air (○) or 100% oxygen (●). (From Barer *et al.* 1970.)

values approaching those of mixed venous blood, the local blood flow was almost abolished.

There are differences among species in the stimulus–response curves. Tucker and Rhodes (2001) carried out an extensive review of a series of species and noted that sheep and dogs typically have small responses whereas cattle and pigs have large increases in pulmonary artery pressure. The response is related to the degree of muscularization of the pulmonary arteries. Species that live at high altitudes including yaks and pikas are typically hyporesponders. In yaks there is evidence that augmented nitric oxide production is partly responsible for the low pulmonary vascular tone (Ishizaki *et al.* 2005).

In humans, the vasoconstrictor response to acute hypoxia shows considerable variation between individuals, leading Read and Fowler (1964) to refer to 'responders' and 'nonresponders'. Indeed, an attractive hypothesis is that hypoxic pulmonary vasoconstriction is vestigial in the adult and that its most important function occurs in the transition from placental to pulmonary gas exchange. Here there is a release of pulmonary vasoconstriction when the newborn baby starts to breathe air, and the circulation rapidly transforms from the fetal placental mode to the adult lung mode. Presumably this is where the primary evolutionary pressure for the phenomenon comes from.

Acclimatized lowlanders exhibit pulmonary hypertension at high altitude with a mean

pulmonary arterial pressure increasing from its sea level value of about 12 mmHg to about 18 mmHg after 1 year at 4540 m (Rotta *et al.* 1956, Sime *et al.* 1974). This resting pulmonary arterial pressure increases considerably more during exercise. Figure 7.10 shows the relationship between mean pulmonary vascular pressure gradient across the lung (mean pulmonary arterial pressure minus pulmonary wedge pressure) and cardiac output in the subjects of Operation Everest II (Groves *et al.* 1987). Note that the resting values of the gradient (determined primarily by the mean pulmonary artery pressure) increased, but the most dramatic change was in the slope of the pressure gradient with respect to cardiac output. This indicates the striking increase in pulmonary vascular resistance at these great simulated altitudes.

High altitude natives also show a substantial increase in mean pulmonary artery pressure during exercise. In one study, mean pulmonary artery pressure increased from 26 to 60 mmHg during exercise at an altitude of 4500 m (Sime *et al.* 1974). This was a greater increase than that found in acclimatized lowlanders.

In contrast to the dramatic effect of oxygen breathing in acute hypoxia, which causes pulmonary vascular resistance to return to its pre-hypoxic level, oxygen breathing has relatively little effect in acclimatized lowlanders and high altitude natives. For example, after the subjects had been exposed to low pressure for 2–3 weeks in Operation Everest II, 100%

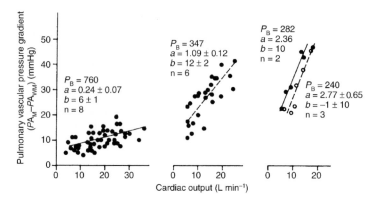

Figure 7.10 Mean pulmonary artery pressure (PA_m) minus mean pulmonary wedge pressure (PA_{WM}) plotted against cardiac output (by thermodilution) at various barometric pressures (P_B) during Operation Everest II. For the measurements at 240 mmHg, the subjects breathed an oxygen mixture to give an inspired Po_2 of 43 mmHg; ●, 282 mmHg; ○, 240 mmHg. (From Groves *et al.* 1987.)

oxygen breathing resulted in a lower cardiac output and pulmonary artery pressure but there was no significant fall in pulmonary vascular resistance (Groves *et al.* 1987). In interpreting this result it should be recognized that a fall in cardiac output normally results in an *increase* in pulmonary vascular resistance because the reduction in capillary pressure causes derecruitment of capillaries and a reduction in caliber of those which remain open (Glazier *et al.* 1969). Thus the fact that pulmonary vascular resistance did not change when it was expected to rise indicated that oxygen breathing probably reduced vascular resistance to some extent. Nevertheless, it is remarkable that the subjects who were hypoxic for only 2–3 weeks when the measurements were made had a substantial degree of irreversibility of the increased pulmonary vascular resistance. This implies that there were structural changes in the pulmonary blood vessels, in addition to simple contraction of vascular smooth muscle, and is consistent with more recent studies on rapid remodeling of the pulmonary circulation (Tozzi *et al.* 1989).

High altitude natives also show little response of their increased pulmonary vascular resistance to 100% breathing. In this case it is known that there are substantial structural changes in the lungs including a large increase in smooth muscle in the small pulmonary arteries (section 7.5.2).

A study of a small sample of Tibetans showed that they have an unusually small degree of hypoxic pulmonary vasoconstriction compared with other high altitude natives (Groves *et al.* 1993). Five normal male residents of Lhasa (3658 m) were studied at rest and during near-maximal ergometer exercise. The resting mean pulmonary arterial pressure and

pulmonary vascular resistance were within normal values for sea level. Alveolar hypoxia resulted in a smaller rise of mean pulmonary artery pressure than in other high altitude residents of North and South America (Reeves and Grover 1975) (Fig. 7.11). Exercise increased cardiac output more than three-fold with a reduction in pulmonary vascular resistance; 100% oxygen breathing during exercise did not reduce pulmonary arterial pressure or vascular resistance. The authors argued that elevated pulmonary arterial pressure in high altitude residents may be a maladaptive response to chronic hypoxia, and the findings indicated improved adaptation in a group that has been at high altitude for a very long period.

7.5.2 Mechanisms of hypoxic pulmonary vasoconstriction

The mechanism of hypoxic pulmonary vasoconstriction is not fully understood despite a great deal of research. Since the phenomenon occurs in excised isolated lungs, it clearly does not depend on central nervous connections. Furthermore, excised segments of pulmonary artery can be shown to constrict if their environment is made hypoxic (Lloyd 1965), so the response is due to local action of the hypoxia on the artery itself. It is also known that it is the Po_2 of the alveolar gas, not the pulmonary arterial blood, which chiefly determines the response (Duke 1954, Lloyd 1965). This can be proved by perfusing a lung with blood of a high Po_2 while keeping the alveolar Po_2 low. Under these conditions the response is well seen.

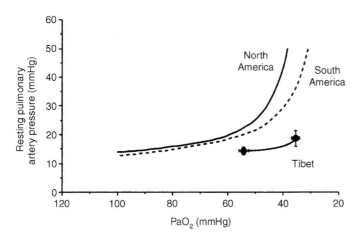

Figure 7.11 Change in mean pulmonary artery pressure during alveolar hypoxia in five Tibetans compared with high altitude residents of North and South America. (From Groves *et al.* 1993.)

The predominant site of vasoconstriction is in the small pulmonary arteries (Kato and Staub 1966, Glazier and Murray 1971). Some studies suggest that the alveolar vessels may be partly responsible for the increased resistance, and contractile cells have been described in the interstitium of the alveolar wall, which could conceivably distort capillaries and increase their resistance (Kapanci *et al.* 1974). However, the fact that the pulmonary arterial pressure can increase to levels of 50 mmHg or more in subjects at high altitude without the occurrence of pulmonary edema is evidence that the main site of constriction is upstream of the pulmonary capillaries from which the fluid leaks.

Having said this, it is also true that pulmonary edema does occur at high altitude from time to time (Chapter 20) and a likely mechanism is that the hypoxic pulmonary vasoconstriction is uneven (Hultgren 1978), with the result that those capillaries which are not protected from the increased pulmonary arterial pressure develop ultrastructural damage to their walls. This results in a high permeability type of edema and this topic is considered in more detail in section 20.7.5.

As indicated earlier, the exact mechanism of hypoxic pulmonary vasoconstriction is still an active area of research. Chemical mediators which have been studied in the past include catecholamines, histamine, angiotensin and prostaglandins (Fishman 1985). Recently, a great deal of interest has been generated by the observation that inhaled nitric oxide reverses hypoxic pulmonary vasoconstriction.

Nitric oxide is an endothelium-derived relaxing factor for blood vessels (Ignarro *et al.* 1987). It is formed from L-arginine via catalysis by endothelial nitric oxide synthase (eNOS) and is a final common pathway for a variety of biological processes (Moncada *et al.* 1991). Nitric oxide activates soluble guanylate cyclase, which leads to smooth muscle relaxation through the synthesis of cyclic GMP. Several studies suggest that potassium ion channels in smooth muscle cells may be involved, leading to increased intracellular concentration of calcium ions. Nitrovasodilators, such as nitroprusside and glycerol trinitrate, which have been used clinically for many years, are thought to act by these same mechanisms.

Inhibitors of nitric oxide synthesis have been shown to augment hypoxic pulmonary vasoconstriction in isolated pulmonary artery rings (Archer *et al.* 1989), and attenuate pulmonary vasodilatation in intact lambs (Fineman *et al.* 1991). Inhaled nitric oxide reduces hypoxic pulmonary vasoconstriction in humans (Frostell *et al.* 1993) and sheep (Pison *et al.* 1993), and lowers pulmonary vascular resistance in patients with high altitude pulmonary edema (HAPE) (Anand *et al.* 1998). The required inhaled concentration of nitric oxide is extremely low (about 20 ppm), and the gas is highly toxic at high concentrations. The recognition of the role of nitric oxide has opened up a new era in our understanding of hypoxic pulmonary vasoconstriction.

Calcium and potassium channels in the vascular smooth muscle have an important role in the development of vasoconstriction. This is a rapidly developing area of research and a recent review can be found in Remillard and Yuan (2005). Hypoxia decreases K^+ channel activity causing membrane depolarization which leads to increased Ca^{2+} influx and so to contraction of smooth muscle cells. Thus

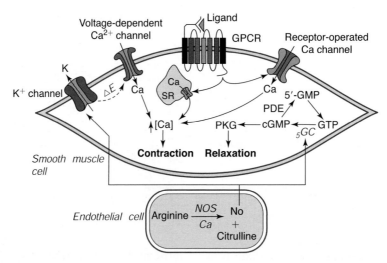

Figure 7.12   Role of ion channel function and intracellular Ca^{2+} in the regulation of pulmonary vasoconstriction. Ca^{2+} influx via voltage-dependent (VDCC) or receptor-operated (ROC) Ca^{2+} channels, and Ca^{2+} release from the endoplasmic or sarcoplasmic reticulum (SR) stores cause the rise in cytosolic free [Ca^{2+}] ([Ca^{2+}]$_{cyt}$) that acts as the major trigger for pulmonary artery smooth muscle cell (PASMC) contraction. VDCC activity is modulated by a change in membrane potential (ΔE_m), which is tightly regulated by the activity of K$^+$ channels. In quiescent cells, normal K$^+$ channel activity maintains resting E_m at negative potentials. During acute hypoxia, the protein expression and function of K$^+$ channels are decreased and cells are depolarized (i.e. E_m becomes less negative), causing activation of VDCC, and thereby increases [Ca^{2+}] in the cytosol ([Ca^{2+}]$_{cyt}$). Binding of vasoconstrictors (e.g. norepinephrine) to membrane receptors (e.g. G protein-coupled receptors, GPCR) can promote both Ca^{2+} release from the SR and Ca^{2+} influx via ROC. Hypoxia also enhances Ca^{2+} release from the SR and Ca^{2+} influx via ROC. Ca^{2+} channel blockers (e.g. nifedipine, verapamil or diltiazem), by attenuating Ca^{2+} influx in PASMC, have been used clinically to treat patients with pulmonary arterial hypertension. Nitric oxide (NO) produced in adjacent endothelial cells diffuses into PASMC to activate soluble guanylate cyclase (sGC), which catalyzes the formation of cyclic GMP (cGMP) from GTP. Catabolism of cGMP into inactive 5′-GMP is promoted by phosphodiesterases (PDE); PDE inhibitors, such as sildenafil, prevent this step and increase cytosolic cGMP concentration in PASMC. cGMP promotes and prolongs smooth muscle relaxation via a mechanism involving cGMP-dependent protein kinase (PKG). NO, which has been used therapeutically for patients with pulmonary hypertension, can also promote PASMC relaxation (a) by directly activating plasma membrane K$^+$ channels (shown here) to attenuate VDCC activity, (b) by directly blocking Ca^{2+} channels, and/or (c) by enhancing Ca^{2+} re-uptake into the SR, all of which result in decreased [Ca^{2+}]$_{cyt}$. Diagram and caption are courtesy of Jason Yuan.

the resulting transmembrane ion flux modulates excitation–contraction coupling in the smooth muscle cells. This flux also regulates cell volume, apoptosis and proliferation which results in remodeling of the blood vessels.

Pulmonary vascular vasodilators can be used to reduce the degree of pulmonary hypertension under some conditions. Calcium channel blockers such as nifedipine reduce the pulmonary artery pressure and are useful in both the treatment and prevention of high altitude pulmonary edema (Bärtsch *et al.* 1991b, Hackett and Roach 2001). More recently 5-phosphodiesterase inhibitors such

as sildenafil have been shown to reduce the pulmonary hypertension at high altitude both during rest and during exercise, and they may also be useful in the treatment and prophylaxis of high altitude pulmonary edema (Zhao *et al.* 2001, Ricart *et al.* 2005, Richalet *et al.* 2005a). Figure 7.12 summarizes some of the mechanisms responsible for hypoxic pulmonary vasoconstriction.

Hypoxic pulmonary vasoconstriction has the effect of directing blood flow away from hypoxic regions of lung, caused, for example, by partial obstruction of an airway. Other things being equal, this will reduce the amount of ventilation/perfusion inequality in a diseased lung and limit the depression of the arterial P_{O_2}. This is a valuable mechanism in some patients with asthma and chronic obstructive pulmonary disease. However, the pulmonary hypertension that is seen at high altitude has no value except to cause a more uniform topographical distribution of blood flow (Dawson 1972). The improvement in ventilation/perfusion relationships resulting from this more uniform distribution of blood flow is trivial in terms of overall gas exchange (West 1962b) and we must conclude that the pulmonary hypertension of high altitude has no useful function, but in fact is deleterious because it can be responsible for the occurrence of HAPE. As stated earlier, the evolutionary pressure for the mechanism of hypoxic pulmonary vasoconstriction presumably comes from its value in the perinatal period.

7.5.3 Remodeling

The lungs of long-term residents at high altitude show marked changes related to pulmonary hypertension (Heath and Williams 1995). Bands of smooth muscle develop in the small pulmonary arteries (arterioles) of approximately 500 µm diameter which normally have a wall consisting only of a single elastic lamina. The result is that these small vessels develop a media of circularly oriented smooth muscle bonded by internal and external elastic laminae (Fig. 7.13). These changes are associated with narrowing of the lumen and an increase in pulmonary vascular resistance. Medial hypertrophy of the parent muscular pulmonary arteries is not a common feature (Arias-Stella and Saldaña 1963), though it occurs in some individuals (Wagenvoort and Wagenvoort 1973). Occlusive intimal fibrosis apparently does not occur. However, longitudinal muscle fibers developing in the intima of pulmonary arterioles in highlanders have been described (Wagenvoort and Wagenvoort 1973). Some authors have also described an increase in mast cell density in experimental animals exposed to long-term hypoxia (Kay et al. 1974). This is of interest because at one stage it was thought that mediators from mast cells, for example histamine, might be involved in the vasoconstrictor response.

These structural changes are consistent with the fact that the pulmonary arterial pressure of high altitude natives falls only slightly (by 15–20%)

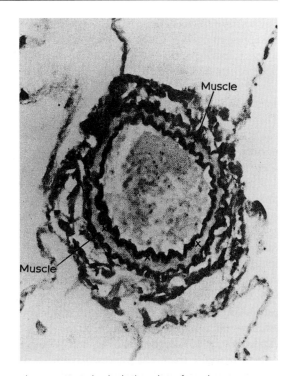

Figure 7.13 Histological section of a pulmonary arteriole from a Quechua Indian living at high altitude in the Peruvian Andes. Muscle tissue is seen between the internal and external elastic laminae. Normally there is a single elastic lamina and no muscle tissue in a vessel of this size at sea level. (Elastic van Gieson stain, ×375.) (From Heath and Williams 1995.)

when oxygen is breathed (Peñaloza et al. 1962). These authors showed that inhabitants of Cerro de Pasco (4330 m) who moved to sea level had their mean pulmonary arterial pressure halved from 24 to 12 mmHg after 2 years of residence at sea level. The fact that lowlanders who are exposed to high altitude for 2–3 weeks develop pulmonary hypertension which is not completely reversed by 100% oxygen breathing (Groves et al. 1987) suggests that their pulmonary blood vessels may also have developed some increased smooth muscle.

The structural changes that occur in pulmonary arteries when the pulmonary arterial pressure is raised as a result of exposing an animal to hypoxia are referred to as vascular remodeling (Riley 1991). This was studied by Meyrick and Reid (1978, 1980) who exposed rats to half the normal barometric pressure for 1–52 days. The result was an increase in pulmonary artery pressure as a result of hypoxic pulmonary vasoconstriction. After 2 days they saw the appearance of new smooth muscle in small pulmonary arteries, and after 10 days there was doubling of the thickness of the media and adventitia of the main pulmonary artery due to increased smooth muscle, collagen and elastin, and also edema. There was some recovery after 3 days of normoxia, and after 14–28 days the thickness of the media was normal. However, some increase in collagen persisted up to 70 days.

The molecular biology of the responses of the pulmonary blood vessels has been studied by several groups. Mecham *et al.* (1987) looked at the response of the pulmonary arteries of newborn calves to alveolar hypoxia. There was a two- to four-fold increase in elastin production in pulmonary arterial wall and medial smooth muscle cells. This was accompanied by a corresponding increase in elastin messenger RNA consistent with regulation at the transcriptional level. Poiani *et al.* (1990) exposed rats to 10% oxygen for 1–14 days. Within 3 days of exposure there was increased synthesis of collagen and elastin, and an increase in mRNA for $\alpha_1(I)$ procollagen.

A particularly interesting study was done by Tozzi *et al.* (1989) who placed rat main pulmonary artery rings in Krebs–Ringer bicarbonate as explants. The investigators then applied mechanical tension equivalent to a transmural pressure of 50 mmHg for 4 h, and found increases in collagen synthesis (incorporation of ^{14}C-proline), elastin synthesis (incorporation of ^{14}C-valine), mRNA for $\alpha_1(I)$ procollagen, and mRNA for protooncogene v-*sis*. The last may implicate platelet-derived growth factor (PDGF) or transforming growth factor (TGF)-β as a mediator. They were able to show that these changes were endothelium-dependent because they did not occur when the endothelium was removed from the arterial rings.

It is possible that this vascular remodeling is a general property of pulmonary vascular endothelium. It has been pointed out that the capillary wall has a dilemma in that it must be extremely thin for gas exchange but immensely strong to withstand the wall stresses that develop when the capillary pressure rises during heavy exercise (West and Mathieu-Costello 1992b). There is good evidence that the extracellular matrix of the blood-gas barrier, at least on the thin side, is responsible for its strength, and it is known that in mitral stenosis,

where the capillary pressure rises over long periods of time, there is an increase in thickness of the extracellular matrix (Kay and Edwards 1973). Thus it may be that the capillary is continually regulating the structure of the wall in response to the capillary pressure which is sensed by the endothelium. The capillaries appear to be the most vulnerable vessels in the pulmonary circulation when the pressure rises. Thus vascular remodeling, which has been chiefly studied in larger blood vessels, may be a general property of the pulmonary vasculature, and its evolutionary advantage may be primarily to protect the walls of the capillaries.

The mechanism of capillary wall remodeling in response to increased wall stress has been the subject of several studies. Berg *et al.* (1997) exposed rabbit lungs to high levels of lung inflation because this is known to increase the wall stress of pulmonary capillaries (Fu *et al.* 1992). Increased gene expression for $\alpha_1(III)$ and $\alpha_2(IV)$ procollagens, fibronectin, basic fibroblast growth factor (bFGF), and TGF-β1 was found in peripheral lung parenchyma compared with control animals in normal states of lung inflation. However, mRNA levels for $\alpha_1(I)$ procollagen and vascular endothelial growth factor (VEGF) were unchanged. Parker *et al.* (1997) raised capillary transmural pressure by intermittently increasing the venous pressure in isolated perfused rat lungs. There were significant increases in gene expression for $\alpha_1(I)$ and $\alpha_1(III)$ procollagens, fibronectin and laminin compared with controls in which the venous pressure was normal. Berg *et al.* (1998) placed rats in 10% oxygen for periods from 6 h up to 10 days. Here the hypothesis was that because the pulmonary vasoconstriction caused by alveolar hypoxia is uneven, some capillaries will be exposed to a high transmural pressure, and therefore have increased wall stress. Levels of mRNA for $\alpha_2(IV)$ procollagen increased six-fold after 6 h of hypoxia, and seven-fold after 3 days of hypoxia. However, the levels decreased after 10 days of exposure. mRNA levels for PDGF-B, $\alpha_1(I)$ and $\alpha_3(III)$ procollagens and fibronectin also increased. All the above results are consistent with capillary wall remodeling in response to increased wall stress, but the overall picture is still far from clear.

The environment of the human fetus is similar in some respects to that of the high altitude dweller in that the arterial P_{O_2} is less than 30 mmHg, based on measurements on experimental animals (Itskovitz *et al.* 1987). The fetus also has pulmonary hypertension because the pulmonary artery is connected to the systemic arterial system through the patent ductus arteriosus. In keeping with this, the fetal lung shows a high degree of muscularization of the pulmonary arteries. Babies born at a high altitude show persistence of this muscularization, whereas the pulmonary arteries of those born at sea level assume the adult appearance after only a few weeks (Heath and Williams 1995).

7.5.4 Right ventricular hypertrophy

The pulmonary hypertension of high altitude causes right ventricular hypertrophy both in acclimatized lowlanders and in high altitude natives. In one study of children of 2–10 years of age it was shown that at sea level the ratio of left to right ventricular weights was about 1.8, whereas at high altitude (3700–4260 m) it was less than 1.3 (Arias-Stella and Recavarren 1962). Experimental studies on rats exposed to an altitude of 5500 m showed that they developed right ventricular hypertrophy within 5 weeks (Heath *et al.* 1973).

Data on acclimatized lowlanders are not generally available, but there is abundant indirect evidence of right ventricular hypertrophy from electrocardiographic changes (section 7.5.4). Occasionally, climbers returning from high altitude have shown evidence of right heart enlargement on the chest radiograph (Pugh 1962a).

7.5.5 Electrocardiographic changes

Electrocardiographic changes are considered here because most of the changes are attributable to pulmonary hypertension. An extensive study was carried out during the 1981 American Medical Research Expedition to Everest (Karliner *et al.* 1985) when recordings were made at sea level, 5400 m, 6300 m, and again at sea level. A total of 19 subjects were studied, although complete data were not obtained from all. Resting heart rate increased from a mean of 57 at sea level to 70 at 5400 m and 80 at 6300 m (compare section 7.3.2). The amplitude of the P wave in standard lead 2 of the electrocardiogram increased by over 40% from sea level to 6300 m, consistent with right atrial enlargement. Right axis deviation of the QRS axis was seen. The mean frontal plane QRS axis increased from +64° to +78° at 5400 m and +85° at 6300 m. Three subjects showed abnormalities of right bundle branch conduction at the highest altitude and three others showed changes consistent with right ventricular hypertrophy (posterior displacement of the QRS vector in the horizontal plane). Seven subjects developed flattened T waves and four showed T-wave inversions (Fig. 7.14). All the changes returned to normal in tracings obtained at sea level after the expedition.

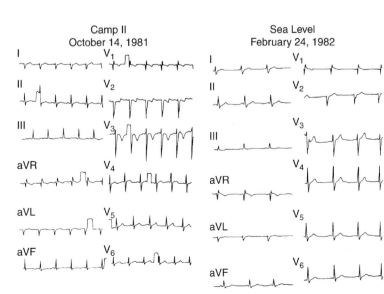

Figure 7.14 Twelve-lead electrocardiogram obtained at Camp 2 (6300 m) and about 3 months after return of the subject to sea level. Sinus tachycardia and diffuse T-wave flattening present at altitude; the T waves in leads V_2 and V_3 exhibit terminal inversion. (From Karliner *et al.* 1985.)

Other investigators have reported similar findings in acclimatized lowlanders, though generally on smaller numbers or at lower altitudes. Milledge (1963) made measurements during the 1960–61 Silver Hut expedition and reported data on subjects who spent several months at an altitude of 5800 m. In addition some recordings were made as high as 7440 m in climbers who never used supplemental oxygen. He found T-wave inversions on the right pre-cordial leads in six subjects; two had left pre-cordial T-wave inversion as well. Oxygen breathing had no effect on these changes. Das *et al.* (1983) reported on over 40 subjects who were rapidly transported to either 3200 or 3771 m. There was a tendency for a rightward axis shift which, interestingly, tended to resolve in most subjects after 10 days at high altitude.

A particularly remarkable measurement was made on Ms Phantog, deputy leader of the successful 1975 Chinese ascent of Mount Everest. She lay down on the summit under the newly erected tripod while her standard lead 1 was telemetered down to Base Camp. However, there were no changes from sea level to 8848 m and back again (Zhongyuan *et al.* 1980). Other electrocardiographic studies at high altitude include those made by Peñaloza and Echevarria (1957), Jackson and Davies (1960), Aigner *et al.* (1980), Kapoor (1984), Malconian *et al.* (1990), Chandrashekhar *et al.* (1992) and Halperin *et al.* (1998).

8

Hematology

SUMMARY

The best-known aspects of altitude acclimatization are the increase in red cell numbers per unit volume and the increase in hemoglobin concentration. These are achieved, initially, by a reduction in plasma volume (PV) and later by an increase in red cell mass (RCM). The mechanism for PV reduction on ascent to altitude is probably via carotid body stimulation by hypoxia, which reduces the reabsorption of sodium by the kidney via neural pathways. Hypoxia causes an increase in erythropoietin (EPO), which stimulates the bone marrow to increase red cell output. The EPO gene is induced by hypoxia through a nuclear factor, the hypoxia-inducible factor-1 alpha (HIF-1α). Although EPO levels rise within a few hours, the increase in RCM takes weeks and only reaches a steady state after some 6 months. Plasma volume is restored to near sea level values after a few weeks. The rise in hemoglobin concentration is roughly linear with altitude up to about 5500 m and is similar in acclimatized lowlanders and residents of high altitude throughout most of the world, though with wide individual variation. However, Tibetan (and possibly Ethiopian) highlanders have lower hemoglobin levels than other high altitude residents at similar altitudes. Extreme polycythemia among residents or lowlanders staying at altitude for many years is considered pathological and termed chronic mountain sickness (Chapter 21).

The effect of altitude on white cells has been little studied. Changes are variable, though increase in CD16 natural killer cells has been reported.

The effects of altitude on platelets and clotting are considered in Chapter 22.

8.1 INTRODUCTION

Probably the best-known adaptation to high altitude is the increase in the number of red cells per unit volume of blood. Paul Bert suggested in his book *La Pression Barométrique* (1878) that adaptation to high altitude might include an increase in the number of red cells and in the quantity of hemoglobin. Thus the blood would be able to carry more oxygen. A few years later he was sent samples of blood from a number of domestic animals from La Paz, Bolivia (3500 m). He showed that these samples combined with 16.2–21.6 volumes of oxygen per 100 volumes of blood compared with 10–12 volumes percent in the blood of animals in France (West 1981).

Viault, in 1890, made the first blood counts of men at high altitude. His own blood count at sea level in Lima was 5 million mL^{-1} and after 3 weeks at Morococha, a mining township at 4372 m in the

Andes, the value had increased to 7.1 million mL^{-1}. We now know that most of this increase, early in altitude exposure, is due to reduced plasma volume rather than an increase in RCM. Viault found these elevated counts present in a companion doctor from Lima and also in a number of the local Indian residents at altitude. He also noted that in a male llama the value was 16 million mL^{-3}. He called the llama, 'l'animal par excellence des grandes altitudes', although, in fact, since the llama has very small red cells, the hemoglobin concentration of the blood is the same as in humans. In 1891 Viault published further observations which confirmed Bert's work on the oxygen-carrying capacity of high altitude animals. He showed in two sheep and one dog that their oxygen-carrying capacity was increased compared with similar animals in France.

Since then, almost all expeditions with any pretense at carrying out physiological research at high altitude have observed this increase in red cell count, packed cell volume, or hemoglobin concentration.

The increase in red cell number and hemoglobin concentration increases the oxygen-carrying capacity in such a way that, up to about 5300 m, fully acclimatized humans have the same oxygen content in their blood as at sea level (Fig. 8.1).

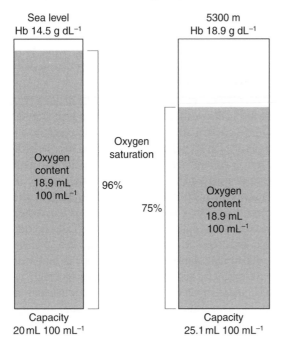

Figure 8.1 The oxygen content of arterial blood in an acclimatized subject at 5300 m and at sea level.

The increased carrying capacity compensates for the reduced oxygen saturation. This affords physiology teachers a classical example of beneficial adaptation. However, it is unlikely that the mechanism of this adaptation evolved primarily to serve humans at high altitude (section 8.2.1). The extent to which benefit can be gained by increasing hemoglobin concentration is fairly limited and indeed has been questioned as beneficial at all (Winslow and Monge 1987, p. 203; section 8.5.4). The conclusion of a recent study that addressed this topic was that

> Under conditions where O$_2$ supply limits maximal exercise, the increase in [Hb] with altitude acclimatization does not improve maximal exercise capacity or VO$_2$max. (Calbet *et al.* 2002).

8.2 REGULATION OF HEMOGLOBIN CONCENTRATION

The hemoglobin concentration and packed cell volume (PCV) depend upon the ratio of the RCM to plasma volume (PV). These two variables are regulated by different mechanisms. The rate of formation of red cells (erythropoiesis) and their rate of loss determine the RCM.

Red blood cells are lost by death (their natural length of survival is about 120 days), or by hemorrhage. Their death can be hastened by a variety of pathological states such as hemolytic anemia. Erythropoiesis can be impaired by various deficiencies, such as iron or vitamin B$_{12}$ (needed for hemoglobin synthesis), or by disorders of the bone marrow. In the absence of these, erythropoiesis is controlled by the level of the hormone of erythropoietin (EPO).

8.2.1 EPO and its regulation

EPO is produced mainly in the kidney, though 10–15% of total production is in the liver (Erslev 1987). The gene coding for the hormone has been cloned and expressed in cultured cells, allowing for sufficient material to be produced for clinical studies. It has been shown to stimulate erythropoiesis in patients anemic with end-stage renal failure (Winearls *et al.* 1986) and is now part of standard management for these patients.

The two classical stimuli for EPO secretion are hypoxia and blood loss, both of which result in tissue hypoxia. Of the two, blood loss is probably more important in evolutionary terms of survival of the organism. Blood loss is a far more common danger than is chronic hypoxia, and of course this system is no defense against acute hypoxia. The stimulus to EPO secretion is hypoxia at some tissue site, probably in the kidney, possibly identical with the site of production of the hormone. It is instructive to compare this system with another hypoxia-sensitive system in the body, the hypoxic ventilatory response (HVR), mediated mainly via the carotid body:

- The HVR appears in seconds after a step change in arterial P_{O_2} whereas there is no detectable rise in EPO concentration for over an hour, 114 min when exposed suddenly to 3000 m or 84 min at 4000 m (Eckardt *et al.* 1989).
- The carotid body is sensitive to reduction in P_{O_2} rather than oxygen content of the blood. Therefore it does not respond to anemia, whereas anemia stimulates EPO secretion.

From these observations it is assumed that, whereas the carotid body response is to arterial P_{O_2}, the sensing of P_{O_2} for EPO secretion is at the venous or tissue level. In patients with a reversed flow through a patent ductus arteriosus, there is cyanosis (hypoxia) in the lower half of the body only. These patients have high hemoglobin concentration, indicating that the P_{O_2} sensor is in the lower half of the body, presumably in the kidney. Fisher and Langston (1967) showed that EPO was produced in the juxtaglomerular apparatus in the kidney and that hypoxia was sensed there, since the isolated dog kidney increased its output of EPO when perfused with hypoxic blood. The EPO gene is switched on by the hypoxia inducible factor, HIF-1α, discussed below (section 8.4.1). It now seems that all cells are capable of sensing hypoxia via HIF-1α and probably other mechanisms (see section 10.4).

8.2.2 Regulation of plasma volume

The central control of PV is probably by a feedback loop involving atrial natriuretic peptide (ANP) and the right atrium (Laragh 1985). ANP is released in response to stretching of the right atrium. Physiologically, this is produced by increased right atrial pressure. This in turn may be due to shifts of blood volume from the periphery, mainly the lower body, or by increase in the total blood volume (i.e. PV). ANP causes the kidney to excrete sodium and with it water, thus reducing the PV. This simple feedback loop is shown in Fig. 8.2.

We can add on to this simple system a host of other factors which affect PV (Fig. 8.3).

HYDRATION

Hydration and dehydration will obviously affect PV, along with all other body fluid compartments.

VASCULAR CAPACITY

The vascular capacity is determined by the tone of the vessels, especially the venous capacitance vessels and vessels in the skin. Vessel tone, in turn, depends on a number of factors, such as temperature and catecholamine levels. Peripheral vasoconstriction shifts blood from the periphery to the center, raising right atrial pressure and stimulating ANP release. Vasodilatation has the opposite effect. A change in vascular capacity also has a more direct effect on PV by shifting the balance of forces in the Starling equation. Vasodilatation will tend to reduce the intravascular pressure, favoring inward movement of fluid at the tissue level; vasoconstriction has the opposite effect. It is this direct effect that is depicted in Fig. 8.3.

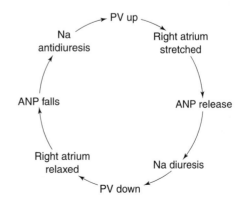

Figure 8.2 The regulation of plasma volume (PV) by atrial natriuretic peptide (ANP).

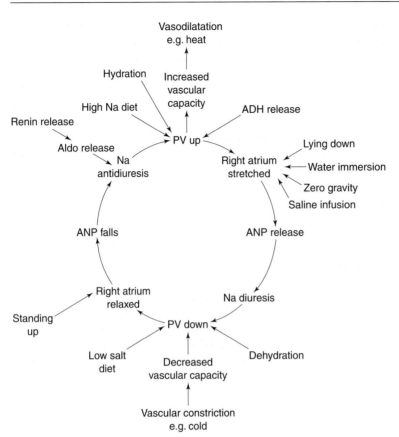

Figure 8.3   Some of the factors affecting plasma volume (PV) and its regulation by atrial natriuretic peptide (ANP), antidiuretic hormone (ADH), aldosterone (Aldo) and vascular capacity.

OTHER FACTORS

Other factors that cause a shift of blood volume to the center include lying down, lower body immersion and G-suits. Zero gravity experienced by astronauts has a similar effect. Right atrial pressure is raised and ANP excretion is increased. Conversely, the upright position tends to shift volume away from the center to the lower body, reducing right atrial pressure and inhibiting ANP release.

ANTIDIURETIC HORMONE

Secretion of antidiuretic hormone (ADH) will result in increased PV by retaining water, but there is another feedback loop involving plasma osmolality and ADH. If plasma volume increase is caused by hydration, osmolality falls and secretion of ADH is inhibited. A water diuresis then follows which restores the osmolality and ADH levels rise again. This loop is not shown in Fig. 8.3, to avoid overloading the diagram.

SODIUM STATUS

The sodium status is important in determining the PV. A high sodium intake will tend to cause water retention and increase PV. Increase in ANP will then compensate for this. Stimulation of the rennin–angiotensin–aldosterone system causes sodium retention with the same result. Renin is stimulated by posture (the upright position) and by exercise; though posture and exercise have effects on PV via other mechanisms (section 8.2.3).

8.2.3 Posture and plasma volume

Seventy percent of the blood volume is below the heart in the upright position and, of this, 75% is in the distensible veins. On standing up, 500 mL of additional blood enters the legs, so that reflex tachycardia and vasoconstriction are essential to prevent fainting. Vasoconstriction maintains the blood pressure and reduces flow, especially to the skin, muscles, kidneys and viscera. The capillaries are exposed to the hydrostatic pressure of the column of venous blood. This will tend to increase filtration of fluid out of the vascular compartment, and hemoconcentration would be expected. Numerous investigators from Thompson *et al.* (1928) onwards have confirmed these theoretical expectations. Thompson *et al.* found a reduction of plasma volume of 15% on assuming the upright position, but the magnitude of this effect is variable and is influenced by many factors, including environmental and subject temperature, state of hydration, etc.

The effect of posture is therefore significant and needs to be taken into account when considering the effect of other variables such as hypoxia or exercise on plasma volume.

8.2.4 Exercise and plasma volume

Exercise can have an important effect on plasma volume and hence on hemoglobin concentration and PCV, but the effect varies according to the intensity, duration and type of exercise. The temperatures of the environment and the subject modify the effect. It is also modified by posture (section 8.2.3). This is because temperature and posture affect the skin blood flow and hence the distribution of cardiac output to skin, working muscles, kidneys, splanchnic area, etc. This, in turn, affects the capillary and venous pressures in these areas and hence the balance of forces in the Starling equation. Many studies on the effect of exercise have ignored the effect of posture and have taken control samples in a different posture from exercise samples.

Harrison (1985) has reviewed the literature and, with a number of reservations, comes to the conclusion that, for bicycle ergometer exercise, there is a reduction in the PV soon after starting exercise. This reduction is proportional to the intensity of exercise or, more precisely, to the rise in atrial pressure. Thereafter there is little change with continued exercise at normal room temperature but in high temperatures there is a further reduction in PV with time. However, these laboratory studies tend to look at fairly high intensity exercise (greater than 50% $V_{O_{2,max}}$) for periods of up to an hour or two.

Exercise on mountains is taken over periods of many hours and may go on day after day. The availability of fluid for drinking will obviously make a difference. If this is not available, dehydration will certainly reduce PV, but usually fluid is available to climbers and exercise heat stress can usually be avoided. Under these circumstances of exercise of 8 h or more at normal climbing rates (i.e. up to about 50% $V_{O_{2,max}}$ but averaging much less) an increase in PV is found. Pugh (1969) found an increase in blood volume of 7% after a 28 mile hill walk. Williams *et al.* (1979) found PV increased progressively for 5 days of strenuous daily hill walking to reach a 22% expansion. Both these studies were carried out under cold conditions and subjects avoided both overheating and cold stress. The changes in PV, interstitial and intracellular volumes are shown in Fig. 8.4.

The mechanism is probably via activation of the renin–angiotensin–aldosterone system, which results in sodium retention and thus a general expansion of the extracellular fluid (ECF) volume including the PV (Milledge *et al.* 1982). Under these circumstances the PCV decreased from a mean of 43.5–37.9% after 5 days of exercise.

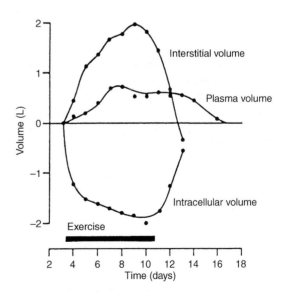

Figure 8.4 The effect of five consecutive days' strenuous hill walking on body fluid compartments. The changes are calculated from changes in packed cell volume, and sodium and water balances. (Reproduced with permission from Williams *et al.* 1979.)

8.3 EFFECT OF ALTITUDE ON PLASMA VOLUME

8.3.1 Acute hypoxia and plasma volume

During the first few hours of altitude exposure the effect on PV is variable and data are scanty. In the field, the effect of hypoxia may be overshadowed by that of cold, dehydration and exercise but it seems that those subjects free from acute mountain sickness (AMS) have a diuresis and contract their PV. Singh et al. (1990) found a reduction in PV from 40.4 mL kg^{-1} at sea level to 37.7 mL kg^{-1} on day 2 at 3500 m, and 37.0 mL kg^{-1} on day 12. Wolfel et al. (1991) reported similar changes in PV on ascent to 4300 m; PV fell from 48.8 mL kg^{-1} to 42.5 mL kg^{-1} on arrival at altitude and to 40.2 mL kg^{-1} by day 21. Some caution must be exercised in the interpretation of these studies in the light of a later study by Poulson et al. (1998). They measured the change in PV of 10 subjects on being airlifted to the Vallot observatory (4350 m) using both the Evans' blue and the carbon monoxide methods. Twenty-four hours after arrival at altitude they found the expected reduction in PV with the carbon monoxide method (350 mL reduction) but not with the Evans' blue method (30 mL reduction). A possible explanation is that, since the Evans' blue labels albumin, and hypoxia induced an increase in capillary permeability to albumin, the Evans' blue method would have included this extravascular pool of albumin and thus have given a falsely high result.

Subjects with AMS have an antidiuresis and probably expand their PV. Vigorous exercise taken on getting up to altitude or on arrival will also result in expansion of the PV, as it does at sea level, via the renin–aldosterone system along with expansion of the extravascular space. Withey et al. (1983) found that subjects who hiked up to the Kulm Hotel on the Gornergrat (3100 m) and continued to exercise with hill walking thereafter, had an increased PV and decreased haematocrit on the second day after ascent. In this particular situation the effect of exercise overrode the effect of hypoxia.

Honig (1983) has reviewed the effect of acute hypoxia on body fluid volumes, especially in animal experiments. With exposure to moderate hypoxia equivalent to altitudes of 3000–6000 m there is a diuresis and natriuresis. After reviewing possible mechanisms via effects on the cardiovascular system,

Honig presents evidence, from his own work, that the carotid body, stimulated by hypoxia, reduces the reabsorption of sodium by the kidney via neural pathways. (This comprehensive review antedates the recognition of the importance of atrial natriuretic peptide.) From the same group a study in humans have shown similar results (Brauer et al. 1996). They found that after 3 h of breathing 12% oxygen, there was the expected increase in ventilation and heart rate but also there was an increase in filtration fraction and in renal vascular resistance. There was increased proximal and reduced distal tubular sodium reabsorption.

8.3.2 Chronic hypoxia and plasma volume

After this early phase of altitude exposure, there is a definite reduction in PV over the next few weeks. Pugh (1964b) found a 21% reduction in PV after 18 weeks at altitudes above 4000 m in four members of the 1960–61 Silver Hut Expedition (Fig. 8.5). During the following 7–14 weeks the PV returned towards control levels, values being on average 10% less than control when corrected for changes in body weight. Sanchez et al. (1970) found altitude residents at Cerro de Pasco (4370 m) in Peru to have a mean PV two-thirds that of a group of students at Lima

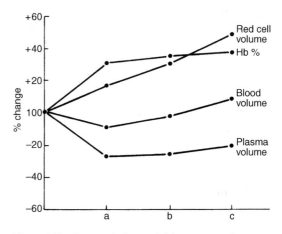

Figure 8.5 Changes in hemoglobin concentration (Hb%), red cell volume, blood volume and plasma volume in four subjects during the Silver Hut Expedition: (a) after 18 weeks at between 4000 and 5800 m; (b) after a further 3–6 weeks at 5800 m; (c) after a further 9–14 weeks at or above 5800 m. (After Pugh 1964b.)

(sea level). When allowance was made for the weight difference of the groups they still had a PV 27% less in a blood volume that was 14% greater.

8.3.3 Plasma volume on return to sea level

The PV is rapidly restored on return to sea level. In Operation Everest III by 1–3 days after return to sea level the PV was, on average, higher than before altitude exposure (Robarch *et al.* 2000). A later study by the same group (Robach *et al.* 2002) studied subjects at 4350 m and found a PV reduction of 13.6% after 7 days which was restored to control values by the second day after return to sea level. The mechanism was thought to be due to decreased diuresis on return.

8.3.4 Effect of plasma volume decrease on cardiac function and $V_{O_2,max}$

The result of a decrease in PV is a reduction in blood volume until the RCM increases sufficiently to restore it. The possibility that this reduced blood volume might contribute to the lower maximum cardiac output and lower $V_{O_2,max}$ was explored in two recent studies, Operation Everest III (Robach *et al.* 2000) and a Danish study at Chacaltaya (5260 m) in Chile (Calbet *et al.* 2004). In the earlier study, subjects were studied after 10–12 days having reached at altitude of 6000 m by a progressive increase in simulated altitude in a chamber. PV had decreased by 26%. A maximal exercise test decreased PV further and the intervention was to infuse a plasma expander during the progressive exercise both at sea level (SL) and at altitude. This lessened the PV reduction though did not prevent it totally. There was no effect of this intervention on $V_{O_2,max}$ at SL but the infusion did result in a 9% increase in V_{O_2} at altitude with the greatest effect being seen in subjects with the greatest PV reduction, suggesting that the reduced PV had some effect in reducing performance. In the Danish study plasma volume was expanded by 1 L of dextran in subjects acclimatized for 9 weeks at 5260 m. There was no effect on maximum cardiac output or $V_{O_2,max}$ despite maximum oxygen transport being reduced by 19% due to hemodilution. The same work rate and V_{O_2} was achieved by greater oxygen extraction by the working muscles after PV expansion. The difference in effect of PV expansion may be due to the longer period at altitude in the later study when perhaps the PV had already increased. However, the result does add evidence against any great advantage of a high hemoglobin concentration, [Hb].

8.4 ALTITUDE AND ERYTHROPOIESIS

8.4.1 Erythropoietin, HIF-1, hypoxia and other stimuli to production

EPO is a hormone secreted by peritubular cells in the kidney. It is one of a number of gene products whose transcription is stimulated by hypoxia. These include aldolase A, enolase-1 glucose transporter-1, lactate dehydroginase and fosphofructokinase, all involved with glycolysis; inducible nitric oxide synthase and heme oxygenase, involved with vasodilatation; and vascular endothelial growth factor which promotes angiogenesis. The link between hypoxia and the induction of the genes for all these proteins involves HIF-1α. HIF-1α is a nuclear factor normally produced and rapidly degraded in normoxia. In hypoxia it accumulates and binds to the promoter part of these genes. It was first identified as a nuclear factor that bound to the hypoxia response element of the EPO gene (Semenza *et al.* 1998). The other hypoxia-induced genes all have similar core binding sites for HIF-1α. For an overview of this important topic see section 10.4.

Although hypoxia is the major stimulus to EPO production, other stimuli have been investigated. Exercise has been reported to increase serum eryth-ropoietin (SiEp) (Schwandt *et al.* 1991) but others have found no effect (Schmidt *et al.* 1991, Bodary *et al.* 1999). Some forms of severe exercise are associated with a reduction in plasma volume. The possibility that plasma volume contraction may stimulate EPO production was studied by Roberts *et al.* (2000). They measured SiEp before and after supramaximal exercise and after plasma volume reduction (5%) by plasmapheresis. Exercise resulted in a nonsignificant rise in SiEp but after plasma volume reduction there was a significant (34%) rise in SiEp peaking 7–24 h after plasmapheresis, despite a small (4%) rise in hematocrit. They suggest that changes in plasma volume may modulate the production of EPO. Another stimulant to EPO production may be the plasma thiol–disulfide redox state. Hildebrandt *et al.* (2002) showed, in a crossover trial, that subjects when treated with *N*-acetyl-cysteine, which affects the redox state, had a much greater EPO response to 2 h of hypoxia than after placebo treatment.

8.4.2 Altitude and serum EPO concentration

Until about 1980, measurements of EPO in blood were by bioassays which could not detect the hormone until its concentration was above normal sea level values. Therefore, earlier work often relied on more indirect indices of erythropoietic activity such as intestinal iron absorption or reticulocyte counts. The latter is a rather late effect. Intestinal iron absorption has been shown to be independent of EPO and to be promoted as a direct effect of hypoxia rather than secondary to plasma iron turnover or erythropoietic activity (Raja *et al.* 1986).

On going to altitude there is an elevation of EPO concentration in the first 24–48 h (Siri *et al.* 1966, Albrecht and Little 1972). Newer methods of EPO estimation using radioimmunoassay are sensitive to levels of EPO well below the normal range (13–37 mIU mL^{-1}). Using this type of assay it has been found that serum immunoreactive EPO concentration (SiEp) begins to rise within 2 h of hypoxic exposure, depending on the altitude (Eckardt *et al.* 1989), and reaches a maximum at about 24–48 h. Thereafter, it declines to reach values not measurably different from controls after about 3 weeks (Milledge and Cotes 1985). This is shown in Fig. 8.6, which also shows the rise in PCV on going to altitude. A similar rapid rise and decline was found by Gunga *et al.* (1994) at the modest altitude of 2315 m.

Intermittent hypoxia is increasingly being used by athletes as part of their training programs. Koistinen *et al.* (2000) studied the effect of 12 h hypoxia (normobaric, 15% O$_2$) at night for a week on various indices of erythropoiesis and compared it with similar but continuous hypoxia. They found it had the same effect as continuous hypoxia, on SiEp, reticulocyte count and transferrin receptor levels.

The rise in SiEp with altitude shows great individual variability. In a study in the Andes, Richalet *et al.* (1994) found the increase to range from threefold to

134-fold in their group of subjects 1 week after arrival at 6540 m.

Figure 8.6 also shows that, even after 3 weeks above 4500 m, a rise in altitude to 5500 m caused another rise in SiEp. Quite a short pulse of hypoxia initiates a rise in SiEp, which continues after normoxia is restored. For instance, 120 min breathing 10% oxygen caused SiEp to rise just after normoxia was restored and the rise continued for a further 120 min (Knaupp *et al.* 1992).

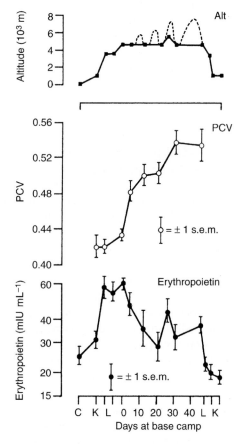

Figure 8.6 The effect of going to altitude on the serum erythropoietin concentration. The top panel shows the altitude/time profile for the eight subjects. The dotted line indicates ascent above base camp between blood samples. Note, the samples at 30 days were taken at 5500 m after four sample times at Base Camp (4500 m). Mean packed cell volume (PCV) is shown in the center panel and mean erythropoietin concentration in the lower panel. C, control, sea level; K, Kashgar (1200 m); L, Karakol lakes (3500 m). (Reproduced with permission from Milledge and Cotes 1985.)

It will be seen from Fig. 8.6 that PCV continues to rise after SiEp falls to near control values. The rise in RCM continues even longer (section 8.4.3). In patients with polycythemia secondary to hypoxic lung disease the SiEp was found to be within the normal range in over 50% of patients (Wedzicha *et al.* 1985). A continued erythropoiesis when levels of SiEp have fallen to near control values is unexplained.

A recent study in mice at simulated altitude found that if the increased in [Hb] is prevented by either blood removal or treatment with a hemolytic drug, phenylhydrazine, SiEp remained elevated for the 10 days of the study whereas in control mice there was the usual fall on the second and subsequent days to levels about twice that of baseline values (Bozzini *et al.* 2005). This suggests that the normal increase in [Hb] on ascent to altitude is sufficient to relieve, to a degree at least, the hypoxia causing the rise in SiEp. This confirms, in very controlled conditions, an incidental finding from the Sajama Expedition (Richalet *et al.* 1994) that two women in the team who, during their 10 day stay on the 6542 m summit, showed no increase in [Hb], had a large increase SiEp compared with the other subjects.

8.4.3 Altitude and red cell mass

The result of increased erythropoiesis at altitude is an increase in RCM since the life span of the red cell is unchanged (Berlin *et al.* 1954). Figure 8.5 shows the rise in RCM, which is quite slow but continues for a long time. After about 6 months at altitudes above 4000 m it had increased by a mean of 50% in absolute terms or 67.5% when corrected for loss of body weight. By this time the blood volume had increased over control by 7.3% or 22.8% corrected for body weight (Pugh 1964a) (Fig. 8.5). Sanchez *et al.* (1970) found altitude residents in the Andes to have a RCM 83% greater than sea level residents when corrected for weight difference.

8.5 ALTITUDE AND HEMOGLOBIN CONCENTRATION

8.5.1 Lowlanders going from sea level to altitude

The combined effect of changes in PV and RCM results in an increase in hemoglobin concentration [Hb]. This increase allows more oxygen to be carried per liter of blood at any given oxygen saturation. The price paid for this gain in oxygen capacity, however, is an increase in viscosity of the blood with the attendant increased risk of thrombosis (Chapter 22).

As discussed in section 8.3, the initial rise in [Hb] during the first few days and weeks at altitude is largely a result of reduction in PV. The [Hb] rise is roughly exponential with time, leveling out at about 6 weeks at a given altitude. However, after that, the RCM continues to rise but so does the PV so that [Hb] remains approximately constant (Fig. 8.5).

Pugh (1964c) reviewed results from five expeditions (51 observations in 40 subjects) and concluded that the [Hb] after about 6 weeks at altitude averaged 20.5 g dL^{-1}; there was no correlation between [Hb] and performance on the mountain. Winslow *et al.* (1984), reviewing [Hb] values from the 1981 American Everest expeditions and two previous Everest expeditions, found the range of mean values was 17.8–20.6 g dL^{-1} at altitudes of 5350–6300 m, with no correlation between altitude and [Hb] within this altitude range.

8.5.2 Residents at altitude

Figure 8.7 shows the rise in [Hb] with altitude in residents of high altitude from North and South America and Asia. Andean subjects have been reported to have values in the region of 22 g dL^{-1} at altitudes of 4300–4500 m (Talbott and Dill 1936, Dill *et al.* 1937, Merino 1950). However, these studies may include subjects who would now be considered to have chronic mountain sickness. More recent publications from South America give mean values nearer 20 g dL^{-1} (Peñaloza *et al.* 1971).

In Sherpa subjects [Hb] is lower; a mean of 17 g dL^{-1} at 4000 m is given by Adams and Strang (1975) and of 16.2 g dL^{-1} by Morpurgo *et al.* (1976). In this case the possibility that some subjects may be iron deficient cannot be ruled out. Morpurgo *et al.* argue that it represents greater adaptation. It is estimated that Tibetans have been resident at high altitude for at lease 100 000 years, compared with about 14 000 years for Andean highlanders. However, results in residents of the Tien Shan and Pamirs by Son (1979) give values closer to those from South America (Fig. 8.7) and would seem not to support

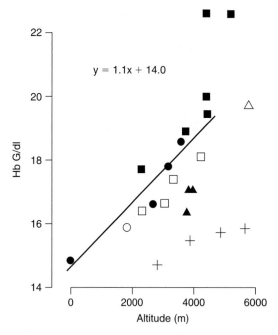

Figure 8.7 The effect of altitude on hemoglobin concentration in male residents at altitude: ●, from the Tien Shan; □, from Colorado mining camps; ○, from south Indian hill towns; ■, from the Andes; ▲, from Nepal (Sherpas); △, climbers after 3 months or more at altitude. Data from Altman and Dittmer (1966) + from Tibetans. The line is the best fit line from the literature for males at various altitudes in North and South America (from Wu *et al.* 2005).

this hypothesis. A possible explanation for the difference between Andean residents on the one hand and Sherpas and Tien Shan/Pamir residents on the other is that the latter move up and down in altitude more frequently than do Andean altitude dwellers on the altiplano. However, recent studies (below) showing Tibetan populations to have lower [Hb] than Andean populations suggest there may be a genetic explanation.

A study from Tibet (Beall *et al.* 1987) demonstrated a hemoglobin concentration of 18.2 g dL^{-1} in male and 16.7 g dL^{-1} in female subjects resident at an altitude of 4850–5450 m, a value substantially lower than most results from the Andes at comparable altitude. A later study by the same group (Beall *et al.* 1998) confirms this impression. In this study the same investigators using the same methods studied highland populations at altitude in Tibet and

Bolivia. They found Tibetans had significantly lower hemoglobin concentration than the Bolivian highlanders (15.6 compared to 19.2 g dL^{-1}). They found that genetic factors accounted for a very high proportion of the phenotypic variance in hemoglobin concentration in both samples. This more recent study is in line with that of Winslow *et al.* (1989) who compared Himalayan natives (Sherpas) to high altitude Andean natives at similar altitudes in Khundi, Nepal and Ollague (Chile) at 3700 m. Mean PCV values in Nepal were significantly lower than in Chile (48.4 compared with 52.2 g dL^{-1}). They also found serum Epo concentrations to be higher in the Andean population, indicating that they were functionally anemic even with the higher PCV!

White people resident in high altitude towns in Colorado and acclimatized climbers tend to have lower hemoglobin concentration than Andeans but higher than Central Asian residents (Fig. 8.7).

A recent very large study ($n = 5887$) by Wu *et al.* (2005) from north-west China and Tibet confirmed previous work that showed differences between lowlanders, Han Chinese, at altitude for many years and Tibetans (Fig 8.7). The rise in [Hb] with altitude in Han Chinese follows the same line as that given by a regression equation derived from the literature for North and South American populations at various altitudes. This rise is 1 g dL^{-1} for every 1100 m increase in altitude ($y = 1.1x + 14.0$ when altitude is given in kilometers). The Tibetans on the other hand had significantly lower [Hb] showing only a very small rise with altitude increase from 3813 to 5200 m. Wu *et al.* also looked at the difference between men and women and the effect of age on [Hb]. These aspects will be discussed in Chapters 25 and 26, respectively. It seems therefore that Tibetans do have significantly lower [Hb] than other populations at altitude presumably due to genetic adaptation over many generations.

Ethiopian residents at an altitude of 3530 m were studied by Beall *et al.* (2002) and found to have [Hb] of 15.9 and 15 g dL^{-1} for males and females respectively, similar to or slightly higher than Tibetan values at that altitude.

8.5.3 Polycythemia of high altitude

Excessive rise of [Hb] (i.e. above 22 g dL^{-1}) is generally considered to be pathological and diagnostic of chronic mountain sickness (Chapter 21). Both people native to high altitude and lowlanders resident at high altitude for some years are at risk of developing this condition. Huang *et al.* (1984) report that Han Chinese lowlanders resident on the Tibetan plateau have a higher incidence of this polycythemia than Tibetans.

8.5.4 Optimum hemoglobin concentration

An increase in [Hb] increases the oxygen-carrying capacity of blood. The oxygen content of the blood is the product of capacity and saturation (Sa,O_2) plus the dissolved oxygen. Thus the increase in [Hb] with altitude compensates for a reduction in arterial Sa,O_2. At altitudes up to about 5300 m this compensation results in an arterial oxygen content approximately equal to that at sea level in those who are acclimatized (Fig. 8.1). However, increasing [Hb] results in increasing viscosity (Guyton *et al.* 1973). This increase in viscosity is curvilinear so that, with [Hb] above about 18 g dL^{-1}, viscosity increases rapidly. Eventually, this increased viscosity increases resistance in both systemic and pulmonary circulation, so impeding blood flow, and cardiac output falls. Oxygen supply to the tissues depends upon oxygen delivery, which is the product of arterial oxygen content and cardiac output.

These considerations result in the concept of an optimum [Hb] below which oxygen delivery is reduced because of reduction in oxygen content, and above which it is reduced because the great increase in viscosity causes a reduction in cardiac output which more than offsets the increase in content. The major problem in calculating what should be the value of this optimum [Hb] is the viscosity of blood and its effect on cardiac output. Since blood is a non-Newtonian fluid (a fluid whose viscosity is not constant at all shear rates), a single value for viscosity cannot be assigned to it at any given [Hb]. The value will vary according to the way it is measured *in vitro*. *In vivo* the effect on resistance will vary according to the diameter of the vessel under consideration as well as to whether flow is streamlined or turbulent. Apparent resistance will also vary with flow. If we ignore the physics and just look at the effect of changing [Hb] on cardiac output in acute animal experiments, these may not reflect the human situation at altitude where the vascular system has time to adapt to the polycythemia. The situation is so complex that it is clearly impossible, on theoretical grounds, to predict an optimum [Hb]. Another factor affecting the apparent viscosity is the deformability, or filterability, of the red cells. A study by Simon-Schnass and Korniszewski (1990) addressed this and concluded that altitude exposure resulted in an impaired filterability of red cells which was prevented by the administration of vitamin E.

From clinical experience, it seems that the extremely high [Hb] found in chronic mountain sickness (Chapter 21) and in some patients with chronic hypoxic lung disease is deleterious. Hemodilution by venesection alone or with intravenous fluid replacement results in clinical improvement. In such patients reduction of PCV from 61 to 50% resulted in a decrease in pulmonary artery pressure and resistance (Weisse *et al.* 1975). Similarly, Winslow *et al.* (1985) found in Andean high altitude residents that reduction of PCV from 62 to 42% resulted in increased cardiac output and mixed venous Po_2. Willison *et al.* (1980) found that reducing the PCV from 54 to 48% in patients resulted in an increase of cerebral blood flow from 44 to 57 mL min^{-1} 100 g^{-1} brain tissue. This would increase oxygen delivery to the brain by 15% and was accompanied by an increase in alertness.

In a study of climbers at altitude by Sarnquist *et al.* (1986) it was found that hemodilution produced no improvement or deterioration in measured physical performance, though there was a small, significant improvement in psychomotor tests. However, the subjects studied, though having the highest PCV in the expedition, were not very polycythemic. Their PCV ranged from 57 to 60% before hemodilution.

There is no obvious correlation between climbing performance and [Hb] within the range of values common on an expedition, at about 17–22 g dL^{-1} (Pugh 1964c). Indeed it is usual to find that climbers who perform best are at the lower end of this range, suggesting that the optimum [Hb] at altitudes above about 5000 m is in the region of 18 g dL^{-1}. Winslow and Monge (1987, p. 203) conclude that 'Excessive polycythemia serves no useful purpose. Indeed, it is doubtful whether there is any physiologic value in "normal" polycythemia.'

A recent study using mathematical modeling techniques even came to the conclusion that, at moderate altitude, at rest, a [Hb] of 14.7 was optimum (Villafuerte *et al.* 2004). Of course, a rather higher value may be better for exercise performance. The problem of excessive erythropoiesis in chronic mountain sickness is further discussed in Chapter 21.

8.5.5 Effect of blood boosting on performance at sea level and altitude

At sea level there is little doubt that blood boosting (doping) by auto or hetero-infusion or by use of EPO has a significant effect in improving performance, as measured by $V_{O_{2,max}}$, and endurance. This is due to the increased oxygen-carrying capacity achieved by increasing the red cell mass by these maneuvers and hence the [Hb]. There have been numerous studies to show this improved athletic performance in middle distance running, cycling and skiing, of which that by Ekblom *et al.* (1972) was probably the first. He showed that increasing the [Hb] by 13% by re-infusion of autologous blood, there was an increase in physical performance capacity (work time at a standard rate) of 23% and an increase in $V_{O_{2,max}}$ of 9%. The improvement in performance correlated with the increase in [Hb]. Buick *et al.* (1980) found similar results in their subjects who had genuine re-infusions but not in the group who had sham infusions thus eliminating the possibility of a psychological effect. Of course, the practice is illegal in sport. A recent review of the topic (Leigh-Smith 2004) summarizes the history, techniques, effects and side effects of the practice. After discussing the measures to combat this illegal practice, he concludes that, 'Far from being consigned to the history books, blood boosting may still be a current topic worthy of a sports physician's attention'.

However, at altitude the situation is less clear. Young *et al.* (1996) found no significant benefit from re-infusion of 700 mL of autologous blood in subjects at 4300 m, though mean values for $V_{O_{2,max}}$ were slightly higher on day 1 at altitude in the test subjects. In a further study by Pandolf *et al.* (1998) they found no significant improvement in time for a 3.2 km run in subjects infused with 700 mL of autologous blood. They suggest that the effect diminishes with increasing altitude and quote earlier work supporting that concept. More recently, Lundby and Damsgaard (2006) increased [Hb] by 16% by treating their subjects with a new form of Epo. They tested them whilst breathing 12.4% oxygen mixture (altitude equivalent 4100 m) before and after the month long treatment. They thus produced raised [Hb] without other changes in acclimatization. The treatment increased oxygen-carrying capacity as expected but did not increase $V_{O_{2,max}}$. They point out that, at least at altitudes above about 3500 m, it has been shown that acclimatization does not increase $V_{O_{2,max}}$ despite a rise in [Hb]. At submaximal exercise acclimatization may well result in an increase in performance, in that endurance may be increased (Maher *et al.* 1974). This is certainly felt to be true by climbers at altitude. It is not at all clear why submaximal exercise performance is increased by acclimatization, whilst $V_{O_{2,max}}$ is unchanged.

8.5.6 Hemoglobin concentration on descent from altitude

On descent from altitude arterial oxygen saturation will return to the normal 96–98% and this, together with the now raised [Hb], might be expected to inhibit EPO secretion. However, Milledge and Cotes (1985) reported that levels were 66% of control values 8 h and 20 h after descent following 2 months at or above 4500 m. This reduced EPO level presumably is sufficient to reduce erythropoiesis since [Hb] declines after descent and [Hb] reaches normal sea level values after about 6 weeks (Heath and Williams 1995, pp. 61–3). However, as well as low EPO levels reducing the rate of red cell production, a recent study (Rice *et al.* 2001) of hematological values of high altitude residents descending to sea level found evidence of neocytolysis. Neocytolysis is the process by which young red blood cells are selectively hemolyzed, allowing rapid reduction in RCM. The process was first observed in astronauts. On entering micro gravity their plasma volume decreases and the haematocrit rises, erythropoietin decreases and reduction of red cell mass follows with neocytolusis. The process may be triggered by the fall in EPO concentration below a critical threshold.

8.6 PLATELETS AND CLOTTING AT ALTITUDE

The physiological response to hypoxia does not seem to involve any important changes in platelet count or adhesiveness, or in clotting factors. However, there may be changes associated with acute mountain sickness (AMS), high altitude pulmonary or cerebral edema. If there are changes in clotting factors, they may represent an effect or a complication of the altitude illness rather than being essential in its genesis.

8.7 WHITE BLOOD CELLS

There seem to be variable changes in total white cell and differential count on going to altitude. One study reported a rise in granulocyte count on ascent to 4300 m (Simon-Schnass and Korniszewski 1990) and another, an increase in certain lymphocyte subsets. CD16[+] or natural killer cells were particularly increased in seven subjects in a decompression chamber at 380 mmHg (Klokker et al. 1993). There is anecdotal evidence that infections in the skin and subcutaneous tissues are slow to clear at altitude. One could speculate that the above finding might have a bearing on this.

9

Blood-gas transport and acid–base balance

SUMMARY

Alterations of the oxygen affinity of hemoglobin can alter the oxygen dissociation curve at high altitude and therefore affect oxygen transport by the blood. Many animals that live in oxygen deprived environments have high oxygen affinities of their hemoglobin. This is the case in the human fetus. It is interesting that climbers at extreme altitude increase their oxygen affinity by extreme hyperventilation which causes a marked respiratory alkalosis. The effect of the alkalosis overwhelms the small decrease in oxygen affinity caused by the increased concentration of 2,3-diphosphoglycerate in the red blood cells. The P_{50} of high altitude natives is essentially the same as the sea level value according to most studies. However, lowlanders living at high altitude for weeks tend to have a reduced P_{50}, indicating an increased oxygen affinity of hemoglobin. An increased oxygen affinity is advantageous at high altitude because it assists in the loading of oxygen by the pulmonary capillaries. The acid–base status of high altitude natives is a little controversial but many studies have found a normal arterial pH, indicating a fully compensated respiratory alkalosis. However, acclimatized lowlanders usually have a slightly alkaline pH, indicating that metabolic compensation is not complete. There is evidence that at extreme altitude, metabolic compensation for the respiratory alkalosis is slow, possibly because of chronic volume depletion caused by dehydration.

9.1 INTRODUCTION

Physiological changes in the blood play an important role in acclimatization and adaptation to high altitude. In this chapter, the main topics considered are the changes in oxygen affinity of hemoglobin, and the alterations of the acid–base status of the blood. The increase in red cell concentration of the blood was discussed in Chapter 8, where the regulation of erythropoiesis was described. Some of the consequences of an altered oxygen affinity of hemoglobin are alluded to in other chapters, especially Chapter 6 on diffusion of oxygen across the blood-gas barrier, and Chapter 12 on limiting factors at extreme altitude.

9.2 HISTORICAL

9.2.1 Oxygen dissociation curve

The honor of plotting the first oxygen and carbon dioxide dissociation curves apparently belongs to Paul Bert. In his monumental book *La Pression Barométrique* he reported the relationships between partial pressure and blood gas concentration for both oxygen and carbon dioxide as experimental animals were exposed to lower and lower barometric pressures, or as they were gradually asphyxiated by rebreathing in a closed space (Bert 1878, pp. 135–8 in the 1943 translation). However, he did not discover the S-shaped curve for oxygen because he did not reduce the P_{O_2} far enough.

The first oxygen dissociation curve over its whole range was published by Christian Bohr in 1885. The measurements were made on dilute solutions of hemoglobin and showed precise hyperbolas (Bohr 1885). They were clearly not compatible with the data obtained by Bert in experimental animals, although Bohr did not comment on this. Hüfner (1890) published similar curves for hemoglobin solutions and argued that a hyperbolic shape would be expected from the simple equation

$$Hb + O_2 \rightarrow HbO_2$$

An important advance was made by Bohr when he used whole blood rather than hemoglobin solutions and this led him to the discovery of the now familiar S-shaped curve. In the following year he showed, in collaboration with Hasselbalch and Krogh, that the dissociation curve was shifted to the right when the P_{CO_2} of the blood was increased, a phenomenon which came to be known as the Bohr effect (Bohr et al. 1904). A few years later, Barcroft found that the addition of acid displaced the dissociation curve to the right (Barcroft and Orbeli 1910), and also that an increase in temperature had the same effect (Barcroft and King 1909). Astrup and Severinghaus (1986) wrote a valuable historical review of blood gases and acid–base balance.

Soon after these important modulators of the oxygen affinity of hemoglobin were discovered, physiologists wondered about their importance at high altitude. For example, when Barcroft accompanied the first international high altitude expedition to Tenerife in 1910 he made a special study of the position of the oxygen dissociation curve, expecting it to be displaced to the left by the low arterial P_{CO_2}. In the event, he found that the oxygen dissociation curves of some members of the expedition at 2130 and 3000 m were shifted to the right when measured at the normal sea level P_{CO_2} of 40 mmHg. However, when he repeated the equilibrations at the subjects' actual P_{CO_2} at altitude, the positions of the curves were essentially the same as at sea level (Barcroft 1911). He concluded that the decrease in carbonic acid in the blood was compensated for by an increase in some other acid, possibly lactic acid. One year later Barcroft went to Mosso's laboratory, the Capanna Regina Margherita on Monte Rosa (4559 m), and

reported a slight excess acidity of the blood at that altitude (Barcroft et al. 1914).

Some 10 years later, during the 1921–22 International High Altitude Expedition to Cerro de Pasco in Peru, Barcroft and his colleagues found an increased oxygen affinity in acclimatized lowlanders as a result of the increased alkalinity of the blood. It also appeared that the increase in affinity was greater than could be explained by the change in acid–base status (Barcroft et al. 1923).

The question of oxygen affinity of hemoglobin was examined again on the International High Altitude Expedition to Chile in 1935. It was found that the 'physiological' dissociation curves (that is, measured at a subject's own P_{CO_2}) were displaced slightly to the left of the sea level values up to about 4270 m, but above that altitude, the curves were displaced increasingly to the right of the sea level positions (Keys et al. 1936). Measurements of oxygen affinity of the hemoglobin were also made at constant pH and these showed a uniform tendency to a decreased affinity. The investigators argued that this rightward shift of the curve might be advantageous at high altitude because it would facilitate oxygen unloading to the tissues.

An important discovery was made in 1967 by two groups working independently (Benesch and Benesch 1967, Chanutin and Curnish 1967) that a fourth factor (in addition to P_{CO_2}, pH and temperature) had an important effect on the oxygen affinity of hemoglobin. This was the concentration of 2,3-diphosphoglycerate (2,3-DPG) within the red cells. This unexpected development raised doubts about much of the earlier work where this important factor had not been controlled, and it was shown that 2,3-DPG was depleted when blood was stored. It was subsequently shown that 2,3-DPG increased at high altitude (Lenfant et al. 1968) and it was argued that the resulting decrease in oxygen affinity, which facilitated unloading of oxygen in the tissues, was an important part of the adaptation process (Lenfant and Sullivan 1971).

Until recently, relatively little information was available on the oxygen affinity of hemoglobin at extreme altitudes. A few measurements from the Silver Hut expedition of 1960–61 showed that lowlanders who were well acclimatized to 5800 m had an almost fully compensated respiratory alkalosis (West et al. 1962). Data above this altitude did not exist. It was therefore astonishing to find on the 1981

American Medical Research Expedition to Everest that climbers near the summit apparently had an extreme degree of respiratory alkalosis which greatly increased the oxygen affinity of their hemoglobin. The arterial pH of Pizzo on the Everest summit exceeded 7.7 as determined from the alveolar P_{CO_2} and base excess, both of which were measured (section 9.4.4).

9.2.2 Acid–base balance

Turning now to the early history of acid–base balance at high altitude, it is clear from the above that this overlaps considerably with a discussion of oxygen affinity of hemoglobin. However, the reaction of the blood (as it was called) at high altitude created a great deal of interest in its own right. Indeed, the acid–base status of the blood played an important role in early theories of the control of breathing at high altitude (Kellogg 1980). As long ago as 1903, Galeotti studied various experimental animals taken to Mosso's Capanna Margherita laboratory on Monte Rosa, and found that the amount of acid needed to bring their hemolyzed blood to a standard pH (determined from litmus paper) was decreased compared with sea level (Galeotti 1904). He interpreted this decrease in titratable alkalinity to mean that there was an increase in some acid substance in the blood. It was known that hypoxia caused lactic acid production (Araki 1891) and that acid blood stimulated breathing (Zuntz *et al.* 1906). It was therefore natural to conclude that this explained the hyperventilation of high altitude, and that the P_{CO_2} fell as a consequence (Boycott and Haldane 1908). Winterstein (1911) formulated what became known as the 'reaction theory' of breathing, which stated that the effects of both hypoxia and carbon dioxide as stimulants of ventilation could be explained by the fact that they both acidified the blood.

The correct explanation of how hypoxia stimulates ventilation at high altitude had to wait for discovery of the peripheral chemoreceptors by Heymans and Heymans (1925). Meanwhile Winterstein (1915) provided evidence against his own theory when he showed that, in acute hypoxia, the blood becomes alkaline rather than acid. A few years later, Henderson (1919) and Haldane *et al.* (1919) correctly explained the alkalinity as being secondary to the lowered P_{CO_2} caused by hyperventilation. Nevertheless, it is true

that even today the control of ventilation during chronic hypoxia is a subject of intense research (Chapter 5) and interest still remains in the acid–base status of the extracellular fluid (ECF) which forms the environment of the central chemoreceptors.

9.3 OXYGEN AFFINITY OF HEMOGLOBIN

9.3.1 Basic physiology

Figure 9.1 shows the oxygen dissociation curve of human whole blood and the four factors that shift the curve to the right, that is decrease the affinity of hemoglobin for oxygen. These four factors are increases in P_{CO_2}, hydrogen ion concentration, temperature and the concentration of 2,3-DPG in the red cells. Increasing the ionic concentration of the plasma also reduces oxygen affinity.

Almost all of the change in oxygen affinity caused by P_{CO_2} can be ascribed to its effect on hydrogen ion concentration, although a change in P_{CO_2} has a small effect in its own right (Margaria 1957). The mechanism of the alteration of oxygen affinity through hydrogen ion concentration (Bohr effect) is by a

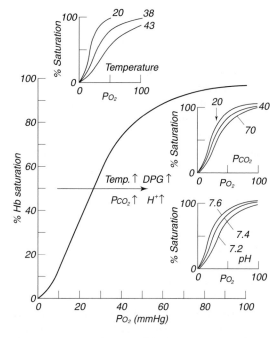

Figure 9.1 Normal oxygen dissociation curve and its displacement by increases in H^+, P_{CO_2}, temperature and 2,3-diphosphoglycerate (DPG). (From West 1994.)

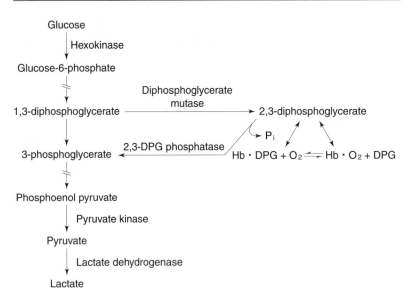

Figure 9.2 Formation of 2,3-DPG in erythrocytes. The vertical chain at the left shows the glycolytic pathway in cells other than red blood cells. In red cells the enzyme DPG mutase catalyses the conversion of much of the 1,3-DPG to 2,3-DPG. (Modified from Mines 1981.)

change in configuration of the hemoglobin molecule which makes the binding site less accessible to molecular oxygen as the hydrogen ion concentration is raised. The molecule exists in two forms: one in which the chemical subunits are maximally chemically bonded (T form), and another in which some bonds are ruptured and the structure is relaxed (R form). The R form has a higher affinity for oxygen because the molecule can more easily enter the region of the heme. The approximate magnitudes of the effects of change in P_{CO_2} and pH on the oxygen dissociation curve are shown in the right insets of Fig. 9.1.

An increase in temperature has a large effect on the oxygen affinity of hemoglobin, as shown in the top inset of Fig. 9.1. The temperature effect follows from thermodynamic considerations: the combination of oxygen with hemoglobin is exothermic so that an increase in temperature favors the reverse reaction, that is dissociation of the oxyhemoglobin.

The compound 2,3-DPG is a product of red cell metabolism, as shown in Fig. 9.2. An increased concentration of this material within the red cell reduces the oxygen affinity of the hemoglobin by increasing the chemical binding of the subunits and converting more hemoglobin to the low affinity T form.

A useful number to describe the oxygen affinity of hemoglobin is the P_{50}, that is the P_{O_2} when 50% of the binding sites are attached to oxygen. The normal value for adult whole blood at a P_{CO_2} of 40 mmHg, pH 7.4, temperature 37°C, and normal 2,3-DPG concentration is 26–27 mmHg. Human fetal blood has a P_{50} of about 19 mmHg mainly

because the substitution of serine for histidine in one of the globin chains reduces the affinity for 2,3-DPG. An increase of 2,3-DPG within the red cell increases the P_{50} by about 0.5 mmHg mol^{-1} of 2,3-DPG. The magnitude of the Bohr effect is usually given in terms of the increase in log P_{50} per pH unit. The normal value for human blood is 0.4 at constant P_{CO_2}. Note that although historically the 'Bohr effect' referred to the change in affinity caused by P_{CO_2}, in modern usage the term is restricted to the effect of pH. The temperature effect is 0.24 for the change in log P_{50} (mmHg °C^{-1}).

Much can be learned about the effect of changes in the oxygen affinity of hemoglobin on the physiology of high altitude by modeling the oxygen transport system using computer subroutines for the oxygen and carbon dioxide dissociation curves (Bencowitz *et al.* 1982). Kelman described useful subroutines for the oxygen dissociation curve (Kelman 1966a,b) and the carbon dioxide dissociation curve (Kelman 1967). The practical use of these procedures has been described (West and Wagner 1977). These procedures are able to accommodate changes in P_{CO_2}, pH, temperature and 2,3-DPG concentration, and allow the investigator to answer questions about the interactions of these variables which would otherwise be impossibly complicated.

9.3.2 Animals native to high altitude

It has been known for many years that animals that live at high altitude tend to have an increased oxygen affinity of their hemoglobin. Figure 6.6 shows part of the oxygen dissociation curves of the vicuna and llama which are native to high altitude in the South American Andes (Hall *et al.* 1936). The diagram also shows the range of dissociation curves for eight lowland animals including humans, horse, dog, rabbit, pig, peccary, ox and sheep. It can be seen that the hemoglobin of high altitude native animals has a substantially increased oxygen affinity. This adaptation to high altitude is of genetic origin, as is shown by the fact that a llama brought up in a zoo at sea level has the same high oxygen affinity.

High altitude birds also have high oxygen affinities for hemoglobin. Hall and his colleagues (1936), during the 1935 International High Altitude Expedition to Chile, reported that the high altitude ostrich and huallaga have higher oxygen affinities than a group of six lowland birds including the pigeon, muscovy duck, domestic goose, domestic duck, Chinese pheasant and domestic fowl. A particularly interesting example is the bar-headed goose which is known to fly over the Himalayan ranges as it migrates between its breeding grounds in Siberia and its wintering grounds in India. This remarkable animal has a blood P_{50} about 10 mmHg lower than its close relatives from moderate altitudes (Black and Tenney 1980).

Deer mice, *Peromyscus maniculatus*, show the same relationships. A study was carried out on 10 subspecies that live at altitudes from below sea level in Death Valley in California to the high mountains of the nearby Sierra Nevada (4350 m), and it was found that there was a strong correlation between the habitat altitude and the oxygen affinity of the blood. The genetic source of this relationship was proved by moving one subspecies to another location and showing that the oxygen affinity was unchanged. Moreover, the relationship persisted in second generation animals (Snyder *et al.* 1982).

9.3.3 Animals in other oxygen deprived environments

High altitude is just one of the oxygen deprived environments in which animals are found, and it is interesting to consider the variety of strategies that have been adopted to mitigate the problems posed by oxygen deficiency. Table 6.1 shows examples of some of the strategies that have been adopted through genetic adaptation. The change in amino acid sequence in the globin chain of hemoglobin in

the human fetus has already been referred to. This is also seen in the bar-headed goose. The next two groups increase the oxygen affinity of their hemoglobin by decreasing the concentration of organic phosphates. This is done with 2,3-DPG in the fetus of the dog, horse and pig, and by decreasing the concentration of ATP in the trout and eel.

Some species of tadpoles that frequently live in stagnant pools have a high oxygen affinity hemoglobin, whereas the adult frogs produce a different type of hemoglobin with a lower affinity that fits their higher oxygen environment. Note also that the tadpole blood shows a smaller Bohr effect. This is useful because low oxygen and high carbon dioxide pressures are likely to occur together in stagnant water, and a large Bohr effect would be disadvantageous because it would decrease the oxygen affinity of the blood when a high affinity was most needed.

As indicated earlier, the human fetus also has a high oxygen affinity by virtue of its fetal hemoglobin. This is essential because the arterial P_{O_2} of the fetus is less than 30 mmHg. Indeed the human fetus and the adult climber on the summit of Mount Everest have some similar features in that in both cases the arterial P_{O_2} is extremely low, and the P_{50} of the arterial blood (at the prevailing pH) is also very low (section 9.4.4).

A particularly interesting example of an unusual human hemoglobin was described by Hebbel *et al.* (1978). The authors studied a family in which two of the siblings had a mutant hemoglobin (Andrew-Minneapolis) with a P_{50} of 17.1 mmHg. They showed that the siblings with the abnormal hemoglobin tolerated exercise at an altitude of 3100 m better than the normal siblings.

The last row in Table 6.1 refers to the climber at extreme altitude who has a marked respiratory alkalosis which greatly increases the oxygen affinity of the hemoglobin. This is discussed in detail below.

9.3.4 High altitude natives

Barcroft *et al.* (1923) measured the oxygen dissociation curves of three natives of Cerro de Pasco (4330 m) in Peru at the prevailing P_{CO_2} (25–30 mmHg) and showed that the curves were displaced to the left, i.e. there was an increased oxygen affinity. A similar result was found in acclimatized members of the expedition. Barcroft (1925) believed that part of the leftward shift was caused by increased alkalinity of the blood, but part was also due to an intrinsic change in the affinity of hemoglobin.

During the International High Altitude Expedition to Chile in 1935, a number of measurements were made on high altitude natives who were living at 5340 m (P_B 401 mmHg). Some of the men were accustomed to working each day at 5700 m. The dissociation curves were found to be within normal limits for men at sea level, or perhaps shifted slightly to the right (Keys *et al.* 1936). Measurements were also made on dilute solutions of hemoglobin taken both from high altitude residents and from acclimatized lowlanders (Hall 1936). The results were very similar to those obtained at sea level but the high altitude residents seemed to have a slightly reduced oxygen affinity.

Aste-Salazar and Hurtado (1944) measured the oxygen dissociation curves of 17 healthy Peruvians in Lima at sea level and 12 other permanent residents of Morococha (4550 m). These studies were subsequently extended to a total of 40 subjects in Lima and 30 in Morococha (Hurtado 1964). The mean value of the P_{50} at pH 7.4 was 24.7 mmHg at sea level and 26.9 mmHg at high altitude (Fig. 9.3). It was argued that the rightward displacement of the curve would enhance the unloading of oxygen from the peripheral capillaries.

More recently Winslow and his colleagues (1981) reported oxygen dissociation curves on 46 native Peruvians in Morococha (4550 m, P_B 432 mmHg) and confirmed that at pH 7.4 the P_{50} was significantly higher in the high altitude population than in the sea level controls (31.2 mmHg as opposed to 29.2 mmHg, $p < 0.001$). However, these investigators also found that the acid–base status of the high altitude subjects was that of a partially compensated respiratory alkalosis with a mean plasma pH of 7.44. When the P_{50} values were corrected to the subjects' actual plasma pH, the mean value of 30.1 mmHg could no longer be distinguished from that of the sea level controls (Fig. 9.4). The conclusion was that the small increase in P_{50} resulting from the increased concentration of 2,3-DPG in the red cells was offset by the mild degree of respiratory alkalosis, with the net result that the position of the oxygen dissociation curve was essentially the same as that in sea level controls.

In a controversial study Morpurgo *et al.* (1976) reported that Sherpas living permanently at an

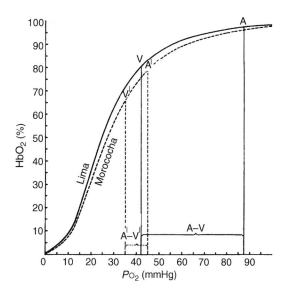

Figure 9.3 Mean positions of the oxygen dissociation curves of Peruvians in Lima (sea level) and Morococha (4540 m). Note that the high altitude natives have a slightly reduced oxygen affinity. Mean values of the P_{O_2} in arterial (A) and mixed venous (V) blood for the two groups are also shown. (From Hurtado 1964.)

altitude of 4000 m in the Nepalese Himalayas had a substantially increased oxygen affinity at standard pH. However a subsequent study by Samaja *et al.* (1979) failed to confirm this provocative finding. Samaja *et al.* also showed that the oxygen affinity could be completely accounted for by the known effectors of hemoglobin function: pH, P_{CO_2}, 2,3-DPG and temperature.

9.3.5 Acclimatized lowlanders

As discussed in section 9.2, Barcroft (1911) was perhaps the first person to measure the position of the oxygen dissociation curve in acclimatized lowlanders. This was done at altitudes of 2130 and 3000 m on Tenerife, and he reported that the curve was shifted to the right if measured at the normal P_{CO_2} of 40 mmHg, but if the P_{CO_2} for those altitudes was used, the curves had the same position as at sea level. Barcroft made additional measurements on Monte Rosa in 1911 (Barcroft *et al.* 1914) and reported a slight rightward shift of the curves at the prevailing P_{CO_2}. However, during the expedition to Cerro de Pasco in 1922, a leftward shift was observed at the

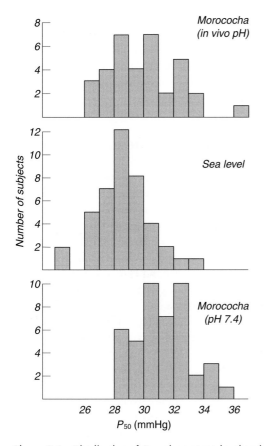

Figure 9.4   Distribution of P_{50} values at sea level and high altitude. In the top panel, values are expressed at the *in vivo* pH; in the bottom at pH 7.4. When corrected for the subjects' plasma pH, the *in vivo* P_{50} at high altitude falls in the sea level range in all but one subject. (From Winslow *et al.* 1981.)

prevailing arterial $P\text{CO}_2$ of 25–30 mmHg (Barcroft *et al.* 1923). They made the point that this might be beneficial because of enhanced oxygen uptake in the lung owing to the increased oxygen affinity of the hemoglobin.

During the International High Altitude Expedition to Chile 1935, three ways of measuring the oxygen affinity of the hemoglobin were employed: whole blood at a normal pH, whole blood at the prevailing pH, and dilute solutions of hemoglobin. At constant pH, Keys *et al.* (1936) reported that the oxygen affinity of the hemoglobin was apparently slightly reduced with a change in P_{50} of approximately 3.5 mmHg. However, the 'physiological' dissociation curves were displaced to the left from sea

level up to an altitude of approximately 4270 m, though above that they were displaced increasingly to the right of the sea level positions. On dilute hemoglobin solutions, Hall (1936) showed that the oxygen affinity of the hemoglobin was essentially unchanged compared with sea level.

These somewhat confusing results were clarified when the role of 2,3-DPG in the red cell was appreciated (Benesch and Benesch 1967, Chanutin and Curnish 1967). It was shown that this normal product of red cell metabolism reduced the oxygen affinity of hemoglobin, and it was then clear that many previous measurements were unreliable because of ignorance of this factor. Lenfant and his colleagues (Lenfant *et al.* 1968, 1969, 1971) showed that the concentration of 2,3-DPG was increased in lowlanders when they became acclimatized to high altitude. The primary cause of the increase in 2,3-DPG was the increase in plasma pH above the normal sea level value as a result of the respiratory alkalosis. When subjects were made acidotic with acetazolamide there was no increase in plasma pH or red cell 2,3-DPG concentration at high altitude, and the oxygen dissociation curve did not shift to the right. It was argued that the increase in 2,3-DPG was an important feature of the acclimatization process of lowlanders and of the adaptation to high altitude of highlanders (Lenfant and Sullivan 1971). Treatment with erythropoietin is known to increase 2,3-DPG levels in red cells at sea level (Birgegard and Sandhagen 2001).

Subsequent measurements on lowlanders at high altitude have confirmed these changes, although there is still some uncertainty about whether acclimatized lowlanders develop complete metabolic compensation for their respiratory alkalosis (that is, whether the pH returns to 7.4). Certainly this does not happen at extremely high altitudes. During the 1981 American Medical Research Expedition to Everest, Winslow *et al.* (1984) made an extensive series of measurements on acclimatized lowlanders at an altitude of 6300 m. They also obtained data on two subjects who reached the summit (8848 m). These measurements were made on venous blood samples taken at an altitude of 8050 m the morning after the summit climb. Winslow and his colleagues found that the red cell concentration of 2,3-DPG increased with altitude (Fig. 9.5) and that this was associated with a slightly increased P_{50} value when expressed at pH 7.4. However, because the

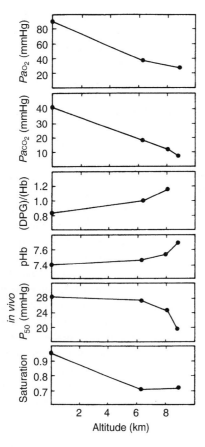

Figure 9.5 Blood variables measured on the 1981 American Medical Research Expedition to Everest at sea level, 6300 m, 8050 m and 8848 m (summit). pHb, pH blood. (From Winslow *et al.* 1984.)

respiratory alkalosis was not fully compensated, the subjects' *in vivo* P_{50} at 6300 m (27.6 mmHg) was slightly less than at sea level (28.1 mmHg). The estimated *in vivo* P_{50} was found to become progressively lower at 8050 m (24.9 mmHg), and on the summit at 8848 m it was as low as 19.4 mmHg in one subject. Thus these data show that, at extreme altitudes, the blood oxygen dissociation curve shifts progressively leftward (increased oxygen affinity of hemoglobin) primarily because of the respiratory alkalosis. Indeed this effect completely overwhelms the relatively small tendency for the curve to shift to the right because of the increase in red cell 2,3-DPG.

The results obtained on Operation Everest II were generally in agreement with these (Sutton *et al.* 1988) except that the P_{CO_2} values at extreme altitude were higher, and the blood pH values therefore

lower. These differences can probably be explained by the smaller degree of acclimatization because of the limited time available in the low pressure chamber. Another factor may be differences in hypoxic ventilatory responses which may affect ventilation at high altitude.

9.3.6 Physiological effects of changes in oxygen affinity

As indicated above, there have been differences of opinion on whether a decreased or an increased oxygen affinity is beneficial at high altitude. Barcroft *et al.* (1923) found a slightly increased affinity and argued that this would enhance oxygen loading in the lung. However, Aste-Salazar and Hurtado (1944) reported a slight decrease in oxygen affinity in high altitude natives at Morococha and reasoned that this would enhance oxygen unloading in peripheral capillaries. The same argument was used by Lenfant and Sullivan (1971) when the influence of the increased red cell concentration of 2,3-DPG on the oxygen dissociation curve was appreciated. They stated that the decreased oxygen affinity would help the peripheral unloading of oxygen, and that this was one of the many features both of acclimatization of lowlanders to high altitude and of the genetic adaptation of highlanders.

However, there is now strong evidence that an increased oxygen affinity (left-shifted oxygen dissociation curve) is beneficial, especially at higher altitudes, and particularly on exercise (Bencowitz *et al.* 1982). Indeed this should not come as a surprise when it is appreciated that many animals increase the oxygen affinity of their blood in oxygen-deprived environments by a variety of strategies (section 9.3.3 and Table 6.1). In addition, Eaton *et al.* (1974) reported that rats whose oxygen dissociation curve had been left-shifted by cyanate administration showed an increased survival when they were decompressed to a barometric pressure of 233 mmHg. The controls were rats with a normal oxygen affinity. Turek *et al.* (1978) also studied cyanate-treated rats and found that they maintained better oxygen transfer to tissues during severe hypoxia than normal animals. In addition, we have already referred to the studies of Hebbel *et al.* (1978) who found a family with two members who had a hemoglobin with a very high affinity (Hb Andrew-Minneapolis, P_{50}

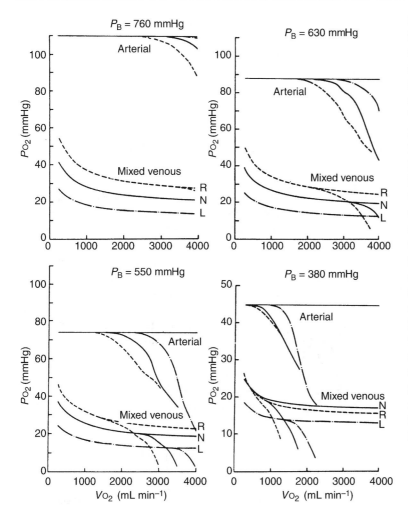

Figure 9.6   Results of a theoretical study showing changes in calculated arterial and mixed venous P_{O_2} with increasing oxygen uptake at four altitudes for three values of P_{50}. The P_{50} values are normal (N, 26.8 mmHg), right-shifted (R, 36.8 mmHg), and left-shifted (L, 16.8 mmHg). The nearly horizontal lines labeled 'mixed venous' show the P_{O_2} values for an infinitely high pulmonary oxygen diffusing capacity. The curved lines peeling away from these lines show the results of diffusion limitation. In this example, the diffusing capacity of the membrane for oxygen (DM_{O_2}) is 80 mL min^{-1} mmHg^{-1}. Note that at the highest level of exercise, and especially at high altitude, the left-shifted curve gives the highest values of P_{O_2} in mixed venous blood and therefore the tissues. (From Bencowitz *et al.* 1982.)

17.1 mmHg). These two members performed better during exercise at an altitude of 3100 m than two siblings with normal hemoglobin.

Theoretical studies show that a high oxygen affinity is beneficial at high altitude, especially on exercise (Turek *et al.* 1973, Bencowitz *et al.* 1982). In one study, oxygen transfer from air to tissues was modeled for a variety of altitudes and a range of oxygen uptakes (Bencowitz *et al.* 1982). The oxygen dissociation curve was shifted both to the left and right with P_{50} of 16.8 mmHg (left-shifted), 26.8 mmHg (normal) and 36.8 mmHg (right-shifted). The pulmonary diffusing capacity for oxygen was varied over a wide range and all the determinants of oxygen transport, including temperature, base excess, hemoglobin concentration and hematocrit, were taken into account.

The results showed that in the presence of diffusion limitation of oxygen transfer across the blood-gas barrier in the lung, a left-shifted curve resulted in the highest P_{O_2} of mixed venous blood (which was taken as an index of tissue P_{O_2}) (Fig. 9.6). In other words, in the presence of diffusion limitation, an increased oxygen affinity of hemoglobin results in a higher tissue P_{O_2}. The explanation is that the increased affinity enhances the loading of oxygen in the lung more than it interferes with unloading in peripheral capillaries. This appears to be the physiological justification for the increased oxygen affinity so frequently seen among animals that live in low oxygen environments (Table 6.1).

An analysis of the effects of changes in hemoglobin–oxygen affinity at high altitude was carried out by Samaja *et al.* (2003). They concluded that a reduction in affinity was advantageous at altitudes up to about 5000 m because it reduces the cardiac output necessary for adequate tissue oxygenation. However, at higher altitudes an increased oxygen affinity was more advantageous in agreement with Turek *et al.* (1978) and Bencowitz *et al.* (1982). Samaja *et al.* (2003) noted that some of the experimental evidence is contradictory, and they raised the possibility of other confounding factors such as changes in body temperature, especially differences between the muscles and lungs, changes in the Bohr effect within capillaries, heterogeneity of oxygen affinity between different red cells, possible vasodilator effects of nitric oxide carried by hemoglobin, and the effect of different red cell transit times in capillaries.

The role of an increased oxygen affinity is seen dramatically in a climber on the summit of Mount Everest. Despite some increase of 2,3-DPG concentration within the red cell, the extremely low P_{CO_2} of 7–8 mmHg as a result of the enormous increase in ventilation causes a dramatic degree of respiratory alkalosis with an arterial pH calculated to exceed 7.7 (West *et al.* 1983b). As a result, the *in vivo* P_{50} is about 19 mmHg, which is very similar to that of the human fetus *in utero*. The resulting striking increase in oxygen affinity of hemoglobin plays a major role in allowing the climber to survive this extremely hypoxic environment (Chapter 12).

9.4 ACID–BASE BALANCE

9.4.1 Introduction

This topic overlaps with that of the previous section, oxygen affinity of hemoglobin, because the affinity at high altitude is primarily determined by the pH of the blood together with the concentration of 2,3-DPG in the red cells. However, for convenience, available information on acid–base status is set out here.

9.4.2 During acclimatization

When a lowlander goes to high altitude, hyperventilation occurs as a result of stimulation of the peripheral chemoreceptors by the hypoxemia (Chapters 4

and 5), the arterial P_{CO_2} falls, and the arterial pH rises in accordance with the Henderson–Hasselbalch equation:

$$pH = pK + \log \frac{[HCO_3^-]}{0.03 P_{CO_2}}$$

where $[HCO_3^-]$ is the bicarbonate concentration in millimoles per liter and the P_{CO_2} is in mmHg. However, the kidney responds by eliminating bicarbonate ion, being prompted to do this by the decreased P_{CO_2} in the renal tubular cells. The result is a more alkaline urine because of decreased reabsorption of bicarbonate ions. The resulting decrease in plasma bicarbonate then moves the bicarbonate/P_{CO_2} ratio back towards its normal level. This is known as metabolic compensation for the respiratory alkalosis. The compensation may be complete, in which case the arterial pH returns to 7.4 or, more usually, incomplete with a steady-state pH that exceeds 7.4.

The time course of the changes in arterial pH when normal subjects are taken abruptly to high altitude has been studied by several investigators (Severinghaus *et al.* 1963, Lenfant *et al.* 1971, Dempsey *et al.* 1978). In one study, lowlanders were taken from sea level to an altitude of 4509 m (P_B 446 mmHg) in less than 5 h, and remained there for 4 days. The arterial pH rose to a mean of about 7.47 within 24 h and then apparently slowly declined but was still about 7.45 at the end of the 4-day period. On return to sea level the pH fell steadily to reach the normal value of 7.4 after about 48 h (Lenfant *et al.* 1971).

In another study, four normal subjects were taken abruptly to 3800 m for 8 days. The arterial pH rapidly rose from a mean of 7.424 at sea level to 7.485 after 2 days, and remained essentially constant, being 7.484 at the end of 8 days (Severinghaus *et al.* 1963). In a further study, 11 lowlanders moved to 3200 m altitude where they remained for 10 days (Dempsey *et al.* 1978). The arterial pH rose by 0.03–0.04 unit within 2 days and then remained essentially unchanged. In all instances, the arterial P_{CO_2} continued to fall as did the plasma bicarbonate concentration. However, it appears that the return of the arterial pH to (or near to) its sea level value is very slow.

9.4.3 High altitude natives

Most authors have reported a fully compensated respiratory alkalosis in high altitude natives with arterial pH values close to 7.4. Table 9.1 shows a summary of a number of published papers prepared by Winslow and Monge (1987). This is perhaps the expected finding. The body generally maintains the arterial pH within very narrow limits in health, and it seems reasonable that people who are born and live at high altitude would fully compensate for their reduced P_{CO_2} by eliminating bicarbonate and restoring the pH to the normal sea level value.

However, Winslow et al. (1981) measured the arterial pH in 46 high altitude natives of Morococha (4550 m, P_B 432 mmHg) and reported that the mean plasma pH was 7.439 ± 0.065. In other words these highlanders did not have a fully compensated respiratory alkalosis but their blood lay slightly on the alkaline side of normal. As pointed out in section 9.3.4, the result of this mild respiratory alkalosis was to restore the oxygen dissociation curve to the normal sea level position because there was an increase in red cell 2,3-DPG concentration which tended to move the curve to the right.

The interpretation of these results is complicated by the fact that Winslow et al. (1981) believed that the increased red cell concentration that is seen at high altitude had an effect on the glass electrode for measuring pH (Whittembury et al. 1968). If the observed pH is corrected for this effect of increased red cell concentration, the calculated plasma pH becomes 7.395, as shown in the bottom row of Table 9.1. However, no other investigators have corrected the pH in this way and the conclusion from the work of Winslow and his colleagues is that high altitude natives have a mildly uncompensated respiratory alkalosis with an arterial pH that exceeds 7.4.

Table 9.1   Blood-gas and pH values in high altitude natives

Altitude (m)	n	Hb[a]	Pa,o_2 (mmHg)	Sa,o_2 (%)	Pa,co_2 (mmHg)	pH	Source
4300	3	–	46.7	84.6	–	–	Barcroft et al. (1923)
4300	12	–	–	–	–	7.360	Aste-Salazar and Hurtado (1944)
4500	40	20.6[a]	45.1	80.1	33.3	7.370	Hurtado et al. (1956)
4515	22	19.5[a]	–	82.8	33.8	7.400	Chiodi (1957)
4300	6	56.0	–	–	32.5	7.431[b]	Monge et al. (1964)
4300	5	73.8	–	–	39.0	7.429[b]	Monge et al. (1964)
3700	–	–	–	–	3.0	7.431[b]	Monge et al. (1964)
4545	–	–	–	–	–	7.424[b]	Monge et al. (1964)
4820	–	–	–	–	–	7.426[b]	Monge et al. (1964)
3960	3	–	–	–	–		Lahiri et al. (1967)
4880	4	–	–	–	–	7.399	Lahiri et al. (1967)
4500	6	73.4	–	–	–	–	Lenfant et al. (1969)
4500	10	65.5	–	–	–	–	Lenfant et al. (1969)
4300	6	54.4	45.2	74.7	31.6	7.414	Torrance (1970)[c]
4500	4	63.3	44.1	73.3	32.2	7.405	Torrance (1970)[c]
4300	4	–	50.8	–	32.9	7.405	Rennie (1971)
4500	35	61.0	51.7	85.7	34.0	7.395	Winslow et al. (1981)

N:See Winslow and Monge (1987) for details and sources.

–, no data available.

[a]Hemoglobin concentration (g dL^{-1}).

[b]Plasma pH.

[c]Himalayan subjects.

9.4.4 Acclimatized lowlanders

When sufficient time is allowed for extended acclimatization to high altitude, the arterial pH returns close to the normal value of 7.4, at least up to altitudes of 3000 m. For example, during the 1935 International High Altitude Expedition to Chile, Dill and his colleagues (1937) found that the arterial pH increased little if at all up to this altitude, but above 3000 m higher values of pH were found, with a mean of about 7.45 at an altitude of 5340 m. A few measurements on acclimatized subjects at an altitude of 5800 m during the 1960–61 Silver Hut expedition indicated values of between 7.41 and 7.46 (West *et al.* 1962).

Extensive measurements were made by Winslow *et al.* (1984) during the 1981 American Medical Research Expedition to Everest. The mean arterial pH of acclimatized lowlanders living at an altitude of 6300 m was 7.47 (Fig. 9.7). It was also possible to calculate the arterial pH at an altitude of 8050 m (Camp 5) and the Everest summit (8848 m). The calculations were made from the base excess measured on venous blood samples taken at 8050 m and measurements of alveolar P_{CO_2} on sealed samples of alveolar gas brought back to the USA. It was assumed that the arterial and alveolar P_{CO_2} values were the same, and

also that base excess did not change over the 24 h between the summit and Camp 5. As discussed in section 9.4.5, there is evidence that base excess was changing very slowly at this great altitude. The mean arterial pH of two climbers at 8050 m was 7.55, and the one subject whose alveolar P_{CO_2} was measured as 7.5 mmHg on the summit gave a calculated arterial pH of over 7.7.

These climbers were not 'acclimatized' to 8050 or 8848 m in the sense that they had spent long periods at these great altitudes. However, it is not possible to spend an extended time at an altitude such as 8000 m because high altitude deterioration occurs so rapidly. Thus the values probably represent the inevitable respiratory alkalosis which occurs in climbers who go so high.

Samaja and colleagues (1997) measured the pH and blood gases from arterialized earlobe blood in lowlanders and Sherpas at altitudes of 3400, 5050 and 6450 m in the Everest region. In the lowlanders the blood pH increased progressively with altitude from 7.46 to about 7.50 but interestingly it remained nearly constant in the Sherpas in the range of 7.45–7.46. The more marked alkalosis in the lowlanders than Sherpas was consistent with a higher P_{CO_2} in the latter group. Paradoxically however the P_{O_2} and O_2 saturation were the same in the two groups at all altitudes, a finding that was not fully explained.

Another study was carried out by Wagner *et al.* (2002) in which they compared the acid–base status in lowlanders and native Bolivian residents of La Paz (3600–4100 m) when both groups ascended to 5260 m. Measurements were made both at rest and maximal exercise. After 9 weeks' residence at 5260 m, the resting arterial pH in the lowlanders was 7.48. In the highlanders it was only 7.43 two hours after ascent. During exercise the arterial P_{CO_2} was 8 mmHg lower in the lowlanders than the highlanders, but again, as in the study of Samaja *et al.* (1997) the P_{O_2} values were the same in the two groups. The calculated diffusing capacity for oxygen was substantially higher in the highlanders than lowlanders.

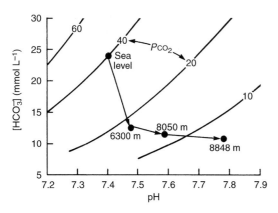

Figure 9.7   Davenport diagram showing the pH, P_{CO_2} and plasma bicarbonate concentration of arterial blood during the 1981 American Medical Research Expedition to Everest at altitudes of 6300 m, 8050 m and 8848 m (summit). Note the increasingly severe respiratory alkalosis at the extreme altitudes. The points for 8050 and 8848 m are from Pizzo. (Data from Winslow *et al.* 1984.)

9.4.5 Metabolic compensation for respiratory alkalosis

An interesting feature of the studies at extreme altitude referred to above (Winslow *et al.* 1984) is that metabolic compensation for the respiratory alkalosis appears to be extremely slow. The mean base excess measured on three subjects who were living at an altitude of 6300 m was -7.9 mmol L^{-1}. The measurements made on venous blood taken from two climbers at 8050 m gave a mean value of -7.2 mmol L^{-1}, essentially the same. The 8050 m measurements were taken several days after the climbers had left Camp 2 at 6300 m, and the data therefore suggest that metabolic compensation was proceeding extremely slowly despite the fact that the P_{CO_2} had fallen considerably. For example, the mean P_{CO_2} at 6300 m was 18.4 mmHg, at 8050 m 11.0 mmHg, and at 8848 m (summit) 7.5 mmHg. The last value was obtained from only one subject.

The reason for the very slow change in bicarbonate concentration at these great altitudes is unclear. One possible factor is chronic dehydration. Blume et al. (1984) measured serum osmolality at sea level, 5400 m and 6300 m in 13 subjects of the expedition and showed that the mean value rose from 290 ± 1 mmol kg^{-1} at sea level to 295 ± 2 at 5400 m, and to 302 ± 4 at 6300 m. This volume depletion occurred despite adequate fluids to drink and a reasonably normal lifestyle. An interesting feature of the fluid balance studies was that plasma arginine vasopressin (AVP) concentrations remained unchanged from sea level to 6300 m despite the hyperosmolality. A possible factor in the volume depletion was the increased insensible loss of fluid at these great altitudes as a result of hyperventilation. However, the failure of the vasopressin levels to change suggests that there was some abnormality of body fluid regulation.

It is known that the kidney is slow to correct an alkalosis in the presence of volume depletion. It appears that when given the option of correcting fluid balance or correcting acid–base balance, the kidney gives a higher priority to fluid balance. In order to correct the respiratory alkalosis, bicarbonate ion excretion must be increased (or reabsorption decreased) and this entails the loss of a cation which inevitably aggravates the hyperosmolality. This would explain the reluctance of the kidney to correct a respiratory alkalosis in the presence of volume depletion.

A different explanation was offered by Gonzalez et al. (1990) when they studied the slow metabolic compensation of respiratory alkalosis in a chronically hypoxic rat model. They found that the rate of metabolic compensation was indeed slower than in acute hypoxia, and they attributed this to the lower plasma bicarbonate concentration resulting from chronic hypoxia. They argued that, because proton secretion and reabsorption of bicarbonate are functions of the bicarbonate load offered to the renal proximal tubule, it is probable that the slower increase in bicarbonate excretion of the chronically hypoxic animals was ultimately the result of the lower plasma bicarbonate concentration.

10

Peripheral tissues

SUMMARY

The movement of oxygen from the peripheral capillaries to the mitochondria is the final link in the oxygen cascade. In muscle cells, the diffusion of oxygen may be facilitated by the presence of myoglobin, and it is possible that convection also occurs in the cytoplasm of some cells. There is good evidence that the P_{O_2} in the immediate vicinity of the mitochondria of many cells is very low, of the order of 1 mmHg. Many investigators believe that much of the pressure drop from the capillary to the mitochondria occurs very close to the capillary wall because of the limited surface area available for diffusion. This leads to the conclusion that the diffusion distance from the capillary wall to the mitochondria is relatively unimportant as a barrier to oxygen transport. This diffusion distance is decreased at high altitude, mainly because of the reduction in diameter of the muscle fibers. There is also an increase in myoglobin concentration and mitochondrial density at moderate altitudes. At extreme altitudes, mitochondrial volume in human skeletal muscle is decreased. Increases in the concentration of oxidative enzymes are seen at moderate altitudes, as is the case following training at sea level. The reverse occurs at extreme altitudes, where oxidative enzymes are decreased.

10.1 INTRODUCTION

The diffusion of oxygen from the peripheral capillaries to the mitochondria, and its subsequent utilization by these organelles, constitutes the final link of the oxygen cascade which begins with the inspiration of air. Despite its critical importance, many uncertainties remain concerning the changes that occur in peripheral tissues both in acclimatized lowlanders and in the adaptation of high altitude natives. An obvious reason for this paucity of knowledge is the difficulty of studying peripheral tissues in intact humans. Much of our information necessarily comes from measurements on experimental animals exposed to low barometric pressures, though some additional studies have been made on tissue biopsies in humans.

It is probable that tissue factors play an important role in the remarkable tolerance of high altitude natives to exercise at high altitude. As was pointed out in Chapter 5, people born at high altitude often have a reduced ('blunted') ventilatory response to hypoxia. At first sight this is counterproductive because it will result in a lower alveolar P_{O_2}, and therefore a lower arterial P_{O_2}, other things being equal. However, Samaja *et al.* (1997) found that the arterial P_{O_2} and oxygen saturation (estimated from earlobe blood) were the same in a group of Caucasians and Sherpas at altitudes of 3400 m, 5050 m and 6450 m, despite the fact that the Sherpas had a higher arterial P_{CO_2}. Similar findings were reported in Bolivian highlanders who were studied at an altitude of 5260 m by Wagner *et al.* (2002) who sampled arterial blood directly. This suggests an improved efficiency of oxygen transfer in the lung, and may be linked to the higher pulmonary diffusing capacity of high altitude natives. However, even if the arterial P_{O_2} is the same in highlanders as lowlanders, the better exercise performance of the former at high altitude suggests that there are important adaptations within the tissues of which we are ignorant.

The present chapter overlaps with others to some extent. The principles of diffusion of gases through tissues were dealt with in Chapter 6, and there is a discussion in Chapter 11 of how diffusion limitation in peripheral tissues may limit oxygen delivery during exercise. This topic is also alluded to in Chapter 12 in the discussion of limiting factors at extreme altitudes.

10.2 HISTORICAL

Early physiologists interested in high altitude did not attach much importance to tissue changes. For example, Paul Bert in *La Pression Barométrique* hardly refers to the possibility of tissue acclimatization, although he deals at some length with changes in respiration and circulation. At one point he speculates with his dry wit on whether the metabolism of high altitude natives is different from that of lowlanders:

> . . . just as a Basque mountaineer furnished with a piece of bread and a few onions makes expeditions which require of the member of the Alpine Club who accompanies him the absorption of a pound of meat, so it may be that the dwellers in high places finally lessen the consumption of oxygen in their organism, while keeping at their disposal the same quantity of vital force, either for the equilibrium of temperature, or the production of work. Thus we could explain the acclimatization of individuals, of generations, of races. (Bert 1878, p. 1004 in the 1943 translation)

Incidentally, we now know that the oxygen requirements of a given amount of work are no different at high altitude compared with sea level, or in high altitude natives compared with lowlanders. Bert goes on,

> But we should consider not only the acts of nutrition, but also the stimulation, perhaps less, which an insufficiently oxygenated blood causes in the muscles, the nerves, and the nervous centers. . . .

However, he does not carry these speculations any further.

There is a delightful section where Bert suggests that there may be changes in the blood at high altitude:

> We might ask first whether, by a harmonious compensation of which general natural history gives us many examples, either by a modification in the nature or the quantity of hemoglobin or by an increase in the number of red corpuscles, his blood has become qualified to absorb more oxygen under the same volume, and thus to return to the usual standard of the seashore. (Bert 1878, p. 1000 in the 1943 translation)

He goes on to say that this hypothesis would be very easy to test, since it had recently been shown:

> that the capacity of the blood to absorb oxygen does not change after putrefaction, nothing would be easier than to collect the venous blood of a healthy vigorous man (an acclimated European or an Indian) or of an animal, defibrinate it, and send it in a well-corked flask; it would then be sufficient to shake it vigorously in the air to judge its capacity of absorption during life. (Bert 1878, p. 1008 in the 1943 translation)

This beautiful research project handed to the research community on a silver plate was taken up by Viault (1890) with exactly the results predicted by Bert. However, this project studied a change in the blood compartment of the body rather than in the peripheral tissues with which this chapter is chiefly concerned.

Following the work of Krogh (1919, 1929) on the increase in the number of open capillaries in muscle when the oxygen demands were raised by exercise, it was natural to wonder whether increased capillarization was a feature of tissue acclimatization in response to chronic hypoxia. It was subsequently reported that capillaries in the brain, heart and liver were significantly dilated and that their number was apparently increased after hypoxic exposure (Mercker and Schneider 1949, Opitz 1951). As we shall see later, some more recent measurements confirm these findings. However, other studies show that in some situations the actual number of capillaries in muscle tissue does not increase as a result of chronic hypoxia, but the intercapillary diffusion distance lessens because the muscle fibers become smaller.

Hurtado and his co-workers (1937) reported an increase in the intracellular concentration of the oxygen-carrying pigment, myoglobin, in high altitude animals. The measurements were made on dogs born and raised in Morococha (4550 m) and the increased concentrations were found in the diaphragm, myocardium and muscles of the chest wall and leg. The controls were dogs from Lima, at sea level. Since then a number of other investigators have reported increased tissue myoglobin levels at high altitude.

An increase in mitochondrial density was shown in the myocardium of cattle born and raised at high altitude by Ou and Tenney (1970). Changes in mitochondrial enzymes in muscle of high altitude natives were reported by Reynafarje (1962). He found alterations in the enzyme systems NADH-oxidase, NADPH-cytochrome c-reductase, $NAD[P]^+$ transhydrogenase and others. These measurements were made on muscle biopsies taken from permanent residents of Cerro de Pasco in Peru at an altitude of 4400 m. The sea level controls were residents of Lima.

10.3 DIFFUSION IN PERIPHERAL TISSUES

10.3.1 Principles

Oxygen moves from the peripheral capillaries to the mitochondria, and carbon dioxide moves in the opposite direction by the process of diffusion. Fick's law of diffusion was discussed in section

6.4.1. It states that the rate of transfer of a gas through a sheet of tissue is proportional to the area of the tissue and to the difference in gas partial pressure between the two sides, and inversely proportional to the tissue thickness.

In discussing the lung, it was pointed out that the blood-gas barrier of the human lung is extremely thin, being only 0.2–0.3 mm in many places. By contrast, the diffusion distances in peripheral tissues are typically much greater. For example, the distance between open capillaries in resting muscle is of the order of 50 mm. However, during exercise, when the oxygen consumption of the muscle increases, additional capillaries open up, thus reducing the diffusion distance and increasing the capillary surface area available for diffusion. As discussed in section 6.4.1, carbon dioxide diffuses about 20 times faster than oxygen through tissues because of its much higher solubility, and therefore the elimination of carbon dioxide poses less of a problem than oxygen delivery.

Early workers believed that the movement of oxygen through tissues was by simple passive diffusion. However, it is now believed that facilitated diffusion of oxygen probably occurs in muscle cells as a result of the presence of myoglobin. This hemeprotein has a structure which resembles hemoglobin but the dissociation curve is a hyperbola, as opposed to the S-shape of the oxygen dissociation curve of whole blood (Fig. 10.1). Another major difference

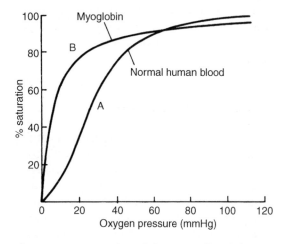

Figure 10.1 Comparison of the oxygen dissociation curves for normal human blood (curve A) and myoglobin (curve B). The P_{50} values are approximately 27 and 3 mmHg respectively. (From Roughton 1964.)

is that myoglobin takes up oxygen at a much lower Po_2 than hemoglobin, that is, it has a very low P_{50} of about 5 mmHg. This is a necessary property if the myoglobin is to be of any use in muscle cells where the tissue Po_2 is very low. Scholander (1960) and Wittenberg (1959) have shown experimentally that myoglobin can facilitate oxygen diffusion.

Other modes of oxygen transport are possible within cells. Streaming movements of cytoplasm have been observed and it is conceivable that such movements, known as 'stirring,' enhance the transport of oxygen by convection. Another hypothesis is that oxygen moves into some cells along invaginations of the lipid cell membrane in which it has a high solubility (Longmuir and Betts 1987).

There is good evidence that the Po_2 in the immediate vicinity of the mitochondria is very low in some tissues, being of the order of 1 mmHg. In fact models of oxygen transfer in tissues often assume that the mitochondrial Po_2 is so low that it can be neglected in the context of the Po_2 of the capillary blood, which is of the order of 30–50 mmHg. In measurements of suspensions of liver mitochondria *in vitro*, oxygen consumption has been shown to continue at the same rate until the Po_2 of the surrounding fluid falls to the region of 3 mmHg. Measurements of Po_2 at the sites of oxygen utilization based on the spectral characteristics of cytochromes also indicate that the Po_2 is probably less than 1 mmHg (Chance 1957, Chance *et al.* 1962). Thus it appears that the purpose of the much higher Po_2 of capillary blood is to ensure an adequate pressure for diffusion of oxygen to the mitochondria and that, at the actual sites of oxygen utilization, the Po_2 is extremely low.

10.3.2 Tissue partial pressures

A classical model to analyze the distribution of Po_2 values in tissue was described by August Krogh (1919). He considered a hypothetical cylinder of tissue around a straight, thin capillary into which blood entered with a known Po_2. As oxygen diffuses away from the capillary, oxygen is consumed by the tissue and the Po_2 falls. If simplifying assumptions are made, such as uniform consumption rate of oxygen in every part of the tissue, an equation can be written to describe the Po_2 profile (Krogh 1919, Piiper and Scheid 1986).

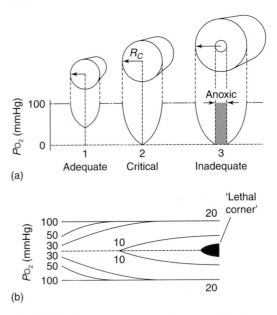

Figure 10.2   Fall in Po_2 between adjacent capillaries. In (a) three hypothetical cylinders of tissue are shown and oxygen is diffusing into these cylinders from capillaries at the periphery. In (2) the cylinder had a critical radius (R_c), and in (3) the radius of the cylinder is so large that there is an anoxic zone in the middle of the cylinder. (b) shows a section along the hypothetical cylinder of tissue. The Po_2 in the blood adjacent to the tissue is assumed to fall from 100 to 20 mmHg along the capillary. Lines of equal Po_2 are shown. Note the possibility of a 'lethal corner' in the middle of the cylinder at the venous end. (From West 1985b.)

Another model is shown in Fig. 10.2 (Hill 1928). In (a) we see a cylinder of tissue which is supplied with oxygen by capillaries at its periphery: in (1) the balance between oxygen consumption and delivery (determined by the capillary Po_2, the intercapillary distance R_c, and the oxygen consumption rate of the tissue) results in an adequate Po_2 throughout the cylinder; in (2) the intercapillary distance or the oxygen consumption has been increased until the Po_2 at one point in the tissue falls to zero. This is referred to as a critical situation. In (3) there is an anoxic region where aerobic (that is, oxygen-utilizing) metabolism is impossible. Under anoxic conditions the tissue energy requirements must be met by obligatory anaerobic glycolysis with the consequent formation of lactic acid.

The situation *along* the tissue cylinder is shown in (b). It is assumed that the Po_2 in the capillaries at the periphery of the tissue cylinder falls from 100 to 20 mmHg as shown from left to right. As a consequence the P_{O_2} in the center of the tissue cylinder falls towards the venous end of the capillary. It is clear that, on the basis of this model, the most vulnerable tissue is that furthest from the capillary at its downstream end. This was referred to as the 'lethal corner.' It is possible that this pattern of focal anoxia is responsible for some tissue damage at high altitude. For example, it may explain how some nerve cells of the brain are damaged at great altitudes causing the residual impairment of central nervous system function. This is discussed in Chapter 16.

Figure 10.2 assumes that the blood in adjacent capillaries runs in the same direction but there is evidence that this is not always the case, and that rather there is a network of capillaries with various directions of flow and many intercommunications. This concept of a network of capillaries is supported by studies emphasizing the tortuosity of capillaries around skeletal muscle cells (Potter and Groom 1983, Mathieu-Costello 1987). Although in some histological sections the capillaries of skeletal muscle appear at first sight to run chiefly parallel to the muscle fibers, this is an oversimplification. Furthermore the density of the connections increases considerably when the muscle shortens (Mathieu-Costello 1987). Thus a reasonable model of oxygen delivery to muscle is a syncytium of capillaries surrounding a tubular muscle cell.

Studies by Honig and his associates (1991) have indicated that the P_{O_2} profiles shown in Fig. 10.2 may be misleading in skeletal muscle. These investigators rapidly froze working muscles of experimental animals and then measured the degree of oxygen saturation of the intracellular myoglobin using a spectrometer with a narrow light beam. The intracellular P_{O_2} was inferred from the myoglobin oxygen saturation. These data and theoretical work by the same group suggest that the major resistance to oxygen diffusion from capillary to muscle fiber mitochondria is at the capillary–fiber interface, i.e. the thin carrier-free region including plasma, endothelium and interstitium. This in turn necessitates a large driving force (P_{O_2} difference) at that site to deliver oxygen to the muscle fibers. Some of the results of this group are shown in Fig. 10.3 where it can be seen that most of the fall of P_{O_2} apparently occurs in the immediate vicinity of the peripheral capillary and that, throughout the muscle

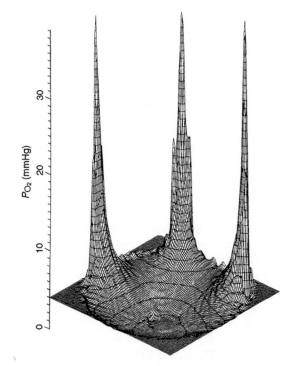

Figure 10.3 Calculated distribution of P_{O_2} around three capillaries in a heavily working red fiber of skeletal muscle. P_{O_2} contours are at intervals of 1 mmHg. There is a rapid fall of P_{O_2} in the immediate vicinity of the capillary, and within the muscle cell the P_{O_2} is relatively uniform and very low. (From Honig et al. 1991.)

cell, the P_{O_2} is remarkably uniform and very low (of the order of 1–3 mmHg). This pattern results in part from the presence of myoglobin which facilitates the diffusion of oxygen within the muscle fibers.

Evidence that the P_{O_2} in human skeletal muscle is low and remains constant in the face of increasing work levels was reported by Richardson et al. (2001). These investigators studied oxygenation in leg muscle during knee extensor exercise of a single leg. They used magnetic resonance spectroscopy of myoglobin as a measure of tissue oxygenation exploiting the fact that the P_{50} of myoglobin is about 3.2 mmHg. They found that although the calculated P_{O_2} was relatively high up to a maximal work rate of 60%, above that the intracellular P_{O_2} fell to a relatively uniform and constant value of about 3.8 mmHg in all subjects. This ingenious technique provides evidence that during relatively high levels of work, the intracellular P_{O_2} in human leg muscle is very low and remains relatively constant.

10.4 CAPILLARY DENSITY

One way to improve tissue diffusion under conditions of oxygen deprivation such as high altitude is to reduce the intercapillary distance. The technical name for the number of capillaries per unit volume of tissue is capillary volume density. It has been known since the time of Krogh (1919) that the number of open capillaries in a muscle depends on the degree of metabolic activity. During exercise additional capillaries open up, thus reducing the diffusing distance and increasing the diffusing surface area. It has been known for many years that exercise training increases the number of capillaries in skeletal muscle (Saltin and Gollnick 1983).

The effects of high altitude exposure on capillary volume density is complicated and the subject of continuing research. Early studies apparently showed increased vascularization of the brain, retina, skeletal muscle and liver of experimental animals exposed to low barometric pressures over several weeks (Mercker and Schneider 1949, Opitz 1951, Valdivia 1958, Cassin *et al.* 1971). Tenney and Ou (1970) measured the rate of loss of carbon monoxide from subcutaneous gas pockets in rats after 3 weeks of simulated exposure to 5600 m and concluded that there was a 50% increase in capillary number.

However, some of these studies were questioned by Banchero (1982) who argued that the results obtained by Valdivia (1958) and Cassin *et al.* (1971) might be influenced by technical errors. Many investigators now believe that although capillary volume density increases in skeletal muscles with exposure to high altitude, this is not caused by the formation of new capillaries, but by a reduction in size of the muscle fibers. This result has been found in guinea-pigs (Fig. 10.4) which were studied at sea level, in Denver at 1610 m, at 3900 m (in a species native to the Andes) and at a simulated altitude of 5100 m (Banchero 1982).

The same pattern has been described in acclimatized humans where muscle samples were obtained by biopsy. For example, Cerretelli and his co-workers obtained muscle biopsies on climbers immediately after they had spent several weeks attempting to climb Lhotse Shar (8398 m) in Nepal and showed that, although the capillary volume density was somewhat raised, the increase could be wholly accounted for by a reduction of muscle fiber size (Boutellier *et al.* 1983, Cerretelli *et al.*

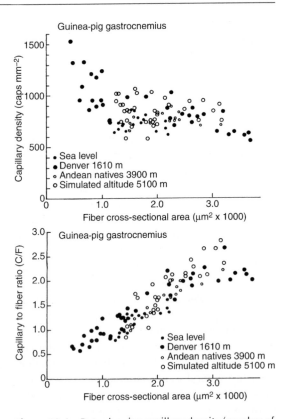

Figure 10.4 Data showing capillary density (number of capillaries per square millimeter of cross-section) and capillary/fiber ratio (number of capillaries per muscle fiber) in gastrocnemius muscle of four groups of guinea-pigs. These were studied at sea level, in Denver at 1610 m, at 3900 m (Andean natives) and at simulated altitude of 5100 m. The data are consistent with the increase in capillary/fiber ratio being explained by a decrease in cross-sectional area of the muscle fibers. (From Banchero 1982.)

1984). A similar result was found in Operation Everest II in six volunteers who were gradually decompressed to the simulated altitude of Mount Everest over a period of 40 days. Needle biopsies from the vastus lateralis showed a significant (25%) decrease in cross-sectional area of type I fibers, and a 26% decrease (nonsignificant) for type II fibers. Capillary to fiber ratios were unchanged and there was a trend (nonsignificant) towards an increase in capillary density (Green *et al.* 1989, MacDougall *et al.* 1991). Lundby *et al.* (2004b) showed that there was no change in the volume density of capillaries in skeletal muscle of lowlanders after acclimatization

Table 10.1 Comparison of tissue changes caused by training and those associated with exposure to high altitude

Tissue changes	Endurance training	High altitude
Capillary density in skeletal muscle	Increased due to new capillaries	Increased due to reduction in diameter of muscle fibers
Fiber diameter of skeletal muscle	May be increased	Decreased
Myoglobin concentration	No change in humans	Increased in skeletal, heart muscle
Muscle enzymes	No change in glycolytic, increase in oxidative	Similar changes at moderate altitudes; at extreme altitudes, increase in glycolytic and decrease in oxidative
Mitochondria	Increased volume density	Increased volume density in some animals at moderate altitude but reduced density in humans at extreme altitude Different intracellular distribution, e.g. loss of subsarcolemmal mitochondria in comparison to training

to an altitude of 4100 m. In addition there was no increase in expression of HIF 1-α or vascular endothelial growth factor (VEGF) mRNA in biopsies of skeletal muscle.

In contrast to the studies showing that new capillaries in skeletal muscle do not develop as a result of exposure to high altitude, some recent reports do find increased capillarization. For example, Mathieu-Costello et al. (1998) reported increases in the number of capillaries in flight muscles of finches at high altitude, and increased capillarity was also found in leg muscles of finches living at high altitude (Hepple et al. 1998). These investigators believe that whether increased capillary number (and mitochondrial density) occur at high altitude depends on the level of metabolic stress on the muscle, and this links with the issue of training at altitude where similar changes are seen.

Although many studies show that the number of new capillaries in skeletal muscle does not increase as a result of exposure to prolonged hypoxia, it has been suggested that there are changes in the configuration of the capillaries with increased tortuosity that would effectively increase capillary surface area and enhance gas diffusion (Appell 1978). However, this result has not been confirmed by Mathieu-Costello and Poole (Mathieu-Costello 1989, Poole and Mathieu-Costello 1990), who showed that muscle capillary tortuosity does not increase with chronic exposure to hypoxia when account is taken

of sarcomere length. These investigators believe that Appell's results may be explained by failure to control the state of contraction of the muscle. It is known that the degree of capillary tortuosity increases during muscle shortening (Mathieu-Costello 1987).

This lack of increase in the number of capillaries per muscle fiber at high altitude found in some studies should be contrasted with the increase in muscle capillarity which occurs with training. Longitudinal studies in humans have shown that exercise training increases muscle capillarity including both the capillary/fiber ratio and number of capillaries per square millimeter within several weeks (Andersen and Henriksson 1977, Brodal et al. 1977, Ingjer and Brodal 1978). Furthermore, it has been demonstrated that the increased capillary supply is proportional to the increased maximum oxygen uptake (Andersen and Henriksson 1977). The increase in capillaries is found in all fiber types provided that they are recruited during training (Andersen and Henriksson 1977, Nygaard and Nielsen 1978). If studies of acclimatization to high altitude involve increased levels of exercise, it is important to take account of this effect. Table 10.1 compares some of the tissue changes caused by training with those resulting from exposure to high altitude.

Recently there has been considerable interest in the possible role of VEGF at high altitude. VEGF is an endothelial cell-specific mitogen which is an

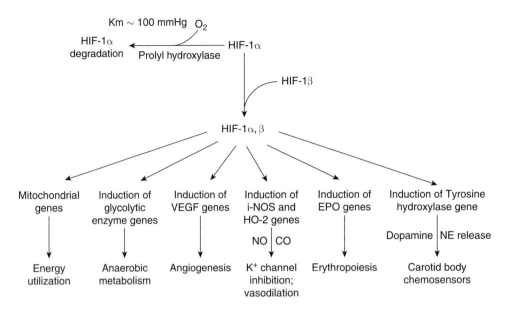

Figure 10.5 Scheme showing the functions of HIF-1α. This is continually produced but in normoxia is rapidly degraded by proline hydroxylation. In hypoxia the rate of degradation is reduced leading to the accumulation of HIF-1α. This binds to HIF-1β and activates the expression of various genes shown in the diagram. HIF-1α is therefore a master switch in hypoxia. (From Wilson *et al.* 2005.)

important mediator of hypoxia-induced angiogenesis. Hypoxia increases transcriptional induction of VEGF and also increases post-transcriptional stabilization of VEGF mRNA. VEGF increases endothelial cell proliferation and migration, and also vascular permeability. It is known to be important in the angiogenesis of embryonic development, wound healing and tumor growth (Ferrara and Davis-Smyth 1997).

Both acute hypoxia and exercise have been shown to increase VEGF mRNA in skeletal muscle of humans (Gustafsen *et al.* 1999, Hoppeler 1999) and animals (Breen *et al.* 1996). As discussed above and in Table 10.1, endurance exercise training is known to increase muscle capillarity, mitochondrial density and oxidative enzyme activity, and local tissue hypoxia has been suggested as the stimulus for these changes. Therefore induction of VEGF may be the mechanism. However, whether chronic hypoxia has a similar effect on VEGF is debated. Indeed whereas acute hypoxia increases VEGF mRNA in animal skeletal muscle, some studies show that chronic hypoxia reduces the levels below those seen in acute hypoxia. This is also true of another growth factor, TGF-β1 (Olfert *et al.* 2001).

The mechanism by which hypoxia stimulates induction of VEGF genes is through an increase in the transcriptional factor, hypoxia-inducible factor 1α (HIF-1α). This important regulator has already been referred to in Chapters 5 and 8. Its various roles in hypoxia are summarized in Fig. 10.5. In normoxia, HIF-1α is continuously formed in the cytoplasm and degraded as a result of hydroxylation by prolyl hydroxylase. However, this enzyme is inhibited in hypoxia and significant accumulation of HIF-1α occurs within 2 min. The HIF-1α combines with HIF-1β to form HIF-1 which moves into the nucleus to induce gene transcription. As Fig. 10.5 shows, a number of genes are upregulated including VEGF genes resulting in angiogenesis, EPO genes resulting in erythropoiesis, and the genes for tyrosine hydroxylase which increases the sensitivity of the carotid body. HIF-1α is therefore a master switch in the general responses of the body to hypoxia.

10.5 MUSCLE FIBER SIZE

As indicated above, one way to increase capillary density and thus reduce diffusion distance within

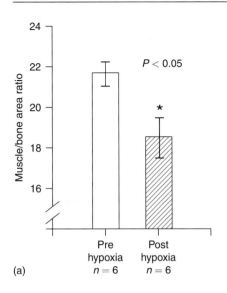

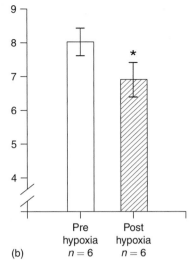

Figure 10.6 Muscle to bone ratio as determined by computed tomography for the subjects of Operation Everest II at the end of 40 days of progressive hypoxia. (a) shows the thigh site and (b) the upper arm. Values are means and SD. (From MacDougall *et al.* 1991.)

skeletal muscle is to reduce the size of the muscle fibers. There is now good evidence that this occurs during high altitude acclimatization and deterioration (Boutellier *et al.* 1983, Cerretelli *et al.* 1984, MacDougall *et al.* 1991). Figure 10.6 shows the reduction in muscle volume as measured by computed tomography in the thigh and upper arm regions of the subjects of Operation Everest II (MacDougall *et al.* 1991). This topic is discussed further in Chapters 4 and 14.

The mechanism of muscle atrophy at high altitude is not well understood. It has been suggested that one contributing factor is lack of muscular activity. Certainly, lowlanders who go to very high altitudes easily become fatigued and often spend much of their time at a reduced level of physical activity. Indeed Tilman (1952, p. 79) once remarked that a hazard of Himalayan expeditions was bedsores!

However, reduced physical activity is unlikely to be the whole story as evidenced by the experience obtained on the 1960–61 Himalayan Scientific and Mountaineering Expedition. During several months at 5800 m, the level of physical activity was well maintained with opportunities for daily skiing and yet the expedition members suffered a relentless and progressive loss of weight which averaged 0.5–1.5 kg per week (Pugh 1964c). Moreover, estimates of energy intake were made and these were apparently more than adequate for the level of activity. It is true that appetite is reduced, and it may be that gastrointestinal absorption is impaired at high altitude (Chapter 14).

However, it seems possible that there is some change in protein metabolism which results in extensive breakdown of muscle protein.

10.6 VOLUME OF MITOCHONDRIA

The muscle mitochondria are the primary sites of oxygen utilization by the body and thus constitute the final link of the oxygen cascade. In general, mitochondrial volume density (volume of mitochondria per unit volume of tissue) in skeletal muscle is related to maximal oxygen uptake and, for example, is greater in highly aerobic animals such as the horse compared with less active animals such as the cow (Hoppeler *et al.* 1987). It is also known that physical training increases mitochondrial volume density (Hollozsy and Coyle 1984).

We might therefore expect that at high altitude where maximal oxygen uptake is reduced (Chapter 11) mitochondrial density would decrease and this is generally the case. It is known that the mitochondrial volume in human skeletal muscle decreases with exposure to very high altitude. In a study on muscle biopsies of climbers returning from two Swiss expeditions to the Himalayas, mitochondrial volume decreased by 20%. This was associated with a decrease of 10% in muscle mass. The net result was a decrease in absolute mitochondrial volume of nearly 30% (Hoppeler *et al.* 1990). A feature of the electron micrographs of muscle biopsies was the presence of poorly defined material known as lipofuscin. This substance is thought to be the consequence of lipid peroxidation related to loss of mitochondria (Howald and Hoppeler 2003). In muscle biopsies of Tibetans, low levels of mitochondrial volume density were demonstrated (Kayser *et al.* 1991) and interestingly, low densities were also seen in second generation Sherpas raised at low altitude (Kayser *et al.* 1996). There was no significant increase in mitochondrial volume density in biopsies of vastus lateralis in subjects of Operation Everest II (MacDougall *et al.* 1991).

Some studies in animals have given different results. In an investigation of the mitochondrial density of the myocardium of rabbits and guinea pigs from Cerro de Pasco (4330 m) in Peru it was found that the values were the same as those at sea level (Kearney 1973). However, Ou and Tenney (1970) showed that the number of mitochondria in samples of myocardium was 40% greater in cattle born and raised at 4250 m compared with cattle at sea level. The size of individual mitochondria was found to be the same and it was argued that the increase in mitochondrial number was advantageous because it reduced the diffusion distance of the intracellular oxygen.

It may be that these discordant results can be explained by the differences between exposure to moderate and very high altitude. The increase in mitochondrial number found by Ou and Tenney (1970) was at an altitude of 4500 m, whereas the decrease in mitochondrial volume reported by Hoppeler *et al.* (1990) was in climbers who had been to altitudes over 6000 m. This is relevant to the discussion of high altitude acclimatization which occurs at moderate altitudes, and high altitude deterioration which occurs at extremely high altitudes, as discussed in Chapter 4. A general review of the response of skeletal muscle mitochondria to hypoxia is in Hoppeler *et al.* (2003).

There is an interesting difference between the mitochondrial density following exposure to high altitude on the one hand, and endurance training at sea level on the other, in their differential effects on subsarcolemmal and interfibrillar mitochondria. There is a greater loss of subsarcolemmal mitochondria at altitude, while subsarcolemmal mitochondria show a greater increase with training at sea level (Desplanches *et al.* 1993, Cerretelli and Hoppeler 1996).

10.7 MYOGLOBIN CONCENTRATION

As stated above, early studies by Hurtado and his colleagues (1937) showed increased concentrations of myoglobin in several muscles of dogs born and raised in Morococha (4550 m) in Peru. The controls were dogs in Lima at sea level. Increased myoglobin concentrations were found in the diaphragm, adductor muscles of the leg, pectoral muscles of the chest and the myocardium.

Reynafarje (1962) measured myoglobin concentrations in the sartorius muscle of healthy humans native to Cerro de Pasco (4400 m) and in other Peruvians native to sea level. Higher concentrations of myoglobin were found in the high altitude natives (7.03 mg g^{-1} tissue) than in the sea level controls (6.07 mg g^{-1}). The result was interpreted as a true high altitude effect because it was accompanied by an increased nitrogen content of the muscle, whereas the lean body mass and body water content were the same as at sea level. This point was important because in another study (Anthony *et al.* 1959), a reported increase in myoglobin content of skeletal muscle in rats could possibly have been caused by a decrease in body weight as a result of dehydration. Other studies which have shown an increase in myoglobin as a result of acclimatization to hypoxia include those of hamster heart muscle (Clark *et al.* 1952), rat heart and diaphragm (Vaughan and Pace 1956) and various guinea-pig tissues (Tappan and Reynafarje 1957).

Moore and colleagues (2002) tested the hypothesis that myoglobin allele frequencies in Tibetans are different from those in a group of sea level residents in Texas. They found that the frequency of the myoglobin 79A allele was higher in high altitude residents compared with those at sea level, although there was no relation between frequency and altitude in Tibetans. Also there was no association between myoglobin genotype and hemoglobin concentration. They concluded that high altitude Tibetans do not show novel polymorphism or selection for specific myoglobin alleles as a function of high altitude residence.

As discussed above, the chief value of myoglobin may be that it facilitates oxygen diffusion through muscle cells. However, it may also serve to buffer regional differences of P_{O_2} (Fig. 10.3) and act as an oxygen store for short periods of very severe oxygen deprivation. It has been shown that increased levels of exercise raise the myoglobin content of muscles in experimental animals (Lawrie 1953, Pattengale and Holloszy 1967). Animals that exhibit large oxygen uptakes in conditions of reduced oxygen availability, such as seals, typically have very large amounts of myoglobin (Castellini and Somero 1981). However, a study comparing trained and untrained human subjects (Jansson *et al.* 1982) and another study of short-term training in humans (Svedenhag *et al.* 1983) both failed to show any effect of training on muscle myoglobin concentration.

10.8 INTRACELLULAR ENZYMES

Enzymes are essential to all aspects of the metabolic pathways involved in energy production. Figure 10.7 summarizes the three main stages in energy metabolism:

- The conversion of glucose units (from either glucose or glycogen, known as glycolysis), amino acids and fatty acids to acetyl CoA
- The citric acid or Krebs cycle
- The electron transport chain

Because oxygen is not required for the glycolytic breakdown of glucose or glycogen, glycolysis represents an important though temporary source of energy under conditions of oxygen shortage or absence. By contrast, neither the Krebs cycle nor the electron transport chain can produce energy in the absence of oxygen.

There is evidence that chronic hypoxia caused by moderate or high altitude increases the concentration or activities of certain important enzymes involved in oxidative metabolism, but hypoxia does not appear to affect enzymes in the glycolytic pathway. However, it must be stressed that endurance exercise training also causes profound changes in the oxidative enzyme systems and it is difficult to maintain a given level of physical activity during exposure to chronic hypoxia. Similarly, it is also difficult to match sea level residents with residents at altitude with respect to physical activity.

One of the first studies of the enzymatic activity of human muscle at high altitude was that by Reynafarje (1962). The measurements were made on biopsies taken from the sartorius muscles of natives

of Cerro de Pasco (4400 m) and these were compared with biopsies from residents of Lima at sea level. Reynafarje measured the activities of enzymes of glycolysis (lactate dehydrogenase), Krebs cycle (isocitrate dehydrogenase), and the electron transport chain (NADH and NADPH-cytochrome c-reductase and $NAD[P]^+$ transhydrogenase). In this study Reynafarje found that the activities of NADH-oxidase, NADPH-cytochrome c-reductase and $NAD[P]^+$ transhydrogenase were significantly increased in the altitude residents.

Harris *et al.* (1970) reported on the levels of succinate dehydrogenase (Krebs cycle) and lactate dehydrogenase (glycolysis) activity in myocardial homogenates from guinea-pigs, rabbits and dogs indigenous to high altitude (4380 m) and compared the measurements with those made on the same species at sea level. They found a consistent increase in the activity of succinate dehydrogenase in the high altitude animals but no significant difference in lactate dehydrogenase. Ou and Tenney (1970) also found increased levels of succinate dehydrogenase and several enzymes of the electron transport chain including cytochrome oxidase, NADH-oxidase and NADH-cytochrome c-reductase in high altitude cattle.

In contrast to the effects of moderately high altitude (4000–5000 m), it appears that extreme altitude (above 6000 m) may cause a reduction in the activity of certain enzymes. The effect of exposure to extreme altitude on muscle enzyme systems has been studied by taking muscle biopsies from climbers before and after the Swiss expeditions to Lhotse Shar in 1981 (Cerretelli 1987) and Mount Everest in 1986 (Howald *et al.* 1990) and also from experimental subjects before and after prolonged decompression during Operation Everest II (Green *et al.* 1989). All of these studies reported decreased activities of oxidative enzymes. Results on three subjects from the Lhotse Shar expedition suggest that extreme altitude reduces the activity of both Krebs cycle (succinate dehydrogenase) and glycolytic (phosphofructokinase and lactate dehydrogenase) enzymes (Cerretelli 1987). In a more comprehensive study of seven climbers from the Swiss 1986 expedition, reduced activity of enzymes of the Krebs cycle (citrate synthase, malate dehydrogenase) and electron transport chain (cytochrome oxidase) were reported (Howald *et al.* 1990). In contrast to the

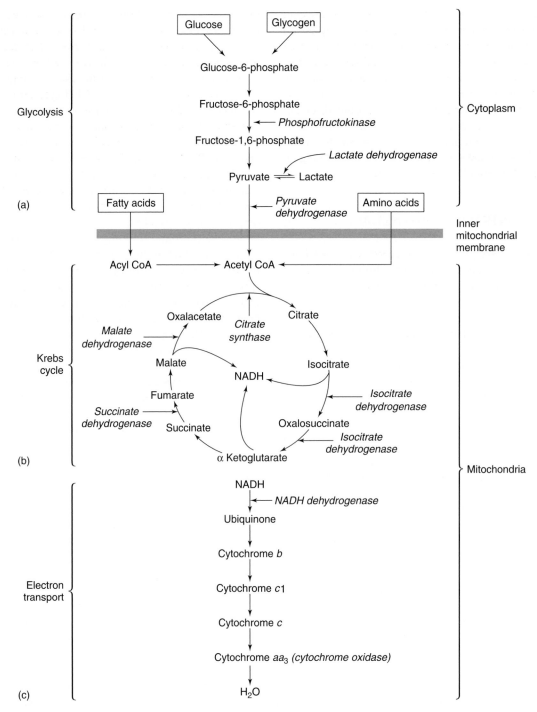

Figure 10.7   Major energy-yielding pathways in muscle. The principal controlling enzymes are indicated. Altitude or hypoxic exposure and exercise training do not affect glycolytic capacity appreciably but cause substantial increases in oxidative capacity as demonstrated by augmented mitochondrial volume in some species and activity of major enzymes of the citric acid cycle and the electron transport chain.

Lhotse Shar study, this latter study found increases in enzyme activities of glycolysis. In Operation Everest II, significant reductions were found in succinate dehydrogenase (21%), citrate synthase (37%) and hexokinase (53%) at extreme altitudes (Green *et al.* 1989).

Interestingly, the enhanced capacity for oxidative metabolism found in the face of an unchanged glycolytic potential after high altitude (below 5000 m) exposure is qualitatively similar to the changes found in skeletal muscle after endurance exercise training (Holloszy and Coyle 1984). This observation supports the notion that tissue hypoxia may be responsible for the changes in mitochondrial density and oxidative enzyme capacity under both conditions. However, as pointed out earlier, there are differences between the two stresses, for example in the intracellular distribution of mitochondria.

It has been argued that the primary importance of an augmented oxidative capacity of skeletal muscle lies not in the ability to achieve a higher maximum oxygen uptake but, rather, to sustain a given submaximal oxygen uptake with less intracellular metabolic disturbance (i.e. change of ADP and inorganic phosphate (P_i), both potent stimulators of glycolysis) (Gollnick and Saltin 1982, Holloszy and Coyle 1984, Dudley *et al.* 1987). Thus, for strenuous exercise where fatigue is associated with depletion of muscle glycogen stores, an augmented muscle oxidative capacity enables a given oxygen uptake to be sustained at lower intracellular ADP and P_i concentrations. Consequently, muscle glycogen stores would be conserved and fat oxidation would contribute proportionally more to the energetic output of the muscle, resulting in an enhanced endurance capacity (Holloszy and Coyle 1984, Dudley *et al.* 1987). In conclusion, these changes in tissue enzymes (with the exception of those at extreme altitudes) are consistent with the assumption that the muscles are improving their ability for oxidative metabolism in the face of oxygen deprivation or deficiency.

Exercise

SUMMARY

In the face of the reduction in the inspired P_{O_2} encountered at high altitude, exercise in this environment makes enormous demands on the transfer of oxygen from the air to the blood in the lung and eventually to the mitochondria of the exercise muscles. Consequently, reduced exercise tolerance is one of the most obvious features of exposure to high altitude. Maximal exercise is accompanied by extremely high ventilations (measured at body temperature and pressure); these can approach $200 \, L \, min^{-1}$ at extreme altitudes, which is close to the maximum voluntary ventilation. Diffusion-limitation of oxygen transfer across the blood-gas barrier is also an important limiting factor. As a result, arterial P_{O_2} levels typically fall greatly as the work rate is increased. Some additional ventilation–perfusion inequality also often develops, possibly because of subclinical pulmonary edema. Maximal cardiac output is reduced at high altitude, although in acclimatized subjects, the relationship between cardiac output and work rate is the same as at sea level, and oxygen consumption for a given work rate is independent of altitude. Maximal oxygen consumption in acclimatized subjects falls from about 4-5 L min^{-1} at sea level to just over 1 L min^{-1} at the Everest summit. Part of the reduction in $\dot{V}_{O_2,max}$ can be ascribed to diffusion limitation within the exercising muscle as well as a limited blood flow to the muscles of locomotion because of the increased demand of the respiratory muscles. Although aerobic performance is greatly impaired at high altitude, there is no change in maximal anaerobic peak power (for example, as measured by a standing jump) unless muscle mass is reduced.

11.1 INTRODUCTION

The hypoxia of high altitude puts stress on the oxygen transfer system of the body even at rest. If the oxygen requirements are further increased by exercise, the problems of oxygen delivery to the mitochondria of the working muscles are correspondingly exaggerated. Indeed, one of the most obvious consequences of going to high altitude is a reduction in both maximal and endurance exercise tolerance.

In this chapter we examine the physiology of oxygen transfer from the air to the mitochondria in the face of the reduced inspired P_{O_2}. The steps in the oxygen cascade involve the convection of air in the airways to the alveoli via pulmonary ventilation, then diffusion of oxygen across the blood-gas barrier, uptake by the pulmonary capillary blood, removal from the lung by the cardiac output, again convection of the oxygenated blood to the tissues, diffusion of oxygen from the blood to the cell to the mitochondria, and then utilization of oxygen by the cellular biochemical reactions. The present chapter synthesizes information, some of which occurs in other chapters. The subject of limitation of oxygen uptake under the conditions of extreme altitude is dealt with in Chapter 12. The literature on exercise at altitude is very extensive, and the present chapter is necessarily selective. Many monographs and reviews have been published including Margaria (1967), Cerretelli and Whipp (1980), Sutton *et al.* (1983), Sutton *et al.* (1987), Cerretelli (1992) and Wagner (1996).

11.2 HISTORICAL

A reduced exercise tolerance at high altitude has been recognized since humans began to climb high mountains. For example, extreme fatigue was often reported in the early climbs of the European Alps which, in fact, led to one of the popular theories of mountain sickness. The argument ran that the normal barometric pressure was necessary to maintain the proper articulation of the head of the femur in the acetabulum of the pelvis, and that at high altitude, when the reduced barometric pressure did not assist this as it should, the muscles became fatigued as a result (Bert 1878, pp. 343–6).

Some of the earliest measurements of exercise at high altitude were made by Zuntz, Durig and their colleagues in the first few years of the twentieth century (Durig 1911, Zuntz *et al.* 1906). For example, Zuntz showed that there was a decline in oxygen consumption but increase in ventilation at high altitude when trekkers walked at the speed that they normally adopted in an Alpine setting. Douglas, Haldane and their colleagues (1913) studied muscular exercise during walking uphill on Pikes Peak during the Anglo-American Expedition of 1911. They made the important observation that a given amount of work required the same amount of oxygen consumption at 4300 m altitude as at sea level.

Vivid descriptions of the great difficulties of exercise at very high altitudes were common in the early Everest expeditions. Indeed the accounts of the 1921 reconnaissance expedition (Howard-Bury 1922), and the expeditions of 1922 (Bruce 1923) and 1924 (Norton 1925) make graphic and compelling reading even today. Typical is E.F. Norton's account of his climb to nearly 8600 m without supplementary oxygen in 1924 (Norton 1925). He wrote

> our pace was wretched. My ambition was to do 20 consecutive paces uphill without a pause to rest and pant elbow on bent knee, yet I never remember achieving it – 13 was nearer the mark.

Norton was accompanied to just below that altitude by the surgeon T.H. Somervell who subsequently wrote 'for every step forward and upward, 7 to 10 complete respirations were required' (Somervell 1925).

Of course, these observations were by lowlanders who were at extreme altitudes after relatively short periods of time for acclimatization. It is interesting to compare the observations of Barcroft who led an expedition at about the same time (winter of 1921–22) to Cerro de Pasco at an altitude of 4330 m in the Peruvian Andes (Barcroft *et al.* 1923). Naturally, this was at a considerably lower altitude than near the summit of Mount Everest. Nevertheless, the lowlanders were amazed at the capacity of the high altitude residents for physical work, and they were astonished at the popularity of energetic sports such as football (soccer), a phenomenon experienced by this author (R.B.S.) while doing research on the high altitude natives of Ollague in Northern Chile in 1986. The contrast between poorly acclimatized lowlanders and native high altitude dwellers, who had been at the same altitude for perhaps generations, was very clear.

Valuable findings on exercise at high altitude were made during the 1935 International High Altitude Expedition to Chile (Keys 1936). The expedition members showed that their own maximal working capacity fell as the altitude increased in spite of acclimatization. Christensen (1937) made measurements up to an altitude of 5340 m using a bicycle ergometer and confirmed the findings of Douglas *et al.* (1913) that the efficiency of muscle exercise was independent of altitude, that is that the oxygen consumption for a given work level was the same. In addition he showed that although exercise ventilation measured at body temperature, ambient pressure, saturated with water vapour (BTPS) was greatly increased at high altitudes, ventilation expressed at standard temperature and pressure, dry gas (STPD) was essentially independent of altitude over a wide range of altitudes and work rates.

An interesting observation was made by Edwards who documented a curious paradox about lactate levels in the blood on exercise. Generally, exhaustive exercise is accompanied by relatively high blood lactate levels, especially in unfit subjects, as the muscles outstrip their capacity for aerobic work and resort to anaerobic glycolysis. It would be natural to expect this to occur to an extreme extent at high altitude, as it does in acute hypoxia, but Edwards found the opposite. Exhaustive work at very high altitude was associated with very low levels of blood lactate (Edwards 1936). Dill and colleagues (1931) had previously seen the same phenomenon in a similar series of measurements.

The expedition members were also surprised by the tolerance of the miners for energetic physical activity at the Aucanquilcha mine which they believed was at an altitude of 5800 m. We now know that the mine is actually higher, the altitude being 5950 m. The exercise level of the miners is indeed astonishing as they break large pieces of sulfur ore (caliche) with sledgehammers (McIntyre 1987). The miners are predominantly Bolivians who were born at moderately high altitudes and since most of them live at Amincha (altitude 4200 m), they have a considerable degree of high altitude acclimatization.

In preparation for the British Mount Everest Expedition of 1953, Pugh measured oxygen uptakes on climbers in the field near Cho Oyu in the Nepal Himalaya in 1952. These data were then used to determine the amount of oxygen to be carried by the 1953 expedition during which Pugh made further measurements of exercise physiology (Pugh 1958). He subsequently extended this program in the ambitious Himalayan Scientific and Mountaineering Expedition (Silver Hut) of 1960–61 in which several physiologists, including authors J.B.W. and J.S.M., spent the winter in a prefabricated hut at an altitude of 5800 m (Pugh 1962). Further measurements of maximal oxygen consumption were carried out in the spring when the expedition moved to Mount Makalu (8481 m) and a bicycle ergometer was erected

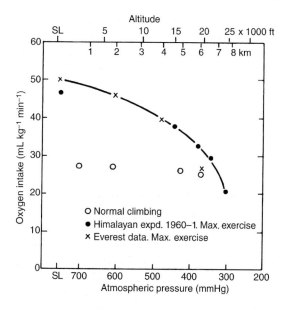

Figure 11.1 $\dot{V}_{O_2,max}$ against barometric pressure in acclimatized subjects (closed circles, crosses) as reported by Pugh et al. (1964). Data from normal climbing rates are also shown (open circles).

on the Makalu Col (altitude 7440 m) (Fig. 1.6). Those measurements of maximal work remain the highest ever made (Pugh et al. 1964). The data assembled by Pugh and his co-workers (Fig. 11.1) were of great interest because they predicted that, near the summit of Mount Everest, the maximal oxygen uptake would be very close to the basal oxygen requirements, and therefore it seemed problematic whether man could ever reach the summit without supplementary oxygen (West and Wagner 1980).

Additional measurements of maximal oxygen consumption were made by Cerretelli during an Italian expedition to Mount Everest in 1973 (Cerretelli 1976a). All the data were obtained at Base Camp (altitude 5350 m) but they included measurements on climbers who had been above 8000 m. One of the many interesting observations was the failure of the maximal oxygen uptake of acclimatized subjects at 5350 m to return to the sea level value when pure oxygen was breathed. The explanation of this finding, also made by Pugh and others, is still controversial but is certainly multifactorial, involving in part some deterioration of oxidative function at the tissue level, as well as a decrease in muscle power from muscle cell atrophy that has long been recognized.

The issue of whether the partial pressure of oxygen at the summit of Mount Everest was sufficient for man to reach it without supplementary oxygen was finally answered in 1978 by Reinhold Messner and Peter Habeler. However, their accounts make it clear that neither had much in reserve (Habeler 1979, Messner 1979). The intriguing question of how the body is just able to transport sufficient oxygen to the exercising muscles under these conditions of profound hypoxia is considered in detail in Chapter 12.

During the 1981 American Medical Research Expedition to Everest (AMREE), extensive measurements of maximal oxygen uptake were made in the main laboratory camp, altitude 6300 m. However, data were also obtained for exercise at higher altitudes by giving the well-acclimatized subjects inspired mixtures containing low concentrations of oxygen. For example, when the inspired P_{O_2} was only 42.5 mmHg, corresponding to that on the summit of Mount Everest, the measured maximal oxygen consumption was just over 1 L min^{-1}; whereas, at sea level in the same subjects the values were around 5 L min^{-1} (West *et al.* 1983a). Although this is very low and equivalent to that of someone walking slowly on the level, it is apparently just sufficient to explain how a climber can reach the summit without supplementary oxygen (Chapter 12).

A further extensive series of exercise measurements were made during Operation Everest II in the autumn of 1985 (Houston *et al.* 1987). The eight subjects spent 40 days in a large low-pressure chamber being gradually decompressed to the barometric pressure existing at the summit of Mount Everest, and a series of measurements of maximal exercise were made using a bicycle ergometer. The measured oxygen consumptions agreed well with those found in the field by the 1981 expedition (Sutton *et al.* 1988), but Operation Everest II had the great additional advantage that many invasive measurements could be made which were impracticable in the field. These included extensive measurements of pulmonary vascular pressures, muscle volume, and muscle biopsies (Sutton *et al.* 1987).

11.3 VENTILATION

Exercise at high altitude is accompanied by very high levels of ventilation. Indeed this was one of

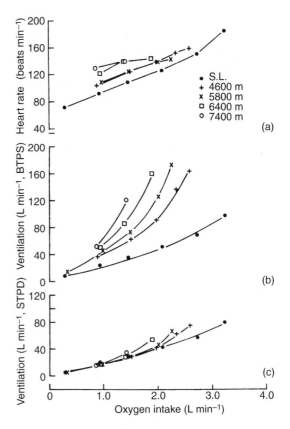

Figure 11.2   Relationship between ventilation, both BTPS and STPD, and oxygen uptake at various altitudes. Heart rate is also shown. (From Pugh *et al.* 1964.)

the most obvious features of climbing at extreme altitudes in the early Everest expeditions as evidenced by the quotations from Norton and Somervell in the preceding section.

Ventilation is normally expressed at body temperature, ambient pressure, and with the gas saturated with water vapour (BTPS). This is because the volumes of gas moved then correspond to the volume excursions of the chest and lungs. Ventilation can also be expressed at standard temperature and pressure for dry gas (STPD). These volumes are very much smaller at high altitude and bear no obvious relationship to the actual chest movements. However, the oxygen consumption and carbon dioxide output are traditionally expressed in these units so that the values are independent of altitude.

For a given work level, the ventilation expressed as BTPS increases at high altitude. Typical results are shown in Fig. 11.2b which shows data obtained during the 1960–61 Silver Hut Expedition (Pugh *et al.* 1964). Figure 11.2c shows ventilations expressed as STPD. Here the values also tend to be somewhat higher than those measured at sea level, especially at work levels approaching the maximum for the altitude, but the differences are clearly much less than for ventilation expressed as BTPS.

Ventilation (BTPS) can reach extremely high levels as evidenced by data obtained during the 1981 AMREE at an altitude of 6300 m (P_B 351 mmHg). In eight subjects who exercised at a work rate of 1200 kg min^{-1} the mean ventilation (BTPS) was 207 L min^{-1} with a mean respiratory frequency of 62 breaths min^{-1}. These values were for a mean oxygen consumption of 2.31 L min^{-1} and correspond to a ventilatory equivalent (V_E/V_{O_2}, i.e. the amount of expired ventilation dedicated to a given metabolic rate) almost four times greater than sea level. In spite of a lower gas density which will decrease the work of breathing a modest amount, this degree of ventilation still results in a much greater work of breathing for any given energy expenditure (Schoene, 2005, Cibella *et al.* 1999). These levels of ventilation are approaching the maximal voluntary ventilation (MVV), that is the maximal amount of air that can be moved per minute by breathing in and out as rapidly and deeply as possible, usually measured over 12 s.

When climbing at high altitude, the body must decide how to apportion its energy output between the muscles of locomotion and those of respiration which require a precise amount of perfusion to deliver oxygen. Cibella *et al.* (1999) demonstrated in subjects that in spite of the lower gas density, there was substantially greater energy expenditure for respiration at high altitude than at sea level. The respiratory muscles in this study, therefore, required a greater proportion of cardiac output for a given workload at high than low altitude, thus depriving the locomotory muscles of perfusion, 5.5% versus 26% at low and high (5000 m) altitude respectively. An increase in resistance of leg muscle blood flow in deference to flow to the respiratory muscles at high levels of work have been shown at low altitude (Barclay 1986, Babcock *et al.* 1995, Harms *et al.* 1997, Wetter *et al.* 1999) and can only be assumed to be greater at higher altitude where respiration is much greater. It is primarily the diaphragm which has been shown both at low and high altitude to compete for the limited blood flow (Marciniuk

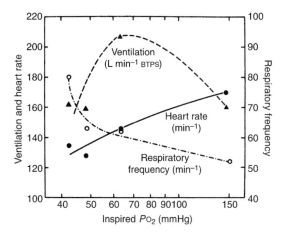

Figure 11.3 Maximal ventilation (BTPS), maximal respiratory frequency, and maximal heart rate plotted against inspired P_{O_2} on a log scale. This scale was chosen only because otherwise the high-altitude points fall very close together. Note that both maximal ventilation and heart rate fall at extreme altitudes because work levels become so low. However, respiratory frequency continues to increase. (From West *et al.* 1983a.) (1 Torr = 1 mmHg)

et al. 1994). Recent work by Lundby *et al.* (2006) demonstrated a persistent decrease in blood flow to the lower extremities in lowlanders even after eight weeks of acclimatization to 4100 m, suggesting this pattern as an important factor in limiting maximal exercise at very high altitudes. Part of this decrease in blood flow can be restored in this same population when hemoglobin and presumed blood viscosity are decreased with isovolumic hemodilution (Calbert *et al.* 2002).

It is interesting that these extremely high levels of ventilation are not seen at the highest altitudes. For example, when two subjects on the 1981 expedition were given a 14% oxygen mixture to breathe at an altitude of 6300 m (inspired P_{O_2} 42.5 mmHg) to simulate the summit of Everest, the maximal exercise ventilation was only 162 L min^{-1}. A reasonable explanation for the lower exercise ventilation is that the work rate was very much lower, being only 450 kg min^{-1} as opposed to 1200 at the altitude of 6300 m while breathing air. Another possibility is that, as mentioned above, the respiratory muscles were limited by the severe hypoxemia and a limitation of blood flow. Figure 11.3 shows maximal exercise ventilation plotted against inspired P_{O_2} (dashed line), and there is a maximal value although there are only four points on the curve. A similar pattern was found during the 1960–61 Silver Hut Expedition. For example, the maximal exercise ventilation at 5800 m had a mean value of 173 L min^{-1}. At an altitude of 6400 m this had fallen to 161, while at an altitude of 7440 m, the value was only 122 L min^{-1}. Corresponding to the fall in maximal exercise ventilation, the $\dot{V}O_{2,max}$ decreased from 1200 kg min^{-1} at 5800 m, to 900 kg min^{-1} at 6400 m, to 600 kg min^{-1} at 7400 m. These extremely high exercise ventilations are facilitated, only in part, by the reduced work of breathing as a result of the lowered density of the air at high altitude. The reduced density also results in an increased maximal voluntary ventilation (or maximum breathing capacity) as altitude is increased (Cotes 1954). For example, Cotes showed that the maximal voluntary ventilation (BTPS) increased from 158 at sea level to 197 L min^{-1} at a simulated altitude of 5180 m in a low-pressure chamber. In a further study, a mean value of 203 L min^{-1} was observed at a simulated altitude of 8250 m (Cotes 1954). The increase in MVV was compatible with the hypothesis that the work of maximum breathing remains constant at high altitude. The reduction in the work of breathing at high altitude caused by the change in gas density was also analyzed by Petit *et al.* (1963).

Oxygen breathing reduces exercise ventilation for a given work rate at high altitude. However, as Fig. 11.4 shows, the ventilations do not return to the sea level values but are intermediate between the high altitude and sea level values for ambient air. This observation is probably secondary to the increased sensitivity of the carotid body which is the primary organ of ventilatory acclimatization (see Chapter 5).

The pattern of breathing during exercise at high altitude is characterized by very high frequencies and relatively small tidal volumes. Somervell's observation referred to in section 11.2 of 7 to 10 complete respirations per step is evidence for that. The highest measurements of respiratory frequency and tidal volume yet made were those on Pizzo during the 1981 Everest expedition (West *et al.* 1983a). He climbed for about 7 min at an altitude of 8300 m (P_B 271 mmHg) while measuring his ventilation with a turbine flow meter, and the output was registered on a slow-running tape recorder. During the middle 4 min of this period, his mean respiratory

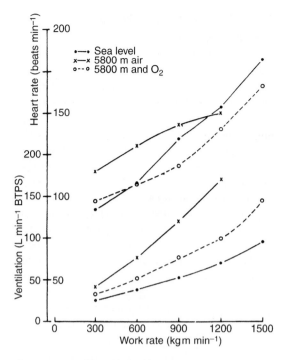

Figure 11.4 Effect of breathing oxygen at sea level pressure on ventilation and heart rate in acclimatized subjects at 5800 m. The points are mean values from two subjects. (From Pugh *et al.* 1964.)

frequency was 86 ± 2.8 (SD) breaths per minute, mean tidal volume was 1.26 L, and mean ventilation was 107 L min^{-1} at BTPS. Thus, his breathing was shallow and extremely rapid. Reference has already been made to the measurements of maximal exercise at an inspired P_{O_2} of 42.5 mmHg corresponding to that on the Everest summit which was obtained by making the subjects inspire 14% oxygen at an altitude of 6300 m. For two subjects, the mean respiratory frequency was 80 breaths min^{-1}. This tachypneic response of a low tidal volume, high frequency pattern is the body's attempt to minimize the overall work of breathing.

This pattern of breathing is consistent with the very powerful hypoxic drive via the peripheral chemoreceptors. As pointed out in Chapter 5, it is remarkable that the hypoxic drive is so strong under these conditions because the arterial P_{CO_2} is less than 10 mmHg and the arterial pH is over 7.7. A very low P_{CO_2} and high pH normally inhibit ventilation, but the over-riding hyperventilatory stimulus is the marked hypoxemia.

11.4 VENTILATION–PERFUSION RELATIONSHIPS

For many years, it was believed that the only change in ventilation–perfusion relationships at high altitude was a more uniform topographical distribution of blood flow. This is caused by the increased pulmonary arterial pressure as a result of hypoxic pulmonary vasoconstriction (Chapter 7). For example, measurements with radioactive xenon have shown that the topographical differences of blood flow between apex and base of the upright lung are reduced at an altitude of 3100 m (Dawson 1972). As discussed in Chapter 12, measurements by Wagner and his co-workers show a broadening of the distribution of ventilation–perfusion ratios during high levels of hypoxic exercise, the cause of which is still uncertain. The change in the distribution of ventilation and perfusion demonstrates an increase in blood flow to poorly ventilated lung units, seen in normal subjects who are exercising while acutely exposed to hypoxia in a low pressure chamber (Gale et al. 1985), exercising normal subjects who are inhaling low oxygen mixtures (Hammond et al. 1986), and normal subjects during a 40-day exposure to low pressure in a chamber during Operation Everest II (Wagner et al. 1988b). Evidence from this last study suggests that the ventilation–perfusion abnormalities are most likely to be seen in poorly acclimatized subjects after a rapid ascent. In general, the abnormalities were most marked at the most severe levels of hypoxia, and at the heaviest exercise levels.

Acclimatization does convey a modest improvement in gas exchange as noted by Wagner et al. (2002) and Lundby et al. (2004). They studied lowlanders before and after ascent and over 8 weeks at 4100 m and found an improvement in exercise Sa,O_2 that was secondary both to a modest improvement in the $(A - a)DO_2$ as well as ongoing ventilatory adaptation. On the other hand, litter greyhounds exposed to high altitude for 5 months had higher diffusion capacities than control dogs, suggesting that actual improvement in pulmonary function and gas exchange from the effect of high altitude requires that the exposure needs to be during the somatic maturation (McDonough et al. 2006.) These findings support previous impressions in humans that actual changes in pulmonary function

and gas exchange can only occur during the formative growth phase. The study by Lundby et al. (2004) supports the findings of improved gas exchange in lowlanders during altitude exposure which still could not achieve that of high altitude natives.

A reasonable hypothesis to explain the impairment in gas exchange is that these changes are caused in some way by subclinical pulmonary edema which results in inequality of ventilation. As discussed in Chapter 19, high altitude pulmonary edema is a well-known complication of going to high altitude. The likely mechanism is uneven hypoxic pulmonary vasoconstriction, which allows some capillaries to be exposed to high pressure with subsequent damage to their walls (West and Mathieu-Costello 1992). The increase in pulmonary artery pressure is exaggerated during heavy exercise (Groves et al. 1987). There is further evidence of microvascular leak in the extremities of unacclimatized individuals which was accentuated during exercise which suggests that a similar process occurs in the lung (Bauer et al. 2006.)

11.5 DIFFUSION

As discussed in Chapter 6, there is strong evidence that diffusion limitation of oxygen transfer in the lung occurs during exercise at high altitude. This is the primary reason for the fall in arterial PO_2 and arterial oxygen saturation which has been consistently observed. Analysis of the situation at extreme altitude indicates that the diffusing capacity of the blood-gas barrier is one of the chief limiting factors for maximal exercise (Chapter 12).

There is no evidence that the diffusing capacity of the blood-gas barrier increases during acclimatization to high altitude in normal subjects, whereas high altitude natives demonstrate higher diffusion capacities compared to lowlanders (Wagner et al. 2002). Measurements from the 1960–61 Silver Hut Expedition showed that the diffusing capacity of the blood-gas barrier for a given level of exercise was the same as at sea level (West 1962). Overall pulmonary diffusing capacity for carbon monoxide increased by 19% at an altitude of 5800 m, but this could be attributed to the more rapid rate of combination of carbon monoxide with oxygen because of the low prevailing PO_2. The volume of blood in the pulmonary capillaries as determined by measuring the diffusing capacity at two values of alveolar Po_2 showed no change or possibly a slight fall. This may have been due to hypoxic pulmonary vasoconstriction.

These results also imply that, in acclimatized subjects, the transit time for red cells in the pulmonary capillaries at a given work level is approximately the same as at sea level. The transit time of the pulmonary capillary blood is given by the pulmonary capillary blood volume divided by the cardiac output (Roughton 1945). As discussed in Chapter 7, there is good evidence that in acclimatized lowlanders at high altitude, the cardiac output for a given work level is the same as at sea level (Pugh 1964, Reeves *et al.* 1987). Thus, since both the pulmonary capillary blood volume and the cardiac output are essentially unchanged, this indicates that the transit time through the pulmonary capillaries will also be the same as at sea level, but because of the lower driving pressure for oxygen from the air to the blood, there is still not enough time for equilibration into the pulmonary capillary blood.

11.6 CARDIOVASCULAR RESPONSES

These were discussed in Chapter 7. In non-acclimatized and poorly acclimatized lowlanders who go acutely to high altitude, cardiac output at rest and during exercise for a given work level is increased compared with sea level values. The same is true of heart rate.

In acclimatized lowlanders, cardiac output for a given work level returns to its sea level value as shown by Pugh (1964) during the 1960–61 Silver Hut Expedition, and more recently during Operation Everest II (Reeves *et al.* 1987). However, heart rate for a given level of exercise remains higher at altitude and therefore stroke volume is less. Maximum heart rate, on the other hand, decreases with duration of stay at high altitude, especially very high altitude (Lundby *et al.* 2001, 2004, 2006, Lundby and van Hall, 2001). Measurements of contractile function of the heart during Operation Everest II in exercising subjects at all altitudes showed remarkable preservation in spite of the very severe hypoxemia (Reeves *et al.* 1987).

Pulmonary artery pressures are increased during exercise at altitude compared with sea level values

at the same work level. The elevated pressures are seen in both unacclimatized (Kronenberg *et al.* 1971) and acclimatized (Groves *et al.* 1987) lowlanders, and in native highlanders (Penaloza *et al.* 1963, Lockhart *et al.* 1976). The basic cause of the pulmonary hypertension is presumably hypoxic pulmonary vasoconstriction. However, it is of considerable interest that in the subjects of Operation Everest II, the pulmonary vascular pressures did not return to normal when 100% oxygen was breathed even though the subjects had been at high altitude only 2 or 3 weeks (Groves *et al.* 1987). This indicates some structural changes (remodeling) in the pulmonary arteries in addition to hypoxic vasoconstriction even in this relatively brief time of exposure to hypobaria.

Interest in the effect of increased pulmonary vascular resistance during altitude exposure on cardiac output and thus exercise performance has generated studies on pharmacologic intervention to minimize that rise. Sildenafil, a phosphodiesterase type 5 inhibitor, potently inhibits hypoxic pulmonary vasoconstriction. Richalet *et al.* (2005a) carried out a randomized, double-blind, placebo-controlled (RDBPC) trial of sildenafil and placebo in subjects exposed for 6 days at 4350 m. Pulmonary artery pressure (PAP) rose 29% upon hypoxic exposure before medication. Sildenafil resulted in a PAP that was 6% less than sea level values, a lower alveolar–arterial oxygen difference, and a decrease on exercise performance that was less than the placebo group (Figs 11.5 and 11.6). At Everest base camp (approx. 5400 m) Ghofrani *et al.* (2004) looked at the effect of acute administration of sildenafil to subjects during exercise in another RDBPC trial and found a lower PAP, a higher Sa,O_2, and greater work capacity than on placebo. Hsu *et al.* (2006) exposed 10 cyclists to normoxia and simulated high altitude (approx. 3874 m, $FI,O_2 = 0.128$) on placebo and three doses (0, 50 and 100 mg) of sildenafil, and studied cardiac performance as well as time trial lengths of 10 km at sea level and 5 km during hypoxia. During hypoxia sildenafil resulted in an increase in stroke volume and cardiac output and a mean decrease of 15% time in the time trial time but no difference with normoxia. Of interest was the finding that there were responders (39% decrease in time trial time) and nonresponders (1% decrease). This latter finding is fascinating and reinforces the notion that, as in most physiologic responses, the PAP response

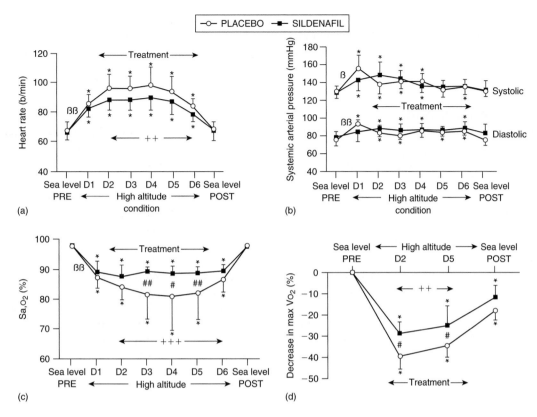

Figure 11.5 Systemic hemodynamic parameters and exercise performance. *$p < 0.05$ versus sea level pre; #$p < 0.05$, ##$p < 0.01$ sildenafil versus placebo; $p < 0.05$, $p < 0.01$ D1 versus sea level pre for the whole group; ++$p < 0.01$, +++$p < 0.001$ sildenafil versus placebo for pooled high altitude with treatment values.

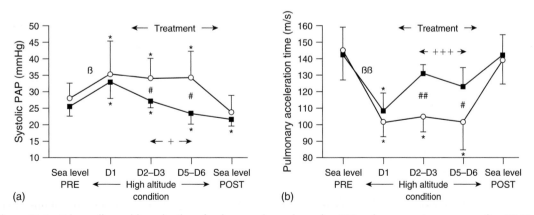

Figure 11.6 Echocardiographic evaluation of pulmonary hemodynamics. PAP: pulmonary artery pressure. *$p < 0.05$ versus sea level pre; #$p < 0.05$, ##$p < 0.01$ sildenafil (filled squares) versus placebo (open circles); $p < 0.05$, $p < 0.01$ D1 versus sea level pre for the whole group; +$p < 0.05$, +++$p < 0.001$ sildenafil versus placebo for pooled high altitude with treatment values.

to hypoxia is a genetically controlled mechanism that is different in each person. These last studies and others will spawn an important area of research in the next few years.

11.7 ARTERIAL BLOOD GASES

At high altitude, the resting pattern of a low arterial P_{O_2} and P_{CO_2} is also seen during exercise. Arterial P_{O_2} typically falls further on exercise because of diffusion limitation. In addition, at high work levels, the arterial P_{CO_2} often falls below the resting value, indicating that alveolar ventilation increases more than CO_2 production. The falling P_{CO_2} is associated with an increased respiratory exchange ratio which may rise to values over 1.2 at the highest work loads at very high altitudes (West $et\ al.$ 1983a). This represents an unsteady state since the respiratory quotient of the metabolizing tissues in a sustainable energy output cannot exceed 1.0. At sea level, such an increase in respiratory exchange ratio is often

associated with lactate production from exercising muscles as a result of anaerobic glycolysis. However, at very high altitude, blood lactate levels remain surprisingly low even following exhausting exercise (Edwards 1936, Cerretelli 1980, West 1986, Lundby $et\ al.$ 2000).

Arterial pH is near normal in well-acclimatized subjects up to altitudes of about 5400 m though Winslow obtained evidence that there is often a small degree of uncompensated respiratory alkalosis, even in native highlanders (Winslow $et\ al.$ 1981, Winslow and Monge 1987). At higher altitudes, the arterial pH at rest tends to increase, and it exceeded 7.7 in one subject on the Everest summit (West $et\ al.$ 1983b). The respiratory alkalosis is exaggerated on exercise because the arterial P_{CO_2} tends to fall and levels of blood lactate are low.

As stated in section 11.2, extensive observations that blood lactate is low in acclimatized subjects at high altitude, even during maximal work, were first made by Edwards (1936) during the 1935 International High Altitude Expedition to Chile,

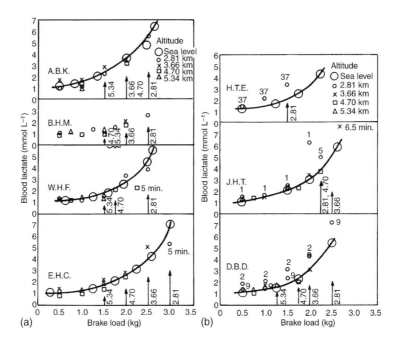

Figure 11.7   Venous blood lactate after exercise as reported by Edwards from the 1935 International High Altitude Expedition to Chile. The lines are drawn through the sea-level values. In general, lactate levels at high altitude lie on the same line, the only obvious exceptions being measurements made at the lowest altitude of 2.81 km. The small figures above these points indicate the number of days spent at that altitude and in most instances this was insufficient for acclimatization. (From Edwards 1936.)

although Dill *et al.* (1931) had obtained some data prior to that. Figure 11.7 is redrawn from Edward's paper and shows that the levels of blood lactate during exercise at high altitude (up to 5340 m) were essentially the same as at sea level. This means that the blood lactate levels for a given work level were apparently independent of tissue P_{O_2}. The only clear exceptions to this were the points shown by the open circles which were obtained at the lowest altitude of 2810 m. The days spent at altitude are shown on the abscissa, and it is clear that in most instances these data were obtained before the subject had had time to become fully acclimatized. Since maximal work capacity declines markedly with increasing altitude, the data of Fig. 11.6 imply that maximal blood lactate falls in acclimatized subjects as altitude increases.

These results have been extended by Cerretelli (1976a,b, 1980) with additional measurements made at an altitude of 6300 m on the 1981 AMREE (West *et al.* 1983a). Figure 12.5 summarizes the data on resting and maximal blood lactate (West 1986) and suggests the surprising conclusion that, after maximal exercise at altitudes exceeding 7500 m, there will be no increase in lactate in the blood at all in spite of the extreme oxygen deprivation. Possible reasons for this are discussed in more detail in Chapter 12.

11.8 PERIPHERAL TISSUES

The changes that occur in peripheral tissues at high altitude were discussed in Chapter 10. Animal studies indicate an increase in capillary density in some tissues as a result of chronic hypoxia. However, data available from human muscle biopsies indicate that the number of capillaries remains constant in acclimatized lowlanders with no increase of mRNA expression of regulatory factors for angiogenesis (VEGF) during acclimatization to 4100 m (Lundby *et al.* 2004). On the other hand, the average distance over which oxygen diffuses is reduced because the muscle fibers become smaller, perhaps secondary to ongoing oxidative damage with prolonged high altitude exposure (Lundby *et al.* 2004b). There are changes in intracellular enzymes, and some studies show an increase in muscle myoglobin which may enhance oxygen diffusion. All these

factors will play an important role in oxygen delivery and utilization during exercise.

Recently, there has been considerable interest in the possible role of oxygen diffusion from capillaries to mitochondria as a factor limiting exercise at high altitude. Traditionally, many physiologists have argued that the power of working muscles at high altitude is determined by the amount of oxygen reaching them via the arterial blood. Oxygen delivery defined as the arterial oxygen concentration multiplied by the blood flow to the muscle has often been regarded as the critical variable.

Wagner and his co-workers have analyzed the relationship between oxygen uptake and the P_{O_2} of muscle capillary blood on the assumption that the uptake is limited by oxygen diffusion from the capillaries to the mitochondria (Hogan *et al.* 1988a). Figure 11.8a shows a diagram relating oxygen uptake to the P_{O_2} of muscle venous blood, taken as an index of muscle capillary P_{O_2}. The line sloping from top left to bottom right shows the amount of oxygen being delivered to the muscle by the capillaries (Fick principle). The line from bottom left to top right shows the pressure gradient available to cause oxygen diffusion from the red cells to the mitochondria (Fick's law) assuming that the mitochondrial P_{O_2} is nearly zero. The slope of this line is the lumped 'diffusing capacity for oxygen' of the tissues. The point where the two diagonal lines cross represents the $\dot{V}_{O_2,max}$. Regions to the left of this indicate situations where ample oxygen is available in the blood but the diffusing head of pressure is inadequate. Regions to the right indicate a more than adequate diffusing head of pressure but inadequate amounts of oxygen in the blood.

Figure 11.8b shows the same diagram with another line added indicating the presumed situation at high altitude. Because the oxygen concentration of the arterial blood is low, the line representing the Fick principle is displaced downwards and to the left. The $\dot{V}_{O_2,max}$ is therefore lower. The diagram assumes that the 'diffusing capacity for oxygen' of the tissue is the same at sea level and at altitude. It could be argued that this is not the case if the diffusing distance is reduced by the appearance of more capillaries, or the size of muscle fibers is reduced. However, experimental evidence indicates that these factors are unimportant and that the diffusing capacity is essentially determined by the number of open capillaries (Hepple *et al.* 2000), congruent

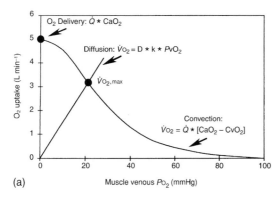 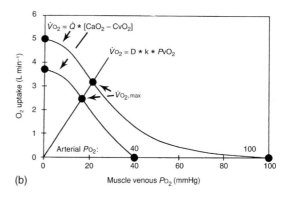

Figure 11.8 (a) Diagram to show how $\dot{V}_{O_2,max}$ is determined assuming that oxygen diffusion from the peripheral capillary to the mitochondria is the limiting factor. The two lines show the oxygen uptake available from the Fick principle on the one hand, and Fick's law of diffusion on the other. The $\dot{V}_{O_2,max}$ is given by the intersection of the two lines. See text for more details. (From Wagner 1988a.) (b) As (a) except an additional line has been added to represent the Fick equation at high altitude. This reduces the $\dot{V}_{O_2,max}$ as shown. See text for further details. (From Wagner 1988a.)

with the fact that most of the fall in P_{O_2} is believed to be at the capillary wall (see Chapter 10), and that the myoglobin or other mechanisms of enhanced intracellular transport make the diffusion distance unimportant.

Several pieces of evidence now support this concept. For example, a retrospective analysis of data from Operation Everest II showed that the points relating the P_{O_2} of mixed venous blood to oxygen uptake tend to lie on a straight line passing through the origin. On the assumption that the P_{O_2} of mixed venous blood reflects the P_{O_2} of the blood in the capillaries of the exercising muscles, this relationship supports the notion. Indeed, it was this observation that prompted the hypothesis.

More direct evidence comes from a prospective study in which normal subjects exercised at high work loads breathing hypoxic mixtures, and samples of femoral venous blood were taken via an indwelling catheter (Roca *et al.* 1989). Again a plot of the P_{O_2} of femoral venous blood against oxygen uptake for different inspired oxygen concentrations showed the points lying close to a straight line passing near to the origin. A similar plot was found when the calculated mean capillary P_{O_2} was substituted for femoral venous P_{O_2}.

Additional studies have been carried out on an isolated dog gastrocnemius preparation where the muscle was supplied with hypoxic blood and stimulated maximally. Again a good relationship was found between the P_{O_2} of the effluent blood

and the maximal oxygen uptake at different levels of hypoxia (Hogan *et al.* 1988a). This preparation allowed a test of two competing hypotheses, that referred to above, and an alternative hypothesis that $\dot{V}_{O_2,max}$ is determined by the amount of oxygen delivered to the muscle via the blood. The test was made by supplying the isolated muscle with the same amounts of oxygen (arterial oxygen concentration × blood flow) but using different blood flows (and therefore oxygen concentrations). The results showed that $\dot{V}_{O_2,max}$ was more closely related to the P_{O_2} of muscle venous blood than to the oxygen delivered via the arterial blood, and therefore the results support the hypothesis of diffusion limitation (Hogan *et al.* 1988b).

The diffusion-limitation hypothesis has also been tested in more recent studies. In one, the oxygen affinity of hemoglobin was increased by feeding dogs sodium cyanate, and it was shown that for the same convective oxygen delivery (cardiac output times arterial oxygen concentration) the maximal oxygen concentration of dog muscle was reduced compared with animals in which the oxygen affinity was normal (Hogan *et al.* 1991). The converse experiment was also carried out by reducing the oxygen affinity of hemoglobin using the allosteric modifier methylpropionic acid. In this case, the dog muscle showed an increased maximal oxygen consumption at a constant blood oxygen delivery compared with an animal with a normal oxygen affinity of hemoglobin (Richardson *et al.* 1998). Therefore, there are considerable experimental data supporting the analysis shown in Fig. 11.8.

11.9 ACE GENE AND ALTITUDE PERFORMANCE

Recently, there has been great interest in the polymorphism of the angiotensin converting enzyme (ACE) gene and deletions or insertions of the I and D alleles. ACE constricts microvascular tone. Insertion of the I allele leads to inhibition of ACE while deletion of the D allele leads to increased ACE activity and vasomotor tone.

Most (Montgomery *et al.* 1999, Myerson *et al.* 1999, Woods, 2000) but not all studies (Rankinen *et al.* 2000 and 2000a) show a strong association of the endurance athletic performance and insertion of the I-allele in the ACE gene, resulting in an inhibition of the microvasoconstrictive response in the tissues. Some studies have shown a similar association between the insertion of the I-allele and performance at very high altitudes (Montgomery *et al.* 1998, Tsianos 2005). This same configuration is also linked with a greater hyperventilatory response to hypoxic exercise (Patel *et al.* 2003). The implications of these findings are not clear but suggest that a better understanding of the genetic signal of physiologic responses is on the horizon.

11.10 MAXIMAL OXYGEN UPTAKE AT HIGH ALTITUDE

Many investigators have documented the fall in maximal oxygen uptake at high altitude since the early studies of Zuntz *et al.* (1906), and the results of Pugh and his co-workers are shown in Fig. 11.1. Figure 11.9 shows data from a number of studies collated by Cerretelli (1980). Note that, even at the very modest altitude of 2500 m, there is already an average decrease of $\dot{V}O_{2,max}$ of 5–10% as compared to sea level. Cerretelli pointed out that these data do not show any consistent differences between subjects exposed to acute hypoxia and those who have had the advantage of acclimatization to high altitude. This conclusion goes against the experience of many climbers who feel that they can work harder at high altitude after acclimatization, and the conclusion cannot presumably be true at the most extreme altitudes where acute exposure to the prevailing

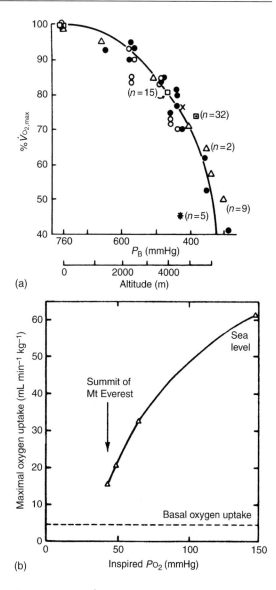

Figure 11.9 (a) $\dot{V}O_{2,max}$ as a percentage of the sea-level value plotted against barometric pressure and altitude. (open circles, triangles), acute hypoxia; (closed circles), chronic hypoxia; (crosses), high-altitude natives. See original text for complete explanation of symbols. (From Cerretelli 1980.) (b) Maximal oxygen uptake against inspired PO_2 as measured on the 1981 American Medical Research Expedition to Everest. The lowest point was obtained by giving well-acclimatized subjects at an altitude of 6300 m an inspired gas mixture containing 14% oxygen. The inspired PO_2 was 42.5 mmHg which is equivalent to that on the Everest summit. Compare Figure 11.2. (Modified from West *et al.* 1983a.) (1 Torr = 1 mmHg)

barometric pressure (for example, on the summit of Mount Everest) results in loss of consciousness within a few minutes in most unacclimatized individuals. It is of interest that some, but not all, elite high altitude climbers have only moderately high levels of maximal oxygen consumption at sea level (Oelz *et al.* 1986).

These data on maximal oxygen uptake were extended by the 1981 AMREE studies, where measurements were made at an altitude of 6300 m on subjects breathing ambient air, but also breathing 16 and 14% oxygen (West *et al.* 1983a). The last gave an inspired P_{O_2} of 42.5 mmHg equivalent to that on the Everest summit. The results are shown in Fig. 11.10 where it can be seen that in these subjects who were well acclimatized to very high altitude, the $\dot{V}_{O_2,max}$ fell to 15.3 mL min^{-1} kg^{-1} O_2 which was equivalent to 1.07 L min^{-1}. Thus at the highest point on Earth, the maximal oxygen uptake is reduced to between 20 and 25% of the sea level value. As pointed out in Chapter 12, this oxygen uptake is equivalent to that seen when a subject walks slowly on the level but nevertheless is apparently sufficient to explain how Messner and Habeler were able to reach the Everest summit without supplementary oxygen in 1978. Indeed Messner's statement that the last 100 m took more than an hour to climb fits with this measured oxygen uptake (Messner 1979).

Measurements of $\dot{V}_{O_2,max}$ at various altitudes were also made during Operation Everest II and the data are almost superimposable on those shown in Fig. 11.9b at the highest altitudes (Sutton *et al.* 1987). This is interesting because the subjects of Operation Everest II were probably not as well acclimatized to the extreme altitudes as the members of the 1981 expedition as judged from their alveolar gas composition and other measurements (West 1993). The values for $\dot{V}_{O_2,max}$ at any given altitude as determined by the 1981 Everest expedition (Fig. 11.9b) are higher than those earlier reported by Pugh *et al.* (1964) based on measurements made during the Silver Hut Expedition and previous measurements on Mount Everest. This can be explained by the higher level of fitness of subjects on the 1981 expedition. For example, several of the AMREE members were competitive marathon runners with very high maximum aerobic capacities as measured at sea level.

Several studies since the early measurements of Douglas *et al.* (1913) have shown that the rela-

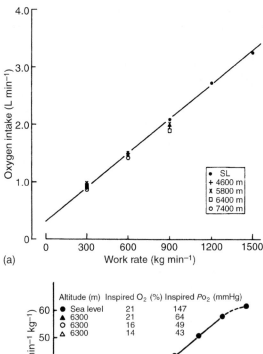

(a)

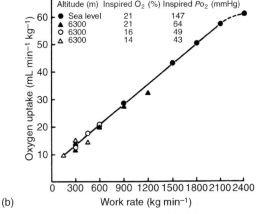

(b)

Figure 11.10 (a) Oxygen uptake plotted against work rate at various altitudes during the Silver Hut Expedition showing that the relationship remains essentially the same as at sea level. (From Pugh *et al.* 1964.) (b) Similar plot as in (a) but showing the much higher work rates at sea level obtained during the 1981 AMREE expedition. (From West *et al.*, 1983a.) (1 Torr = 1 mmHg)

tionship between oxygen uptake and work rate (or power) is independent of altitude. Figure 11.10(a) shows a comparison of data from the 1960–61 Himalayan Scientific and Mountaineering Expedition, and Fig. 11.10b from the 1981 Everest expedition. The message of the two plots is the same but note the much higher work rates at sea level recorded prior to the 1981 expedition which is further evidence of the high level of athletic ability of these subjects.

As indicated earlier, breathing pure oxygen at high altitude does not return the $\dot{V}O_{2,max}$ to the sea level value as shown by Cerretelli (1976a) and others. The reason is unclear; the opposite might be expected since the subjects acclimatized to high altitude have higher blood haemoglobin levels. However, against this are the results of a more recent study showing that when erythrocytes were infused into lowlanders after 1 or 9 days at an altitude of 4300 m, there was no improvement in the decreased $\dot{V}O_{2,max}$ (Young et al. 1996). It has been suggested that the reduced $\dot{V}O_{2,max}$ is caused by the loss of muscle mass at high altitude, and that if $\dot{V}O_{2,max}$ were related to lean body mass, the reduction would not be found. As discussed in Chapter 10, the diameter of muscle fibers decreases during acclimatization. Another possibility is that the increased red blood cell concentration causes uneven blood flow and sludging in peripheral capillaries and this interferes with oxygen unloading.

Does a period of acclimatization at high altitude improve $\dot{V}O_{2,max}$ at sea level? Again the answer is not clear. Cerretelli (1976a) measured $\dot{V}O_{2,max}$ in a group of subjects at sea level shortly before they were exposed to an altitude of 5350 m for 10–12 weeks, and again at sea level about four weeks after return from altitude. Although there was an approximately 11% increase in hemoglobin concentration, this was not accompanied by a statistically significant rise in $\dot{V}O_{2,max}$. On the other hand, more recent studies involving the reinjection of a subject's own red cells in order to raise the hematocrit have shown a small but significant increase in $\dot{V}O_{2,max}$ at sea level (Spriet et al. 1986). This result would suggest that a period at medium altitude (certainly lower than 5350 m) may improve exercise tolerance at sea level. Perhaps the reduction of muscle fiber size at very high altitudes is the

explanation for the failure to see an increase in $\dot{V}O_{2,max}$ after acclimatization at very high altitude. As noted above, erythrocyte infusions into lowlanders exposed to an altitude of 4300 m for 1 or 9 days did not improve the $\dot{V}O_{2,max}$ at that altitude (Young et al. 1996).

It should be pointed out that the $\dot{V}O_{2,max}$ determined at any particular altitude is something of an artificial measurement because climbers, for example, do not ordinarily exercise at that intensity. Pugh (1958) showed that climbers typically select an oxygen uptake of one-half to three-quarters of their maximum for normal climbing at altitudes up to 6000 m. Actual values of oxygen uptake measured by Pugh during normal climbing are included in Fig. 11.1.

11.11 ANAEROBIC PERFORMANCE AT HIGH ALTITUDE

Reference has already been made to the paradoxically low levels of blood lactate following exhaustive exercise at extreme altitude (section 11.7, Fig. 11.5). This phenomenon may be related to the reduced plasma bicarbonate concentration which interferes with buffering of hydrogen ion as discussed in Chapter 12. Cerretelli (1992) has shown that the rate of increase of $\dot{V}O_2$ when exercise is suddenly begun was slower in subjects after return from the 1981 Swiss Lhotse Expedition compared with before departure. This finding may be related to changes in anaerobic performance. However, it was also shown that maximal anaerobic (alactic) 'peak' power as measured by a standing jump was not affected by exposure of up to three weeks at 5200 m. Thereafter it tended to fall along with the reduction of muscle mass.

12

Limiting factors at extreme altitude

SUMMARY

The fact that a well-acclimatized human can just reach the summit of Mount Everest, the highest point on Earth, without breathing supplementary oxygen is an extraordinary coincidence. Several experimental and theoretical studies in the early part of the twentieth century predicted that this would not be possible, and therefore it was of great interest when Messner and Habeler realized the feat in 1978. A critical factor is the higher barometric pressure in the great mountain ranges at latitudes near the equator than that predicted by the Standard Atmosphere. Another critical factor is the extreme hyperventilation that the successful climbers generate, thus forcing their alveolar P_{CO_2} below 10 mmHg and consequently defending their alveolar P_{O_2} at viable levels. Also important is the marked respiratory alkalosis that increases the oxygen affinity of hemoglobin and thus assists in the loading of oxygen by the pulmonary capillary. Even so, the maximal oxygen consumption on the summit of Everest is only just above $1\,L\,min^{-1}$, and the arterial P_{O_2} is less than 30 mmHg during physical work. The analysis of the physiological conditions near the Everest summit explains why tragedies occur when unexpected circumstances arise, such as deterioration of the weather. The fact that normal humans can survive the extreme derangement of blood gases which is necessary for these climbs to extreme altitudes is a graphic reminder of the resilience of the human organism.

12.1 INTRODUCTION

It is a remarkable coincidence that when humans are well acclimatized to high altitude, they can just reach the highest point on Earth without breathing supplementary oxygen. This feat was first realized in 1978 and many physiologists and physicians interested in high altitude had previously predicted that it would not be possible (West 1998). It was truly the end of an era when Messner and Habeler stood on the summit of Mount Everest on 8 May 1978.

This chapter examines the profound physiological changes that are necessary for humans to survive and do small amounts of work at extreme altitudes like the summit of Mount Everest. It includes an analysis of the factors that limit performance at these great altitudes and shows that such ascents are possible only if both the physiological make-up of the climber and physical factors such as barometric pressure are right.

12.2 HISTORICAL

12.2.1 Sixteenth to nineteenth centuries

It has been known for many centuries that very high altitude has a deleterious effect on the human body and that the amount of work that a person can do becomes more and more limited as the altitude increases. One of the first descriptions of the disabling effects of high altitude was given by the Jesuit missionary Joseph de Acosta who accompanied the early Spanish conquistadores to Peru in the sixteenth century. He described how, as he traveled over a high mountain, he 'was suddenly surprised with so mortall and strange a pang, that I was ready to fall from the top to the ground.' His dramatic description was first published in 1590 (Acosta 1590).

In the eighteenth century, climbers in the European Alps reported a variety of disagreeable sensations which now seem to us greatly exaggerated. For example, the physicist De Saussure, who was the third person to reach the summit of Mont Blanc, reported during the climb:

> When I began this ascent, I was quite out of breath from the rarity of the air . . . The kind of fatigue which results from the rarity of the air is absolutely unconquerable; when it is at its height, the most terrible danger would not make you take a single step further.

When he was near the summit he complained of extreme exhaustion:

> This need of rest was absolutely unconquerable; if I tried to overcome it, my legs refused to move, I felt the beginning of a faint, and was seized by dizziness. . . .

On the summit itself he reported:

> When I had to get to work to set out the instruments and observe them, I was constantly forced to interrupt my work and devote myself to breathing.
>
> (de Saussure, 1786–7)

These dramatic complaints at an altitude of only 4807 m or less reflect a combination of almost no acclimatization and the fear of the unknown.

In the nineteenth century numerous ascents were made of higher mountains, including those in the Andes, and there were abundant accounts of the disabling effects of extreme altitude. In 1879, Whymper made the first ascent of Chimborazo and described how, at an altitude of 5079 m (16 664 ft), he was incapacitated by the thin air:

> . . . in about an hour I found myself lying on my back, along with both the Carrels [his guides], placed *hors de combat,* and incapable of making the least exertion. . . . We were unable to satisfy our desire for air, except by breathing with open mouths. . . . Besides having our normal rate of breathing largely accelerated, we found it impossible to sustain life without every now and then giving spasmodic gulps, just like fishes when taken out of water.
>
> (Whymper 1892)

However, Whymper and his two guides gradually recovered their strength and in fact his lively account shows that he was aware of the beneficial effects of high altitude acclimatization.

In the latter part of the nineteenth century, there was considerable interest in the highest altitude that could be tolerated by climbers. Thomas W. Hinchliff, President of the (British) Alpine Club (1875–77), wrote an account of his travels around the world and described his feelings as he looked at the view from Santiago in Chile.

> Lover of mountains as I am, and familiar with such summits as those of Mont Blanc, Monte Rosa, and other Alpine heights, I could not repress a strange feeling as I looked at Tupungato and Aconcagua, and reflected that endless successions of men must in all probability be forever debarred from their lofty crests. . . . Those who, like Major Godwin Austen, have had all the advantages of experience and acclimatization to aid them in attacks upon the higher Himalayas, agree that 21,500 ft [6553 m] is near the limit at which man ceases to be capable of the slightest further exertion.
>
> (Hinchliff 1876)

12.2.2 Twentieth century

In 1909, the Duke of Abruzzi attempted an ascent of K2 in the Karakoram Mountains, and although his party was unsuccessful in reaching the summit, they attained the remarkable altitude of 7500 m without supplementary oxygen. According to the Duke's biographer, one of the reasons given for this expedition was 'to see how high man can go' (de Fillippi 1912), and certainly the climb had a dramatic effect on both the mountaineering and the medical communities interested in high altitude tolerance. In contrast to the florid accounts of paralyzing fatigue and breathlessness given by De Saussure, Whymper and others at much lower altitudes, the Duke made light of the physiological problems associated with this great altitude. However, as we saw earlier (Chapter 6), his feat prompted heated arguments among physiologists about whether the lungs actively secreted oxygen at this previously unheard-of altitude.

Ten years later, a milestone in the history of the physiology of extreme altitude was provided by the British physiologist, Alexander M. Kellas, whose contributions have been largely overlooked. Kellas was lecturer in chemistry at the Middlesex Hospital Medical School in London during the first two decades of the century, but, despite this full-time faculty position, managed to make eight expeditions to the Himalayas, and probably spent more time above 6100 m than anyone else. In 1919 he wrote an extensive paper entitled 'A consideration of the possibility of ascending Mount Everest,' which was not published until 2001 (Kellas 2001). In this he analyzed the physiology of a climber near the Everest summit, including a discussion of the summit altitude, barometric pressure, alveolar P_{O_2}, arterial oxygen saturation, maximal oxygen consumption and maximal ascent rate. On the basis of his study he concluded that:

> Mount Everest could be ascended by a man of excellent physical and mental constitution in first-rate training, without adventitious aids [supplementary oxygen] if the physical difficulties of the mountain are not too great.

The importance of this study was not so much that he reached the correct conclusion. He had so few data that many of his calculations were erroneous. However, Kellas asked all the right questions and he can claim the distinction of being the first physiologist to seriously analyze the limiting factors at the highest point on Earth. It was not until almost 60 years later that all his predictions were fulfilled.

Kellas was a member of the first official reconnaissance expedition to Everest in 1921, but tragically he died during the approach march just as the expedition had its first view of the mountain they came to climb. Three years later, E.F. Norton, who was a member of the third Everest expedition, reached a height of about 8589 m on the north side of Everest without supplementary oxygen. He was accompanied to just below that altitude by Dr T.H. Somervell, who collected alveolar gas samples at an altitude of 7010 m, though unfortunately these were stored in rubber bladders through which the carbon dioxide rapidly diffused (Somervell 1925). Somervell also referred to the extreme breathlessness at that altitude, stating that 'for every step forward and upward, 7 to 10 complete respirations were required.'

The summit of Everest was finally attained in 1953 by Hillary and Tenzing (Hunt 1953). Naturally, this was a landmark event in the physiology of extreme altitude, but the fact that the two climbers used supplementary oxygen still did not answer the question of whether it was possible to reach the summit breathing air. Hillary did remove his oxygen mask on the summit for about 10 min and at the end of the time reported:

> I realized that I was becoming rather clumsy-fingered and slow-moving, so I quickly replaced my oxygen set and experienced once more the stimulating effect of even a few litres of oxygen.

Nevertheless, the fact that he could survive for a few minutes without additional oxygen came as a surprise to some physicians who had predicted that he would lose consciousness.

However, there was a precedent for surviving for this period on the summit in the experiment Operation Everest I, carried out by Houston and Riley in 1945. As briefly described in Chapter 1, four volunteers spent 34 days in a low pressure chamber and two were able to tolerate 20 min without supplementary oxygen on the 'summit.' In fact, the equivalent altitude was even higher because the Standard Atmosphere pressure was inadvertently used (section 12.3.2).

Additional information on whether there was enough oxygen in the air to allow a climber to reach the Everest summit while breathing air was obtained by Pugh and his colleagues during the

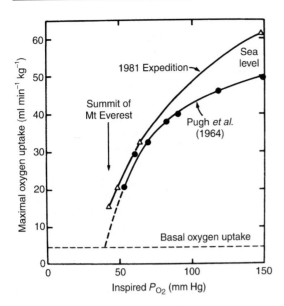

Figure 12.1   Maximal oxygen uptake against inspired P_{O_2}. The lower line shows data from Pugh *et al.* (1964) suggesting that all the oxygen available at the Everest summit would be required for basal oxygen uptake. However, as the upper line shows, the 1981 AMREE measured an oxygen uptake of just over 1 L min^{-1} for an inspired P_{O_2} of 43 mmHg. (From West *et al.* 1983c.)

1960–61 Silver Hut Expedition (Pugh *et al.* 1964). Measurements of maximal oxygen consumption were made using a bicycle ergometer on a group of physiologists who wintered at an altitude of 5800 m and who were therefore extremely well acclimatized to this altitude. Figure 12.1 (lower curve) shows the results of measurements made up to an altitude of 7440 m. Note that extrapolation of the line to a barometric pressure of 250 mmHg on the Everest summit suggested that almost all the oxygen available would be required for the basal oxygen uptake. (For details of the extrapolation procedure, refer to West and Wagner 1980.) Thus these results strongly suggested that a climber who could reach the Everest summit without supplementary oxygen would be very near the limit of human tolerance.

This ultimate climbing achievement occurred when Reinhold Messner and Peter Habeler reached the summit of Everest without supplementary oxygen in May 1978. Messner's account (Messner 1979) makes it clear that he had very little in reserve:

> After every few steps, we huddle over our ice axes, mouths agape, struggling for sufficient

> breath. . . . As we get higher it becomes necessary to lie down to recover our breath. . . . Breathing becomes such a strenuous business that we scarcely have strength to go on.

And when he eventually reaches the summit:

> In my state of spiritual abstraction, I no longer belong to myself and to my eyesight. I am nothing more than a single, narrow gasping lung, floating over the mists and the summits.

The long period of 25 years between the first ascent of Everest in 1953 and this first 'oxygenless' ascent also suggests that we are near the limit of human tolerance. Again, as indicated earlier, Norton ascended to within 300 m of the Everest summit as early as 1924, but it was not until 1978 that climbers reached the top without supplementary oxygen. Thus the last 300 m took 54 years!

Since that historic climb, Messner has further confirmed his outstanding tolerance to the extreme hypoxia of great altitudes. In 1980, he became the first man to ascend Everest alone without supplementary oxygen (Messner 1981), and in 1986 he became the first man to climb all 14 of the 8000 m peaks without supplementary oxygen. These accomplishments assure him a place not only in the history of mountaineering but also in the history of the physiology of extreme altitude.

12.3 PHYSIOLOGY OF EXTREME ALTITUDE

12.3.1 Introduction

This section is devoted to human performance at altitudes over 8000 m. There was renewed interest in this topic when Messner and Habeler climbed Everest without supplementary oxygen in 1978 but, as indicated above, the issue of whether humans would be able to tolerate the highest altitude on Earth was raised early in this century, notably by Kellas in 1919.

The following analysis is based primarily on data from four studies. The first was the 1960–61 Silver Hut Expedition during which data were obtained on maximal oxygen consumptions as high as 7440 m (P_B 300 mmHg) and alveolar gas samples were taken as high as 7830 m (P_B 288 mmHg). These measurements were extended to the Everest summit by the 1981 American Medical Research Expedition to Everest (AMREE), where measurements on the summit included barometric pressure, alveolar gas samples and electrocardiograms, with additional measurements made between the summit and the highest camp situated at 8050 m (P_B 284 mmHg). The third and fourth studies were Operation Everest II and III (COMEX '97) in 1985 and 1997 when several volunteers were gradually decompressed over a period of 31–40 days in low pressure chambers. Although the degree of acclimatization was not as great as in field studies, much valuable data was obtained.

12.3.2 Barometric pressure

Barometric pressure is a critical variable in physiological performance at extreme altitude because it determines the inspired PO_2. This is the first link in the chain of the oxygen cascade from the atmosphere to the mitochondria. As pointed out in Chapter 2, there has been considerable confusion in the past about the relationships between barometric pressure and altitude on high mountains such as the Himalayan chain. The resulting errors are particularly important at extreme altitude because it can be shown that maximal oxygen consumption is exquisitely sensitive to barometric pressure. It is remarkable that Paul Bert gave essentially the correct value of barometric pressure for the Everest summit in Appendix I of his classic book *La Pression Barométrique* (Bert 1878). His figure of 248 mmHg was based on an extrapolation of measurements made by Jourdanet and others at various locations including the Andes (Jourdanet 1875).

However, when the Standard Atmosphere was introduced and used extensively by aviation physiologists in the 1930s and 1940s, it was erroneously applied to Mount Everest, giving a value of 236 mmHg, which is much too low. Nevertheless, this figure was used by several high altitude physiologists. For example, during Operation Everest I when four naval recruits were gradually decompressed to what was thought to be the simulated altitude of Mount Everest, they were exposed to a pressure of 236 mmHg and their alveolar PO_2 fell to as low as 21 mmHg (Riley and Houston 1951)! As

the next section shows, this is about 14 mmHg less than that of a well-acclimatized climber on the summit of Mount Everest.

As described in Chapter 2, Dr Christopher Pizzo measured a barometric pressure of 253 mmHg on the Everest summit on 24 October 1981. This was about 2 mmHg higher than that expected from the mean barometric pressure for that month based on extensive weather balloon data (Fig. 2.4). The discrepancy can be accounted for by normal variation and the high pressure system which made the weather ideal for climbing. The reading of 253 mmHg was within 1 mmHg of the pressure predicted for an altitude of 8848 m from radiosonde balloons released in New Delhi, India, on the same day (West *et al.* 1983a). Several direct measurement on the summit since 1981 have given similar values (see section 2.2.6).

Measurements of $\dot{V}O_{2,max}$ on AMREE (West *et al.* 1983c) and Operation Everest II (Sutton *et al.* 1988) as well as the analysis described in section 12.4 show that exercise performance at these extreme altitudes is exquisitely sensitive to barometric pressure. For example on AMREE, a decrease in inspired PO_2 of only 1 mmHg resulted in a fall of $\dot{V}O_{2,max}$ by about 63 mL min^{-1} (West 1999a). This is partly because the lung is working very low on the oxygen dissociation curve where the slope is steep. As a consequence, a fall of barometric pressure of as little as 3 mmHg (less than twice the daily standard deviation) will apparently cause a reduction of maximal oxygen uptake of about 4%. This means that even the daily variations of barometric pressure caused by weather may affect physical performance.

Seasonal variations of barometric pressure can be expected to have a marked effect on maximal oxygen uptake. As Fig. 2.2 shows, mean barometric pressure falls from nearly 255 mmHg in the summer months to only 243 mmHg in mid-winter. This decrease is predicted to reduce maximal oxygen uptake by some 15%. It is noteworthy that Mount Everest has only once been climbed during winter without supplementary oxygen (in December 1987), despite several attempts, and although the very cold temperatures and high winds are naturally a factor, the reduced barometric pressure must certainly contribute (section 2.2.8).

As pointed out in Chapter 2, the location of Mount Everest at 28°N latitude is fortunate because the barometric pressure at its summit is considerably higher than would be the case if it were at a higher latitude. As an example, if Mount McKinley were 8848 m high, its barometric pressure for May and October (preferred climbing months for Everest) would be only 223 mmHg. It would apparently be impossible to reach the summit without supplementary oxygen under these conditions.

A similar argument would apply if the barometric pressure on the Everest summit were only 236 mmHg, as predicted from the Standard Atmosphere model. The reduction of pressure by 17 mmHg below that measured by Pizzo would reduce the maximal oxygen consumption by over 20%, according to the analysis presented in the present chapter. It seems very probable that climbing Everest without supplementary oxygen under these conditions would be impossible. Thus the higher pressure that Everest enjoys because of its near equatorial latitude makes it just possible for humans to reach the highest point on Earth.

12.3.3 Alveolar gas composition

On ascent to high altitude, the alveolar P_{O_2} falls because of the reduction in the inspired P_{O_2}. At the same time, alveolar P_{CO_2} falls because of increasing hyperventilation. As described in Chapter 5, Rahn and Otis (1949) clarified the differences between unacclimatized and fully acclimatized subjects at high altitude by plotting their alveolar gas P_{O_2} and P_{CO_2} values on an oxygen–carbon dioxide diagram (Fig. 5.6). There are apparently differences between the results obtained in the field, that is on expeditions to high altitude, on the one hand, and simulated ascents in a low pressure chamber on the other. The field studies will be discussed first followed by those using simulated ascents.

Figure 12.2 shows alveolar P_{CO_2} plotted against barometric pressure at extreme altitude from field studies. The closed circles show data reported by Greene (1934), Warren (1939), Pugh (1957) and Gill *et al.* (1962). The triangles show data obtained on the AMREE (West *et al.* 1983b). It can be seen that alveolar P_{CO_2} declines approximately linearly as barometric pressure falls and that the pressure on the summit of Mount Everest is about 7–8 mmHg. The measurements made on the summit itself had high respiratory exchange ratio (R) values, for

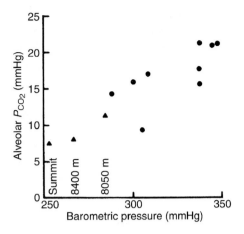

Figure 12.2   Alveolar P_{CO_2} against barometric pressure at extreme altitudes. Triangles show the means of measurements on the AMREE. Circles are results from previous investigators at barometric pressures below 350 mmHg (Table 12.1). (From West *et al.* 1983b.)

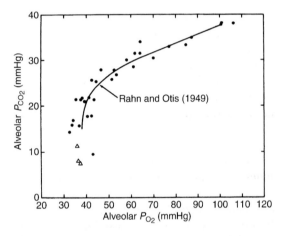

Figure 12.3   Oxygen–carbon dioxide diagram showing alveolar gas values collated by Rahn and Otis (1949) (circles) together with values obtained at extreme altitudes by the AMREE (triangles). (From West *et al.* 1983b.)

reasons which are not clear. However, the data obtained at the slightly lower altitude of 8400 m (P_B 267 mmHg) had a mean R value of 0.82 with a P_{CO_2} of 8.0 mmHg, which means we can be confident of the very low values at this great altitude.

Figure 12.3 shows the line drawn by Rahn and Otis (1949) for fully acclimatized subjects (lower line on Fig. 5.4) together with additional data obtained at barometric pressures below 350 mmHg (Table 12.1). Note that the AMREE data (triangles) fit well with the extrapolation of the line. This

Table 12.1 Alveolar P_{O_2} and P_{CO_2} in acclimatized subjects at barometric pressures below 350 mmHg

Source	Barometric pressure	P_{O_2}	P_{CO_2}	Respiratory exchange ratio (R)
Greene (1934)	337	40.7	17.7	0.87
	305	43.0	9.2	0.79
Warren (1939)	337[a]	37.0	15.6	0.60
Pugh (1957)	347	39.3	21.0	0.87
	337	35.5	21.3	0.87
	308	34.1	16.9	0.77
Gill et al. (1962)	344	38.1	20.7	0.82
	300	33.7	15.8	0.78
	288	32.8	14.3	0.77
West et al. (1983b)	284	36.1	11.0	0.78
	267	36.7	8.0	0.82
	253	37.6	7.5	1.49

All pressure values are given in mmHg.
[a] Barometric pressure estimated from curve of Zuntz et al. (1906).

method of plotting the data shows that as well-acclimatized humans go to higher and higher altitudes, the P_{O_2} falls because of the decreasing inspired P_{O_2}, and the P_{CO_2} falls because of the increasing hyperventilation. However, above an altitude of about 7000 m (P_B 325 mmHg) the alveolar P_{O_2} becomes essentially constant at a value of about 35 mmHg. More recent measurements of alveolar P_{O_2} up to an altitude of 8000 m by Peacock and Jones (1997) are in good agreement with these data. This means that successful climbers are able to defend their alveolar P_{O_2} by the process of extreme hyperventilation. In other words, they insulate the P_{O_2} of their alveolar gas from the falling value in the atmosphere around them. This appears to be the most important feature of acclimatization at extreme altitude.

Not everyone can generate the enormous increase in ventilation required for the very low P_{CO_2} values shown in Figs 12.2 and 12.3. This explains why climbers with a large hypoxic ventilatory response usually tolerate extreme altitude better than those with a more modest response (Schoene et al. 1984). Indeed, experience on the AMREE showed that individuals who had a low hypoxic ventilatory response were not able to remain at the higher camps (West 1985a).

The pattern of alveolar gas values shown in Fig. 12.3 is only obtained if sufficient time is allowed

for full respiratory acclimatization. Figure 12.4 compares the results found in unacclimatized and fully acclimatized subjects at high altitude (Figs 5.4 and 12.3) with alveolar gas data reported from two low pressure chamber experiments in which the simulated rate of ascent was much faster. It can be seen that in Operation Everest I (Riley and Houston 1951) the subjects reached the simulated summit after only 31 days and at the extreme altitudes the data fell close to the region predicted by the line for unacclimatized humans. In Operation Everest II (Malconian et al. 1993) the ascent was a little slower, with the first simulated summit excursion occurring after 36 days. However, the alveolar gas values at extreme altitudes still deviated considerably from those found in fully acclimatized subjects. Little information is available about the time required for full respiratory acclimatization at extreme altitudes, say over 8000 m, but Fig. 12.4 suggests that 36 days is inadequate whereas 77 days is apparently sufficient. However, it may be that other factors such as the level of physical activity are also important.

12.3.4 Acid–base status

BASE EXCESS

Relatively little is known about acid–base changes at extreme altitude, despite the importance of this topic.

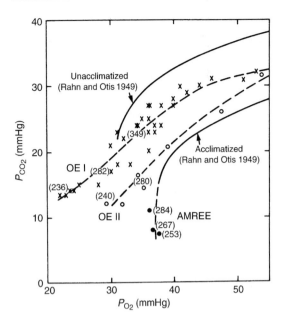

Figure 12.4 Oxygen–carbon dioxide diagram showing the two lines described by Rahn and Otis (1949) for unacclimatized and acclimatized subjects at high altitude (compare Figure 5.4). In addition, data from Operation Everest I (OE I) and Operation Everest II (OE II) are included. Note that the OE I subjects were poorly acclimatized at extreme altitudes whereas the OE II had intermediate values. (From West 1998a.)

Some data are available from two well-acclimatized subjects of the AMREE, based on blood samples removed during the morning after they had reached the summit. Venous blood samples taken at the highest camp (8050 m; P_B 267 mmHg) showed a mean base excess of -7.2 mmol L^{-1}. This was a considerably higher base excess than expected (in other words the base deficit was less than predicted) and the result was an extremely high arterial pH of over 7.7 calculated for the Everest summit (West *et al.* 1983b). This calculation is based on the measured alveolar P_{CO_2} and base excess. It assumes that there was no change in base excess in the previous 24 h and that a climber resting on the summit had a negligible blood lactate concentration (see below). In addition, the measured alveolar P_{CO_2} of 7.5 mmHg is assumed to apply to the arterial blood.

A remarkable feature of these base excess values is that they were essentially unchanged from those measured in 14 subjects living for several weeks at

Camp 2 (6300 m, P_B 351 mmHg) where the mean value was -8.7 ± 1.7 mmol L^{-1} (Winslow *et al.* 1984). This suggests that base excess was changing extremely slowly above an altitude of 6300 m. The reason for this is not known but may be related to the chronic volume depletion which was observed in climbers living at 6300 m. At this altitude the serum osmolality was 302 ± 4 mmol kg^{-1}, which was significantly higher ($p <0.01$) than in the same subjects at sea level, where the value was 290 ± 1 mmol kg^{-1} (Blume *et al.* 1984). It is known that the kidney gives a higher priority to correcting dehydration than acid–base disturbances, and in order to excrete more bicarbonate to reduce the base excess, it would be necessary to lose corresponding cations, which would aggravate the volume depletion. This may be the basis for the slow renal bicarbonate excretion.

These acid–base changes may be part of the explanation of why climbers can spend only a relatively short time at extreme altitudes, say above 8000 m. It was pointed out in Chapter 6 that the marked respiratory alkalosis which increases the oxygen affinity of the hemoglobin at extreme altitude is beneficial because it accelerates the loading of oxygen by the pulmonary capillaries. If a climber remains at extreme altitude for several days, presumably there is some renal excretion of bicarbonate (though this appears to be slow) and the resulting metabolic compensation would move the pH back towards 7.4. Thus the advantage of a left-shifted dissociation curve would tend to be lost.

One way to counter this disadvantage during a climb of Mount Everest would be to put in the high camps and then return to Base Camp at a lower altitude for several days. This period at medium altitude would then allow the body to adjust again to this more moderate oxygen deprivation and enable the blood pH to stabilize nearer its normal value. The final summit assault would then be as rapid as possible to take advantage of the nearly uncompensated respiratory alkalosis. In fact this was the pattern adopted by Messner and Habeler in their first ascent of Mount Everest without supplementary oxygen in 1978.

THE LACTATE PARADOX

Blood lactate is known to be very low in acclimatized subjects at high altitude even during maximal work, an observation made by Edwards (1936)

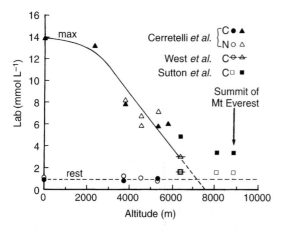

Figure 12.5 Maximal blood lactate (Lab) as a function of altitude. Most of the data are redrawn from Cerretelli (1980). The filled circles and triangles show data for acclimatized Caucasians (C); the open circles and triangles are for high altitude natives (N). The data for 6300 m are from the AMREE for acclimatized lowlanders. (From West 1986.) The points marked Sutton *et al.* are from Operation Everest II (Sutton *et al.* 1988).

during the International High Altitude Expedition to Chile in 1935. Figure 12.5 shows data on resting and maximal blood lactate obtained by Cerretelli (1980). Also shown are measurements made at 6300 m after maximal exercise at the rate of 900 kg min^{-1}, that is, an oxygen uptake of 1.75 L min^{-1} (West 1986c). The mean value after exercise at 6300 m was only 3.0 mmol L^{-1} despite an arterial P_{O_2} of less than 35 mmHg and therefore extreme tissue hypoxia. Note that extrapolation of the line relating maximal blood lactate concentration to altitude suggests that after maximal exercise at altitudes exceeding 7500 m, there will be no increase in lactate in the blood at all despite the extreme oxygen deprivation. This is indeed a paradox.

The blood lactate concentrations after maximal exercise were appreciably higher on Operation Everest II (Sutton *et al.* 1988). For example, at an inspired P_{O_2} of 63 mmHg, the mean lactate concentration following maximal exercise was 4.7 mmol L^{-1}, that is about 56% higher than on the AMREE for the same inspired P_{O_2}. Moreover, the 'summit' measurements on Operation Everest II gave a blood lactate concentration of 3.4 mmol L^{-1}, a higher value than that found at only 6300 m on

the AMREE (Fig. 12.5). It is known that the low lactate concentrations following maximal exercise at high altitude come about as a result of high altitude acclimatization because acute hypoxia causes very high lactate levels. Presumably therefore the higher values seen on Operation Everest II compared with the AMREE and other field studies can be explained by the limited degree of acclimatization.

The reasons for the low blood lactate levels following maximal exercise in well-acclimatized subjects as opposed to poorly acclimatized subjects at high altitude are still unclear. One hypothesis is that on acute exposure to hypoxia, sympathetic stimulation leads to augmented muscle lactate production and blood lactate concentration through a beta-adrenergic mechanism. By contrast, chronic hypoxia causes beta-adrenergic adaptation and the result is a reduced lactate response after acclimatization. However, studies on unacclimatized and acclimatized subjects at 4300 m altitude have not supported this hypothesis (Brooks *et al.* 1998). Another hypothesis is that the bicarbonate depletion that occurs as a result of acclimatization interferes with the buffering of released lactate and hydrogen ions, and the consequent fall in local pH inhibits the enzyme phosphofructokinase in the glycolytic cycle and thus puts a brake on glycolysis (Fig. 10.7). It is known that the activity of phosphofructokinase is reduced as the pH is lowered. Certainly, Cerretelli has shown that the changes in blood hydrogen ion concentration as a result of increases in blood lactate are higher in acclimatized than unacclimatized subjects (Cerretelli 1980). However, many other factors affect blood lactate and the issue is far from settled.

12.3.5 Cardiac output

Intuitively, it would be reasonable to expect an increased cardiac output for a given work level at extreme altitude compared with sea level. It is known that cardiac output increases as a result of acute hypoxia (Chapter 7). Furthermore, the oxygen concentration of the arterial blood is extremely low at very high altitude, and an increase in cardiac output would be expected to help to compensate for the reduced oxygen delivery. Paradoxically however, the relationship between cardiac output and oxygen uptake in acclimatized subjects at an altitude of 5800 m is essentially the same as at sea level

(Fig. 7.2) and this apparently holds true even at extreme altitudes, although data are sparse. Reeves *et al.* (1987) showed that the sea level relationship was maintained down to a barometric pressure of 282 mmHg, and almost maintained at an inspired P_{O_2} equivalent to the summit of Mount Everest, though at that extreme altitude the cardiac output appeared to be slightly higher (Fig. 7.3). Possibly this apparent paradox is related to the fact that when the cardiac output is increased under these very hypoxic conditions, there is increasing diffusion limitation of oxygen transfer, both in the lung and in the muscle. In a theoretical study, Wagner (1996) showed that increasing cardiac output for the conditions on the Everest summit did not improve calculated $\dot{V}_{O_2,max}$ because of diffusion limitation (Fig. 7.5).

12.3.6 Pulmonary diffusing capacity

As discussed in Chapter 6, oxygen transfer during exercise at high altitude is, in part, diffusion limited, and all calculations suggest that this limitation will be exaggerated at the extreme altitudes near the summit of Mount Everest. However, very few data on diffusing capacity at high altitude are available. Available measurements at an altitude of 5800 m (P_B 380 mmHg) indicate that the diffusing capacity for carbon monoxide during exercise is essentially unchanged from the sea level value except for the expected increase caused by the faster rate of combination of carbon monoxide with hemoglobin under the prevailing hypoxic conditions (West 1962a). These data suggest that the diffusing capacity of the pulmonary membrane itself is unaltered by acclimatization.

Measurements of the diffusing capacity for carbon monoxide at different alveolar P_{O_2} values allow calculation of the pulmonary capillary blood volume. Again, in measurements made at 5800 m, there appeared to be little change in capillary blood volume, although there was a suggestion that it was slightly lower, possibly as a result of hypoxic pulmonary vasoconstriction (West 1962a). If we accept the conclusion that capillary blood volume is unchanged, and that the cardiac output/oxygen consumption relationship is the same as at sea level (section 12.3.5), this implies that capillary transit time in the lung is normal since this is given by

capillary blood volume divided by cardiac output (Roughton 1945).

Using these data it is possible to calculate the changes in P_{O_2} along the pulmonary capillary for a climber at rest on the summit of Mount Everest (Fig. 6.5). This shows that the rate of oxygenation is extremely slow and that the end-capillary P_{O_2} is much lower than the alveolar value, indicating severe diffusion limitation of oxygen transfer. This topic is discussed further in section 6.7.

12.3.7 P_{O_2} of venous blood

During maximal exercise at extreme altitude, the extraction of oxygen by the peripheral tissues results in very low values of venous P_{O_2} in the exercising muscles. This in turn reduces the P_{O_2} of mixed venous blood. In order to analyze the relationships between the many variables and determine what limits exercise performance at extreme altitude, one possible assumption is that the body will not tolerate a P_{O_2} of mixed venous blood below a certain value, for example 15 mmHg (West and Wagner 1980, West 1983). This assumption received strong support from Operation Everest II, where direct measurements of the P_{O_2} in mixed venous blood gave similar values (Sutton *et al.* 1988). For example, on the 'summit' during 60 W of exercise, the P_{O_2} of mixed venous blood had a mean value of 14.8 mmHg, and at 120 W, which was the highest work level, the mean P_{O_2} was 13.8 mmHg.

12.3.8 Heat loss by hyperventilation

Matthews (1932) argued that tolerance to extreme altitude might be limited by the high rate of heat loss from the lungs as a result of the extreme hyperventilation. However, subsequent experience has not borne this out. Calculations of net heat loss are complex because the upper respiratory tract acts as a heat exchanger. During expiration, expired gas warms the respiratory tract, and this heat is then available to warm the cold inspired gas. Climbers who have reached the summit of Mount Everest without supplementary oxygen have not been affected by cold beyond the extent expected from the very low temperatures of the environment. When Pizzo reached the summit to take his alveolar gas samples during the course of the AMREE, he became overheated during the climb and photographs taken on the summit when he was breathing air show that he was not even wearing his down jacket, which he carried with him in his backpack (West 1985a, facing p. 51).

12.3.9 Oxygen cost of ventilation

A climber at extreme altitude has considerable hyperventilation at rest, and even more during moderate exercise. An alveolar PCO_2 of 7–8 mmHg was measured on the Everest summit and, since it is known that the carbon dioxide production both at rest and for a given work level is independent of altitude, we can conclude that the alveolar ventilation on the summit was at least five times the resting value. Even small amounts of physical activity will greatly increase this. If we take the normal resting ventilation to be 7–8 L min^{-1}, this means that the resting ventilation on the summit is at least 40 L min^{-1}.

Cibella *et al.* (1999) studied the oxygen cost of ventilation in four normal subjects during exercise at sea level and after a 1-month sojourn at 5050 m. From simultaneous measurements of esophageal pressure and lung volume, the mechanical power (work rate) of breathing was determined. As expected, maximal exercise ventilation and maximal power of breathing were higher at high altitude than at sea level, whereas maximal oxygen uptake was reduced in all subjects at high altitude. Interestingly, in three subjects the relationship between mechanical power of breathing and minute ventilation was the same at sea level and high altitude, whereas in only one individual was it lower at high altitude for a given ventilation. It might have been expected that the mechanical power of breathing would be reduced at high altitude in all subjects because of the reduced density of the air.

Assuming a mechanical efficiency of 5%, the oxygen cost of breathing at high altitude and sea level amounted to 26 and 5.5% of $\dot{V}O_{2,max}$, respectively. The authors concluded that, at high altitude, the mechanical power of breathing may substantially limit the ability to do external work. They also calculated what they called the 'critical ventilation,' that is the ventilation at which the mechanical power of breathing was so high that increasing ventilation above this level did not provide additional oxygen

for external work. At the altitude of 5050 m the maximal exercise ventilation exceeded the critical ventilation even when the efficiency was assumed to be as high as 20% (Fig. 12.6).

12.3.10 Studies using low pressure chambers

A question that is frequently asked is why perform field studies, for example on Mount Everest, when the low pressure conditions can be simulated in a high altitude chamber. Three extensive studies have been carried out in this way and they have certainly produced important information on how humans respond to low pressure. However, for some unclear reason the results from low pressure chambers are different from field studies.

OPERATION EVEREST I

This was carried out in 1944 under the leadership of Charles Houston and Richard Riley at the U.S. Naval School of Aviation Medicine in Pensacola, Florida (Riley and Houston 1951). Four volunteers were placed in a small chamber for a period of 35 days and the pressure was gradually reduced to that believed to occur on the summit of Mount Everest. However, as indicated earlier, the Standard Atmosphere was used and the chamber pressure was reduced to as low as 234 mmHg which actually corresponds to an altitude of about 9400 m, some 550 m above the Everest summit. The small chamber measured only about 3.0 × 3.0 × 2.1 m and contained four bunks. After 29 days the pressure was reduced to that at the 'summit' and two of the subjects were able to tolerate the severe hypoxia at rest during air breathing, while the other two needed oxygen. During these studies alveolar PO_2 values in the low 20s were measured (Riley and Houston 1951, Table 2). These were presumably the lowest values of alveolar PO_2 ever recorded for periods of several minutes. As indicated earlier (Fig. 12.4) the subjects of Operation Everest I showed almost no acclimatization at the extreme altitudes as judged from their alveolar gas values.

OPERATION EVEREST II

This took place in 1985 and again was spearheaded by Charles Houston (Houston *et al.* 1987). A

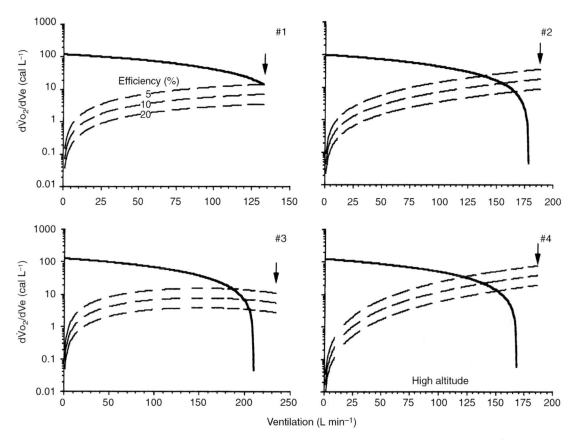

Figure 12.6 Increase in oxygen consumption divided by the increase in ventilation for four subjects at an altitude of 5050 m. The solid line shows the relationship for total oxygen consumption; the dashed lines show the relationship for the oxygen consumption of the respiratory muscles, assuming mechanical efficiencies of 5, 10 and 20%. Arrows show the maximal exercise ventilation. The intersection of the solid and dashed lines shows the critical ventilation above which no increase in external work was possible because the oxygen consumption of the respiratory muscles was so high. In three of the subjects, the maximum ventilation exceeded the critical ventilation for all assumed mechanical efficiencies, though in one of the subjects this was only the case for an efficiency of 5%. (From Cibella *et al.* 1999.)

sophisticated low pressure chamber at the U.S. Army Research Institute of Environmental Medicine in Natick, Massachusetts was used, and eight subjects aged 21 to 29 years spent 40 days and nights in the chamber. The subjects were gradually decompressed over a period of about 35 days followed by excursions to the 'summit' where the inspired P_{O_2} was 43 mmHg which this time was the correct value. Not all the subjects made it to the 'summit' but nevertheless very valuable physiological information was obtained. An advantage of a chamber study over a field study is that much more invasive procedures can be carried out because if a subject gets into difficulties he can rapidly be removed to a medical facility.

Some of the most important studies were on the pulmonary circulation, and these were referred to in Chapter 7. Cardiac catheterization was carried out using a Swan–Ganz catheter at barometric pressures of 760, 347, 282 and 240 mmHg. For the last measurement the oxygen concentration in the chamber was 22% giving an inspired P_{O_2} of 43 mmHg. The mean pulmonary arterial pressure at rest at sea level was 15 $\pm$ 0.9 mmHg but this increased to 34 $\pm$ 3 mmHg at a barometric pressure of 282 mmHg (Groves *et al.* 1987). At the same time the pulmonary vascular resistance increased from 1.2 to 4.3 mmHg L^{-1} min^{-1}. When the subjects performed maximal exercise, the increases in

Table 12.2 Barometric pressures, equivalent altitudes, and arterial blood gases during rest and maximal exercise on Operation Everest II (from Houston *et al.* 1987, and Sutton *et al.* 1988)

Barometric pressure (mmHg)	Inspired P_{O_2} (mmHg)	Altitude on Mount Everest (m)	Rest			Maximum exercise		
			P_{O_2} (mmHg)	P_{CO_2} (mmHg)	pH	P_{O_2} (mmHg)	P_{CO_2} (mmHg)	pH
760	149	0	99	34	7.43	87	35	7.30
429	80	4825	52	25	7.46	42	20	7.42
347	63	6482	41	20	7.50	34	17	7.44
282	49	8043	37	13	7.53	33	11	7.49
253*	43	8848	30	11	7.56	28	10	7.52

*Actual chamber pressure was 240 mmHg but because of oxygen contamination of the chamber air, the oxygen concentration was 22%. Therefore the inspired P_{O_2} was 43 mmHg corresponding to a barometric pressure of 253 mmHg for 21% oxygen. From West (1996a).

mean pulmonary artery pressure were even more remarkable, rising from 33 ± 1 mmHg at sea level to 54 ± 2 mmHg at a barometric pressure of 282 mmHg (Fig. 7.10). However, the pulmonary arterial wedge pressure was unchanged with the increase in simulated altitude.

Cardiac output was measured and shown to have the same relationship with oxygen consumption as at sea level (Fig. 7.3), confirming earlier measurements made on the Silver Hut Expedition (Pugh 1964). However, heart rate as a function of work level was higher as altitude increased. A particularly interesting finding was that when the subjects breathed 100% oxygen at the high altitudes, pulmonary vascular resistance did not return to the sea level values. This indicated a substantial degree of irreversibility in pulmonary vascular resistance after 2 or 3 weeks of hypoxia indicating vascular remodeling.

Additional information was found in the area of pulmonary gas exchange where it was possible to use the multiple inert gas elimination technique to separate the effects of ventilation–perfusion inequality from those of diffusion limitation. These studies were referred to in Chapter 6. Diffusion limitation of oxygen transfer across the blood-gas barrier occurred at oxygen uptakes greater than 3 L min^{-1} at sea level, and at less than 1 L min^{-1} on the 'summit.' This is a graphic demonstration of diffusion limitation at extreme altitude. A new finding was the increasing ventilation–perfusion inequality from rest to exercise at all altitudes. There was indirect

evidence that this may have been caused by interstitial pulmonary edema. Table 12.2 summarizes the arterial blood gases during rest and maximal exercise on Operation Everest II.

Another invasive study that would be extremely difficult to perform in the field was the analysis of skeletal muscle taken by needle biopsies. Skeletal muscle volume was also inferred from computer tomography scans of the arms and legs. Muscle area decreased by about 14% during the 'ascent.' The biopsies showed that this could be accounted for by a significant decrease in the cross-sectional area of both type I and type II fibers. As a result there was an increase in capillary volume density although this was not significant. Muscle enzymes were also measured and showed that at the highest altitude of 282 mmHg where biopsies were taken, there were significant reductions in succinic dehydrogenase, citrate synthetase, and hexokinase compared with measurements made after returning to sea level. Finally the biopsies showed significant reductions in muscle lactate concentrations at the higher altitudes consistent with the low blood lactate concentrations referred to in section 12.3.4.

OPERATION EVEREST III

This low pressure chamber experiment in 1997 was carried out at the COMEX facility in Toulouse, France, and had a number of similarities with Operation Everest II (Richalet *et al.* 1999). However, an innovative feature was that the eight volunteers pre-acclimatized in the Vallot Observatory (4350 m) for several days before spending a total of 31 days in the low pressure chamber, ultimately reaching the 'summit' barometric pressure of 253 mmHg. The arterial blood-gas values were similar to those found on Operation Everest II (Table 12.2) with a 'summit' arterial P_{O_2} of 31 mmHg, P_{CO_2} of 12 mmHg and pH of 7.58. The fact that the P_{CO_2} was higher than on AMREE in both of the chamber studies is consistent with a lesser degree of acclimatizing (compare Fig. 12.4). Body weight fell by an average of 5.4 kg, again in line with Operation Everest II and AMREE. Cardiovascular measurements largely confirmed those made on Operation Everest II (Boussuges *et al.* 2000). An interesting new finding was transient neurological disorders which were attributed to gas emboli, and there were also marked changes in mood of some of the subjects (Nicholas *et al.* 2000).

12.4 WHAT LIMITS EXERCISE PERFORMANCE AT EXTREME ALTITUDE?

12.4.1 Concept of limitation

The oxygen cascade from the atmosphere to the mitochondria includes the processes of convective ventilation of oxygen to the alveoli, diffusion of oxygen across the blood-gas barrier, uptake of oxygen by the hemoglobin in the pulmonary capillaries, convective flow of the blood to the peripheral capillaries, unloading of the oxygen from the hemoglobin, diffusion to the mitochondria and utilization of oxygen by the electron transport system. How can we determine to what extent each of these factors is limiting exercise at extreme altitude?

One approach is to use the analogy of a turbine that is fed by water flowing through a pipe which has a series of constrictions in it. Clearly, all sections of the pipe limit the flow of water to some extent. However, a useful description of the extent to which flow is limited by any particular section of the pipe can be found by calculating the percentage change in total flow for a given (say 5%) change in diameter at that point. In carrying out this calculation, we assume that all other factors remain unchanged. Such an analysis can only be carried out if the whole system is modeled using a computer.

Table 12.3 Key variables for the analysis of factors limiting oxygen uptake on the summit of Mount Everest

Measured	
Barometric pressure	253 mmHg
Alveolar P_{CO_2}	7.5 mmHg
Hemoglobin concentration	18.4 g dL^{-1}
P_{50} at pH 7.4	29.6 mmHg
Base excess	-7.2 mmol L^{-1}

Assumed	
Respiratory exchange ratio	1.0
Cardiac output/oxygen uptake	Same as sea level
Maximal DM_{O_2}[a]	100 mL min^{-1} $mmHg^{-1}$
Capillary transit time	0.75 s
Minimum P_{O_2} in mixed venous blood	15 mmHg

[a] DM_{O_2}, diffusing capacity of the membrane for oxygen.

12.4.2 Limitations to oxygen uptake on the summit of Mount Everest

The model analysis described above has been carried out for a hypothetical subject exercising on the summit of Mount Everest (West 1983). Some assumptions and extrapolations are necessary because so few data have yet been obtained at these great altitudes. In general, the physiological variables were those set out in section 12.3 and Table 12.3 summarizes these. The whole oxygen transport system was modeled using numerical procedures previously described (West and Wagner 1977, 1980). The details of a model analysis like this are not important because of uncertainties in the assumptions. However, some interesting predictions emerge (Fig. 12.7).

The most important variable affecting the maximal oxygen consumption ($\dot{V}_{O_2,max}$) is the barometric pressure. In this analysis a 5% increase in pressure increased the $\dot{V}_{O_2,max}$ by over 20% when all other variables were held constant. Other important variables were the alveolar ventilation and the membrane diffusing capacity of the lung.

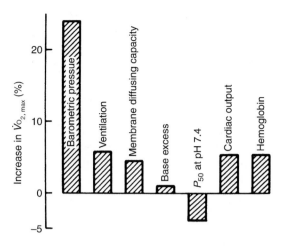

Figure 12.7 Sensitivity of calculated maximal oxygen consumption ($\dot{V}_{O_2,max}$) to changes in variables for a climber on the summit of Mount Everest. The initial conditions are those shown in Table 12.3, and each variable was increased by 5% leaving all the others constant. See text for details. (From West 1983.)

The first increased the $\dot{V}_{O_2,max}$ by raising the alveolar P_{O_2} whereas the second improved the arterial P_{O_2} because of the marked diffusion limitation of oxygen across the blood-gas barrier. An increase in oxygen affinity for hemoglobin as a result of increasing respiratory alkalosis also improved $\dot{V}_{O_2,max}$. In this analysis an increase in cardiac output was also beneficial but in another theoretical analysis which took account of diffusion limitation of oxygen transfer in the exercising muscles, this improvement was not seen (Fig. 7.5).

The chief conclusions from the analysis are as follows:

- A climber attempting an ascent of Mount Everest without supplementary oxygen should ideally choose a day with a relatively high barometric pressure. Indeed, this appears to be

the most critical variable. Fortunately, climbers generally try to make a summit assault when the weather is fine and usually this means a high pressure. Note, however, that this factor makes a winter ascent of Mount Everest without supplementary oxygen particularly difficult.
- The climber should not have a low hypoxic ventilatory response because a high ventilation is critical in maintaining an adequate alveolar P_{O_2}.
- It is advantageous to have a high oxygen diffusing capacity at a moderate work level.
- The climber should have as high a base excess as possible. Presumably one way to ensure this is to avoid prolonged stays at extreme altitudes.

12.4.3 How high can humans climb without supplementary oxygen?

We have seen that the $\dot{V}_{O_2,max}$ in acclimatized subjects with an inspired P_{O_2} of 43 mmHg, equivalent to that on the Everest summit, is only a little over $1\,L\,min^{-1}$. This oxygen uptake is equivalent to walking slowly on level ground. Clearly, humans at the highest point on Earth are very close to the limit of hypoxic tolerance.

Nevertheless, it is interesting to speculate on how much higher humans could climb without supplementary oxygen. The answer from the available data is very little. For example, as indicated earlier, a reduction of barometric pressure by 17 mmHg from 253 to 236 mmHg (the value for the Everest summit given by the Standard Atmosphere), would reduce the $\dot{V}_{O_2,max}$ by about 21% (West 1999a). It seems unlikely that the mountain could be climbed under these conditions emphasizing again that it is only the equatorial bulge in barometric pressure (Figs 2.3 and 2.5) which allows humans to reach the highest mountain top without supplementary oxygen.

13

Sleep

SUMMARY

Sleep is very commonly impaired at high altitude. Typically, people complain that they wake frequently, have unpleasant dreams and do not feel refreshed in the morning. Polysomnographic studies confirm the increased frequency of arousals. Electrencephalograms show changes in the architecture of sleep, usually with a great reduction in time spent in rapid eye movement (REM) sleep. Periodic breathing is almost universal at high altitude, and is accompanied by apneic periods which may be as much as 10–15 s long. The mechanism of the periodic breathing is probably related to the strong hypoxic ventilatory drive. High altitude natives who have a blunted ventilatory response to hypoxia show less or no periodic breathing compared with lowlanders at high altitude. The severe arterial hypoxemia which follows the long apneic periods may reduce the arterial P_{O_2} to its lowest levels of the 24-h period. Acetazolamide stimulates ventilation at high altitude, reduces the time spent in periodic breathing, and improves the arterial oxygen saturation during sleep. Benzodiazepines also reduce periodic breathing. Oxygen enrichment of room air at high altitude results in fewer apneas, less time spent in periodic breathing, and an improved subjective assessment of sleep quality.

13.1 INTRODUCTION

Everyone who has been to high altitude knows that sleeping is often impaired. This ubiquitous problem affects the skier or trekker who sleeps at altitudes of 2500–3000 m, as well as the well-acclimatized climber who spends a night as high as 8000 m. The altitude of many modern skiing resorts is over 2700 m and many people who move rapidly from sea level to that altitude have difficulties with sleep for the first two or three nights. Often they cannot get to sleep for a long period, or they wake frequently, and often they complain that they do not feel refreshed in the morning. This last comment is also frequently heard from climbers at great altitudes on expeditions (Pugh and Ward 1956). Some people trying to sleep at high altitude complain that the mind races with a kaleidoscope of thoughts tumbling through it; this is certainly the case with the writer, who recognizes this as a very characteristic feature of the first night or two at high altitude.

Climbers at high altitude are often urged to climb high during the day but sleep low during the night. This advice acknowledges the increased incidence of difficulties during sleep. Many climbers over an altitude of about 7000 m find that a very low flow of supplementary oxygen of perhaps 1 L min^{-1} greatly improves the quality of sleep.

Periodic breathing during sleep at high altitude has been recognized since the nineteenth century. It is extremely common and may pose a hazard at extreme altitude because of the severe arterial hypoxemia which follows the apneic periods (West *et al.* 1986). Indeed, this may be one of the factors that influences tolerance to very great altitudes. From a scientific point of view, periodic breathing during sleep at high altitude throws light on the control of breathing under these special conditions.

The present chapter overlaps the material of Chapter 5 on the control of ventilation, and also has some links with Chapter 7 on cardiovascular responses because of the alterations in heart rate that occur with periodic breathing.

13.2 HISTORICAL

13.2.1 Quality of sleep

There have been a number of anecdotal references to the poor quality of sleep at high altitude. A particularly colorful description was given by Barcroft when he recounted his experiences during the glass chamber experiment carried out at Cambridge, UK (Barcroft *et al.* 1920). On that occasion he spent 6 days in a closed chamber in which the concentration of oxygen was regulated so that the initial equivalent altitude was 10 000 ft (3048 m) and the final altitude 16 000 ft (4877 m). He wrote:

> In the glass case experiment I had the opportunity of judging a little more exactly of anoxaemic sleeplessness than is usually the case. A committee of undergraduate pupils of mine made up their minds that I was never to be left alone, two of them therefore sat up each night outside the case lest help of any sort should be required. I used to ask them in the morning how I had slept, and each morning except perhaps the last they said I had slept well. My own view of the matter was quite otherwise. I thought I had been awake half the night and was unrefreshed in the morning. I was conscious of their moving about and looking in through the glass to see whether or not I was awake. I used to count my pulse at intervals. The two opinions can only be

reconciled on the hypothesis that whilst I spent most of the night in sleep, the slumber was very light and fitful with incessant dreams. Even some low degree of consciousness which fell short of wakefulness. At Cerro it was the same: measured in hours we slept well, but the quality of the sleep in most cases was of an inferior order. The night seemed long and we woke unrefreshed.

> (Barcroft 1925, p. 166)

It is interesting that more recent studies confirm Barcroft's impression that although total sleep time at altitude may be nearly normal, the increased frequency of awakenings ('fitful' sleep) causes sleep to be less refreshing than normal (Reite *et al.* 1975, Zielinski *et al.* 2000).

13.2.2 Periodic breathing

Various references to the uneven pattern of breathing during sleep at high altitude were made during the nineteenth century. One was by the eminent English physicist Tyndall who was one of the most ardent Alpine mountaineers in the middle of the century. Paul Bert commented that 'every year sees him planting his alpenstock on some new summit' (Bert 1878). During Tyndall's first ascent of Mont Blanc in 1857, he became very fatigued.

> I stretched myself upon a composite couch of snow and granite, and immediately fell asleep. My friend, however, soon aroused me. 'You quite frighten me' he said, 'I listened for some minutes and have not heard you breathe once.'

On renewing the ascent, Tyndall complained of palpitations.

> At each pause my heart throbbed audibly, as I leaned upon my staff, and the subsidence of this action was always the signal for further advance.

> (Tyndall 1860)

Another early comment on periodic breathing was made by Egli-Sinclair (1894) in an article on mountain sickness. He noted that, at an altitude of 4400 m, respiration had the Stokes character, that is, it seemed regular during a certain time, after which a few rapid and profound breaths were drawn, a total suspension of a few seconds then following.

Here he was referring to the Irish physician, Dr William Stokes, who described the pattern of breathing which

consists in the occurrence of a series of inspirations, increasing to a maximum and then declining in force and length until a state of apparent apnoea is established.

(Stokes 1854)

Another Irish physician, John Cheyne, had described the same pattern in 1818 (Cheyne 1818) and so the breathing pattern is often known as Cheyne–Stokes breathing. However, Ward (1973) pointed out that John Hunter had given a lucid and succinct description of the same condition in 1781 (Hunter 1781).

The first extensive studies of periodic breathing at high altitude were made by Angelo Mosso, Professor of Physiology at the University of Turin, Italy. As mentioned earlier, he was one of the first people to use the Capanna Regina Margherita on the Monte Rosa at an altitude of 4559 m for scientific work. He measured the breathing movements by means of a lever which rested on the chest. An example of one of his measurements on his brother, Ugolino Mosso, is shown in Fig. 13.1a. The periods of apnea lasted about 12 s. Note that, in this instance, the first breath after the apneic period was the largest. A more

typical pattern is that shown in Fig. 13.1b which was measured on Francioli, keeper of the Regina Margherita hut. In this instance the waxing and waning of breathing movements are clearly seen and the periods of apnea are shorter (Mosso 1898, pp. 42–7).

A curious feature of Mosso's measurements was that he concluded that ventilation was actually decreased at high altitude, apparently because he converted his readings to standard conditions (0°C and 1000 mmHg in his case) rather than BTPS (body temperature and pressure saturated). Interestingly, Paul Bert also believed that hyperventilation did not occur at high altitude (Bert 1878, p. 106 in the 1943 translation). He wrote

What is really certain is that . . . a dweller in lofty altitudes, does not even try to struggle against the decrease of oxygen in his arterial blood by speeding up his respirations excessively, as was first supposed. The observations of Dr. Jourdanet are conclusive.

Bert probably reached this conclusion because he worked exclusively with low pressure chambers that only allowed short-term observations. It was not until Mosso could work in the Capanna Regina Margherita a few years later that measurements were easily made on subjects exposed to high altitude for several days although, as indicated above, he thought that ventilation was decreased.

Mosso realized that the alveolar P_{CO_2} was reduced in people living in the Capanna Regina Margherita at 4559 m, but instead of attributing this to an increased ventilation, he argued that the low pressure at high altitude extracted carbon dioxide from

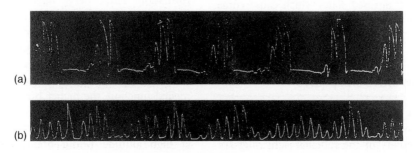

Figure 13.1   Earliest tracings showing periodic breathing at an altitude of 4560 m: (a) a record from Ugolino Mosso, brother of Angelo Mosso. Note the apneic periods of approximately 12 s; (b) a tracing from Francioli, keeper of the Regina Margherita hut. Note the waxing and waning of respiration. (From Mosso 1898.)

the blood just as does a mercury pump in a blood-gas analysis apparatus. Barcroft (1925) could not follow Mosso's argument and remarked:

> I speak with all deference, but Mosso seems to me to have overlooked the fact that the body is exposed to what is practically a vacuum of carbon dioxide, whether it be at the Capanna Margherita or in his own laboratory at Turin.

Mosso introduced the term 'acapnia' to refer to the reduction of P_{CO_2} and believed that this was an important factor in the development of acute mountain sickness (AMS). Indeed, it may well be that the symptoms of this condition are related in part to the respiratory alkalosis. However, Barcroft (1925) pointed out that Mosso's theory was not supported by the experience at the Alta Vista hut (3350 m) on Tenerife during the First International High Altitude Expedition of 1910. Barcroft had an almost normal alveolar P_{CO_2} (38 mmHg) but was incapacitated by the altitude, whereas Douglas, whose P_{CO_2} was only 32 mmHg, was 'perfectly free from all symptoms.' Thus hypoxia (which was more severe in Barcroft because he did not increase his ventilation) rather than the low P_{CO_2} was implicated in the etiology of mountain sickness.

13.3 PHYSIOLOGY OF SLEEP

Despite the fact that we spend up to one-third of our lives in the sleeping state, some aspects of the physiology of sleep are poorly understood. Sleep can be defined as a state of unconsciousness from which the subject can be aroused by sensory or other stimuli. As such it can be distinguished from deep anesthesia and diseased states which cause coma, though these have some features in common with true sleep. Two major types of sleep are recognized.

13.3.1 Slow wave sleep (SWS)

This is often called non-REM or NREM sleep, or sometimes normal sleep. It is characterized by decreased activity of the reticular activating system, and is called slow wave sleep (SWS) because of the predominance of slow delta waves in the electroencephalogram (EEG). These slow waves have a high voltage and occur at a rate of 1 or $2\,s^{-1}$. In the early stages of sleep, the alpha rhythm (8–13 Hz), which is always present during wakefulness, becomes more obvious. In addition, sleep spindles (14–16 Hz) may appear. These features can be used to divide SWS into four stages (I–IV). The delta waves probably originate in the cortex of the brain when it is not driven from below because of the reduced level of activity of the reticular activating system. SWS is dreamless, very restful and associated with a decreased peripheral vascular tone, blood pressure, respiratory rate and basal metabolic rate.

13.3.2 Rapid eye movement (REM) sleep

This is called REM sleep because, although the eyes remain closed, there are rapid horizontal eye movements. In a normal night of sleep, bouts of REM sleep lasting 5–20 min usually appear on the average about every 90 min. Often the first such period occurs 80–100 min after the subject falls asleep. The EEG tracing resembles the waking state, but the person is actually more difficult to arouse than during NREM sleep. REM sleep is usually associated with active dreaming; the muscle tone throughout the body is greatly depressed, but there may be occasional muscular twitching and limb jerking. The heart rate and respiration usually become irregular. Thus, in this type of sleep, the brain is quite active but the activity is not channeled in the proper direction for the person to be aware of his or her surroundings.

In experimental animals, sleep can be produced by electrically stimulating the raphe nuclei in the pons and medulla. There are extensive nerve fiber connections between these nuclei and the reticular formation. These nerve fibers secrete serotonin and some physiologists believe that this is a major transmitter substance associated with the production of sleep. However, other possible transmitter substances may play a role in the onset of sleep.

Sleep deprivation or fragmentation impairs mental function, the higher brain functions being the most susceptible. There are similarities between the behavior of sleep-deprived subjects and people at high altitude whose brains are affected by hypoxia. In both instances, mental activities which are 'mechanical' in nature, such as tabulating a set of data, can be accurately accomplished, whereas activities that require problem solving and initiative are seriously affected (Chapter 16). It may be that some of the impairment of CNS function in individuals living at high altitude can be ascribed to the poor quality of sleep, but the direct effects of hypoxia on the brain also clearly play a role.

13.4 CHARACTERISTICS OF SLEEP AT HIGH ALTITUDE

13.4.1 Increased frequency of arousals

People at high altitude often report that they wake more frequently during the night than at sea level, and this has been confirmed by careful studies (Reite *et al.* 1975, Weil *et al.* 1978, Salvaggio *et al.* 1998, Zielinski *et al.* 2000). The subjects had continuous recordings of the EEG, electromyogram (EMG) and eye movements, and an arousal was recognized by the occurrence of EMG activation, eye movements and alpha wave activity on the EEG. In one study an average of 36 arousals per night occurred at an altitude of 4300 m compared with 20 at sea level (Weil *et al.* 1978). Administration of the drug acetazolamide, which is known to stimulate

ventilation at high altitude, reduced the frequency of arousals. An example of frequent arousals is shown in Fig. 13.2.

Some investigators believe that the arousals are caused in some way by periodic breathing. There is some evidence that arousals are more frequent when the strength of periodic breathing is high. It is easy to imagine that the strenuous muscular activity required to generate large breaths after a prolonged period of apnea could contribute to an arousal. A common nightmare at high altitude is that the tent has been covered with snow by an avalanche and the subject wakes violently feeling suffocated and very short of breath. This may be associated with the air hunger caused by a long apneic period as part of periodic breathing. However, arousals are more frequent at high altitude, even in individuals who do not have periodic breathing (Reite *et al.* 1975, Wickramasinghe and Anholm 1999).

13.4.2 Changes of sleep state

EEG studies confirm that there is a deterioration in the quality of sleep at high altitude. Light sleep

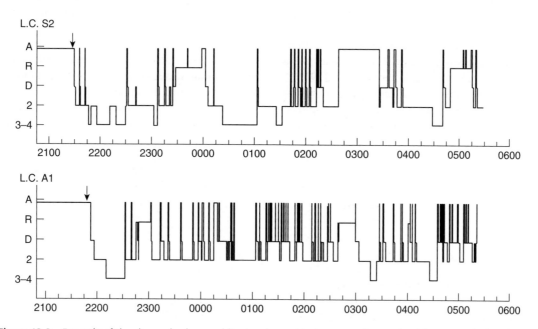

Figure 13.2 Example of the change in sleep architecture in a subject measured at sea level (upper tracing) and on the first night at an altitude of 4300 m (lower tracing). Time is on the horizontal axis and sleep stages are shown on the vertical axis. A, awake; R, REM; D, stage I; 2, stage II; 3–4, stages and 4. At altitude there was greatly increased sleep fragmentation and a reduction in slow wave sleep. (From Reite *et al.* 1975.)

(stages I and II of NREM) is increased, whereas there are decreases both in deep sleep (stages III and IV of NREM) and in REM sleep. In some studies, REM sleep is virtually abolished (Pappenheimer 1977, Megirian *et al.* 1980). These studies of the electrical activity of the brain support the subjective conclusions of climbers that sleep at high altitude is often of poor quality, and not as refreshing as sleep at sea level.

An early study of EEG changes in sleep at altitude was performed in Antarctica where near the South Pole the barometric pressure is reduced because of the actual altitude and also the very high latitude (see section 2.2.4). At this location Joern *et al.* (1970) reported a near absence of sleep stages III and IV coupled with an approximately 50% reduction in REM sleep. Although the light–dark cycle was unusual in this setting, their findings have been confirmed at more moderate latitudes.

An extensive study by Reite *et al.* (1975) studied sleep patterns in subjects following a rapid ascent to Pikes Peak (4300 m). Again there was a shift from deeper to lighter sleep stages and a great reduction in REM sleep. They reported that periodic breathing was common but that it disappeared during REM sleep. The changes in the pattern of sleep and respiration were greatest on the first night at high altitude and then declined. Other investigators have generally confirmed these changes in sleep pattern at high altitude (Anholm *et al.* 1992, Goldenberg *et al.* 1992, Wickramasinghe and Anholm 1999).

Studies in experimental animals have shown similar findings. Pappenheimer (1977, 1984) studied rats with chronically implanted cortical electrodes

and found that there were decreases in deep sleep stages while in some studies REM sleep was virtually abolished. In a more recent study, Lovering *et al.* (2003) showed that sleeping cats had a marked reduction in REM sleep when they were exposed to hypoxia. Interestingly, here the mechanism appeared to be hypocapnia because the reduced REM sleep could also be caused by mechanical hyperventilation.

13.5 PERIODIC BREATHING

13.5.1 Characteristics

Early records of chest movements during periodic breathing are shown in Fig. 13.1. This pattern has now been confirmed in many studies carried out at various altitudes from sea level up to 8050 m (Douglas and Haldane 1909, Douglas *et al.* 1913, Weil *et al.* 1978, Sutton *et al.* 1979, Berssenbrugge *et al.* 1983, Lahiri *et al.* 1983, West *et al.* 1986).

A typical pattern recorded at an altitude of 6300 m (P_B 351 mmHg) in a well-acclimatized lowlander using modern equipment is shown in Fig. 13.3 (West *et al.* 1986). Note that the tidal volume waxed and waned during each burst of breathing, with apneic periods of about 8 s. Arterial oxygen saturation as measured by ear oximeter fluctuated with the same frequency as the periodic breathing. Note the phase difference; the highest arterial oxygen saturation (inverted scale) occurred at approximately the end of the apneic period. This can be accounted for by the circulation time from the lung capillaries to the ear where the oxygen saturation

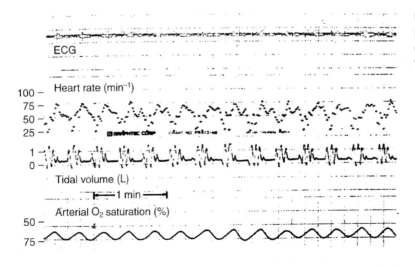

Figure 13.3 Example of periodic breathing at altitude 6300 m (P_B 351 mmHg). (From West *et al.* 1986.)

was measured. Heart rate was measured from the electrocardiogram (ECG) and showed marked fluctuations with the same frequency as the periodic breathing. Note that the highest heart rate appeared at the end of the burst of ventilation.

Nocturnal periodic breathing is extremely common in lowlanders who ascend to high altitude. In the study from which Fig. 13.3 is taken, all eight subjects who were living at an altitude of 6300 m showed obvious periodic breathing during the several weeks over which the measurements were made. Studies were conducted over a period of about 1–3.5 h late at night and the proportion of the study period during which periodic breathing was seen varied between 57 and 90%. In general, the percentage of time occupied by periodic breathing increases with altitude. For example, Waggener et al. (1984) reported that periodic breathing with apnea occupied 24% of the time at 2440 m, and that the percentage increased to 40% at 4270 m. This increase in proportion of time is consistent with a theoretical model discussed below (Khoo et al. 1982) and with the fact that periodic breathing is occasionally observed during sleep at sea level but the proportion of time spent in periodic breathing is small (Priban 1963, Goodman 1964, Lenfant 1967).

In the AMREE study from which Fig. 13.3 is taken, it was not possible to determine how much of the time the subjects were actually asleep. However, other studies have shown that periodic breathing is very common during NREM sleep at high altitude, but that it is uncommon during REM periods (Reite et al. 1975, Berssenbrugge et al. 1983). Of course, as indicated above, REM sleep itself is uncommon at high altitude. The periodic breathing cycle in the AMREE study had a mean of 20.5 s. This was the same as the cycle length measured in a companion study at 5400 m (Lahiri et al. 1983). There is evidence that cycle length decreases with increasing altitude (Waggener et al. 1984) and studies at sea level indicate a cycle period of about 30 s (Douglas and Haldane 1909, Specht and Fruhmann 1972, Lugaresi et al. 1978). Figure 13.4 shows a plot of cycle time against altitude for several experimental studies and the theoretical model developed by Khoo et al. (1982). It can be seen that the cycle times from the AMREE studies were somewhat greater than predicted by the model.

There is strong evidence that the apneic periods are of central nervous origin rather than being caused by airway obstruction. This is supported by the absence of rib cage and abdominal movements as determined from an inductance plethysmograph, a device used for detecting changes in circumference of the chest and abdomen. There was no evidence that the percentage of time during which periodic breathing was observed was altered by the duration of acclimatization. All subjects showed obvious periodic breathing but all were well acclimatized. Some studies suggest that periodic breathing tends to decrease over successive nights of moderate altitudes as acclimatization progresses, but that it persists at altitudes above about 4500 m (Wickramasinghe and Anholm 1999, Weil 2004).

Changes of heart rate during the periodic breathing cycle were seen in all subjects and Fig. 13.3 is a good example. In general, the maximum heart rate appeared shortly after the peak of the hyperpnea. Cardiac rhythm abnormalities were infrequent. In one subject, ventricular premature contractions occurred mainly during the apneic periods. However, this subject had a history of occasional ventricular premature contractions at sea level. There were no other observable changes in ECG pattern except for minor alterations that could be attributed to changes in the position of the heart caused by breathing movements.

In four subjects, evidence of periodic breathing was obtained at an altitude of 8050 m (P_B 282 mmHg). In these studies, breathing movements

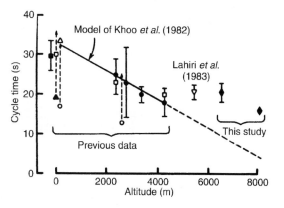

Figure 13.4 Variation of cycle time of periodic breathing with altitude. Points marked 'Previous data' were originally published as Figure 8 in the paper by Khoo et al. (1982), the solid line being results predicted by their model (d). Vertical broken lines indicate differences caused by scaling between neonates and adults. For sources of data see Khoo et al. (1982). 'This study' refers to West et al. (1986). (From West et al. 1986.)

were not recorded directly because of the very remote location of the camp. However, continuous ECG tracings were obtained during the night using a Holter-type monitor, and the occurrence of periodic breathing was inferred from the variations in heart rate as described by Guilleminault *et al.* (1984). An example is shown in Fig. 13.5. This particular subject showed extremely regular cyclic regulation of heart rate over long periods of time (up to 40 min). It was easy to distinguish between this type of cyclic variation caused by periodic breathing and sinus arrhythmia.

13.5.2 Control of breathing

The control of breathing during sleep has been extensively studied: for a review see Phillipson *et al.* (1978). The ventilatory response to carbon dioxide is reduced, at least in NREM sleep (Bulow 1963). However, there is more uncertainty about the hypoxic ventilatory response; some studies indicate that it is increased in NREM sleep (Pappenheimer

1977, Phillipson *et al.* 1978). Responses to pulmonary stretch receptor stimulation appear to be intact during NREM sleep but may be decreased in REM sleep (Phillipson *et al.* 1978).

The control of ventilation during hypoxic sleep has been less well studied and there are some unanswered questions (Dempsey 1983, Weil 2004). Lahiri *et al.* (1983) studied the role of added oxygen and carbon dioxide, and also the importance of the hypoxic ventilatory response to periodic breathing in both well-acclimatized lowlanders and native Sherpas at an altitude of 5400 m.

Figure 13.6 shows the effect of adding oxygen to the inspired air. It can be seen that there was an immediate increase in the apneic period from about 10 to 17 s. Subsequently, the apneic period shortened and shallow rhythmic breathing resumed as the arterial P_{CO_2} increased because of the fall in alveolar ventilation. In most subjects, the periodicity of breathing did not totally disappear following the addition of oxygen, but the strength of the periodic breathing was clearly greatly diminished. The

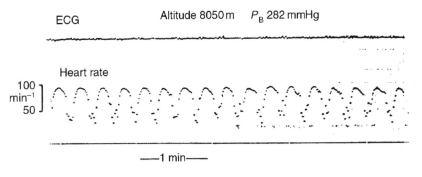

Figure 13.5   Cyclic variation of heart rate caused by periodic breathing in a climber at 8050 m altitude. $P_B = 282$ mmHg. (From West *et al.* 1986.)

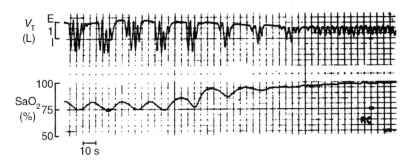

Figure 13.6   Effect of increasing the inspired P_{O_2} on periodic breathing in a lowlander during sleep at 5400 m. Note that adding oxygen to the inspired gas raised the arterial oxygen saturation, eliminated the apneic periods, and reduced the strength of periodic breathing. V_T, tidal volume; Sa_{O_2}, arterial oxygen saturation; E, expiration; I, inspiration. (From Lahiri and Barnard 1983.)

changes can be partly explained by the reduction in respiratory drive from the peripheral chemoreceptors when the arterial P_{O_2} was raised.

Adding carbon dioxide to the inspired gas did not totally abolish the periodic breathing, although it did eliminate the periods of apnea. Withdrawal of carbon dioxide from the inspired gas was followed by a prompt reappearance of apnea, and the rapidity of the response suggested a dominant role for the peripheral chemoreceptors.

An interesting finding was that although the lowlanders showed marked periodic breathing at 5400 m, the Sherpas often did not. The only exception was one Sherpa who had spent long periods of time at low altitudes. As discussed in Chapter 5, the Sherpas often show low ventilatory responses to hypoxia, although the low altitude Sherpa referred to here had an intermediate value. Figure 13.7 shows the relationship between the frequency of apnea during sleep at 5400 m and the hypoxic ventilatory response. This indicates that a high hypoxic ventilatory response predisposes to periodic breathing.

13.5.3 Mechanism

It is profitable to discuss the mechanism of periodic breathing in terms of control theory, and a

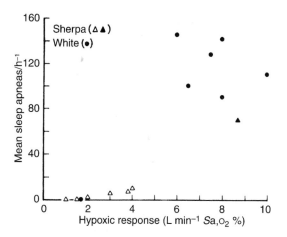

Figure 13.7 Relationship between frequency of sleep apnea and ventilatory response to hypoxia (awake). d, acclimatized lowlanders; n, high altitude Sherpas; m, lower altitude Sherpa. One lowlander did not have periods of apnea, and the low altitude Sherpa showed periodic breathing. (From Lahiri *et al.* 1983.)

particularly useful analysis was presented by Khoo *et al.* (1982). They pointed out that two factors are necessary for self-sustained oscillatory behavior in a control system. In such a system we can identify a 'disturbance', for example a change in alveolar ventilation caused by some adventitious factor such as a sigh or alteration of body position. This is followed by a 'corrective action' which tends to suppress the disturbance. In the case of an increase in alveolar ventilation (caused by a sigh, for example) the corrective action would be a lowering of P_{CO_2}, which would tend to reduce ventilation by its action on central and peripheral chemoreceptors and thus constitute negative feedback. The first necessary requirement for sustained oscillatory behavior is that the magnitude of the corrective action exceeds that of the disturbance, this ratio being known as the loop gain.

The second necessary condition is that the corrective action be presented 180° out of phase with the disturbance, so that what would otherwise inhibit the change in ventilation now augments it. This sustained oscillatory behavior occurs when the loop gain exceeds unity at a phase difference of 180°.

This theory predicts that the higher the loop gain at a phase angle of 180°, the more likely periodic breathing is to occur, the more marked the pattern of periodic breathing, and the shorter the cycle length of the periodic breathing. The main factor increasing loop gain in acclimatized lowlanders at high altitude is the increased chemoreceptor gain, particularly the response to severe hypoxia (Chapter 5). Other contributing factors may be the hyperventilation, which increases the rate of washout of carbon dioxide and wash-in of oxygen in the lungs, and the reduction of functional residual capacity in supine subjects.

This analysis explains why there is a difference between acclimatized lowlanders and Sherpas in periodic breathing. Because native highlanders often have a blunted hypoxic ventilatory response (Severinghaus *et al.* 1966a, Milledge and Lahiri 1967), the loop gain of the control system is reduced and the factors promoting periodicity are weak. Lahiri *et al.* (1983) have argued that this represents an important feature of the true adaptation of native highlanders such as Sherpas to high altitude. Periodic breathing is disadvantageous because of the very low levels of arterial P_{O_2} following the apneic periods (section 13.5.4). Having said this, some studies show that ventilation and oxygenation are actually improved during episodes of periodic breathing, and that the incidence of AMS may be reduced in subjects with increased periodicity (Fujimoto *et al.* 1989, Masuyama *et al.* 1989, Normand *et al.* 1990).

In the analysis discussed above, a disturbance, for example an arousal, is postulated to play an important role in the genesis of periodic breathing. However, Khoo *et al.* (1996) looked at the relationship between arousals and the initiation of periodic breathing in healthy volunteers at simulated altitudes of 4572, 6100 and 7620 m. They found that although arousals promoted the development of periodic breathing with apnea in some instances, arousals were not necessary for the initiation of periodic breathing in all circumstances.

In another study of periodic breathing at high altitude, measurements were made on nine Japanese climbers who participated in an expedition to the Kunlun mountains (7167 m) in China (Matsuyama *et al.* 1989). There was a significant correlation between the degree of periodic breathing during sleep and both the hypoxic ventilatory response and hypercapnic ventilatory response measured at sea level ($p < 0.05$). Although all climbers showed desaturation during sleep, there was a negative correlation between the degree of desaturation and the hypoxic ventilation response (HVR) ($p < 0.05$). The authors concluded that the high HVR helped to maintain the arterial oxygenation during sleep, and that it was therefore advantageous.

In a further study, subjects with early high altitude pulmonary edema (HAPE) showed a trend towards more periodic breathing than subjects without HAPE, probably because of lower values of arterial oxygen saturation (Eichenberger *et al.* 1996). In a study of patients with chronic mountain sickness at 3658 m altitude, sleep-disordered breathing was more common than in a control group (Sun *et al.* 1996).

13.5.4 Gas exchange

Periodic breathing causes marked fluctuations in the arterial P_{O_2}, which is not surprising considering the long periods of apnea that sometimes occur. Figure 13.3 shows a typical record of fluctuations in arterial oxygen saturation as recorded by ear oximeter. Another example is seen in Fig. 13.6.

In the study of nocturnal periodic breathing carried out at an altitude of 6300 m during the 1981 AMREE expedition, the mean fluctuation in arterial oxygen saturation between subjects was approximately 10% (West *et al.* 1986). In order to determine the proportion of the time during which the arterial oxygen saturation fell below a particular value, the analysis described by Slutsky and Strohl (1980) was carried out. This showed that the arterial oxygen saturation below which the subjects spent 50% of their time varied from a minimal value of 64.5% to a maximum of 74.5% with a mean of 68.8%.

Since it is not usually feasible to sample arterial blood over prolonged periods of time, most investigators of periodic breathing have relied on the arterial oxygen saturation measured by ear oximetry. However, based on spot measurements of arterial P_{O_2} it was calculated that the maximum and minimum values of saturation of 73.0% and 63.4% from the AMREE study corresponded to arterial P_{O_2} values of approximately 39 and 33 mmHg, respectively. The conclusion was that the minimal arterial P_{O_2} during sleep was approximately 6 mmHg lower than the resting daytime value, a substantial difference on this very steep part of the oxygen dissociation curve. It should be pointed out that, at high work rates, the arterial P_{O_2} falls considerably below the resting value. However, climbers during their normal activity do not generally work at more than two-thirds of their maximal power (Pugh 1958; section 11.9) so it was concluded that the most severe arterial hypoxemia over the course of the 24 h probably occurred during sleep as a result of the periodic breathing.

Another factor which may exaggerate the effects of this arterial hypoxemia is the augmented cardiac output during the periods when the arterial P_{O_2} is near its lowest value. As Figs 13.3 and 13.6 show, the lowest arterial oxygen saturation typically occurs just after the peak of ventilation during the periodic breathing cycle. If venous return and thus cardiac output are enhanced during this hyperpneic phase, this would lead to enhanced delivery of this poorly oxygenated blood. Thus it may be that the phasing of arterial P_{O_2} and cardiac output aggravate the resulting impairment of oxygen delivery.

It is possible that the severe arterial hypoxemia during periodic breathing affects tolerance to extreme altitude. This leads to a paradox. As Fig. 13.7 shows, there is a correlation between hypoxic ventilatory response and the strength of the periodic breathing, as would be expected from the control theory discussed in section 13.5.3. This would suggest that climbers with a high hypoxic ventilatory response would tolerate altitude poorly. However, the opposite is generally found to be the case (Schoene *et al.* 1984; also see Chapter 5). This can be explained by the better ability of these climbers to defend their alveolar P_{O_2} against the low inspired value by hyperventilation (Chapter 12). However, it is clear that some elite mountain climbers have, in fact, a relatively low hypoxic ventilatory response (Milledge *et al.* 1983c, Schoene *et al.* 1987). One possible explanation is that these climbers maintain a higher arterial P_{O_2} during the night, and this is a factor in their tolerance to extreme altitude.

13.5.5 Effects of drugs

Because of the poor quality of sleep at high altitude and the suspicion that this is sometimes related to periodic breathing, there has been considerable interest in the use of drugs to promote a normal breathing pattern. Sutton *et al.* (1979) showed that the administration of acetazolamide at a dose of 250 mg three times per day decreased the time spent in periodic breathing from 80 to 35% at an altitude of 5360 m. This was associated with an improvement in arterial P_{O_2} as judged by the arterial oxygen saturation measured by ear oximetry. Weil *et al.* (1978) used acetazolamide at an altitude of 4400 m and found that the duration of periodic breathing decreased from 35 to 18%. Hackett *et al.* (1987a) found a decrease from 41 to 17% at 4400 m in four subjects with the same drug (Fig. 13.8).

The mode of action of acetazolamide is not fully understood, but it stimulates ventilation possibly because it induces a metabolic acidosis. At any event, its value at high altitude is now generally accepted in that it reduces the incidence of acute mountain sickness (Hackett and Rennie 1976), maintains a higher alveolar P_{O_2} and lower P_{CO_2}, and may even prevent some of the weight loss which normally occurs as a result of muscle protein breakdown (Birmingham study 1981).

Other drugs have also been studied in an attempt to improve the quality of sleep at high altitude. There have been several studies of the benzodiazepine family. Dubowitz (1998) studied acclimatized subjects

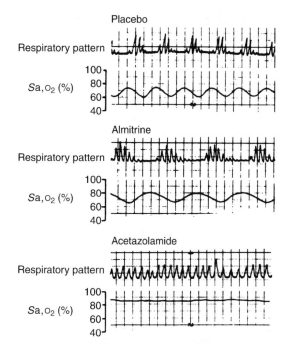

Figure 13.8 Effects of a placebo, almitrine and acetazolamide on periodic breathing and arterial oxygen saturation (Sa_{O_2}) at an altitude of 4400 m. Note that acetazolamide abolished the apneic periods whereas almitrine exaggerated them. (From Hackett *et al.* 1987.)

at an altitude of 5300 m and reported that the number and severity of changes in arterial oxygen saturation during sleep were decreased, and the quality of sleep was improved following administration of temazepam. He found no significant drop in mean oxygen saturation values during sleep. However, in acclimatized subjects Röggla *et al.* (1994) found that low dose sedation with diazepam reduced the ventilatory response at moderate altitude. In a subsequent study of temazepam, Röggla *et al.* (2000) showed that, at an altitude of 3000 m, the arterial P_{CO_2} (determined from earlobe blood) was significantly increased and the arterial P_{O_2} significantly decreased after 10 mg of temazepam.

In a study of zolpidem, an imidazopyridine hypnotic drug, on sleep and respiratory patterns at a simulated altitude of 4000 m in a low pressure chamber, Beaumont *et al.* (1996) reported improved sleep quality at high altitude without adverse effects on respiration. Blood gases were not looked at in this study.

13.5.6 Effect of oxygen enrichment of room air

Adding oxygen to the ventilation of a room shows promise as a way of combating the hypoxia of high altitude, particularly for people who commute to high altitude to work (see Chapter 27 where the technology is discussed). Luks *et al.* (1998) carried out a randomized, double-blind trial at an altitude of 3800 m to determine whether oxygen enrichment of room air to 24% at night improved sleep quality and performance and well being the following day. They found that, with oxygen enrichment, the subjects had significantly fewer apneas and spent significantly less time in periodic breathing with apneas than when they slept in ambient air (Fig. 13.9). Subjective assessments of sleep quality were also significantly improved. There was a lower acute mountain sickness score in the morning after oxygen-enriched sleep, using the Lake Louise criteria. Of particular interest, subjects who slept in the oxygen-enriched atmosphere had a significantly greater increase in arterial oxygen saturation from evening to morning compared with subjects who slept in ambient air. This latter finding suggested either that the control of breathing may have been altered by sleeping in an oxygen-enriched atmosphere, or that there was less subclinical pulmonary edema.

The study described above was conducted at an altitude of 3800 m which is higher than most recreational skiers and trekkers go. However, it is possible that oxygen enrichment of room air might be useful at lower altitudes, for example 2000–3000 m, where many skiing resorts are located. A common complaint of people who typically arrive in a day from near sea level is that sleeping is very unpleasant for the first two or three nights. Oxygen enrichment of room air is perfectly feasible for such resorts (West 2002b) and can be expected to greatly improve the quality of sleep. The provision of oxygen-enriched bedrooms would not be a major undertaking although careful attention has to be given to the ventilation of the rooms. At least one hotel, the Monasterio in Cusco, Peru (3399 m) offers special oxygen-enriched rooms.

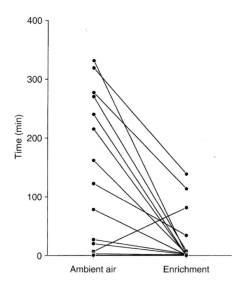

Figure 13.9 Comparison of the time spent by 18 subjects in periodic breathing with apneas during sleep in ambient air, compared with an atmosphere of 24% oxygen at an altitude of 3800 m. The paired differences were significant ($p < 0.01$). (From Luks *et al.* 1998.)

14

Nutrition, metabolism and intestinal function

SUMMARY

Loss of appetite and loss of weight are common at altitude. Initially these may be due to acute mountain sickness (AMS). At heights below about 4500 m appetite returns after a few days but at more extreme altitudes anorexia persists and may get worse. Weight loss on an altitude trip can have many causes. On trek, initial weight loss may be the shedding of excess fat caused by a sedentary lifestyle. Intestinal infections can cause diarrhea and weight loss. High on the mountain, unavailability of food and liquid can be the cause but even in the absence of these factors weight loss is seen, as in long-term chamber studies.

In considering energy balance at altitude, basal metabolic rate is increased 10–17% at 4000–6000 m and possibly more at extreme altitudes. Exercise increases energy needs, though the reduction in maximum work rate would be expected to reduce the energy requirement of climbing. However, the use of new techniques has given values of energy expenditure when climbing at extreme altitudes that are at least as high as in the Alps, if not higher, so daily energy needs are high while intake is often reduced because of anorexia. This anorexia may be mediated by the hormones such as leptin or by cholecystokinin.

Weight loss results in a change of body composition; fat tends to be lost preferentially at low elevations but muscle at higher altitudes.

Apart from calorie imbalance, there is some evidence that at altitudes above about 5500 m there may be malabsorption of food and an increase in intestinal permeability. This effect of hypoxia on the gut will increase the weight loss. But almost certainly the main cause of weight loss is calorie imbalance due to anorexia.

Diet is important on treks and expeditions. There are good physiological reasons to advise a high carbohydrate, low fat diet and many, though not all climbers seem to favor this. However, palatability is more important than composition in combating the loss of appetite. Taste is dulled and most find that they want more highly flavored, spicy foods. A craving for fresh rather than preserved food develops. Fluids remain acceptable and many calories can be taken in sweet milky drinks. Supplements such as vitamins and minerals are probably not necessary if a balanced diet is taken, with the possible exception of iron supplements for pre-menopausal women.

14.1 INTRODUCTION

Anorexia and weight loss are well-known features of life at high altitude, especially extreme altitudes. The mechanism of this anorexia is not known. During the first few days after a rapid ascent, anorexia may be part of the symptomatology of acute mountain sickness (AMS), but after this, when all other symptoms of AMS are gone, anorexia may remain. Studies have suggested that the anorexia of AMS may be mediated by the hormone leptin (Techop et al. 1998) though others have suggested this not to be the case (Zaccaria et al. 2004). Other appetite hormones may be involved such as cholecystokinin (Bailey et al. 2000). This continuing anorexia is not common below about 5000 m but is almost universal above 6000 m and becomes worse at even higher altitudes, though the severity varies considerably between individuals.

Weight loss is also common, though not inevitable, even at extreme altitudes (see below) and is largely due to the reduced energy intake consequent on the anorexia, but the possibility that other factors may contribute, such as malabsorption, is reviewed in this chapter. This chapter also considers diet at altitude and the evidence for the value of a high carbohydrate diet.

14.2 ENERGY BALANCE AT ALTITUDE

14.2.1 Energy output

Energy expenditure can be divided into three components:

- Basal metabolism during sleep and lying or sitting quietly
- Energy expenditure during periods of activity
- Food-induced energy expenditure

The metabolic rate during basal conditions is the basal metabolic rate (BMR) whilst during activity, the active metabolic rate may be increased up to many times the BMR during maximal exercise.

Mountaineers hardly ever use maximal work rate in climbing. Their preferred up-hill climbing rate is typically about 50% of maximum (Pugh et al. 1964) and this occupies only a part of the total time out 'climbing'; the rest being resting, walking down hill etc. Any periods of intense activity are usually of short duration so that under normal conditions it is the basal metabolic rate that is the largest component of daily energy expenditure. This is determined mainly by body size or more exactly the fat-free mass. Food induced energy expenditure is the energy required to digest the food eaten and is about 10% of the energy intake on a normal mixed diet.

BASAL METABOLIC RATE AT ALTITUDE

Nair et al. (1971) found that after a week at 3300 m the basal metabolic rate (BMR) was elevated by about 12%. Exposure to cold as well as hypoxia (in a second group of subjects) made no difference to this effect compared with hypoxia alone. By week 2, BMR was back to control values and was below control by week 3. Cold exposure at this time resulted in elevation of BMR to above sea level values by week 5 and it remained elevated a week after return to sea level. Butterfield et al. (1992) found BMR to be elevated by 27% on day 2 at Pikes Peak (4300 m) in Colorado. The BMR then decreased over the next few days to plateau at +17% compared with sea level by day 10. The metabolism of a group of fit women was studied at 4300 m by Mawson et al. (2000). The BMR was elevated after 3 days at altitude but had returned to sea level values by day 6. However, the energy requirements remained 6% elevated above control values giving rise to an apparent 'energy requirement excess' of about 670 MJ day^{-1} whilst at high altitude. They also found that the phase of the menstrual cycle had no effect on energy requirement at altitude.

After acclimatization, BMR measured at 5800 m was found to be elevated by about 10% in subjects who had been at altitude for 82–113 days (Gill and Pugh 1964). It is likely that BMR rises again if subjects climb to altitudes to which they are not acclimatized and we have no data on BMR at altitudes above 6000 m when weight loss becomes even more rapid, but its elevation might well be a factor.

BMR was found to be high at altitude in altitude residents (Ladakhis and Sherpas) compared with lowlanders and with predicted values (Gill and Pugh

1964, Nair *et al.* 1971). This elevation of BMR remained even when allowance was made for the fact that these people generally have less fat in their body composition. Picon-Reategui (1961) also reported elevated BMR in Andean miners at 4540 m. The mechanism for this rise in BMR is uncertain. Fecal and urinary excretion of energy nitrogen and volatile acids are not altered in the early days at altitude (Butterfield *et al.* 1992). There is increase in sympathetic activity at this time (section 15.6) and the finding that this increase in metabolic rate can be inhibited by a beta-blocker (Moore *et al.* 1987) suggests it is a likely factor. Increased thyroid activity may also play a part, especially in the longer-term elevation of BMR (section 15.7).

ACTIVITY ENERGY EXPENDITURE AT ALTITUDE

Work in absolute terms requires the same oxygen intake at altitude as at sea level until near-maximum work rate is reached (Pugh *et al.* 1964, West *et al.* 1983c, Wolfel *et al.* 1991). At altitude the maximum work rate is reduced (Chapter 11) and all activity seems disproportionately fatiguing. At 8000 m, even rolling over in a sleeping bag demands a great effort. Thus, energy expenditure for normal activities of daily living might be expected to be reduced at extreme altitude. Another fact of life at extreme altitudes is that often the only warm place is a sleeping bag and much of the 24 h of the day is spent lying down. However, the increased work of breathing has a small opposite effect, as does the increase in BMR, so that the daily energy expenditure is probably about the same as, or slightly above that at sea level (see below). At intermediate altitudes (2500–4500 m), although maximum work rate is reduced, energy expenditure on normal daily activities of short duration is probably not much altered. For longer-term work such as hill climbing, much will depend upon the degree of acclimatization and fitness. Pugh *et al.* (1964) found V_{O_2} intake on climbers climbing at their 'preferred' rate to decline very little up to about 5000 m (Fig. 11.1), whereas Butterfield *et al.* (1992) found a 37% reduction in energy expenditure for exercise 'more strenuous than walking'. But the overall requirement for energy to maintain body weight increased from 13.22 MJ at sea level to 14.64 MJ a day at 4300 m due to the increase in BMR.

Before about 1990 it had been impossible to measure energy expenditure over long periods, but a doubly labeled water technique was then developed which made this possible. Water is labeled with both deuterium and ^{18}O. The deuterium is eliminated as water while the oxygen is eliminated as both water and carbon dioxide. Thus carbon dioxide production can be calculated from the different elimination rates (Schoeller and van Santen 1982, Coward 1991). Using this technique, Westerterp *et al.* (1992) found average daily energy expenditure in the Alps (2500–4800 m) to be 14.7 MJ and on Mount Everest (5300–8848 m) it was not significantly different at 13.6 MJ. Very similar daily results were obtained in the 1992 British Winter Everest Expedition of 11.7–15.4 MJ (Travis *et al.* 1993). Pulfrey and Jones (1996), using the same technique at altitudes of 5900–8046 m, found the very high mean values of 19.4 MJ day^{-1} and a negative energy balance of 5.1 MJ day^{-1}. Reynolds *et al.* (1999) found the same high mean value of 20.6 MJ day^{-1} above Base Camp with a dietary intake of only 10.5 MJ, giving a deficit of 10 MJ day^{-1}! On the other hand, in a chamber experiment simulating an ascent of Everest over 31 days (Operation Everest III), there was a small reduction in energy expenditure from a mean of 13.6 in normoxia to 13.3 and 12.1 MJ day^{-1} in the early and late phases of the study (Westerterp *et al.* 2000). This suggests that hypoxia per se does not elevate BMR sufficiently to balance the effect of reduced daily activity in hypoxic subjects confined to a chamber, whereas on a mountaineering expedition high energy outputs and large calorie deficits can be expected.

14.2.2 Energy intake and caloric balance

Up to about 4500 m, people who have acclimatized have normal appetites and normal food intake (Consolazio *et al.* 1968). Above 6000 m most climbers experience anorexia. This tends to become more pronounced the longer one stays at these altitudes. Climbers complain about the food available and feel that the preserved nature of food increases the anorexia and reduces their intake. There are few data on actual calorie intake under these circumstances. Those that there are, rely on diary cards and estimates of portion size. On Cho Oyu in Nepal in 1952 food eaten at between 5250 and 6750 m was only about 13.4 MJ a day compared with 17.6 MJ on the march out, and on Everest in 1953, above 7250 m, the intake was only about 6.3 MJ (Pugh and Band 1953). On the Silver Hut Expedition (1960–61), in four climbers at 5800 m whose living conditions were excellent and where a good variety and quantity of food was available, a daily intake of 12.6–13.4 MJ day^{-1} was estimated (Pugh 1962a). Boyer and Blume (1984) reported that on the American Medical Expedition to Everest (AMREE) in 1981, over 3 days, four subjects had a mean intake of 9.34 MJ at 6300 m compared with 12.5 MJ at sea level. Dinmore *et al.* (1994) found intakes similar during the march in (1500–2000 m) and above 5500 m (10.8 and 10.3 MJ). However, Westerterp *et al.* (1992) and Travis *et al.* (1993) estimated intakes high on Everest of 7.5 MJ and 8.6 MJ, respectively, indicating the expected reduction in intake above 6300 m.

Clearly, high on major mountains (above 6000 m), when actively climbing, it is not possible to maintain caloric balance even when acclimatized. Westerterp *et al.* (1994) on Mount Sajama (6542 m) in Bolivia found an energy deficit of 3.5 MJ day^{-1} in 10 subjects camped on the summit for 21 days. The average weight loss was 4.9 kg (1.6 kg week^{-1}), 74% of it being due to loss of fat. In Everest climbers studied by Westerterp *et al.* (1992) there was a daily negative balance of 5.7 MJ. Clearly, more studies using the labeled water technique are needed to answer the question of whether acclimatized subjects can maintain energy balance at intermediate altitudes (4500–6000 m) when semi-sedentary.

14.3 WEIGHT LOSS ON ALTITUDE EXPEDITIONS

14.3.1 Weight loss on the march out

Most climbing and trekking groups experience weight loss in the initial 1–3 weeks of an expedition, even when walking below 3000 m. This is probably due to the change in lifestyle for most subjects from an urban semi-sedentary existence to the more active lifestyle of walking 16 km (10 miles) a day with some considerable ascents and descents. In addition, gastrointestinal infections are common.

Boyer and Blume (1984) found that 13 AMREE members, during the march out to the Everest region, lost an average of 2 kg (range 0–6 kg). Those with the highest percentage of body fat to start with lost most weight, the correlation being significant; 70% of this weight loss was due to loss of fat. Two subjects with less than 13% of body fat lost no weight. Dinmore *et al.* (1994) similarly found an average loss of 1.3 kg during the first week of trekking but only a further 0.5 kg in the next week.

Weight loss during this phase of an expedition or trek can be considered as shedding unnecessary fat.

14.3.2 Weight loss at altitude

On first arrival at altitude, AMS may cause anorexia and vomiting with resultant weight loss, though usually the duration is not long enough to do this. Also, fluid may be retained and subjects with AMS often gain weight (Hackett *et al.* 1982). Consolazio *et al.* (1972) found a small gain in weight on the first day at altitude followed by a loss of weight of about 1 kg over the next 5 days at 4300 m.

The mechanism of the anorexia as a symptom of AMS is not clear. A few humoral factors which are known to affect appetite or satiety have been investigated.

LEPTIN

Leptin is a hormone which suppresses appetite. In subjects taken to 4559 m by helicopter, Tschop *et al.* (1998) found that the leptin levels were raised and in those who complained of anorexia levels were higher than those with no loss of appetite (Fig. 14.1). This work suggested that leptin might be involved in the mechanism of appetite loss at altitude but recent studies have found a reduction of leptin levels at altitude (Bailey *et al.* 2004, Vats *et al.* 2004, Zaccaria *et al.* 2004) and no correlation between leptin levels and AMS scores in the first few days after arrival at 5050 m (Zaccaria *et al.* 2004). However, one further study did find an increase (Shukla *et al.* 2005).

CHOLECYSTOKININ, GHRELIN AND NEUROPEPTIDE Y

Apart from leptin there is now a whole list of new hormones, neurotransmitters and receptors which

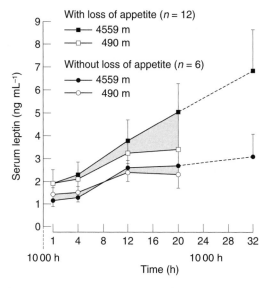

Figure 14.1 Serum leptin concentrations at 490 and 4559 m (Capanna Margherita) in 18 subjects with and without loss of appetite. The increase in leptin from low to high altitude (area between curves) was significant for subjects with loss of appetite ($p = 0.008$) but not for those with no appetite loss ($p = 0.35$). From Tschop *et al.* (1998) with permission.

are thought to influence appetite. A few of these have been assayed in subjects going to altitude. Cholecystokinin induces a sense of satiety. It is increased by exercise. Bailey *et al.* (2000) found significantly elevated resting cholecystokinin levels in subjects who had AMS on arrival at 5100 m compared with those without AMS. Ghrelin is an appetite-stimulating peptide produced in the stomach (Wren *et al.* 2001). Shukla *et al.* (2005) found ghrelin levels to be reduced by 30% in subjects at an altitude of 4300 m compared with baseline levels. NPY is another peptide affecting appetite but Vats *et al.* (2004) found no significant change in NPY levels in subjects at 3600 and 4580 m. These results should be considered as preliminary and clearly more work is needed to try to elucidate the mechanisms involved in the loss of appetite in both AMS before acclimatization and, at higher altitudes, the increasing aversion to food after acclimatization.

WEIGHT LOSS AFTER ACCLIMATIZATION

After acclimatization, weight loss is usually seen only above about 5000 m. Dinmore *et al.* (1994)

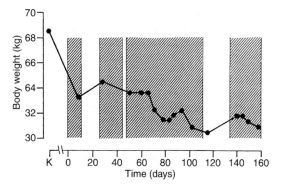

Figure 14.2 Record of body weight of one subject during the Silver Hut Expedition 1960–61. After the march out from Kathmandu (K) and the initial period of preparation, he was in residence at 5800 m (hatched areas) or at Base Camp at 4500 m. Note the loss of weight at 5800 m but weight gain during two breaks at 4500 m.

found an average loss of 3.9 kg during 2 weeks' climbing above 5000 m; on the 1992 British Winter Everest Expedition a mean weight loss of 5 kg was observed above 5400 m out of a total loss of 7.8 kg (Travis *et al.* 1993). Figure 14.2 shows the crucial effect of altitude on body weight on one well-acclimatized subject. The combined effects of the march out and early residence at the Silver Hut, at 5800 m, produced a weight loss of 5.3 kg. Thereafter, during time spent at the Silver Hut the subject lost weight steadily at a weekly rate of just under 400 g week^{-1} but, on two occasions, on descent to altitudes of 4000–4500 m, he began to gain weight. Most subjects in the Silver Hut lost between 0.5 and 1.5 kg week^{-1} (Pugh 1962a).

Rai *et al.* (1975) found no weight loss in their subjects living at 3500–4700 m, even though they were working quite hard at road building and digging. Indeed, on a high fat diet (232 g daily) they actually gained an average of 1.4 kg during 3 weeks at 4700 m. Butterfield *et al.* (1992) also found that it was possible to attenuate weight loss at 4300 m by increasing dietary intake in proportion to the increase in BMR. However, at Advanced Base Camp (6300 m) in the Western Cwm on Everest most subjects lost weight. Boyer and Blume (1984) documented this weight loss as an average of 4 kg (range 0–8 kg) over a mean of 47 days in 13 subjects. Again, there was considerable individual variation in the amount of weight lost which correlated with initial percentage of body fat. Boyer and Blume also found that Sherpas, who averaged only half as much body fat as the Western climbers, lost no weight during the time spent above Base Camp, mostly at or above 6300 m (see also section 14.9).

A possible reason for differences in weight loss response to altitude is the athletic fitness of subjects. Westerterp (2001), in a review of the limits to sustainable human metabolic rate, points out that whereas normal, healthy, untrained men, at sea level, can sustain a physical activity level (PAL) of about 1.5 times their average daily metabolic rate, trained endurance athletes can sustain a PAL of 3.0–4.5 without losing weight! This they do by increasing their food intake enormously, especially of carbohydrates. In the case of Scandinavian athletes studied, this was by frequent meals and the use of high energy carbohydrate drinks. An alternative strategy seems to be used by Sherpas and Nepali porters accustomed to long-term high energy expenditure. For logistical reasons they can only eat two meals a day (they have to stop, light a fire and cook) but Westerners are impressed at the huge quantities of rice or tsampa that they can put away at a sitting.

Women seem to lose less weight than men do. Hannon et al. (1976) found their female subjects lost an average of only 1.8% of body weight during 7 days at 4300 m whereas studies, previously reported, of men at this altitude had found losses of 3.5 and 5.0%. Collier et al. (1997b) found changes in body mass index at Everest Base Camp (5340 m) over a median of 15 days: 22 men lost $110 \, g \, m^{-2} \, day^{-1}$ compared with $20 \, g \, m^{-2} \, day^{-1}$ in eight women, a significant difference ($p = 0.03$). The seven male climbers who climbed to between 7100 and 8848 m, using oxygen at extreme altitude, all lost weight, averaging $150 \, g \, m^{-2} \, day^{-1}$. The one female climber who spent 4 nights above 8000 m without supplementary oxygen lost no weight between leaving and arriving back at Base Camp!

14.3.3 Weight loss in chamber experiments

It could be argued that some of the weight loss on expeditions is due to cold, limited food supplies, and the increased energy expenditure of climbing. This may often be the case, although not so in a number of the studies quoted above. Chamber studies avoid this potential criticism; most are of

too short a duration to be relevant, but Operation Everest I and II, studies of 40 days' duration, showed that, despite good environmental conditions of temperature, humidity and diet *ad libitum*, subjects lost weight (Rose et al. 1988). In Operation Everest II the six subjects lost an average of 7.4 kg during the 38 days of observations as they ascended the simulated height of the summit of Everest. Energy intake fell by 43% and, interestingly, the subjects chose a diet that resulted in a reduction of carbohydrate from 62 to 53% of the total diet. The authors considered that the weight loss could not be accounted for totally by the reduction in intake and considered that malabsorption or increase in energy expenditure due to increased BMR must be invoked (section 14.2.1). The exercise taken in this chamber study would probably be less than on a climbing expedition. On Operation Everest III (COMEX '97) there was a similar loss of weight, averaging 5 kg during the 31 day chamber study taking eight subjects to the simulated height of the Everest summit. Intake was reduced by $4.2 \, MJ \, day^{-1}$ due to subjects feeling satiated sooner (Westerterp-Plantenga 1999).

14.4 BODY COMPOSITION AND WEIGHT LOSS

Assuming much of the weight loss is due to negative energy balance, a simplistic view would be that the body would use up fat stores first and then start using protein from the lean body mass, principally the muscles. However, even with a most carefully controlled diet aimed at fat reduction, it is never possible to lose fat exclusively and retain all the lean body mass (Garrow 1987). The best that can be achieved is that, of the weight lost, 75% is fat and 25% lean body tissue. This compares with the situation during a complete fast when fat and lean body tissues are lost in roughly equal proportions (Forbes and Drenick 1979).

Boyer and Blume (1984) used skinfold measurements to estimate body fat. There are uncertainties about the absolute results of this method, but relative changes probably can be reliable. They found that, of the average 2 kg loss during the march out to Base Camp, 70% was due to loss of fat, which is a figure close to the most efficient muscle sparing regimen available. However, above 5400 m, mainly at or above

6300 m, of the 4 kg average weight loss only 27% was due to loss of fat and 73% due to loss of lean body tissue, despite the fact that subjects still had at least 10% of their body weight as fat. This percentage loss of muscle, greater than that seen in starvation, suggests that at this altitude hypoxia may be interfering with protein metabolism (section 14.5).

In the Operation Everest II study (Rose *et al.* 1988) there was loss of 2.5 kg of fat (1.6% body weight) and 4.9 kg of lean body tissue. Computerized tomographic examination of the thigh showed a 17% loss of muscle and a 34% loss of subcutaneous fat. Although loss of muscle mass must be a disadvantage, one beneficial effect is to increase the density of muscle capillaries. This is because the loss of muscle mass is achieved by reducing fiber diameter rather than number, with the number of capillaries per fiber remaining constant. Thus the intercapillary distance decreases with an improvement in oxygenation of the muscles (Chapter 10). Evidence in support of this speculation is found in the work of Oelz *et al.* (1986), who studied muscle biopsies from six elite climbers at sea level some months after return from altitude. It was found that their muscle fibers were smaller and the capillary density greater than controls. Another explanation for the loss of muscle mass is that with decreased overall activity at altitude there is some disuse atrophy which would similarly reduce muscle fiber diameter. These two explanations are not mutually exclusive. Results of muscle biopsy studies during Operation Everest II (MacDougall *et al.* 1991) showed similar histological changes in muscle fiber size (Chapter 10 contains a fuller discussion of changes in muscle histology).

14.5 INTESTINAL ABSORPTION AND HYPOXIA

In view of the continued weight loss at altitudes above 5000 m with, in some cases, adequate intake and reduced energy output, the possibility of malabsorption and malutilization of food must be considered. Pugh (1962a) reported that members of the Silver Hut Expedition noted that stools tended to be greasy and bulky, suggesting possible steatorrhea due to malabsorption of fat.

As mentioned in section 14.3, weight loss is not a feature of living at altitudes below about 5000 m,

and the fact that most altitude research is conducted below this level may explain why so little work has been carried out on the topic of intestinal absorption. Other reasons for the neglect of this field may be that the methods involved are either too sophisticated for easy use in the field (e.g. absorption of radioactive materials), or are unattractive to investigators (e.g. fecal collection, liquidization and aliquot sampling, etc.). Finally, few altitude physiologists have a background in gastroenterology.

14.5.1 Carbohydrate absorption and hypoxia

Milledge (1972) studied patients who were hypoxic either because of congenital heart disease or chronic obstructive lung disease. Xylose absorption decreased with decreasing arterial oxygen saturation (Fig. 14.3).

On relieving the hypoxia by surgery in the cardiac cases, or by 13 h of supplementary oxygen breathing in the respiratory cases, there was improvement in xylose absorption in all patients. The xylose absorption test has a rather uncertain lower normal limit, especially in a population in which intestinal parasitic infection is common (the study was carried out in South India). However, the results suggest that, below an arterial saturation of about 70%, absorption was impaired (Fig. 14.3); improvement on relief of hypoxia supports this view.

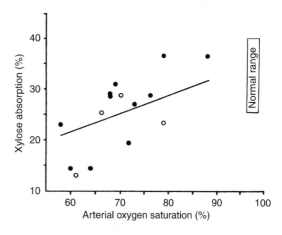

Figure 14.3 Xylose absorption in patients hypoxic because of either congenital cyanotic heart disease (s), or chronic respiratory disease (d), plotted against their arterial oxygen saturation.

Pritchard and Lane (1974) did not find malabsorption in 26 patients with chronic obstructive lung disease. However, the lowest arterial P_{O_2} was 48 mmHg, equivalent to about 78% saturation. Chesner *et al.* (1987) found no malabsorption of xylose in 11 subjects up to 4846 m. However, 60-min plasma xylose concentrations were reduced in subjects who ascended to 5600 m, confirming that absorption is not affected until hypoxia is severe. Boyer and Blume (1984), who studied subjects at 6300 m, found xylose absorption decreased by 24% in six out of seven subjects, compared with sea level controls.

However, absorption measured by xylose has the drawback that the result is influenced by factors such as gastric emptying time, absorption area, intestinal transit and renal function. Dinmore *et al.* (1994) used a double carbohydrate test; the two nonmetabolized carbohydrates used undergo different forms of mediated absorption but are otherwise subject to the same external influences which cancel out when results are expressed as a ratio (Menzies 1984). D-xylose is absorbed by passive mediated transport, whereas 3-*O*-methyl-D-glucose is absorbed by active mediated, sodium-dependent transport. Dinmore *et al.* found that at 6300 m there was 34% decrease in D-xylose (Fig. 14.4) and a 15% decrease in 3-*O*-methyl-D-glucose absorption. The ratio was consistently decreased at altitude and in a subsequent study the 60-min serum xylose/3-*O*-methyl-D-glucose ratio was 17% lower at 5400 m than at sea level (Travis *et al.* 1993). These more sophisticated studies therefore support the hypothesis that at these high altitudes carbohydrate absorption is impaired.

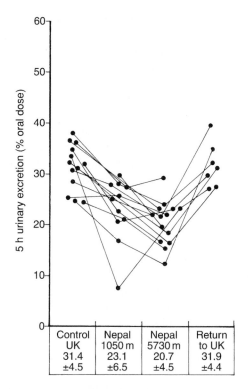

Figure 14.4 D-xylose absorption tested in a group of climbers at sea level (UK), at altitudes indicated in Nepal and after return to UK (with mean and S.D. values at each location). (Data from Dinmore *et al.* 1994.)

14.5.3 Protein absorption and hypoxia

Kayser *et al.* (1992) measured protein absorption using urinary and fecal ^{15}N excretion after ingestion of ^{15}N-labeled soya protein. They found no reduction in absorption in subjects after 3 weeks at 5000 m.

14.5.4 Summary: malabsorption at altitude

There is no evidence of malabsorption up to an altitude of about 5000 m and this has been confirmed by measurements of fecal energy excretion which have shown that 96% of energy intake is assimilated (Kayser *et al.* 1992), a normal sea level value for subjects on a western low residue diet. This test of overall food digestibility is measured over a 3-day period; the total energy values of both food and feces

14.5.2 Fat absorption and hypoxia

Rai *et al.* (1975) found no malabsorption for fat at 4700 m; neither did Chesner *et al.* (1987) at 3100 m and 4800 m. Imray *et al.* (1992), using the ^{14}C-triolein breath test, found no malabsorption of fat at 5500 m on Aconcagua in Argentina, and Butterfield *et al.* (1992) found no increase in fecal excretion of volatile fatty acids at 4300 m. However, Boyer and Blume (1984) found fat absorption decreased by 49% at 6300 m compared with sea level results in three acclimatized subjects.

are measured in a bomb calorimeter and the energy of the food digested expressed as a percentage of the food eaten. Above 5000 m there may be malabsorption of carbohydrate, fat and protein though the evidence is not compelling. There is always the possibility that intestinal infections, at the time of the study or in the previous few days or weeks, may have caused some malabsorption since many of these field studies were undertaken in countries where such infections are all too common. Westerterp *et al.* (1994) on Mount Sajama (6542 m) found that gross energy digestibility decreased to 85%, indicating some malabsorption, though most of the weight loss was attributable to low food intake. On the other hand in Operation Everest III, Westerterp *et al.* (2000) found a normal energy digestibility of 94% at 7000 m simulated altitude.

It now seems likely that malabsorption, due to hypoxia, if it exists, is only a minor factor in the weight loss seen at altitude which is predominantly due to a negative energy balance.

14.6 PROTEIN METABOLISM AT ALTITUDE

The obvious muscle wasting seen especially in climbers returning from extreme altitude prompts the question of whether hypoxia affects protein metabolism directly. There are very few data on this topic in humans.

Consolazio *et al.* (1968) studied protein balance at altitude and found no difference between subjects there and at sea level, but the altitude station was Pikes Peak (4300 m), below the crucial height at which continued weight loss is observed.

Rennie *et al.* (1983) studied the effect of acute hypoxia in a chamber (equivalent altitude 4550 m) on leucine metabolism in forearm muscles. They found that acute hypoxia resulted in a net loss of amino acids from the muscles, probably due to a fall in muscle protein synthesis. If this finding can be extrapolated to the situation of chronic hypoxia at altitudes of above 5000–6000 m (where hypoxia in acclimatized subjects would be similar to that in the above study), then it provides a further contributing factor to the loss of muscle mass described above. It has been suggested that protein or branched-chain amino acid (BCAA) supplementation might be helpful in reducing the muscle loss. Bigard and

colleagues (1996b) gave one group of skiers BCAA supplementation while participating in six sessions of ski mountaineering at altitudes of 2500–4100 m. They found that they did no better than a control group given 98% carbohydrate supplement with respect to changes in body composition or performance of isometric contraction. However, body weight loss was possibly less in the BCAA group. In another study (Bigard *et al.* 1996a) they found that adding protein to the diet of growing rats did not affect the depression of muscle growth caused by altitude.

A recent study of 8–9-year-old children resident at altitude (La Paz, 3600 m) by San Miguel *et al.* (2002) found that protein absorption or utilization was significantly reduced as compared with a group of children at low altitude. The high altitude group had only oxidized 19% of the casein after 6 h, compared with 25% in the low altitude group ($p < 0.02$) The method used was ingestion of ^{13}C-labeled leucine incorporated into casein. Expired $^{13}CO_2$ was then analyzed. However, this method does not distinguish between reduced absorption and increased utilization of protein.

14.7 WATER BALANCE AT ALTITUDE

There is no doubt that dehydration was common amongst early high altitude climbers and one of Pugh's contributions to the success of the 1953 Everest Expedition was his insistence on the importance of planning for adequate fluid intake of climbers high on the mountain. Pugh writes:

> For men climbing seven hours a day [at altitude] 3–5 litres of fluid, in the form of beverages and soup, were required in order to maintain a urine output of 1.5 l/day. This high fluid requirement was partly explained by the high rate of fluid loss from the lungs associated with increased ventilation and the dry cold air, and partly by sweating.
>
> (Pugh 1964a)

Since then all those involved with advice to trekkers and mountaineers have emphasized the importance of adequate hydration. Dehydration certainly impairs performance and it has been suggested that it may be a risk factor for acute mountain sickness, though there is not a lot of evidence for this (see Chapter 18). Whilst not denying the importance of hydration, it is possible to overstate the case and be too enthusiastic about pushing fluids, especially electrolyte-free water which can lead to hyponatremia. Cases have been described in hot environments (Backer *et al.* 1993, four cases), in a cold environment (Zafren 1998) and in the mountains (Basnyat *et al.* 2000a). At altitude this condition is easily misdiagnosed as acute mountain sickness.

Water balance is the difference between intake and output of water. Water intake may well be restricted because of unavailability of water especially at high altitude where it can only be obtained by melting snow or ice; hence the need to plan for adequate fuel to achieve adequate fluid intake. Water is also derived from metabolism of food as well as the water content of food, so if food intake is reduced at altitude, as it often is, that will increase the requirement for fluids.

Fluid output is the sum of fluid loss in urine and feces and insensible loss. The latter consists of loss by sweat and respiratory loss. There may be considerable sweat loss. Although the air is cold, climbers are dressed for it and the solar load may be high because of the reduced filtering effect of air and the effect of reflection of heat from snow. Because the air is so dry, sweat evaporates very efficiently, and the climber is unaware that he is sweating, perhaps profusely. Of course, in really cold conditions sweat loss may be minimal. The effect of altitude hypoxia alone on insensible water loss was found to be unchanged from control conditions in the chamber study, Operation Everest III (Westerterp *et al.* 2000).

14.7.1 Respiratory water loss and its calculation

As mentioned, it has been assumed that hyperventilating in the cold dry air of high altitude must result in considerable respiratory water loss. Respiratory water loss is the loss in the expired gas minus any water in the inspired air. The latter depends upon the temperature and relative humidity. At sea level typical indoor conditions of 22°C and 50% humidity the inspired water vapor pressure (PI,H_2O) is 10 Torr and each liter of inspired air contains 10.6 mg of water. At altitude both temperature and humidity

are low and the water content of the air is close to zero. On inspiration air is warmed and wetted so that by the time the gas reaches the alveoli it is fully saturated and warmed to body temperature. The PI,H_2O is 47 Torr and the water content 49.7 mg L^{-1}. On the assumption that expired gas is at body temperature and fully saturated there would be an estimated net loss of 49.7 mg of water for each liter expired, when dry air is breathed, or 39.1 mg L^{-1} under typical indoor conditions. At rest, assuming a ventilation of 6 L min^{-1}, the loss would be 234.7 mg min^{-1} or 338 mL day^{-1} and if the air was completely dry, 298.1 mg min^{-1} or 429 mL day^{-1}.

Exercise, by increasing the minute ventilation, will increase this figure. From studies of daylong (8 h) hill walking at altitudes up to 1000 m, total 24 h oxygen consumptions of 596 and 928 L have been reported for rest and exercise days respectively (Williams *et al.* 1979). This represents a total ventilation of about 14 900 and 23 200 L in 24 h and respiratory loss of 584 and 909 mL water.

At altitude, the increased ventilation and dry air will increase these figures. With a barometric pressure at half an atmosphere (about 5800 m) the acclimatized subject roughly doubles his ventilation both at rest and at sub-maximal work rates so that on these assumptions the 24 h respiratory losses work out at 859 mL on rest days and 1.718 L on climbing days. If we consider a climber spending a day climbing above 8000 m and assume an average minute ventilation over the 24 h of 40 L min^{-1} (an extreme value), the water loss would be 2.863 L.

However, it has been known for many years (though often forgotten and rediscovered) that the temperature of expired gas is below body temperature and probably is not fully saturated with water at even this lower temperature (Loewy and Gerhartz 1914, Burch 1945, Webb 1951, Ferrus *et al.* 1984). Therefore the actual respiratory water loss will be less than figures calculated using our starting assumptions.

As cold dry air is inhaled the mucosal surfaces are cooled and partially dried. During expiration the temperature of the initial portion of the expirate, the dead-space gas, is well below body temperature and less than fully saturated. The next portion of the expirate, leaving the alveoli is fully saturated and at body temperature. It warms and wets the mucosal surfaces of the upper airways but is itself cooled and loses water to the airways surface. The final portion of the expirate may or may not be expired at body temperature, fully saturated, depending on the inspired gas conditions and respiratory factors. In either case the total, mixed expirate will be well below body temperature and not fully saturated.

Ferrus *et al.* (1984) have studied a number of factors which affect the temperature and water saturation of mixed expired gas. These include:

- Temperature of inspired air
- Partial pressure of inspired water
- Respiratory frequency
- Tidal volume
- Density of inspired gas

They found that the mass of water per liter of expired gas was affected by all the above, although tidal volume and gas density have only a small effect. They proposed an equation linking them which allows a calculation of how much respiratory loss is saved by this mechanism under a variety of conditions. The lower the inspired temperature and the higher the respiratory frequency (and ventilation) the greater the saving in respiratory water loss. Thus if we consider the extreme case (above) of the climber above 8000 m with a calculated respiratory water loss of almost 3 L, and apply the Ferrus equation, we find the loss reduced to just under a liter, a saving of 65%. For full details of such calculations and their effect of respiratory water loss see Milledge (1992).

In conclusion, water loss in the expired gas is not great. Under extreme conditions of exercise at extreme altitude, when minute ventilation is very high and when water loss is greatest, the conservation of water has its greatest effect. This is due to the expirate being at a lower than body temperature and less than fully saturated. Even assuming an average ventilation of 40 L min^{-1} for 24 h in dry air at minus 15°C, the respiratory water loss is calculated to be less than one liter suggesting that water loss due to sweating is more important than respiratory loss.

14.8 DIET FOR HIGH ALTITUDE

Views on diets (not only at altitude) are strongly held, often the strength of opinion being inversely related to the strength of scientific evidence.

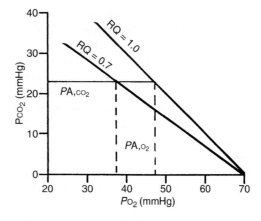

Figure 14.5   Oxygen–carbon dioxide diagram showing the effect of the respiratory quotient (RQ) on alveolar P_{O_2} at a given $PA,_{O_2}$. By changing from an RQ of 0.7 (the RQ when utilizing fat) to 1.0 (the RQ when using carbohydrate) the $PA,_{O_2}$ is increased from 37.2 to 47.0 mmHg.

14.8.1 High carbohydrate diet

There is sometimes a preference amongst climbers for a high carbohydrate, low fat diet at altitude and there are good physiological reasons for this. Figure 14.5 shows the basis for advising a high carbohydrate diet, which moves the respiratory quotient (RQ) from 0.7, if one uses fat exclusively for energy, to 1.0 when carbohydrate (or protein) is used.

The result of such a change of RQ is that for any given $PA,_{CO_2}$ the $PA,_{O_2}$ is increased. In the case illustrated in Fig. 14.5, the subject is considered to be at 5800 m in the Himalayas or Andes when the barometric pressure is half that at sea level and the $PI,_{O_2}$ is 70 mmHg. $PA,_{CO_2}$ is assumed to be 23 mmHg. With an RQ of 0.7 the $PA,_{O_2}$ would be 37.2 mmHg, whereas with an RQ of 1.0 it would be 47 mmHg; this is an important gain in arterial oxygen saturation. This represents the extreme case of a switch from pure fat to pure carbohydrate utilization, but even a partial switch in this direction would be helpful to the climber at extreme altitudes.

Consolazio *et al.* (1969) compared a normal with a high carbohydrate diet in two groups of subjects at 4300 m. The performance of the group on a high carbohydrate diet was superior in that they had a greater endurance for heavy work, though $V_{O_2,max}$ was not significantly better. Also, the symptoms of AMS were less in the high carbohydrate group.

Another reason for recommending a high carbo-hydrate diet is that it has been suggested that the body becomes more dependent upon glucose as a fuel at altitude after acclimatization (Brooks *et al.* 1991, Roberts *et al.* 1996). Lundby and van Hall (2002) in a more recent study addressed this question in subjects acutely exposed to an altitude of 4100 m and after 4 weeks' acclimatization to this altitude. When the same absolute rates of exercise were compared there was a shift towards more glucose and less free fatty acid use but this change disappeared when the same relative work rates were compared. It could be argued that, in practice, climbers at altitude are often exercising at higher relative rates than they would adopt at sea level, though lower than the same absolute work rate. Hence they would be shifting to more glucose utilization.

However, Reynolds *et al.* (1998) in a study on Everest found that subjects did not shift their food selections from high fat towards high carbohydrate items as they ascended from Base Camp to camps higher up the mountain though they may have already changed their diet to a higher carbohydrate one before the study began at Everest Base Camp.

14.8.2 Low fat diet

Many climbers find fatty foods become distasteful at altitude, in contrast to the preference shown by Arctic and Antarctic travelers. Tilman, who was experienced in both Arctic and mountain travel, writes:

> If you do succeed in getting outside a richly concentrated food like pemmican a great effort of will is required to keep it down – absolute quiescence in a prone position and a little sugar are useful aids. Eating a large mug of pemmican soup at 27,200 feet as Peter Lloyd and I did in '38 is, I think, an unparalleled feat and shows what can be done by dogged greed
> (Tilman 1975).

There are good physiological reasons for a low fat diet at altitude: the effect of fat as an energy source on the RQ (as discussed above) and the possible effect of fat malabsorption on the absorption of sugars and amino acids. This fat intolerance is unfortunate because fat provides more calories weight for weight than carbohydrate or proteins.

In conclusion: the main problem of nutrition at high altitude is the deficit in energy intake due to loss of appetite. Any diet that helps climbers take in more calories is beneficial and should be encouraged.

14.8.3 Other dietary constituents

IRON

Since the red cell mass is increased at altitude it has been suggested that extra iron should be taken. Unless there is pre-existing iron deficiency the iron stores of the body and the iron content of a normal diet will be adequate. However, in pre-menopausal women there may be a degree of deficient iron stores and the addition of iron may be indicated (Richalet *et al.* 1994). A rapid response to hypoxia is an increase in intestinal iron absorption from the gut before any change in plasma iron turnover, at least in rats and mice (Hathorn 1971, Raja *et al.* 1986). Thus the iron stores of the body are replenished even before they begin to be depleted.

VITAMINS

It is common for expedition and trekking parties to take added vitamins, but although such dietary supplements probably do no harm, there is no evidence that they are needed provided that a normal, balanced diet is taken.

14.8.4 Fresh food, flavor and variety

The appetite becomes jaded at high altitude and the most common complaints on expeditions are about the drab sameness of the flavor of preserved foods. More experienced climbers tend to adopt a policy of eating local fresh foods, supplemented by the minimum of imported preserved foods. The sense of taste seems to be dulled at altitude, and Western food tastes insipid. The addition of strong flavors such as curries and herbs is increasingly appreciated. There is great individual variation in likes and dislikes, even more than at sea level. The wise quartermaster of an expedition will attempt to meet this by providing as wide a variety of foods and flavors as possible. However, the task is unenviable since, whatever the quartermaster provides, fellow expedition members will yearn for what is unavailable.

14.9 NUTRITION AND METABOLISM IN HIGH ALTITUDE RESIDENTS

Little work has been done on nutrition in peoples native to high altitude. There is the impression that Sherpas do better than lowland climbers with respect to weight loss, and Boyer and Blume (1984), as mentioned in section 14.3.2, documented this. There are caretakers who live at the Aucanquilcha mine in Chile (5950 m) for 1–2 years. Presumably they do not lose weight in the relentless way we did

in the Silver Hut (5800 m), though it must be added that only a subset of miners is able to stay at this altitude indefinitely (West 1998, p. 227).

Holden *et al.* (1995) studied the cardiac metabolism of Quecha (Andean natives) and found they relied on glucose as a fuel to a greater extent than lowlanders. Hochachka *et al.* (1996) studied the metabolism of Sherpas under normoxic and hypoxic conditions. They too found that, compared to lowlanders, the Sherpas made greater use of carbohydrate substrates for cardiac function and less use of free fatty acids. This metabolic organization is advantageous in hypoxic conditions because the ATP yield per molecule of oxygen is 25–60% greater with glucose than with free fatty acids.

Endocrine and renal systems at altitude

SUMMARY

The chronic hypoxia of altitude has an effect on many endocrine systems. Among those most studied are hormones that affect the salt and water balance of the body and are involved in cardiovascular function. Exercise affects many hormonal systems and is an important activity at altitude; both altitude and exercise, therefore, need to be considered. The possible role of certain hormones in the mechanism of acute mountain sickness (AMS) has to be addressed by comparing levels in subjects with and without AMS.

Levels of antidiuretic hormone (ADH) are not affected by altitude or exercise. Previously it seemed that AMS was not associated with changes in ADH except in cases with severe nausea when levels are elevated. However, a recent study suggests that in AMS-resistant subjects there is a reduction in ADH levels within an hour of exposure leading to a water diuresis whilst AMS-susceptible subjects have a rise in ADH and water retention. After full acclimatization and at more extreme altitudes there is high osmolality with inappropriately low levels of ADH.

The change in response of ADH to osmolality with altitude acclimatization appears to be both in the slope and intercept of the response line.

The rennin–angiotensin–aldosterone system is activated by exercise and, in the case of the long continued exercise involved in mountaineering, can produce sodium and some water retention. Altitude in the absence of exercise results in lower levels of aldosterone, but exercise involved with ascent to altitude results in raised levels of aldosterone.

On first arrival at altitude, corticosteroids are elevated by ACTH then decline to baseline levels over 5–7 days. Even in subjects who had spent some weeks above 6000 m, corticosteroid levels were normal, but one report of subjects who spent months at this altitude did show high levels.

The sympathoadrenal system is stimulated during the first few days at altitude with high levels of urinary catecholamines. These decline with acclimatization in line with the changes in resting heart rate.

Thyroid function is enhanced in humans at altitude, unlike in animals in which it is depressed by hypoxia. Because of this and the increased sympathetic activity, basal metabolic rate (BMR) is increased on going to altitude and remains elevated after acclimatization.

Insulin sensitivity is reduced on first arrival at altitude but with acclimatization insulin sensitivity becomes enhanced.

Plasma endothelin levels are raised by hypoxia in line with the raised pulmonary artery pressure and are high in high altitude pulmonary edema (HAPE) patients and subjects susceptible to HAPE.

Glucagon, growth hormone, bradykinin and the sex hormones are little affected by hypoxia except that the exercise response to growth hormone is enhanced and sex hormones tend to be decreased.

Renal function is remarkably little affected by altitude. At extreme altitude, above 6500 m, renal compensation for further respiratory alkalosis seems to be incomplete. There is an increase in microproteinuria, especially on first going to altitude, which is greater in subjects with AMS.

15.1 INTRODUCTION

Endocrinology comprises many systems controlling a great variety of bodily functions and the effect of altitude has been studied on only a fraction of these. The areas studied reflect the interests of scientists going to altitude. Thus hormones that play a part in fluid and electrolyte balance have been widely studied because of their possible relevance to AMS and its complications, as have thyroid hormones because of their effect on metabolic rate. Another factor in the selection of systems for study has, of course, been the availability and ease of relevant assays. This chapter surveys the principal systems studied to date but clearly there are great areas of endocrinology in which the effects of acute and chronic hypoxia have yet to be explored.

The study of endocrinology at altitude is perfectly feasible, but attention to details of sampling, such as time of day, subject's posture, diet and exercise is required, as it is in studies at sea level. Practical aspects of collection and storage of samples are discussed in Chapter 30.

15.2 ANTIDIURETIC HORMONE

There is considerable evidence that ascent to altitude is associated with changes in body fluid compartments both in those with AMS and in asymptomatic subjects. Not surprisingly, therefore, investigators have studied the role of antidiuretic hormone (ADH) (arginine vasopressin) in both the normal (healthy) response to hypoxia and AMS. Reports on the effect of hypoxia on ADH have given conflicting results.

15.2.1 Exercise and ADH

Williams et al. (1979) studied exercise in the absence of hypoxia. They studied the effect of daylong hill walking over 7 consecutive days and found no alteration in ADH concentration, despite the fact that their subjects developed peripheral (exercise) edema associated with sodium retention (section 15.3.3).

15.2.2 Acute hypoxia and ADH

Forsling and Milledge (1977) found that breathing 10–10.5% oxygen for 4 h had no effect on ADH levels in samples taken at intervals of from 3 min to 4 h of hypoxia. In a chamber experiment, where subjects were taken to an equivalent altitude of 4000 m for 14 h, there was no significant change in ADH plasma concentration until subjects began to feel nauseated, when levels rose markedly (Forsling and Milledge 1980). Claybaugh et al. (1982) took subjects to various equivalent altitudes in a chamber and found an initial increase of urinary ADH at 8–12 h of hypoxia with subsequent return to sea level values. In two subjects with AMS there was a rise in urinary excretion of ADH at 2–4 h of hypoxia. De Angelis et al. (1996) studied 26 young pilots in a chamber at an altitude of 5000 m equivalent for 3 h. They found a significant increase in ADH as a result of this quite severe hypoxic stress. Loeppky et al. (2005) studied a group of subjects in a chamber with, on one occasion, normobaric hypoxia and on another, hypobaric hypoxia for 12 h. The latter resulted in more AMS and significant rise in ADH whilst the former produced little AMS and a nonsignificant fall in ADH. It would seem, therefore, that acute hypoxia alone has very little effect but nausea due to AMS is associated with a rise in ADH, analogous to that seen in motion sickness (Eversman et al. 1978).

Bocqueraz et al. (2004), in a chamber study of cyclists at an altitude equivalent of approx. 4200 m, found no change in ADH during 60 min of exercise at 50 and 75% of $V_{O_2,max}$.

15.2.3 Chronic hypoxia and ADH

Studies conducted in the field include one by Singh *et al.* (1974), who measured a number of hormones in a group of subjects who had a history of HAPE. In those who remained free of symptoms on going to altitude, there was no change in ADH concentration. In subjects who became sick there was a tendency to higher levels but this was mainly seen after a few days at altitude and was not statistically significant. Harber *et al.* (1981) found no significant change in urinary ADH concentration on going to altitudes up to 5400 m; nor was there any relationship with AMS. Even in a fatal case of high altitude cerebral edema there was no significant rise in ADH. Cosby *et al.* (1988) found higher levels of ADH in five skiers with HAPE compared with controls at the same altitude, but the difference did not reach statistical significance. Ramirez *et al.* (1992) found no change in ADH with altitude.

Hackett *et al.* (1978) found normal levels in trekkers at 4300 m, including those with and without symptoms of AMS; the only exceptions were higher concentrations in two cases of HAPE.

The conclusion from this work would seem to be that hypoxia per se has no significant effect on ADH concentration. High values may be associated with AMS but not all cases have high values (Claybaugh *et al.* 1982). Where high concentrations are found they may be an effect of AMS rather than its cause.

However, a recent large chamber study produced evidence that the ADH response to hypoxia may be important in the mechanism of AMS (Loeppky *et al.* 2005). These workers studied 51 subjects in a chamber at 4880 m equivalent altitude for 8–12 h and then compared the 16 subjects most affected and 16 least affected by AMS. The non-AMS subjects showed a drop in ADH at 1 h whereas the AMS group showed a small rise. Thereafter both groups showed a rise, the non-AMS back to baseline and the AMS to almost double baseline values. Free water clearance showed reciprocal changes. The diuresis in the non-AMS group was clearly shown and it was a water diuresis, the sodium excretion being unchanged as were levels of atrial natriuretic peptide and aldosterone. Thus the diuresis was ADH driven (a reduction in ADH level) and, by the end of the altitude exposure, resulted in a cumulative free water balance of 955 mL in the AMS group and 534 mL in the non-AMS. The water balance results

were even more distinct. The AMS group had a positive balance of 1197 mL whilst the non-AMS had a negative balance of 724 mL, a difference of almost 2 L ($p = 0.002$). This suggests that the early diuresis which is ADH driven is crucial in the physiological response to hypoxia and the resistance to AMS.

This early water diuresis was also found by Hildebrandt *et al.* (2000) in a 90 min chamber experiment where the effect of hypoxia (12% O_2) was studied with either iso- or poikilocapnia. It was found with both forms of hypoxia, and was not related to the hypoxic ventilatory response. Swenson *et al.* (1995) had earlier shown that the later sodium diuresis was correlated with HVR.

15.2.4 Alterations in ADH secretion at altitude

Blume *et al.* (1984) presented evidence of inappropriately low secretion of ADH at altitude. They studied 13 subjects after some weeks at 5400 m and 6300 m on Everest during the American Medical Research Expedition to Everest (AMREE) in 1981 and found ADH concentration unchanged from sea level despite a significant increase in plasma osmolality with increasing altitude. At 6300 m the serum osmolality was 302 mosm kg^{-1} compared with 290 mosm kg^{-1} at sea level (normal value 280–295 mosm kg^{-1}). An overnight dehydration test at sea level which might produce this degree of hyperosmolality would result in ADH concentrations of about 7 μU mL^{-1}, whereas subjects on Everest had a mean value of only 0.9 μU mL^{-1}; 12-h urinary ADH showed the same lack of response. Sodium, potassium, calcium and phosphate concentrations were all modestly increased compared with sea level values. A study by Ramirez *et al.* (1992) confirmed these observations. They increased osmolality by intravenous sodium, loading a group of subjects at sea level and at altitude (3000 m). At sea level there was the expected rise in ADH but at altitude there was no significant rise. Thus, at altitude, there seems to be a failure of the osmoregulatory mechanism. This is the converse of the clinical syndrome of inappropriate ADH secretion often associated with small cell carcinoma of the lung (Bayliss 1987). In such cases serum sodium concentration and osmolality are low but ADH secretion is inappropriately high. A later study (Ramirez

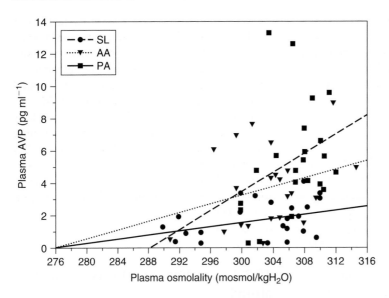

Figure 15.1   Regression analysis describing P_{osm} vs P_{AVP} forced into a linear model. Solid regression line, SL, dotted line, 2 days at altitude, dashed line, 20 days at altitude. (From Maresh *et al.* 2004 with permission.)

et al. 1998) found evidence of reduced sensitivity of the kidney to ADH in acclimatized individuals and that infusion of exogenous ADH caused an increase of urinary arginine vasopressin (AVP) sensitive water channel (aquaporin-2).

A recent study by Maresh *et al.* (2004) explored the response in ADH secretion to a water deprivation test at sea level, on acute altitude exposure (2 days) and more chronic exposure (20 days) on Pikes Peak (4300 m). Like other studies they found higher plasma osmolality at altitude but no change in baseline levels of ADH. With water deprivation the rise in ADH was greater at altitude and more so on day 20 than at day 2 of their altitude stay and the osmolality threshold which stimulated ADH release appeared to rise. This is shown in Fig 15.1.

An 8-day study by Bestle *et al.* (2002) at the Capanna Margherita (4559 m) using a hypertonic saline loading test found the AVP response unchanged from sea level though they too found the set point of plasma osmolality to AVP level elevated at altitude.

15.3 RENIN–ANGIOTENSIN–ALDOSTERONE SYSTEM

This system is depicted in Fig. 15.2. Renin is released in response to a number of stimuli, including posture, exercise and, possibly, hypoxia. The mechanism common to these stimuli is sympathetic

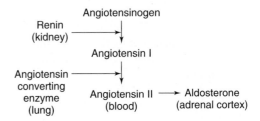

Figure 15.2   Renin–angiotensin–aldosterone system. Renin and angiotensin converting enzyme (ACE) act as enzymes hydrolyzing angiotensinogen and angiotensin I to angiotensin II. The latter stimulates release of aldosterone from adrenocortical cells by a receptor mechanism.

activation, and both circulating catecholamine and direct sympathetic nervous stimulation result in release of renin from the juxtaglomerular apparatus of the kidney.

Renin has no biological activity but acts on its circulating substrate (angiotensinogen), cleaving it to produce the octapeptide angiotensin I, which is also devoid of activity. Angiotensin converting enzyme (ACE), found on the luminal surface of endothelial cells, converts angiotensin I to angiotensin II by cleaving the final two amino acids. The principal site of conversion is in the rich capillary network of the lung where nearly 90% of angiotensin I is converted to angiotensin II in a single passage. Angiotensin II is a powerful vasopressor and also acts on the cells of the adrenal cortex via a receptor mechanism to release aldosterone. Aldosterone acts on the renal tubules, promoting the reabsorption of sodium. In this way the system is important in the salt and water economy of the body, which is why it has been quite intensively studied at altitude.

15.3.1 Aldosterone and altitude

Indirect evidence of the effect of altitude on aldosterone activity was first provided by Williams (1961), who brought back samples of saliva from the Karakoram. The ratio of sodium to potassium in these samples indicated suppression of aldosterone at altitude. This has been confirmed by direct measurements of either plasma aldosterone concentration or urinary metabolites (Tuffley *et al.* 1970, Hogan *et al.* 1973, Frayser *et al.* 1975, Pines *et al.* 1977, Sutton *et al.* 1977, Keynes *et al.* 1982, Ramirez *et al.* 1992, Antezana *et al.* 1995, Zaccaria *et al.* 1998). In one study the secretion rate was shown to be reduced (Slater *et al.* 1969). Milledge *et al.* (1983a) studied the time course of the effect of altitude over a 6-week stay at or above 4500 m. After initial suppression, aldosterone concentration rose to control values after 12–20 days. All these studies were made on resting subjects. In subjects who had been above 6000 m for more than 10 weeks and had expanded fluid compartments (blood volume 85% above normal) the aldosterone concentration was twice normal (Anand *et al.* 1993). These subjects were probably in incipient right heart failure due to high altitude pulmonary hypertension previously known as subacute mountain sickness (Chapter 21).

15.3.2 Renin activity and altitude

The effect of altitude on plasma renin activity (PRA) has been studied by a number of groups with conflicting results. Some have found a rise (Slater *et al.* 1969, Tuffley *et al.* 1970, Frayser *et al.* 1975) and others a fall (Hogan *et al.* 1973, Maher *et al.* 1975a, Keynes *et al.* 1982, Antezana *et al.* 1995, Zaccaria *et al.* 1998) and one group no change (Sutton *et al.* 1977). However, most studies have shown a reduced response of aldosterone to renin. This is obvious where PRA has increased and aldosterone has decreased but even where both have declined, the reduction in aldosterone has usually been greater.

It is not clear why these different studies produced different results. One possibility is that subjects, though sampled at rest, may have been more active in some studies, resulting in a rise in PRA. However, this is unlikely in view of the fact that one study showing a rise in PRA was conducted in a chamber (Tuffley *et al.* 1970) and in another, samples were taken before getting up in the morning after subjects had been flown to altitude in a helicopter (Slater *et al.* 1969). The main stimulus to renin release is thought to be sympathetic drive and this certainly occurs with exercise but is probably also induced by altitude hypoxia alone if sufficiently severe (section 15.4), although with great individual variation.

15.3.3 Exercise and the renin–aldosterone system

Since exercise frequently accompanies ascent to altitude, the effect of exercise needs to be considered in relation to the effect of altitude. Exercise stimulates renin release via activation of the sympathetoadrenal system. The effect can be blocked by beta-blockers (Bonelli *et al.* 1977, Bouissou *et al.* 1989). After intense short-term exercise (3 × 300 m sprints in 10 min), PRA, angiotensin II and aldosterone concentration were elevated at 30 min but measurable elevation was still present up to 6 h later (Kosunen and Pakarinen 1976). The rise in PRA is also proportional to the intensity of the work, both at sea level and at altitude (Maher *et al.* 1975a).

Mountaineers are more concerned with daylong exercise, often continuing for a number of days. Williams *et al.* (1979) showed that this form of exercise resulted in marked sodium retention after 7 days and suggested that this was due to activation of the rennin–aldosterone system. There was a mean cumulative retention of 358 mmol of sodium with a modest retention of 650 mL of water. Since plasma sodium concentration did not change significantly it was argued that the extracellular space must have been expanded by 2.68 L (of which 0.68 L was in the plasma volume), mainly at the expense of the intracellular volume. These calculated changes are shown in Fig. 15.3. This increase in extracellular fluid (ECF) is the probable cause of the dependent edema frequently found after exercise of this sort.

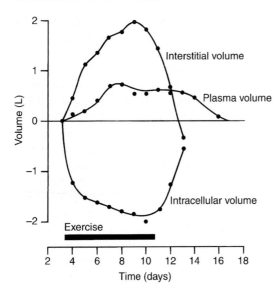

Figure 15.3 Calculated changes in body fluid compartments with exercise at sea level. (From Williams *et al.* 1979.)

The same group (Milledge *et al.* 1982) studied the effect of 5 consecutive days' hill walking on the rennin–aldosterone system and on sodium and water balance, and confirmed the suggestion, from the previous study, that the sodium retention was associated with activation of the rennin–aldosterone system. There was elevation of PRA and aldosterone at the conclusion of each day's exercise. This was maximal on day 2 or 3 and less marked on days 4 and 5, perhaps reflecting a training effect. Values were back to control on day 2 after stopping exercise. The effect of exercise and altitude was studied by repeating the same protocol but on the first exercise day subjects climbed to 3100 m and stayed there for 5 days, exercising for 8 h each day. The results were very similar to sea level results in terms of changes in fluid and sodium balance and hematocrit. Renin and aldosterone also increased, but the aldosterone response to the renin rise was blunted (see section 15.3.5; Milledge *et al.* 1983d).

15.3.4 Control of aldosterone release

The control of aldosterone release via renin and angiotensin has been mentioned above and is shown in Fig. 15.2, but ACTH and the sodium status of the subject also control aldosterone concentration. Salt depletion increases aldosterone release whereas salt loading inhibits it. Anderson *et al.* (1986) have shown that atrial natriuretic peptide (ANP) infusion inhibits the response of aldosterone to angiotensin II.

15.3.5 Effect of altitude on the aldosterone response to renin

Milledge and Catley (1982) showed that, if after 1 h of exercise the inspired oxygen was reduced, renin activity increased while aldosterone levels decreased, indicating that the aldosterone response to renin became blunted. In the chronic situation of hill walking or climbing at altitude compared with sea level the same phenomenon is seen. This is shown in Fig. 15.4, which shows data from three studies, at sea level, at 3100 m and on Mount Everest. This blunting has been confirmed by Shigeoka *et al.* (1985), who found the response completely abolished by hypoxia, by Lawrence *et al.* (1990), and, in acute hypoxia, by De Angelis *et al.* (1996). Antezana *et al.* (1995) also found the response in lowlanders to be blunted in La Paz (3600 m). Andean highlanders with polycythemia showed a reduced response but highlanders without polycythemia had a normal response at this altitude.

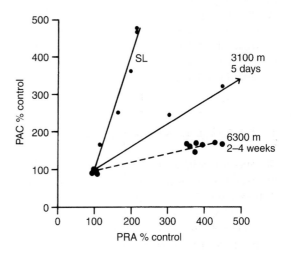

Figure 15.4 Plasma aldosterone concentration (PAC) response to plasma renin activity (PRA) from a sea level (SL) study and from two separate altitude studies. (From Milledge *et al.* 1983b.)

The cause of this blunting is not entirely clear. It had been suggested that ACE activity was reduced by hypoxia, but most workers have found this not to be the case (Milledge and Catley 1987, Bouissou *et al.* 1988). However, Vonmoos *et al.* (1990) have found that, although angiotensin I levels were unchanged with acute hypoxia, levels of angiotensin II were reduced. The next stage in the promotion of aldosterone release is adrenal stimulation by angiotensin II. Colice and Ramirez (1986) studied the effect of angiotensin II infusion on aldosterone release and found that hypoxia had no effect, suggesting that it did not result in an increase of inhibitors of this part of the system. However, Raff and Kohandarvish (1990) found evidence that adrenocortical cells *in vitro* were less responsive to angiotensin II under hypoxic conditions. More recently, Raff *et al.* (1996) have shown that chronic hypoxia in rats (10% oxygen for 3 days) results in a decrease in expression of the steroidogenic enzyme P-450c11AS in adrenocortical cells. This enzyme is unique to the aldosterone pathway. However, with less severe hypoxia, 12% oxygen for 3 days, there was no effect.

Aldosterone secretion is stimulated by ACTH as well as by angiotensin II. Ramirez *et al.* (1988) found this effect to be reduced in subjects at altitude whereas the ACTH-induced secretion of cortisol was unaffected. ANP has been found to inhibit aldosterone release (Elliott and Goodfriend 1986). It is therefore possible that the rise in ANP on going to altitude (section 15.4.4) may be a factor in blunting this response at rest (Lawrence *et al.* 1990) and on exercise (Lawrence and Shenker 1991).

15.4 ALTITUDE AND ATRIAL NATRIURETIC PEPTIDE

15.4.1 ANP release and actions

ANP is secreted by the atria of the heart in response to stretching. Atrial stretch is usually caused by an increase in atrial pressure. However, in the case of cardiac tamponade the pressure is high but the atrial wall is not stretched. As the tamponade is relieved the pressure falls and the atrium dilates. It has been found that relief of tamponade results in a rise in ANP plasma levels, indicating that stretch rather than pressure is the stimulus for ANP synthesis and release (Au *et al.* 1990).

Amongst its actions, ANP has the effect of increasing sodium excretion by the kidneys and thus of promoting a natriuresis and diuresis (Morice *et al.* 1988). This provides a homeostatic mechanism for salt and water. If the plasma volume is increased, the raised atrial pressure results in atrial stretch and secretion of ANP, diuresis follows and vascular pressures and volume return to normal. This system is further considered in relation to the regulation of plasma volume in section 8.2.2. ANP possibly also has a role as a vasodilator, countering the pressor effect of hypoxia on the pulmonary artery. It has been shown to have this effect in a dose-dependent manner in the isolated rat lung (Stewart *et al.* 1991b) and in the pig (Adnot *et al.* 1988). Liu *et al.* (1989) infused ANP (20 mg min^{-1} for 10 min) into four patients with HAPE and showed a reduction in pulmonary artery pressure for 1 h after the infusion.

15.4.2 ANP and hypoxia

Since the first edition of this book almost 20 years ago, there have been numerous reports of the effect of hypoxia on the plasma levels of ANP at rest and on exercise. Ten minutes of severe hypoxia on isolated rat and rabbit heart with constant flow perfusion caused a four-fold increase in ANP released (Baertschi *et al.* 1986). The same group found increases in ANP blood levels in the whole animal made hypoxic under anaesthesia. There was great variability in the response, which correlated with the baseline central venous pressure, but not with any other measured variables. Winter *et al.* (1989) also found ANP levels to be increased by hypoxia in the rat after 24 h but not after only 2 h. In patients with chronic hypoxic lung disease, levels of ANP were elevated and varied inversely with the Pa,O_2 (Winter *et al.* 1987b).

In healthy volunteers Kawashima *et al.* (1989) studied the effect of 10 min of hypoxia at two levels: 15% oxygen breathing produced no change, but 10% oxygen breathing increased ANP levels by 15% accompanied by an increase in pulmonary artery pressure. Vonmoos *et al.* (1990) found that 60 min of 12% oxygen breathing produced a small but significant elevation of ANP. Lawrence *et al.* (1990) found that the same hypoxic stimulus produced a 50% increase in ANP levels in subjects on a low salt diet and whose endogenous cortisol was suppressed with dexamethasone. Conversely, Ramirez *et al.* (1992) did not find a significant rise in ANP levels with either acute (60 min) or chronic hypoxia at 3000 m, although the ANP response to a sodium load was greater at altitude. Antezana *et al.* (1995) found a reduction in ANP levels in lowlanders at 3600 m compared with sea level and highlanders had significantly lower ANP than lowlanders at altitude.

15.4.3 Exercise and ANP: normoxia

Somers *et al.* (1986) found that a progressive exercise test to maximum exercise resulted in an almost four-fold increase in plasma ANP with a decline to baseline after 1 h at rest. Similar results have been found for short-term exercise by Schmidt *et al.* (1990) and by Lawrence and Shenker (1991). Hill walking exercise for 5 days also resulted in elevated ANP levels to about twice baseline values (Milledge *et al.* 1991b). It is interesting to note that during this type of exercise, sodium is retained despite elevated ANP levels.

15.4.4 Exercise and ANP: hypoxia

Mountaineers and trekkers going to altitude normally have the double stimulus of exercise and hypoxia. Schmidt *et al.* (1990) studied exercise while breathing air or reduced oxygen (PI,O_2 92 mmHg). With both maximal and submaximal exercise the ANP response to exercise was reduced under hypoxic conditions. In contrast, Lawrence and Shenker (1991), using less severe hypoxia (16% inspired oxygen) and exercise such as to give a heart rate of 70–75% of maximum for 30 min, found that hypoxia enhanced the ANP response. A third study using a decompression chamber to give a simulated altitude of 3000 m and a progressive exercise test to maximum showed a reduced response (Vuolteenaho *et al.* 1992). The reasons for these differing results are not apparent.

Milledge *et al.* (1989) reported levels of plasma ANP in 15 subjects before and after ascent on foot from 3100 m to 4300 m. Values tended to be higher at altitude but were significantly so only in the 4 a.m. sample on the second altitude day, there being no difference on day 1 at altitude or in the 9 a.m. sample on either day. Bärtsch *et al.* (1991a) found,

in blood samples taken on the morning after the ascent to 4559 m on foot, no increase in ANP levels in a group of nine climbers who did not have AMS. Five subjects who did become sick had elevated levels. These subjects had a history of HAPE and were shown by echocardiography to have increased atrial diameters at altitude. The increase in ANP is probably secondary to developing high pulmonary artery pressures. Kawashima *et al.* (1992) showed that, in subjects susceptible to high altitude pulmonary edema, breathing 10% oxygen resulted in a greater rise in ANP levels than in controls, and that the rise correlated with the rise in pulmonary artery pressure.

Later in altitude exposure the effect of maximum exercise in raising ANP levels is reduced (Robarch *et al.* 2000) but then so is maximum work rate.

15.4.5 ANP and AMS

An important motive for the study of the effect of altitude hypoxia on ANP has been the hypothesis that it may play a part in the genesis of AMS. Milledge *et al.* (1989) did not find any correlation between levels of ANP on the morning after arrival at altitude and the AMS symptom score. However, Bärtsch *et al.* (1988) and Cosby *et al.* (1988) found subjects with AMS or HAPE to have higher levels than subjects without AMS. If the rise in ANP in AMS sufferers is related to high pulmonary arterial pressure, elevation would be expected mainly in AMS with pulmonary edema and not in the milder, non-HAPE cases. In the first-mentioned study there was no clinical evidence of pulmonary edema.

15.4.6 ANP and chronic mountain sickness

Antezana *et al.* (1995) have reported higher levels of ANP in patients with chronic mountain sickness (CMS) than in controls in Andean highlanders. In this study pulmonary artery pressure was assessed by Doppler ultrasound and found to be raised. Ge *et al.* (2001) also found raised levels of ANP in patients with CMS (Han Chinese and Tibetans). There was a significant correlation between the hemoglobin concentration, [Hb], and ANP.

In conclusion, it seems that although both exercise and hypoxia cause an elevation of ANP, the combined stimulus does not result in very high levels at altitude. Despite its name, ANP is not a powerful natriuretic hormone. Levels of ANP are elevated in conditions where the pulmonary artery pressure is raised, including HAPE and polycythemia, and this rise is presumably secondary to the raised pressure causing some atrial enlargement. The rise in ANP is probably beneficial in that it tends to reduce the pressure by its vasodilatory function.

15.5 CORTICOSTEROIDS AND ALTITUDE

On ascent to altitude, there is stimulation of the adrenal cortex by ACTH and cortisol is secreted. Early work documented this as a rise in 17-hydroxy-corticosteroids (17-OHCSs) during the first few days at altitude, which decreased to control values by days 5–7 (MacKinnon et al. 1963, Moncloa et al. 1965). This has been confirmed by measurement of plasma cortisol by Frayser et al. (1975) and Sutton et al. (1977), who showed that with the elevation of plasma cortisol there was a decrease in its normal diurnal variation on the first day of altitude exposure. Richalet et al. (1989), in a chamber experiment, also found elevation of plasma cortisol with re-establishment of the diurnal variation after the first altitude day. Many of the subjects of these studies, taken rapidly to an altitude of 4300–5300 m, suffered from AMS, but even those free of symptoms showed this transitory rise in cortisol or its urinary metabolite. It is assumed that this is a nonspecific stress response.

15.5.1 Case report

An interesting case report shows that there is a clinical lesson to be learnt. A 58-year-old man, who had had his pituitary removed 10 years earlier for an adenoma, went trekking in Nepal. On arrival at Menang (3535 m) he complained of fatigue, abdominal pain, nausea and vomiting, but no headache. He was on regular medication with cortisone 25 mg daily and had taken his treatment. Twenty-four h later he had deteriorated and was unable to stand. He was treated with dexamethasone 5 mg i.v., 5 mg i.m. and oral rehydration, and his cortisone dose was quadrupled.

Within 24 h all symptoms had disappeared, and the next day he successfully crossed the Thorong La (5450 m) (Westendorp et al. 1993). Clearly, the lesson is that subjects on corticosteroid replacement therapy should increase their dosage on going to altitude. The authors point out that this does not apply to thyroid replacement therapy since thyroid stimulating hormone (TSH) is not increased by hypoxia.

The effect of prolonged stay at more extreme altitude was studied by Siri et al. (1969). They brought back urine samples from the 1963 Everest expedition from climbers staying at 5400 m and 6500 m. The 17-OHCS levels were not significantly different from sea level values. They also demonstrated a normal response to injected ACTH. Mordes et al. (1983) collected samples from subjects who had been at 5400 m and 6300 m for some weeks and found no change from sea level values in either morning or evening cortisol concentrations.

In animals studied after chronic hypoxia there was some hyperplasia of the adrenal cortex and of the corticotrophic cells in the pituitary. No such morphological changes have been found in humans with long-standing chronic bronchitis (Gosney 1986). However, in subjects who had spent more than 10 weeks above 6000 m, the cortisol level was found to be three times normal (Anand et al. 1993). Marinelli et al. (1994) studied athletes taking part in a marathon race from 3860 m to 5100 m and down to finish at 3400 m. Cortisol levels were similar at altitude before the race but were greatly elevated at the end.

In people resident at the moderate altitude of 2600 m in Colombia, Ramirez et al. (1995) found an enhanced response to corticotrophin releasing hormone, with higher levels of both ACTH and β-endorphin after stimulation than in sea level control subjects. This was true for a number of tropic hormones (sections 15.7.1 and 15.9.2).

15.6 SYMPATHOADRENAL SYSTEM

15.6.1 Acute hypoxia

Acute hypoxia increases heart rate at rest and on exercise (Maher et al. 1975b). This is presumed to be due to increased sympathetic activity stimulating the β-adrenergic receptors on heart muscle cell membrane. Within 4 h of arrival at altitude there is an increase in arterial epinephrine, at rest, due to hypoxia stimulating release from the adrenal medulla (Mazzeo and Reeves 2003). Bouissou et al. (1989) also found a 32% increase in norepinephrine after 48 h at altitude. Levels of epinephrine reach a peak on about days 2–4 and then decline as hypoxia is relieved by increasing ventilation and [Hb] over the next 7–14 days (Mazzeo and Reeves 2003). Norepinephrine is released by sympathetic nerves and about 10–20% spills over into the circulation. This is measured as plasma norepinephrine and, in contrast to epinephrine, values rise only slowly, in line with increasing ventilation, reaching a plateau after 10–14 days at altitude. Exercise results in a further rise in epinephrine depending on the work rate and degree of hypoxia. The two stimuli, hypoxia and exercise, are additive for epinephrine. Norepinephrine levels also rise with exercise depending upon the work load but if work loads relative to $V_{O_{2,max}}$ are compared, the rise at altitude is similar to that seen at sea level (Mazzeo and Reeves 2003).

15.6.2 Chronic hypoxia

Cunningham et al. (1965) reported elevated plasma and 24-h urinary catecholamines during 17 days at 4559 m on Monte Rosa. There was no significant change in epinephrine but the increase in norepinephrine was greater on day 12 at altitude. Pace et al. (1964) found similar results at 3850 m, with urinary norepinephrine excretion rising slowly during 14 days at altitude without change in urinary epinephrine secretion. Maher et al. (1975b) found increased urinary catecholamines at 4300 m. Levels were increased on day 1 compared with sea level and further increased on day 11. On exercise, both light and severe, the effect of chronic hypoxia compared with acute was to increase levels still further. Hoon et al. (1977) found no significant change in urinary catecholamine secretion in a total of 76 subjects who had no symptoms of AMS. However, in 29 symptomatic subjects there was a small but significant rise on the first day at altitude, which was maintained through to day 10 at altitude. Mazzeo et al. (1991) found that, at rest, norepinephrine and epinephrine levels were higher at altitude than at sea level. With submaximal exercise, norepinephrine rose to higher values than expected at sea level, whereas epinephrine levels did not rise, though values remained above

those at sea level. In Operation Everest II at extreme altitude (282 mmHg) after 40 days in the chamber, resting plasma norepinephrine was raised but epinephrine was reduced. On maximum exercise, values for both catecholamines fell with increasing altitude (Young et al. 1989).

In subjects who had spent more than 10 weeks above 6000 m the plasma norepinephrine concentration was found to be almost three times normal (Anand et al. 1993). Gosney et al. (1991) studied the adrenal and pituitary glands of five lifelong residents of La Paz who had lived at 3600–3800 m, and compared their glands with those of controls from sea level. The adrenal glands were significantly bigger, by about 50%. The pituitary glands were not larger but contained more corticotrophs. They surmised that greater amounts of ACTH were required to maintain adrenal function, perhaps because of hypoxic inhibition of adrenocortical sensitivity. However, Ramirez et al. (1988) found no such inhibition.

Calbet (2003) studied nine subjects during 9 weeks' stay at 5260 m and found an increase in arterial blood pressure (measured directly) with increased plasma epinephrine and norepinephrine. He showed that blood norepinephrine spill-over from the leg was increased compared with sea level values. This increase in sympathetic nervous activity was after arterial oxygen content had been restored by the normal rise in [Hb] with time at altitude. Hansen and Sander (2003), on the same expedition, measured sympathetic activity directly by peroneal microneurography after 4 weeks at altitude. They found activity to be about three times sea-level values. They also studied the effect of oxygen breathing and a saline infusion (to reduce baroreflex deactivation). These interventions had only minor effect on sympathetic activity. Three days after returning to sea level sympathetic activity was still significantly higher than pre-expedition values as were results for blood pressure and heart rate.

Bogaard et al. (2002) studied the effect of blocking either the sympathetic or parasympathetic arms of the autonomic system in a group of subjects at 3800 m on the heart rate and cardiac output on exercise. Propranalol had the expected effect of reducing heart rate and glycopyrrolate increased the maximum heart rate to sea level values. But interestingly neither medication had any effect of maximum cardiac output, $V_{O_{2,max}}$, or work rate at altitude, though, of course, these values were lower than sea level. Mazzeo *et al.* (2003) showed that blocking the alpha-adrenergic system in a group of female subjects at 4300 m resulted in increased norepinephrine levels compared with unblocked controls both at rest and exercise.

Women appear to have the same sympathoadrenal response to altitude as men and there is no difference related to the menstrual cycle (Mazzeo and Reeves 2003). However, it is worth noting that this elevated response may be a factor in the increased incidence of pre-eclampsia in pregnant women at altitude.

15.6.3 Adrenergic response and acclimatization

Acute hypoxia causes an increase in heart rate and cardiac output. However, after several days at altitude the heart rate and cardiac output fall back towards sea level values. On exercise the maximum heart rate is limited to well below the sea level maximum, being typically 140–150 beats min^{-1} at 5800 m compared with 180–200 beats min^{-1} at sea level (Chapter 7). This reduction in maximal heart rate and cardiac output takes place at a time when the plasma and urinary catecholamines are higher than at sea level.

Evidently, the heart's response to sympathetic stimulation becomes blunted. This has been demonstrated by Maher *et al.* (1975b), who showed in dogs that the cardio-acceleratory effect of an infusion of isoproterenol was reduced after 10 days' altitude acclimatization. Workers from the same institution (Maher *et al.* 1978) found in cardiac muscle of acclimatized goats that there was a twofold rise of the enzyme *O*-methyltransferase. This enzyme inactivates cardiac norepinephrine, and its induction during acclimatization may account for the blunting of the adrenergic response to exercise. Another possibility is that there may be downregulation, that is, a reduction in the density of adrenergic receptors on the heart muscle. Voelkel *et al.* (1981) have shown this to be the case in rats kept for 5 weeks at a simulated altitude of 4250 m. These two possible mechanisms are not mutually exclusive. Sherpa high altitude residents do not suffer this heart rate limitation on maximal exercise. Their heart rates can go up to 190–198 beats min^{-1} at 4880 m (Lahiri *et al.* 1967).

15.6.4 Autonomic system response and AMS

Duplain and colleagues (1999a) studied eight climbers who were susceptible to HAPE measuring their sympathetic activity directly with intraneural electrodes and compared them to seven subjects resistant to HAPE. Measurements were made at low altitude breathing a hypoxic gas mixture and at high altitude (4599 m). In both situations the HAPE susceptible subjects had significantly higher sympathetic activity than resistant subjects. This increased activity at altitude preceded the onset of lung edema. Also taking both groups together, there was a direct, significant relationship between sympathetic nerve activity and pulmonary artery pressure.

A chamber study was carried out by Loeppky *et al.* (2003) measuring autonomic responses by heart rate variability and plasma catecholamines. There were significantly higher levels of catecholamines and higher low/higher frequency ratios in AMS subjects indicating greater sympathetic activity. These differences became greater with time (over 6–12 h). They also found lower temperature in their AMS subjects which they attributed to greater vasodilatation despite greater sympathetic activity.

Lanfranchi *et al.* (2005) studied 41 mountaineers at the Capanna Margherita (4559 m) using spectral analysis of the R–R interval and blood pressure variability as a measure autonomic system activity. Seventeen subjects had AMS. Measurements were repeated at low altitude 3 months later, breathing air and a hypoxic gas mixture. They found evidence of autonomic dysfunction in subjects with AMS at altitude and claimed that AMS-prone subjects could be identified as those showing marked low-frequency component of systolic BP variability in the field. However, the short-term, acute hypoxia test at sea level did not show a difference between those who were AMS prone and those who were resistant.

15.6.5 Sympathetoadrenal response: Summary

Hypoxia has no effect on epinephrine levels in the blood or urine but there is a modest rise in norepinephrine levels. In the first few days at altitude there is increased sympathetic and parasympathetic activity. This increased sympathetic activity results in increased heart rate but does not affect cardiac output. The increase in sympathetic activity is more marked in subjects with AMS and HAPE. The response of the heart to adrenergic stimulation becomes blunted after a week or 10 days at altitude and this is probably due to down regulation of receptors and induction of the enzyme responsible for catecholamine metabolism. After prolonged altitude exposure the enhanced sympathoadrenal activity continues for some days after return to normoxia.

15.7 THYROID FUNCTION AND THE ALTITUDE ENVIRONMENT

Hypothalamic–pituitary–thyroid axis function is affected by hypoxia and possibly by cold. The effect of cold on thyroid function is considered in Chapter 23. Iodine is essential for synthesis of thyroid hormone and is deficient in the soil and water of some mountainous regions, so that thyroid function in residents of these regions is affected.

15.7.1 Thyroid function and hypoxia

The response of the hypophyseal–thyroid axis to hypoxia seems to be quite different in humans compared with animals. In animals, hypoxia results in depression of thyroid function (Heath and Williams 1995, pp. 265–6). In the pituitary gland the number of thyrotrophs – cells that secrete TSH – is reduced, suggesting a decreased output of TSH (Gosney 1986). In humans, however, thyroid activity is increased at altitude. Surks (1966) found elevated levels of thyroxine binding globulin (TBG) and free thyroxine (T_4) in the first 2 weeks at altitude (4300 m), with a peak at 9 days. Kotchen et al. (1973), in a 3-day chamber experiment (3650 m equivalent), found T_4 elevated (free and bound) but TSH to be unchanged, suggesting a shift of T_4 from extravascular to intravascular compartments rather than increased pituitary activity. Westendorp et al. (1993) also found no increase in TSH in response to a 1-h acute hypoxia equivalent of 4115 m.

These results have been confirmed in a number of field studies (Rastogi et al. 1977, Stock et al. 1978b) which showed levels returning towards control in the third week at altitude. Sawhney and Malhotra (1991) studied both acclimatized lowlanders and high

altitude natives, and found levels of triiodothyronine (T_3) and T_4 to be higher than sea level residents. T_4 concentration in red cells was decreased at high altitude but there was no change in levels of reverse T_3 (rT_3), TBG, and T_4 binding capacity of TBG and thyroxine binding prealbumin. They also found no change in TSH. In L-eltroxine-treated men they still found a rise in T_3 and T_4, suggesting the rise to be independent of pituitary stimulation.

Exercise increases T_3 and T_4 to a greater extent at altitude than at sea level (Stock et al. 1978b). At higher altitudes of 5400 m and 6300 m, Mordes et al. (1983) showed elevated resting T_3, free T_4 and T_3 in subjects who had been at altitude for some weeks. In these subjects TSH was also elevated, in contrast to the finding at lower altitudes.

The basal metabolic rate is elevated during the first 2 weeks at moderate altitude and correlates with the free T_4 (Stock et al. 1978a). At higher altitudes (above 5500 m) it remains elevated for months (Gill and Pugh 1964), as does T_4 (Mordes et al. 1983). Mordes et al. (1983) also found evidence of impaired conversion of T_4 to T_3 at 6300 m. Perhaps there is a change in the set point for the pituitary negative feedback system, resulting in higher levels of TSH. They also found that the response of the pituitary to an injection of thyrotrophin releasing hormone was enhanced at 6300 m compared with sea level. A similar finding has been reported by Ramirez et al. (1995) in resident highlanders at only 2600 m.

15.7.2 Iodine deficiency, goiter and altitude

The frequency of goiter in mountainous areas is well known and is discussed in Chapter 17. In England it was known as 'Derbyshire neck' and it was equally well known in the Pyrenees, the Alps, the Andes and the Himalayas, but it is not confined to the mountains.

The association of iodine deficiency and mountainous areas is mainly due to the geological factors causing iodine deficiency in the soil and hence in the diet but altitude hypoxia stimulates thyroid function (section 15.7.1). Thus the effect of iodine deficiency will result in more exaggerated hyperplasia, which contributes to the extremely high rate of goiter in resident populations at altitude in the past.

15.8 CONTROL OF BLOOD GLUCOSE AT ALTITUDE

15.8.1 Acute hypoxia

On acute exposure to hypoxia there is a rise in fasting blood glucose of about 1.7 mmol L^{-1}, followed by a fall towards control values by the end of a week. At the same time insulin levels are elevated (Williams 1975). This is presumably part of the nonspecific stress response indicated by the concurrent rise in plasma cortisol levels (section 15.5).

15.8.2 Chronic hypoxia

In subjects acclimatized to high altitude, fasting blood glucose was found to be lower than at sea level by some workers (Blume and Pace 1967, Stock et al. 1978b, Blume 1984) but unchanged by others (Sawhney et al. 1986). Singh et al. (1974) found a persistently raised glucose level after 10 months at altitude. Resting insulin levels have also been found to be reduced (Stock et al. 1978b).

Glucose loading increases both blood glucose and insulin levels at altitude as it does at sea level, but the rise in both was found to be less than at sea level in two studies (Stock et al. 1978b, Blume 1984) but greater in one (Sawhney et al. 1986). There are a number of explanations for this blunted response. Glucose may be absorbed less rapidly, though this is probably only true above about 5500 m (section 14.5). Liver glycogen synthesis may be enhanced at altitude and some evidence for this has been found in rats injected with labeled glucose at altitude (Blume and Pace 1971). There may be increased target organ sensitivity to insulin, presumably by upregulation (increased density) of insulin receptors on target cells. This is a feature of athletic training and may well happen as part of altitude acclimatization. A recent study by Lee and colleagues (2003) in healthy subjects found that as little as 3 days' sedentary living at 2400 m resulted in an improvement in the oral glucose tolerance test. That is a faster decline of glucose levels after a similar rise in response to glucose loading, suggesting increased insulin sensitivity.

The effect of the action of insulin at altitude was investigated by Larsen and colleagues (1997) using a euglycemic clamp technique in a group of men,

at sea level and on days 2 and 7 of altitude exposure at 4559 m. They found that insulin action decreased markedly on day 2 but had improved somewhat by day 7 at altitude. More recently, Braun et al. (2001) studied a group of women at an altitude of 4300 m over 12 days. They found the same pattern of initial decrease in insulin sensitivity followed by enhanced sensitivity with acclimatization. They also investigated whether the reduced insulin sensitivity was due to adrenaline secretion early in altitude exposure by using an α-adrenergic antagonist. They concluded that this was not the case. De Glisezinski et al. (1999) studied lipolysis in subcutaneous fat biopsies in subjects exposed to prolonged simulated altitude exposure in a chamber (Operation Everest III). They found that the anti-lipolytic activity of insulin was significantly decreased.

K. Moore et al. (2001) in a group of trekkers attempting Kilimanjaro (5895 m) found that insulin requirements reduced from a mean of 67 to 12 units day^{-1}. This may have been partly due to AMS and reduction in food intake. However, in mountaineers with type 1 diabetes, the insulin requirements during a climb of Cho Oyu (8201 m) increased from a mean of 38 to 51 units day^{-1} (Pavan et al. 2004). Of course insulin requirements depend upon many factors apart from insulin sensitivity. For a discussion of the problems faced by patients with diabetes see Chapter 24.

Braun et al. (1998) studied the glucose response to a standard meal in women at sea level and at 4300 m in the presence of estrogen (E) and estrogen plus progesterone (E+P). The peak of glucose was lower and returned to baseline more slowly at altitude than at sea level although the insulin levels were the same. The response was also lower in E than E+P at sea level but the difference at altitude was not significant. It would seem that at altitude the relative concentration of ovarian hormones does not appear to be important in glucose control.

15.9 ENDOTHELIN

15.9.1 Endothelin family

The endothelins are a family of peptides produced by a wide variety of cells affecting mainly blood vessels. Endothelin-1 (ET-1), clinically the most important member of the family, is the most potent vasoconstrictor yet discovered with about 100 times the activity of norepinephrine. Other members of the family identified are ET-2 and ET-3, which are more localized to certain organs. All three peptides bind to the same two receptors, A and B, though with differing binding affinities. Synthetic inhibitors of these receptors are now available and their use has served to elucidate some of the actions of these peptides. ET-1 is produced by the endothelium and as much as 75% of the production is exported from the side of the cell opposite to the vessel lumen, where it acts on the adjacent smooth muscle without contributing to the plasma pool. In this way it perhaps should be considered as mainly a paracrine, rather than an endocrine, hormone. However, plasma levels probably do reflect the output of ET-1 and parallel the severity of the condition in, for instance, congestive cardiac failure. A good clinical review has been published by Levin (1995), and Holm (1997) has provided a more pharmacological review.

15.9.2 Altitude and endothelin

Horio et al. (1991) showed that ET-1 in rats increased with increasing hypoxia. Since then there have been a number of studies in humans at altitude. Cargill et al. (1995) found that 30 min of acute hypoxia (Sa,O_2 75–80%) raised plasma ET-1 levels to about 2.5 times baseline. A group of hypoxic patients with cor pulmonale had similar levels. Similar results were found by Ferri et al. (1995) in patients with chronic obstructive lung disorder (COLD). They also found that ET-1 levels correlated with pulmonary artery pressure. Morganti et al. (1995) studied 10 subjects on a 2-day ascent of Monte Rosa (4559 m) and eight subjects in the Everest region at 5050 m. They found plasma ET-1 raised progressively with increasing altitude, the level correlating with the fall in Sa,O_2. There was no correlation with blood pressure or hematocrit. Richalet and colleagues (1995) studied 10 subjects on Sajama (6542 m) and found modest increases in ET-1 at both rest and exercise. Levels were highest after 1 week and decreased slightly after 3 weeks' altitude exposure.

Blauw et al. (1995) studied the effect of hypoxia and ET-1 infusion on forearm blood flow. Forearm blood flow was not changed by hypoxia, but the ET-1 plasma increased significantly. They conclude that hypoxia causes release of ET-1 from the pulmonary circulation but that this does not influence peripheral vascular tone. Cruden et al. (1998) measured both ET-1 and big ET-1 in a group of mountaineers. Both were increased on ascent to altitudes above 2500 m, indicating that the increase in ET-1 was due to increased production and not decreased elimination. After 3 weeks at altitude, levels had returned to baseline values. Exercise had no effect on endothelin levels. In a separate study, they also found increases in both ET-1 and big ET-1 with cold exposure (Cruden et al. 1999).

15.9.3 Endothelin and HAPE

A Japanese group (Droma et al. 1996a) reported detailed findings on a single case of HAPE with pulmonary hypertension and found ET-1 levels elevated on admission. The levels reverted to normal as the patient recovered and pulmonary artery pressure fell. The same team (Droma et al. 1996b) studied a group of HAPE-susceptible subjects. Their subjects had a greater hypoxic vascular response than controls but no significant change in ET-1 levels with a hypoxic challenge. However, the hypoxia was only of 5-min duration (10% oxygen).

Sartori et al. (1999b) studied a group of 16 mountaineers prone to HAPE, comparing them with a group resistant to HAPE. At altitude (4559 m) the HAPE prone group had endothelin-1 plasma levels 33% higher than the HAPE resistant group. There was a significant direct relationship between changes ET-1 levels and pulmonary artery pressure from low to high altitude.

In conclusion, it seems likely that ET-1 plays a part in the mechanism of hypoxic pulmonary vasoconstriction, at least in the pig (Holm 1997). The augmented release of ET-1 in HAPE-susceptible subjects suggests that it may have a role in the mechanism of HAPE.

15.9.4 Bradykinin

The levels of bradykinin, a potent vasodilator, are not changed by acute hypoxia (Ashack et al. 1985) and the vasodilatory effect of bradykinin is not altered by high altitude in the guinea pig uterine arteries (White *et al.* 2000).

15.10 ALTITUDE AND OTHER HORMONES

15.10.1 Glucagon

Fasting glucagon levels are the same at altitude and at sea level and are slightly depressed after glucose loading (Blume 1984).

15.10.2 Growth hormone

Levels are unchanged in most subjects but were found to be increased fivefold in two subjects who had lost 15 kg in body weight (Blume 1984). Although acute hypoxia causes no change in growth hormone levels, exercise under acute hypoxic conditions causes a 20-fold increase in this hormone, whereas normoxic exercise causes only a modest rise (Sutton 1977, Raynaud *et al.* 1981). Ramirez *et al.* (1995) studied residents at Pasto, Colombia (2600 m), and found that response of growth hormone to stimulation with growth hormone releasing hormone was greatly enhanced compared with lowland control subjects. On the other hand the *in vitro* lipolytic response to growth hormone (and parathormone) was significantly decreased in biopsies of subcutaneous fat in subjects exposed to simulated altitude in a chamber (Operation Everest III) (de Glisezinski *et al.* 1999).

15.10.3 Testosterone, luteinizing hormone, follicle stimulating hormone and prolactin

Sawhney *et al.* (1985) studied levels of testosterone, luteinizing hormone (LH), follicle stimulating hormone (FSH) and prolactin in lowland men after ascent to 3500 m. On day 1 at altitude there were no significant changes from sea level values, though LH and testosterone levels were already falling. By day 7, LH and testosterone levels were significantly reduced and remained so to day 18; by then prolactin levels were significantly elevated. After 7 days at sea level all values had reverted to control except for some residual depression in LH

levels. These results are in accord with previous work (Guerra-Garcia 1971) which found urinary testosterone excretion to be reduced by 50% on day 3 at 4300 m. Sawhney *et al.* (1985) also found a negative correlation between prolactin and testosterone levels at altitude but no correlation with LH levels. They suggested that the reduction in testosterone is due to an increase in prolactin secretion rather than to a reduction in LH or a direct effect of hypoxia on the testes.

In a separate experiment at sea level Sawhney *et al.* (1985) showed a reduction in LH levels in response to daily cold exposure after 1 and 5 days, and suggested that the reduction in LH found at altitude might be due to cold rather than hypoxia. However, low levels of LH have been found in hypoxia due to chronic lung disease in hospital patients with no cold exposure (Semple 1986); these patients also had low testosterone levels which correlated with their Pa,O_2.

Semple (1986) found normal testosterone levels in patients who were hypoxic because of congenital cardiac defects, presumably because of lifelong adaptation to hypoxemia. He suggests that an alternative mechanism may be that testosterone depression is a response to dips in oxygen saturation at night, due to sleep apnea in patients with chronic obstructive lung disease, and a result of periodic breathing in lowlanders at altitude. In high altitude residents, Bangham and Hackett (1978) found reduced levels of LH after 10 days but no changes in levels of FSH, testosterone or prolactin.

Testosterone is increased in exercise and Bouissou *et al.* (1986) studied the effect of acute hypoxia (14% oxygen, equivalent to 3000 m) on this response. They found that, when the exercise was expressed as a percentage of maximum exercise, there was no effect of acute hypoxia. This is also true for the acute hypoxic effect on the exercise-induced rises of lactate, epinephrine and norepinephrine.

15.11 MALE REPRODUCTIVE FUNCTION AT ALTITUDE

The effect of altitude on male reproductive function at altitude has been little studied. Donayre *et al.* (2003) found, in nine subjects, decreased sperm count, increased abnormal forms and decreased motility during a 4-week stay at an altitude of 4267 m and 15 days after return to sea level. Recently, Okumura *et al.* (2003) studied three members of an expedition to the Karakoram where heights of 7100 m were reached. They did not carry out measurements at altitude but extended the study to results at 1 month, 3 months and 2 years after return to sea level. The sperm count was reduced at 1 and 3 months and had recovered at 2 years. There was also an increase in abnormally shaped sperm which recovered by 3 months. In this study testosterone was low at 1 and 3 months but had recovered by 2 years after return from altitude.

15.12 RENAL FUNCTION AT ALTITUDE

15.12.1 General function

The kidney is remarkably resistant to altitude hypoxia. This is not surprising since it is designed to suffer quite severe reductions in blood flow, and therefore oxygen delivery, during exercise. At 5800 m, after 24-h dehydration, the kidney concentrates urine normally and eliminates a water load as well as it does at sea level. It also responds to ingestion of bicarbonate or ammonium chloride (metabolic alkalosis or acidosis) by producing appropriate changes in pH (Ward, reported by Pugh 1962a). Olsen *et al.* (1993) found a 10% reduction in effective renal plasma flow (ERPF) but normal glomerular filtration rate and sodium clearance in eight normal subjects at 4350 m. Dopamine infusion had less effect on ERPF than at sea level, presumably because of increased adrenergic activity (norepinephrine was increased). The diuretic effect of dopamine was reduced, possibly because of an altitude effect on distal tubular function. High altitude residents at 4300 m showed no evidence of deficient renal oxygenation (Rennie *et al.* 1971a).

However (as discussed in section 9.4.5), at extreme altitude (above 6500 m) the renal compensation for respiratory alkalosis is slow and incomplete; that is, the blood bicarbonate is very little further reduced and the blood pH becomes very alkaline as the P_{CO_2} is reduced by extreme hyperventilation. Whether this represents a degree of renal failure is debatable, since it results in a shift of the oxygen dissociation curve to the left (because of the alkaline pH), which is beneficial for oxygen

transport at extreme altitude (section 9.3.6). A study by Hackett *et al.* (1985) showed that, in acclimatized subjects at 6300 m acetazolamide still resulted in the excretion of bicarbonate producing further base deficit. Exercise performance was not increased and, indeed, in two out of four subjects it was decreased.

There is also fluid volume depletion at altitude and it is known that the kidney gives a higher priority to correcting dehydration than acid–base disturbances. In order to excrete more bicarbonate to reduce the base excess, it would be necessary to lose corresponding cations, which would aggravate the volume depletion. This may be the basis for the slow renal bicarbonate excretion at extreme altitude.

15.12.2 Proteinuria at altitude

Rennie and Joseph (1970) showed that proteinuria became apparent on ascent to altitude. Values rose from 290 to 578 mg mmol^{-1} as their subjects climbed to 5800 m in 12 days. There was a time lag of 1–3 days between peak altitude and peak proteinuria. Figure 15.5 shows that there is a good correlation between the degree of proteinuria and altitude, provided allowance is made for a 24-h time lag between ascent and its effect on the kidney.

In another study, Rennie *et al.* (1972) found no effect of acclimatization on proteinuria but Pines (1978) found less proteinuria on repeat ascents to the same altitude, and also that subjects with AMS had the greatest proteinuria. High altitude residents

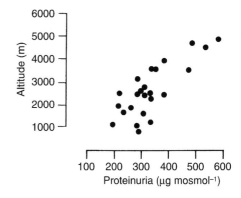

Figure 15.5 Proteinuria at altitude, the altitude being that of the subjects 24 h before urine sampling. (After Rennie 1973).

excrete more protein in the urine than subjects of the same race at sea level (Rennie *et al.* 1971b).

Patients with cyanotic heart disease who are chronically hypoxic from birth also have increased proteinuria, the severity being directly related to the degree of polycythemia (and hypoxia) (Rennie 1973); it is also found in patients with chronic obstructive lung disease (Wilkinson *et al.* 1993).

Bradwell and Delamere (1982) studied the effect of acetazolamide on altitude proteinuria as part of a double blind trial of the drug as a prophylactic for AMS. They found that, at 5000 m, albuminuria was six times greater in subjects on placebo tablets than in those on acetazolamide. They found an inverse correlation between $Pa_{,O_2}$ and percentage increase in urine albumin. The eight subjects on acetazolamide were of course less hypoxic, with $Pa_{,O_2} > 42$ mmHg, than nine subjects on placebo with $Pa_{,O_2} < 42$ mmHg. The authors suggest that the effect of acetazolamide on albuminuria was due to this reduction in hypoxia. The mechanism for altitude proteinuria may be either a reduction in tubular reabsorption of protein or increased glomerular permeability to protein, or both.

A recent study from La Paz, Bolivia, in patients with chronic mountain sickness (CMS) also found significant proteinuria which was improved on treatment with an ACE inhibitor. Twenty-four hour protein excretion fell from 359 to 248 mg. The Hct fell as well from 63.5 to 56.8% (Plata *et al.* 2002). Another recent study from the Andes (Jefferson *et al.* 2002) also found significant proteinuria in CMS patients. There were high levels of urate (and a high incidence of gout) as well, which they attribute mainly to high levels of generation of uric acid, although a relative impairment of renal excretion might also contribute.

16

Central nervous system

SUMMARY

The central nervous system is exquisitely sensitive to hypoxia, so it is not surprising that impairment of neuropsychological function occurs at high altitude. Brain oxygenation is a function of both the arterial P_{O_2} and cerebral blood flow. The latter is regulated in part by the arterial blood gases. Hypoxemia causes cerebral vasodilatation while a reduced arterial P_{CO_2} results in cerebral vasoconstriction. Therefore, these are conflicting factors at high altitude. Some impairment of neuropsychological function, for example slow learning of complex mental tasks, can be demonstrated at altitudes of less than 2000 m. At higher altitudes many aspects of neuropsychological function have been shown to be impaired including reaction time, hand–eye coordination, and higher functions such as memory and language expression. Several studies have documented residual impairment of neuropsychological function after ascents to very high altitude. An interesting finding is that climbers with a high hypoxic ventilatory response tend to have the most severe residual impairment, possibly because the associated reduced arterial P_{CO_2} causes cerebral vasoconstriction and therefore diminished oxygen delivery, and more severe cerebral hypoxia. Oxygen enrichment of room air improves neuropsychological function at an altitude of 5000 m and therefore improves performance in commuters to mines and telescopes.

16.1 INTRODUCTION

Of all the parts of the body, the central nervous system (CNS) is the most vulnerable to hypoxia. It is not surprising, therefore, that people who go to high altitude often have changes in neuropsychological function, including special senses such as vision, higher functions such as memory, and affective behavior such as mood. Such changes have been observed in individuals acutely exposed to hypoxia, in lowlanders sojourning at high altitude, and in high altitude natives.

In addition to the changes in neuropsychological function seen in individuals at high altitude, there is mounting evidence that there may be persistent defects of CNS function upon return to sea level after periods of severe hypoxia at high altitude. These findings are of special interest now because increasing numbers of climbers choose to climb at great altitudes without supplementary oxygen. Many people are concerned about the increase in morbidity and mortality on expeditions to extreme altitude and irrational decisions made by severely hypoxemic climbers probably play an important role. An excellent review gives a detailed account of high altitude, human mental performance, and the biology of hypoxia and the brain (Raichle and Hornbein 2001).

16.2 HISTORICAL

Changes in mood and behavior at high altitude have been recognized from the early days of climbing high mountains. However, the most extreme effects of hypoxia on the central nervous system were seen by the early balloonists where partial paralysis, difficulties with vision, mood changes, and even loss of consciousness are well documented. For example, during the famous flight of the balloon *Zenith* by Tissandier and his two companions (Tissandier 1875),

> towards 7500 meters, the numbness one experiences is extraordinary . . . One does not suffer at all; on the contrary. One experiences inner joy, as if it were an effect of the inundating flood of light. One becomes indifferent. . . .

This lack of appreciation of the dangers of acute hypoxia is well known to aircraft pilots and is the reason why there are stringent regulations on using oxygen above certain altitudes in spite of the fact that the pilot may not feel that he needs it.

The paralyzing effects of hypoxia were vividly described during the balloon ascent by Glaisher and Coxwell in 1862 (Glaisher *et al.* 1871). At the highest altitude, Glaisher collapsed unconscious in the basket, and it was left to Coxwell to vent the hydrogen from the balloon to bring it down. However, Coxwell had apparently lost the use of his hands and instead had to seize the cord that controlled the valve with his teeth and dip his head two or three times. Incidentally, this flight also underscored the rapid recovery from severe acute hypoxia. When the balloon landed, Glaisher stated that he felt 'no inconvenience,' and they both walked between 7 and 8 miles to the nearest village because they had come down in a remote country area.

When climbers began to reach great altitudes, neuropsychological disturbances were frequently reported. For example, there were several descriptions of bizarre changes in perception and mood on the early expeditions to Mount Everest. During the 1933 Everest expedition, Smythe gave a dramatic description of a hallucination when he saw pulsating cloud-like objects in the sky (Ruttledge 1933). Smythe also reported a strong feeling that he was accompanied by a second person; he even divided food to give half to his non-existent companion. On occasions, the changes in CNS function suggest attacks of transient cerebral ischemia. For example, the very experienced mountaineer, Shipton, had a remarkable period of aphasia at an altitude of about 7000 m on the same expedition (Shipton 1943). He reported that

> if I wished to say 'give me a cup of tea', I would say something entirely different – maybe 'tram-car, cat, put' . . . I was perfectly clear-headed . . . but my tongue just refused to perform the required movements. . . .

In the last few years, there has been increasing interest in the neuropsychological effects of high altitude. For example, the Polish climber and psychiatrist Ryn found a range of psychiatric disturbances in mountaineers who had ascended to over 5500 m (Ryn 1971). He also reported that symptoms similar to an organic brain syndrome persisted for several weeks after the expedition. Some climbers had electroencephalogram abnormalities after climbs to great altitudes. Studies made during the war between China and India in the early 1960s, when Indian troops were rapidly airlifted to high altitude, showed residual changes in psychomotor function on return to sea level (Sharma *et al.* 1975, 1976). Townes *et al.* (1984) made measurements on members of the American Medical Research Expedition to Everest (AMREE) after they had returned to sea level following about three months at altitudes of 5400–8848 m and found residual abnormalities of neuropsychological performance. Similar results were found on Operation Everest II, including the additional interesting observation that climbers with the highest hypoxic ventilatory response were more severely affected (Hornbein *et al.* 1989). The authors postulated that in spite of the less severe hypoxemia in the individuals with the higher ventilatory responses, the resultant more profound hypocapnia may have caused a relatively greater vasoconstriction and therefore lower blood flow and thus oxygen delivery to the brain. The findings in the more controlled OE II chamber study were similar to those in the field study on Mount Everest (AMREE 1981), and the results were combined for the Hornbein (1989) publication. There have been steady improvements in the techniques of neuropsychological testing and it is becoming clear that minor changes in function are extremely common at high altitude, and that some residual impairment often remains in some climbers who return to sea level from great altitudes.

16.3 MECHANISMS OF ACTION OF HYPOXIA

16.3.1 Hypoxia and nerve cells

In spite of a great deal of research over the last few decades, a clear understanding of the effect of hypoxia on the brain remains elusive (Siesjo 1992a,b, Haddad and Jiang 1993, Hossmann 1999, Raichle and Hornbein 2001 for recent reviews).

There are three consistent findings from years of research on the effect of hypoxia on the brain. First, whole human brain oxygen consumption remains constant during hypoxia, even severe levels. In order to maintain this equilibrium, a commensurate increase in blood flow has to occur. Second, in spite of no change in oxygen consumption, hypoxia accelerates glucose utilization and lactate production suggesting an increase in glycolytic flux by nerve cells, but utilization is depressed during severe hypoxemia while oxygen consumption remains the same. In clinical states of severe ischemia, the hippocampus, white matter, superior colliculus and lateral geniculates appear particularly sensitive to levels of oxygen. The increase in brain lactate levels in early stages of hypoxia is counter-balanced by an increase in bicarbonate which results in a near normal pH. Third, brain tissue concentrations of ATP, ADP and AMP as markers of the energy state of the tissue remain close to normal even during severe hypoxia, comparable to elevations above 8000 m. While the brain is very sensitive to a decrease in oxygen supply, i.e. blood flow and glucose, examples from nature demonstrate some species' phenomenal resistance to profound hypoxia, such as

the turtle (Perez-Pinon *et al.* 1992), the harbor seal (Kerem and Elsner 1973), and high altitude birds (Faraci 1986, Faraci and Fedde 1986).

IONIC CHANGES IN BRAIN WITH HYPOXIA

Altered ion homeostasis during hypoxia clearly occurs though whether the ionic changes are primary, or whether they are due to altered oxidative or neurotransmitter metabolism, is unclear. Hypoxia interferes with calcium homeostasis. For example, very low oxygen levels diminish calcium uptake at synapses. One hypothesis is that the decrease of calcium in the endoplasmic reticulum is a critical factor in cerebral dysfunction in hypoxic environments (Paschen 1966). Intracellular levels of potassium are increased during severe hypoxia. There is accumulation of free radicals which cause further injury, particularly to the capillaries. Neurotransmitter metabolism is thought to be sensitive to hypoxia although there is conflicting evidence about which transmitter or metabolic step is most sensitive. There is evidence that acetylcholine synthesis by brain is oxygen-dependent as is the biosynthesis of amino acid neurotransmitters. Brain catecholamine concentrations are apparently decreased by hypoxia though the mechanism is unclear. Much of the experimental work has been done on ischemia, and the relationship of the changes to those caused by pure hypoxia is controversial, but it is clear that ischemia is a far more important condition than hypoxia alone in causing brain damage although hypoxia accentuates ischemic injury in rat brains (Miyamoto *et al.* 2000).

VASCULAR ENDOTHELIAL GROWTH FACTOR AND HYPOXIA

As mentioned in Chapter 19, certain factors, such as hypoxia-induced vascular endothelial growth factor are known to induce fluid leak from capillaries in the brain (Fischer *et al.* 1999, Schoch *et al.* 2002), an effect known to occur with acute hypoxic exposure. The mechanism of the stimulation of vascular endothelial growth factor (VEGF) has been elegantly unraveled in the last few years, and the beneficial effects to the brain in terms of improvement of oxygen delivery have been fascinating to observe.

The response of the brain to chronic hypoxia and ischemia is one of survival which takes the forms of angiogenesis and neuroprotection respectively.

The initiation of these events depends on the stimulation of the transcription factor, hypoxia inducible factor 1 (HIF-1) (Semenza 2000). The alpha portion of the heterodimer is the one which acts as an immediate transcription factor for a number of growth factors, one of which is VEGF. HIF-1α is present in many tissues and responds immediately and transiently to hypoxia and/or ischemia. HIF-1α targets mRNA genes and stimulates the induction of the *VEGF* gene which, along with the synergistic effect of glycolytic metabolism, induces angiogenesis in the insulted cerebral tissue (Bergeron *et al.* 2000, Marti *et al.* 2000).

With several weeks exposure to hypoxia, rats demonstrate an immediate and sustained increase in HIF-1α (Chavez *et al.* 2000) which stimulates VEGF. This together with other growth factors results in angiogenesis and vascular remodeling such that there is an increase in capillary density and improvement and maintenance of oxygen delivery (Boero *et al.* 1999, Dor *et al.* 2001, Pichiule and LaManna 2002, LaManna *et al.* 2004). Excellent reviews about this area of research are available (Semenza 2000, LaManna *et al.* 2004, Xu and LaManna 2006). This body of work is an elegant example of the quest to understand down to the genetic level the adaptation to hypoxia which minimizes the decrease in availability of oxygen whether it be from high altitude or disease.

Another fascinating area of investigation recently has been the discovery of the neuroprotective effect of various growth factors, especially erythropoietin, under the conditions of ischemia and/or hypoxia. HIF-1α plays an important role in initiating this process (Semenza 2000, Bergeron *et al.* 2000, Kerendi *et al.* 2005; and see Chapter 7). It is the transcription factor for erythropoietin which has been found to minimize cerebral damage (Sirén *et al.* 2001, Bernaudin *et al.* 2002, Wen *et al.* 2002). Some investigators have hypothesized that 'preconditioning' by sublethal exposure to hypoxia might protect the brain from subsequent damage from ischemic and hypoxic exposure. Hypoxia stimulates HIF-1α which is rapidly inactivated by proline hydroxylation. Inhibition of this proteosome is being investigated as a therapeutic intervention in stroke therapy (Ratan *et al.* 2004). This line of research may have profound implications in clinical medicine, especially in the area of cerebrovascular disease.

HYPOXIA AND THE ELECTROENCEPHALOGRAM

The effects of hypoxia on brain synapses and membrane polarization interfere with the normal electrical activity of the brain and alter the EEG. In cats in which the arterial P_{O_2} is gradually reduced from 80 to 20 mmHg, the EEG amplitude initially increases slightly and then slow waves and sharp spikes appear. Subsequently, the slow waves decrease in amplitude and then disappear. Later these small spikes become sporadic, and finally the EEG flattens. The initial activation which is followed by depression may be due to the effect of hypoxia on the reticular activating system. Since acute exposure to high altitude results in increased cortical activity on EEG, high altitude exposure may increase susceptibility to seizures by decreasing the threshold for the initiation of epileptic discharge (Basynat 2000a, Daleau *et al.* 2006), but this theory is disputed by many who advise patients with seizure disorders who wish to go to high altitude.

EVOKED POTENTIALS AND HYPOXIA

Evoked potentials are also altered by hypoxia. Brain-stem auditory response is abolished by low levels of oxygen. Visually evoked potentials are initially increased and then abolished as the level of oxygen is reduced.

HISTOLOGICAL CHANGES

Histological changes in the brain result from severe hypoxia. The changes are indistinguishable from those due to hypotension and the greatest changes are seen in the cortex and basal ganglia. Microvacuolization of neuronal perikaryon occurs first, the H1 zone (Sommer sector) of the hippocampus being the most vulnerable region.

16.3.2 Cerebral blood flow

The levels of arterial P_{O_2} and P_{CO_2} have crucial effects on cerebral blood flow and since these levels are greatly altered by going to high altitude, the results are important (Xu and LaManna 2006). Arterial hypoxemia dilates cerebral blood vessels and greatly increases cerebral blood flow. Figure 16.1

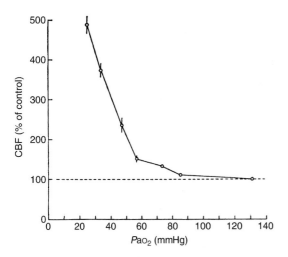

Figure 16.1 Effect of changes of arterial P_{O_2} on cerebral blood flow (CBF) in anesthetized rats. The arterial P_{CO_2} was maintained normal. Note the very sharp rise in blood flow as the arterial P_{O_2} was reduced below 50 mmHg. (From Borgström *et al.* 1975.)

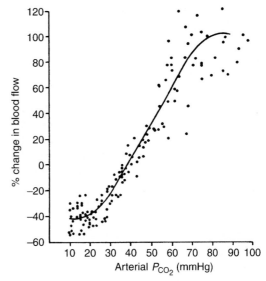

Figure 16.2 Effect of alterations in arterial P_{CO_2} on cerebral cortical blood flow in anesthetized dogs. The zero reference line for blood flow is at an arterial P_{CO_2} of 40 mmHg. Animals were normoxic and normotensive. (From Harper and Glass 1965.)

shows typical results found in anaesthetized normocapnic rats. It can be seen that cerebral blood flow was little changed until the arterial P_{O_2} fell below 60 mmHg but with lower levels of P_{O_2} there was a dramatic increase in cerebral blood flow. Note that at an arterial P_{O_2} of 25 mmHg, cerebral blood flow was approximately five times the normoxic level. As indicated in Chapter 12, the arterial P_{O_2} of a climber resting on the summit of Mount Everest is between 25 and 30 mmHg.

The results shown in Fig. 16.1 were obtained in mechanically ventilated animals where P_{CO_2} was kept constant at the normoxic level. However, in conscious animals and humans, the hyperventilation caused by the hypoxaemia will cause a reduction in arterial P_{CO_2} and an increase in pH which will cause cerebral vasoconstriction. Therefore the results shown in Fig. 16.1 cannot be applied directly to the climber at extreme altitude.

A reduction in arterial P_{CO_2} has a strong vasoconstrictor effect on cerebral blood vessels and consequently reduces cerebral flood flow. Figure 16.2 shows typical results in mechanically ventilated anesthetized dogs which were made hypocapnic by increasing the ventilation, or hypercapnic by adding carbon dioxide to the inspired gas. In every instance the arterial P_{O_2} was maintained at approximately the normal level. Note that when the arterial P_{CO_2}

fell to about 15 mmHg, cerebral blood flow was reduced by about 40% (Harper and Glass 1965).

In humans at high altitude, the two effects of hypoxemia and hypocapnia will clearly have opposing effects on the cerebral circulation, but have been found to balance each other in a way that after 3 weeks' exposure to high altitude and an increase in oxygen-carrying capacity with erythropoiesis and other adaptive mechanisms, cerebral blood flow returns to low-altitude baseline levels (Møller *et al.* 2002).

There have not been systematic studies of cerebral blood flow at various altitudes partly because of the difficulties of measurement. However, Severinghaus *et al.* (1966) measured cerebral blood flow in seven normal subjects by a nitrous oxide method at sea level and after 6–12 h and 3–5 days at an altitude of 3810 m. The blood flow increased by an average of 24% at 6–12 h, and by 13% at 3–5 days at altitude. Acute correction of the hypoxia restored the cerebral blood flow to normal. Extrapolation of additional data suggested that if the P_{CO_2} had not been reduced at high altitude, the cerebral blood flow would have been 60% above the control. An interesting feature of the data obtained by Severinghaus *et al.* (1966) is that the subsequent analysis shows that oxygen delivery to the brain (as calculated from cerebral blood flow multiplied by arterial oxygen concentration) was held essentially constant (Wolff 2000). However, there is no known receptor that responds to oxygen delivery.

Indirect evidence about cerebral blood flow in humans can be obtained by measuring blood flow velocity in the internal carotid artery by Doppler ultrasound. Huang *et al.* (1987) measured flow velocities in the internal carotid and vertebral arteries in six subjects within 2–4 h of arrival on Pikes Peak (4300 m), and found that the velocities in both arteries were slightly increased above sea level values; 18–44 h later, a peak increase of 20% was observed. However, over days 4–12, velocities declined to values similar to those at sea level. In the further study by the same group (Huang *et al.* 1991) the effect of prolonged exercise (45 min at approximately 100 W) on blood flow velocity in the internal carotid artery was studied at sea level and at 4300 m. The velocities at sea level and high altitude were similar. In a low-pressure chamber study, Reeves *et al.* (1985) measured blood flow velocity in the internal carotid artery of 12 subjects at Denver (1600 m) and repeatedly up to 7 h at a simulated altitude of 4800 m. Their hypothesis was that an increase in blood flow velocity might be associated with the development of high altitude headache, but no correlation was found. Other studies by Doppler ultrasound have shown no correlation between cerebral blood flow and acute mountain sickness (Baumgartner *et al.* 1999), or cerebral blood flow and susceptibility to high altitude pulmonary edema (Berre *et al.* 1999). On the other hand, Jansen *et al.* (1999) reported that subjects with acute mountain sickness had higher cerebral blood flows than normals, and also a greater hemodynamic response to hyperventilation.

Huang *et al.* (1992) measured blood flow velocity in the internal carotid arteries of 15 native Tibetans and 11 Han Chinese residents of Lhasa (3658 m) both at rest and during exercise. There were no differences at rest and during submaximal exercise. At peak exercise, the Tibetans showed an increase in flow velocity and cerebral oxygen delivery whereas the Hans did not. Frayser *et al.* (1970) measured the mean circulation time through the retina following fluorescein injection and found that the circulation time decreased from a mean of 4.9 s at Base Camp to 3.4 s at an altitude of 5330 m. This is consistent with an increase in cerebral blood flow.

Another possible factor at high altitude which could influence cerebral blood flow is an increased viscosity of the blood caused by polycythemia. It is known that a blood flow of less than half the normal value can occur in severe polycythemia vera (Kety 1950) and that cerebral blood flow is significantly increased in severe anemia (Heyman *et al.* 1952, Robin and Gardner 1953). Tomiyama *et al.* (2000) altered blood viscosity in rats up and down by hemodilution or transfusion, respectively, and measured cerebral blood flow during hypoxia and hypercapnia. They found that cerebral blood flow correlated with viscosity with the most profound effect being a decrease in the animals with the highest viscosity. Some drugs, including caffeine, reduce cerebral blood flow.

16.4 CENTRAL NERVOUS SYSTEM FUNCTION AT HIGH ALTITUDE

16.4.1 Moderate altitudes

There is general agreement that CNS function is impaired at altitudes over about 4500 m but an interesting question is the lowest altitude at which minor alterations in function occur. This question frequently arises in the aviation industry because it is important in selecting the cabin pressure of commercial aircraft. Most high flying commercial aircraft are pressurized to maintain the cabin pressure at or below an equivalent altitude of about 2500 m. This ceiling was accepted after considering the penalty of extra weight and expense which would have to be paid in order to reduce it further; however, there is some evidence that at a pressure equivalent to an altitude of 2440 m, subjects are slower to learn complex mental tasks than at sea level. There is some pressure to increase the cabin pressure of airplanes to simulate 1800 m in new aircraft such as the Boeing 787 and Airbus 380.

Even at the considerably lower altitude of only 1524 m, eight subjects were slower to learn complex tasks than a matched group breathing an enriched oxygen mixture (Denison *et al.* 1966). The tests here involved recognizing the posture of man-like figures having different orientations and presented in random sequence on a screen. However, Paul and

Fraser (1994) using similar tests, involving the learning of new tasks, found no impairment at altitude equivalent to 1524, 2438 and 3048 m. Thus it appears that even at the cabin altitudes of commercial aircraft, sensitive psychometric tests can pick up minor degrees of impairment.

Interesting problems concerning CNS function at moderate altitudes occur in relation to the operation of optical and infrared telescopes on mountain summits (see also Chapter 29). The reduction in the absorption of optical and infrared radiation because of the reduced thickness of the earth's atmosphere at high altitude makes high mountains ideal locations for astronomical observatories. For example, several telescopes are located on the summit of Mauna Kea, altitude 4200 m, on the island of Hawaii.

The barometric pressure on the summit of Mauna Kea is only about 468 mmHg, giving a moist inspired P_{O_2} of 88 mmHg. The telescope operators frequently live at sea level and ascend rapidly by car to the summit. Forster (1986) measured arterial blood gases on 27 telescope personnel on the first day of reaching 4200 m and reported a mean arterial P_{O_2} of 42 mmHg, P_{CO_2} 29 mmHg and pH 7.49. After 5 days, during which time the nights were spent in dormitories at an altitude of 3000 m, the arterial blood gases at 4200 m showed a mean P_{O_2} of 44 mmHg, P_{CO_2} 27 mmHg and pH of 7.48.

A number of psychometric measurements showed no change on ascending to 4200 m, though performance of the digit symbol backwards test did deteriorate on the first day. At the end of 5 days, however, the scores had returned to sea level values. Numerate memory and psychomotor ability were also reported to be impaired in commuters to Mauna Kea. Several features of acute mountain sickness were noted in shift workers, particularly on their first day at the summit. Headache was the most disabling symptom but others included insomnia, lethargy, poor concentration and poor memory.

16.4.2 High altitudes

A classical series of studies were carried out by McFarland (1937a,b, 1938a,b) in connection with the International High Altitude Expedition to Chile which took place in 1935. In his first study, McFarland reported on the psychophysiological effects of sudden ascents to 5000 m in unpressurized aircraft and compared the results with ascents by train and car to villages as high as 4700 m in Chile. The measurements showed that the rate of ascent was an important variable, with the rapid increase in altitude by aircraft being the most damaging. Both simple and complex psychological functions were significantly impaired at high altitudes including arithmetical tests, writing ability, and the appearance and disappearance time of after-images following exposure of the eye to a bright light. There were increased memory errors, errors in perseverance, and reductions in auditory threshold and words apprehended.

In a second study of sensory and motor responses during acclimatization, when measurements were obtained at altitudes as high as 5330 and 6100 m, significant reductions in audition, vision, and eye–hand coordination were seen. Measurements were made at several altitudes but in general, impairment of function was not significant below an altitude of 5330 m. Again, members of the expedition with the longest periods of acclimatization appeared to suffer less deterioration.

In a further study, mental and psychosomatic tests were also administered at the same altitudes and these showed deterioration. Tests involving the quickness of recognizing the meaning of words, mental flexibility or tendency to perseveration, and immediate memory showed significant impairment. It was noted that complex mental work could be carried out if the subjects increased their concentration but in general there was increased distractibility and lethargy which tended to reduce the ability to concentrate.

In a final series of measurements, sensory and circulatory responses were measured on sulfur miners residing permanently at an altitude of 5330 m at Aucanquilcha. They were compared with a group of workmen at sea level who were similar in age and race, and also with members of the expedition. It was found that the miners at high altitude were slower in simple and choice reaction times and less acute in auditory sensitivity than the workmen at sea level. However, McFarland and his colleagues were impressed by the evidence for circulatory and respiratory adaptation in these permanent residents at an altitude of 5330 m.

Additional studies on the deleterious effects of acute hypoxia on visual perception have been carried out, partly because of the importance of this topic in aviation. For example, Kobrick (1975) documented impaired response times in the detection of flash stimuli at equivalent altitudes of sea level, 4000 m, 4600 m and 5200 m during acute exposure in a low-pressure chamber. The effects of hypoxia on other peripheral stimuli have also been studied (Kobrick 1972).

A special opportunity to study the central nervous system effects of high altitude occurred during the India–China border war in the early 1960s when large numbers of Indian troops were rapidly taken to an altitude of 4000 m and remained there for as long as 2 years. Sharma and his colleagues (1975) measured psychomotor efficiency in 25 young Indians ranging in age from 21 to 30 years. Psychomotor performance including speed and accuracy was determined by administering an eye–hand coordination test in which a stylus was moved in a narrow groove so that it did not touch the sides. The tests were performed at sea level and at an altitude of 4000 m after periods of 1, 10, 13, 18 and 24 months. Figure 16.3 shows how overall psychomotor efficiency declined over the first 10 months of altitude exposure but then recovered somewhat over the ensuing 13 months as a result of acclimatization.

Overall psychomotor efficiency as shown in Figure 16.3 includes both the speed and accuracy scores from the test. Figure 16.4 shows a breakdown of the accuracy and speed of this test of psychomotor performance. Note that the accuracy of the measurement increased substantially after the 10-month period but there was little improvement in speed. This result is consistent with the impression given by many people who have worked at high altitude, namely that thought processes are slowed, but if one concentrates hard enough, accurate procedures can be carried out.

In a related study, Sharma and Malhotra (1976) compared the performance of three groups of Indians drawn from the Corkha, Madrasi and Rajput areas after 10 months' stay at altitude of 4000 m. There were no differences in the scores for eye–hand coordination and social interaction at altitudes for the three ethnic groups. However, the Corkhas showed a better toleration of altitude stress as evidenced by the effects on concentration, anxiety and depression.

In a study of 20 male soldiers exposed to a simulated altitude of 4700 m for 5–7 h, the relationships between symptoms and signs of acute mountain sickness, mood and psychometric performance were studied (Shukitt-Hale *et al.* 1991). It was found that evidence of acute mountain sickness was best correlated with symptoms, then mood changes, and least with performance.

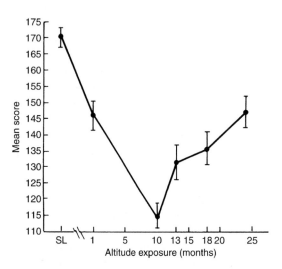

Figure 16.3 Psychomotor efficiency in young adults rapidly taken to an altitude of 4000 m where they remained for 2 years. Psychomotor efficiency was calculated using an eye–hand coordination test which included speed and accuracy. Note the deterioration in psychomotor efficiency over the first 10 months, which then gradually improved. (From Sharma *et al.* 1975.)

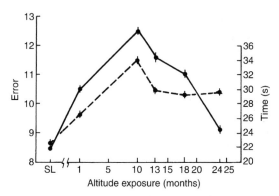

Figure 16.4 Same data as in Fig. 16.3 except that psychomotor efficiency is broken down into accuracy and speed of eye–hand coordination. Note that the accuracy of the measurement increased after 10 months but there was relatively little improvement in speed. (From Sharma *et al.* 1975.)

An unusual opportunity for studying the effects of very high altitude on mental performance was offered by the 1960–61 Silver Hut Expedition when several normal subjects spent up to 3 months at an altitude of 5800 m. Mental efficiency was tested by asking the subjects to sort playing cards into bins using specially designed equipment which recorded events on magnetic tape (Gill *et al.* 1964). It was found that the efficiency of sorting cards was less at the high altitude than at sea level. The inefficiency took the form of a delay in placing the cards into the correct bins rather than errors of sorting. Again these results reinforce the common notion that accurate work can be done at high altitude, but it takes longer, and more effort in concentration is required. Cahoon (1972) also showed a reduced efficiency of card sorting in eight normal subjects exposed to a simulated altitude of 4600 m for 48 h.

During the 1981 AMREE, a series of psychometric tests were carried out prior to the expedition, at the Base Camp (5400 m), at the Main Laboratory Camp (6300 m) and immediately after and 1 year after the expedition (Townes *et al.* 1984). The main emphasis was on a comparison of CNS function before and after exposure to extreme altitude, and only a few of the measurements made at high altitude were reported. However, finger-tapping speed decreased significantly over the course of the expedition. Mean taps of the right hand were 53.7 (pretest), 52.6 (5400 m altitude), 50.8 (6300 m altitude), 48.1 (on subjects returning to 6300 m altitude from 8000 m) and 45.4 (immediately after the expedition). It is not clear from these results whether the reduction in finger-tapping speed was a function of altitude, time at high altitude, or both.

16.4.3 Electroencephalogram

Ryn (1970, 1971) reported EEG abnormalities in 11 of 30 climbers who had been over 5500 m altitude. The predominant abnormality was a decreased frequency of alpha waves and a diminution of their amplitude. He also reported paroxysmal and focal pathology in EEG records performed at high altitude.

Zhongyuan and his colleagues (1983) also reported changes in the EEG at altitudes above 5000 m in members of a Chinese expedition to Mount Everest. There was a reduced amplitude of the alpha rhythm but in this instance there was an increase in its frequency. The EEG changes were less than those observed during acute hypoxia of the same degree in a low-pressure chamber prior to the expedition. Apparently members of the expedition who tolerated the acute hypoxia well tended to show fewer EEG changes on the mountain itself.

Nevison carried out an extensive series of EEG measurements during the Himalayan Scientific and Mountaineering Expedition of 1960–61. Although the results were not written up in the open literature, he apparently found no abnormalities in subjects living at 5800 m. Also the EEG appearances were not altered by hyperventilation or 100% oxygen breathing.

16.5 RESIDUAL CENTRAL NERVOUS SYSTEM IMPAIRMENT FOLLOWING RETURN FROM HIGH ALTITUDE

In view of the known vulnerability of the CNS to hypoxia, it is hardly surprising that neurobehavioral abnormalities can be demonstrated at high altitudes. However, there has been great interest in the possibility of residual impairment of CNS function following return to sea level.

An extensive study was carried out by Townes *et al.* (1984) referred to in section 16.4.2. The subjects were 21 members of the 1981 AMREE, and all were males between 25 and 52 years of age with a mean age of 36.4 years. The general level of education was high with 15 subjects having either an MD or PhD degree. Prior to the expedition, the following psychological tests were administered at the San Diego Veterans Administration Hospital: Halstead–Reitan battery (Reitan and Davison 1974), repeatable cognitive–perceptual–motor battery (Lewis and Rennick 1979), selective reminding test (Buschke 1973) and the Wechsler memory scale (Russell 1975). These same measurements were repeated immediately after the expedition in Kathmandu, Nepal. At an expedition meeting held in Colorado 1 year later, the following tests were re-administered: Halstead–Wepman aphasia screening test, B trials and the finger-tapping test from the Halstead–Reitan battery, the digit vigilance task from the repeatable battery, and a verbal passage from the Wechsler memory scale.

Table 16.1 shows the significant changes found between pre-expedition, post-expedition and

Table 16.1 Wilcoxon signed-rank tests comparing performance before, immediately after (in Kathmandu), and one year after expedition to Mt. Everest (From Townes *et al.*, 1984)

Performance	Results (means ± SE)			Paired responses		
	Before	After	Follow-up	Before and after	After and follow-up	Before and follow-up
Improved performance						
Tactual performance test (right hand)	4.68 ± 1.56	3.86 ± 1.46		2.72*		
Category test	24.29 ± 15.46	11.05 ± 8.39		3.48⁺		
Decline in performance						
Finger tapping test						
Right hand	53.71 ± 4.07	45.40 ± 6.18	48.40 ± 6.60	3.39⁺	1.32	2.20‡
Left hand	47.65 ± 4.60	42.45 ± 5.96	41.73 ± 5.23	2.30‡	0.66	2.93*
Criterion right	1.00 ± 0	0.14 ± 0.36	0.27 ± 0.46	3.06*	0.73	2.67*
Criterion left	1.00 ± 0	0.14 ± 0.36	0.13 ± 0.35	2.93‡	0.54	2.93*
Wechsler memory scale						
Short-term verbal recall	18.12 ± 1.90	15.90 ± 2.15	17.13 ± 2.20	2.60*	2.12‡	0.98
Trials to criterion	1.24 ± 0.44	2.40 ± 1.54	2.27 ± 0.70	2.37‡	0	2.67*
Long-term verbal recall	16.35 ± 2.91	12.70 ± 3.78	14.50 ± 2.85	2.32‡	2.75	0.94
Aphasia screening test	0.59 ± 0.79	1.25 ± 1.25	0.47 ± 0.52	2.22‡	2.31‡	0.47

* *p* 0.01; ⁺ *p* 0.001; ‡ *p* 0.05.

follow-up performance on the neuropsychological tests. It can be seen that verbal learning and memory declined significantly from the beginning to the end of the expedition as measured by the Wechsler memory scale. In the Halstead–Wepman aphasia screening test, the number of expressive language errors increased significantly between pre-test and post-test after the expedition. The number of aphasic errors was significantly related to the altitude attained by the subject.

As indicated in section 16.4.2 finger-tapping speed decreased significantly over the course of the expedition. This was measured by requiring the subject to tap a lever as rapidly as possible over a period of 10 s. For a test to be acceptable, five measurements on each hand gave a difference of less than five taps between trials. Before the expedition all subjects reached this criterion. However, at Kathmandu immediately after the expedition, 15 of 20 subjects could not sustain motor speed, and 13 of 16 subjects could not do so 1 year later.

These findings are of great interest because they provide strong objective evidence for CNS deterioration as a result of exposure to high altitude, a subject which has been debated vigorously in the past. However, other authors have reported similar or consistent findings. Ryn (1970, 1971) also found persistent abnormalities in a group of 20 male and 10 female Polish climbers several weeks after a Himalayan expedition. Half of the male climbers who ascended over 5500 m experienced symptoms similar to the acute organic brain syndrome, and for several weeks after the expedition they had changes in affect and impaired memory. Eleven of the 30 climbers had EEG abnormalities immediately after the climb. Psychological testing (Bender, Benton and Graham–Kendall tests) were reported to be normal in 13 persons, borderline in 12 persons, and indicative of organic pathology in five chambers.

Persistent cognitive impairment was described in five world-class climbers who had reached summits over 8500 m without supplementary oxygen (Regard et al. 1989). The abnormalities were in the ability to concentrate, short-term memory and cognitive flexibility (the ability to shift from one learned concept to another).

In a brief report, Cavaletti et al. (1987) showed residual impairment of memory in seven climbers who returned to sea level after ascending to 7075 m on Mount Satopanth without supplementary oxygen. The measurements were made before leaving Italy, at the base camp after the ascent, and 75 days after the expedition. It was shown that memory performance decreased both at base camp and, to a lesser degree, at sea level 75 days after the climb. However, tests of fluency and 'idiomotor ability' were unaffected by altitude. In a more recent study, persistent changes in memory, reaction time and concentration were reported 75 days after a single ascent over 5000 m (Cavaletti and Tredici 1993).

One study reports cortical atrophy and brain magnetic resonance imaging (MRI) changes in 26 climbers who ascended to over 7000 m without supplementary oxygen (Garrido et al. 1993). No magnetic resonance imaging (MRI) studies were performed prior to the climbs; the measurements were made 26 days to 36 months after return to sea level. The controls were 21 normal subjects, and 46% of the climbers showed MRI abnormalities.

Not everyone has found CNS abnormalities following return after ascent to very high altitude. For example, Clark et al. (1983) tested 22 mountaineers before and 16–221 days after Himalayan climbs above 5100 m with a battery of psychological and neurophysiological tests but found no evidence of cerebral dysfunction. This was a well-designed study and it is not clear why these climbers showed no abnormalities. In another study, Anooshiravani et al. (1999) carried out brain MRI studies and performed neuropsychological testing on eight male climbers before and after ascents to over 6000 m without oxygen. Although they found increases in symptoms of acute mountain sickness, there were no alterations in brain imaging or neuropsychological tests between 5 and 10 days after returning to sea level.

Measurements from the 1985 Operation Everest II confirmed the changes in psychometric function found on the 1981 AMREE, and extended the observations in an interesting and unexpected direction. During Operation Everest II, eight normal subjects spent 40 days in a low-pressure chamber and were gradually decompressed, ultimately being exposed to the simulated altitude of the Everest summit. Impairments in motor speed and persistence, memory, and verbal expressive abilities were found after the simulated ascent just as with the 1981 Everest expedition (Hornbein et al. 1989).

The new finding was a significant negative correlation between hypoxic ventilatory response and neurobehavioral function measured after the expedition. In other words, those climbers with the largest hypoxic ventilatory response showed the greatest decrement in neurobehavioral function. This was unexpected; indeed the prediction might have been that those who increased their ventilation most would protect their CNS function by preserving their alveolar and therefore arterial P_{O_2}.

A hypothesis to explain these unexpected findings was advanced by Hornbein et al. (1989). They argued that the subjects with the highest hypoxic ventilatory response would reduce their arterial P_{CO_2} the most and therefore develop the most cerebral vasoconstriction. This in turn would cause the most severe cerebral hypoxia even though their arterial P_{O_2} would actually be higher than that in the subjects with the smaller ventilatory responses to hypoxia.

Note that this hypothesis is not supported by the measurements of cerebral blood flow against arterial P_{CO_2} in anesthetized dogs shown in Fig. 16.2. Those data show that cerebral blood flow apparently levels off at values of P_{CO_2} below approximately 15 mmHg. However, the situation with acclimatization may be different because the arterial pH returns towards normal and this may improve cerebral blood flow. In addition the scatter in the data is such that this result may not be reliable. It should also be pointed out that the relationship between cerebral blood flow and arterial P_{CO_2} is very sensitive to the systematic arterial pressure (Harper and Glass 1965). Hypotensive dogs show a much smaller change in cerebral blood flow for a given change in P_{CO_2} than normotensive animals. Whether changes in systemic blood pressure occur at extreme altitudes is not known although there are no obvious alterations at 5800 m (Pugh 1964).

The correlation between hypoxic ventilatory response and residual impairment of central nervous system function leads to an interesting paradox. On the one hand, a brisk hypoxic ventilatory response is advantageous for a climber to reach extreme altitudes because otherwise the alveolar P_{O_2} cannot be maintained at the required levels. However, the only way of maintaining the P_{O_2} is by extreme hyperventilation, which reduces the arterial P_{CO_2}, which in turn reduces cerebral blood flow. Thus such a climber is likely to suffer more residual central nervous impairment. In other words, the climber who is endowed by nature to go

the highest is likely to suffer the most severe nervous system damage.

16.6 EFFECT OF OXYGEN ENRICHMENT OF ROOM AIR ON NEUROPSYCHOLOGICAL FUNCTION AT HIGH ALTITUDE

Increasing numbers of people are commuting to high altitude for commercial purposes such as mining, and scientific purposes such as astronomy (see Chapter 29). In order to reduce the neuropsychological impairment that occurs at high altitudes, oxygen enrichment of room air is now being tested. This is remarkably effective because every 1% increase in oxygen concentration (for example, from 21 to 22%) reduces the equivalent altitude by about 300 m. Gerard et al. (2000) evaluated the effectiveness of enriching room air oxygen by 6% at simulated 5000 m altitude. A randomized double-blind study was carried out on 24 subjects who underwent neuropsychological testing in a specially designed facility at 3800 m that could simulate both an ambient 5000 m atmosphere and an atmosphere of 6% oxygen enrichment at 5000 m. The 2-h test battery of 16 tasks assessed various aspects of motor and cognitive performance. Compared with simulated breathing air at 5000 m, oxygen enrichment resulted in higher arterial oxygen saturations, quicker reaction times, improved hand–eye coordination, and a more positive sense of well being, each significant at the $p < 0.05$ level.

It is interesting that other aspects of neuropsychological function were not significantly improved by 6% additional oxygen. One reason may be that short-term concentration may temporarily overcome real underlying deficits. The problem was succinctly stated by Barcroft et al. (1923) reporting on the 1921–22 International High Altitude Expedition to Cerro de Pasco, Peru. He wrote:

Judged by the ordinary standards of efficiency in laboratory work, we were in an obviously lower category at Cerro than at the sea-level. By a curious paradox this was most apparent when it was being least tested, for perhaps what we suffered from chiefly was the difficulty of maintaining concentration. When we knew we were undergoing a test, our concentration could by an effort be maintained over the length of time taken for the test, but under ordinary circumstances it would lapse. It is, perhaps, characteristic that, whilst each individual mental test was done as rapidly at Cerro as at the sea-level, the performance of the series took nearly twice as long for its accomplishment. Time was wasted there in trivialities and 'bungling,' which would not take place at sea-level. (Barcroft *et al.* 1923)

A more recent study after 30 days at 3700 m showed that sleep quality, especially deep sleep stages, total sleep time, and efficient sleep index were all improved with oxygen enrichment. Sleep latency and arousals were not significantly better, but the over-all effect of enrichment was felt to be beneficial.

In view of the above, it would be very interesting to develop neuropsychological tests which were embedded in the normal daily activities of the subject. In other words, it would be valuable to be able to measure the mental efficiency of the subjects when they were unaware of being tested. A formal study along these lines has not yet been carried out at high altitude.

The addition of extra oxygen to any environment also may carry some hazards, such as increased fire risk. John West who has pioneered much of this work discussed what is felt to be a 'safe' amount of oxygen enrichment without incurring undue fire hazard (West 2001). The intervention of supplemental oxygen may be beneficial not only in professional settings where mental acuity is essential but also in areas of recreation where altitude illness can be a limiting factor to enjoyment of the sojourn (West 2002).

High altitude populations

SUMMARY

Many people live permanently at high altitudes which have a significant effect on their physiology (see Chapter 3 for numbers and world distribution). Studies of such populations are hampered by the problem of appropriate comparison groups. Often a group of high altitude residents is compared with a group of lowlanders from a different ethnic, socio-economic and genetic background so that it is difficult to know to what factors any differences may be attributed. Also it is becoming clear that not all high altitude residents are the same. Recent studies have found interesting differences between South American and central Asian high altitude residents.

Altitude residence does not seem to have important demographic effects; economic factors are of greater importance. Fertility, which is reduced in newcomers to altitude, seems to be normal in peoples resident for generations, especially on the Tibetan plateau. Fetal growth in the last stages of pregnancy is retarded, and birth weight falls with increasing altitude of residence. Growth in childhood has been claimed to be retarded but continues for longer, though again this could be due, in part at least, to economic or nutritional factors rather than altitude per se.

The physiology of high altitude residents differs from that of lowlanders at altitude in some respects. The former have lower total ventilation at rest and exercise and blunted hypoxic ventilatory response (though in Tibetans this is less so than in South American highlanders). Despite lower ventilation their oxygen saturation and P_{O_2} are similar to those of lowlanders at altitude. They have higher lung diffusing capacities than lowlanders, an important advantage at altitude where work rate is limited by diffusion. They have slightly larger lungs. Animals adapted to high altitude have very little pulmonary artery pressor response to hypoxia. Tibetans show a degree of this adaptation, but not South American high altitude residents. There are also differences in hemoglobin concentration and oxygen saturation between these populations, all suggesting that the Tibetans, with their longer lineage at altitude, have undergone a greater degree of altitude adaptation.

Certain diseases are found commonly among altitude residents. Again some are the result of socio-economic factors and are common in poor populations at sea level. Cold and cold injury are more common at altitude but, of course, not confined to it. The commonest disease due to altitude hypoxia is chronic mountain sickness and high altitude pulmonary edema. This is covered in Chapter 21. Others include chemodectoma, a benign tumor of the carotid body, and a high incidence of patent ductus arteriosus in infants. Goiter, though not strictly confined to high altitude, is much more prevalent there since iodine-deficient soils are more common at high elevations and possibly the demands for iodine are greater at altitude. Finally, sickle cell disease, though not caused by altitude, is more serious there.

17.1 INTRODUCTION

This chapter considers the characteristics of people born and raised at high altitude and whose ancestors have resided at high altitude for many generations. In Chapter 3 the locations of these populations have been discussed. In general the altitude considered is above 3000 m. The duration of residence of the population is impossible to determine; it ranges from perhaps 50 000 to 100 000 years in Tibet and perhaps 15 000 years in the Andes to a few generations in the high mining towns of Colorado, USA.

Our knowledge of the effect of lifelong residence at altitude has come from studies of particular peoples. A major problem in interpreting results is to decide whether the characteristics found to differ from lowland populations are really due to the high altitude environment (hypoxia or cold) or due to racial, nutritional or economic factors.

Some studies have sought to eliminate racial factors by using low altitude residents of the same ethnic background as controls. It is difficult to control for nutritional factors since high altitude residents may well be economically disadvantaged when compared with their low altitude controls. This seems to be the case in the Andes. The effects of poor nutrition and chronic hypoxia are similar on factors such as growth and development, thus confounding the interpretation of results. The economic advantage may be reversed, as in Ethiopia, where the highland regions are free from malaria and the residents more wealthy and better fed. The result is that studies from this part of the world do not show the differences between high and low altitude residents that are reported from the Andes. There are fewer studies from the Himalayas and Tibet than from the Andes, though this has been redressed in recent years with a number of studies from Lhasa.

However, if these reservations are kept in mind, some conclusions can be drawn from the many surveys about the effects of lifelong residence at high altitude, especially on birth weight and childhood development. Recent studies have addressed the question of differences between South American and Tibetan high altitude residents and the related one of whether there has been natural selection for giving a biological advantage to either of these populations. Moore reviewed some of these areas of interest (Moore 2001).

17.2 DEMOGRAPHIC ASPECTS

17.2.1 Population age and sex distribution

A few high altitude groups have been analyzed in some detail and the population of the Nunoa district (4000 m) of Peru showed some differences compared with the total Peruvian population (Baker and Dutt 1972). The high altitude population was somewhat younger, and the ratio of females to males was larger during infancy and childhood, but in addition there appeared to be more elderly people among the high altitude than the general population.

The explanation seems to be that, in the high altitude population, there was a high birth rate and high adult emigration rate. Male mortality was higher than female in infancy, childhood and early adolescence. The larger number of older individuals may have been due to the prestige associated with telling observers that they were of a great age. Claims to longevity are hard to substantiate because birth certificates and baptismal registers are seldom kept, and some individuals lie outrageously about their age. Areas noted for longevity, the Villcambamba region of Ecuador, the state of Georgia in Russia, and the Hunzas of Northern Pakistan all claimed inordinant longevity, but many of these claims are insubstantiated. For instance, in north Bhutan the oldest individuals were over 80 but not above 90 years old as claimed (Jackson et al. 1966, p. 99), and some Tibetan lamas claim to have lived to a great age. There seems to be little concrete evidence for unusual longevity at high altitude.

In the Khumbu region of north-eastern Nepal, male infant mortality was higher than female. There was little permanent emigration but a higher percentage of males was involved in accidents. In north-west Nepal the number of males born relative to females was higher but mortality in male infants was increased (Baker 1978).

17.2.2 Fertility

Adaptation to the environment must include the ability of the species to reproduce. The Spanish who occupied the high altitude regions of South America in the sixteenth and seventeenth centuries found that neither their animals nor their womenfolk had live offspring. This was in contrast to the indigenous animals and peoples. Clegg (1978) quotes two well-observed Spanish accounts of La Calancha (1639) and Cobo (1653). The former recounts the early history of the city of Potosí (4060 m) in present day Bolivia with a population of 20 000 Spaniards and 100 000 Indians. Children born to Spanish couples died either at birth or within 2 weeks. Pregnant Spanish women developed the habit of returning to low altitude for their pregnancy and delivery and keeping their babies there until a year old. Han Chinese women living in Tibet follow a similar pattern. The cause of failure to thrive in these infants may well have been high altitude pulmonary hypertension (Chapter 21). The Amerindians, of course, had no such problems nor do the indigenous Tibetans. It was not until 53 years after its foundation that the first Spanish child was born and reared in the city. Cobo says that Jauja (3500 m), the early capital of Peru, was considered 'a sterile place' where horses, pigs or fowl could not be raised, whereas 100 years later it was a principal area producing pigs and poultry and supplying Lima with these products. Cobo also pointed out that infant survival depended upon the proportion of Indian blood in the child, with pure-blooded Spanish children mostly dying, children of mixed blood faring rather better, and pure-blooded Indian children having the lowest mortality, despite much poorer living conditions.

What is the cause of this lack of fertility in lowlanders at altitude? Sperm counts in lowland men fall temporarily on going to altitude but then recover. Testosterone levels also fall and then recover after a week or two (section 15.10.3). In the female, on going to altitude, there may be temporary disturbances in menstruation (Sobrevilla *et al.* 1967). Conception rates are virtually impossible to measure, especially since chronic hypoxia may increase the frequency of early abortions. The reduced fertility may be due to a number of factors, possibly reduced conception, probably increased numbers of early abortions, stillbirths and neonatal deaths.

In altitude residents fertility was thought to be reduced. Hoff and Abelson (1976), using aggregate data from Peru, found that fertility, measured as the number of children under the age of 5 divided by the number of women aged 15–49 years, fell linearly with altitude ($p < 0.01$) but they were cautious when interpreting the data on which this was based. They also found that high altitude women who migrate to low altitude increase their fertility. However, both Carrillo (1996) and Gonzales *et al.* (1996) found global fecundity rates higher than at sea level.

Determining the factors which affect fertility in populations with many socio-economic variables has been extremely difficult. Vitzthum *et al.* (2000) studied progesterone levels in Andean woman to determine menstrual and thus ovarian function and concluded that hypoxia per se did not alter ovarian function compared to low altitude patterns. This goup (2000) also found that bias in the data may arise from the low rate of conception in nonlactating women. Kapoor *et al.* (2003) studied Himalayan populations and found that since the high altitude populations are in such socio-economic flux, there were few variables which were solely responsible for an apparent decrease in fertility in these groups. Coital frequency, late age of menarche, prolonged lactation and thus slower restoration of post-partum fecundity, rural versus urban habitation are all factors which play a role in fertility, and most investigators do not find specific variables which result from hypoxia, per se, which impair conception (Vitzhum 2001, Crognier *et al.* 2002, Vitzhum and Wiley 2003).

17.3 FETAL AND CHILDHOOD DEVELOPMENT

17.3.1 Pregnancy

ABORTION

Abortion rates are notoriously difficult to measure, but Clegg (1978) quotes a number of Andean studies giving incredibly low rates ranging from 0 to 1% (compared with worldwide rates of about 15%). He suggested this might be due to a high rate of very early abortions (before 2 weeks) which would be unrecognized and would help to account for the low fertility. In Ethiopian women, Harrison *et al.* (1969) reported a rather higher rate (9.1%) at 3000 m compared with less than 1% in an ethnically similar population at low altitude; however, both rates are low compared with rates in many populations. Beall *et al.* (2004) studied Tibetan women with hemoglobin with high and low affinity for oxygen and found a lower offspring mortality in women with alleles for high affinity characteristics and suggested that hemoglobin affinity may be an agent for natural selection in this population. Non-B haplogroups, as compared to B groups, had a higher adverse outcomes (fetal demise and neonatal deaths), but the molecular basis for these events is not known (Myres *et al.* 2000).

PLACENTAL GROWTH

Placentas are not significantly heavier at high altitude but since birth weights are low the placental/birth weight ratio is significantly increased (McClung 1969, Mayhew 1986), clearly an adaptation which would benefit fetal oxygenation. Villous vascularization is increased in the placentas from high altitude women; this increases the surface area for diffusion (Clegg 1978), although Mayhew (1986) found a smaller surface area of villi but a thinner diffusion barrier, thus resulting in an increase in the membrane diffusing capacity (Zamudio 2003). Placental infarcts are more common in altitude placentas and more frequent in women with a European admixture of genes (McClung 1969).

There is a decrease in nutrient transporters in placenta under hypoxia (Zamudio 2006). In this study while there was an increase in EPO and other growth factors and thus vascularization, a decrease in glucose and other nutrient transporters could account for intra-uterine growth retardation (IUGR).

FETAL GROWTH

The evidence suggests that, after the hazards of the first few weeks of pregnancy, growth is probably normal until the last trimester, when it slows to produce a lighter baby at term. The cause of this growth retardation is not clear, since the evidence reviewed by Clegg (1978) suggests that the fetus at this altitude is not hypoxic compared with lowland fetuses. Possibly this is a genetic adaptive change with elimination, over generations, of genes which

produce a larger baby. This would be advantageous since smaller babies are less likely to outgrow the placental capacity for oxygen transfer.

There does appear to be different adaptation strategies in high altitude populations in the Andes versus the Himalaya. Moore *et al.* (2001) studied Tibetan and Han Chinese woman at 3658 m and found that Tibetan women had a higher percentage of common iliac blood flow contributed to the uterine artery. They felt that the higher birth weight of the Tibetan babies may be attributable to a compensation for a lower hemoglobin level by a higher oxygen delivery from a greater blood flow. On the other hand, in the Andes, Tissot van Patot *et al.* (2003) found a marked increase in vascular remodeling in placentas of women at 3100 versus 1600 m; but since these infants are of lower birth weight than low altitude ones, the investigators felt that this degree of angiogenesis was not adequate to restore the normal degree of oxygen delivery.

Another factor in the regulation of blood flow and thus oxygen delivery is the vasomotor regulators of flow. Moore *et al.* (2004) compared the HIF-1 targeted vasoconstrictor, endothelin-1 (ET-1) in European and Andean women. Andean women were found to have a lower level of ET-1 suggesting less vasoconstriction and thus increased blood flow in the high altitude-adapted women. The mechanism of this phenomenon is thought to be related to a single nucleotide polymorphism in the ET-1 gene and may be a model for identifying women at any altitude prone to vascular problems such as pre-eclampsia.

17.3.2 Birth weight and infant mortality

Results from a number of studies in the Andes and Tibet showed lower birth weight at altitude (Haas 1976, Li 1985). The mean weight declined from about 3.5 kg in Lima to 2.8 kg at Cerro de Pasco (4300 m) and, although there is the possibility that the nutritional status of mothers may be a factor, it is unlikely to account for more than a proportion of this difference. Andean infants at 4340 m also had a marked delay in equilibration of Sa,O_2 and lower Apgar scores compared to babies in Lima at 150 m (Gonzales and Salirrosas 2005). In Bolivia, where infant mortality and stillbirth rates are high, there is also a high prevalence of IUGR, pre-eclampsia and miscarriage (Keyes *et al.* 2003).

A similar effect of altitude has been reported from the USA (Lichty *et al.* 1957, Grahn and Kratchman 1963, Unger *et al.* 1988). Women native to high altitude who descend to low altitude have heavier babies at low altitude (Hoff and Abelson 1976). These studies include women from both indigenous high altitude populations and low altitude stock, and indicate that it is the high altitude environment rather than genetics which result in low birth weights. A study from Colorado also concludes that altitude is an independent factor in causing low birth weights. The authors obtained data from 3836 birth certificates and found that none of the characteristics associated with low birth weight – gestational age, maternal weight gain, parity, smoking, hypertension, etc. – interacted with the effect of altitude; the decline in birth weight averaged 102 g per 1000 m (Jensen and Moore 1997). However, genetic factors may play a role.

In a study in Lhasa (3658 m) Niermeyer *et al.* (1995) reported that Han Chinese infants had lower birth weights than Tibetan babies born at the same altitude. They also had lower $Sa_{,}O_2$ and higher hemoglobin levels. Possibly the genetic factors work through giving better oxygenation to Tibetan mothers (see section 17.5.2). Not all investigators have found that Tibetan fetuses are spared from IUGR (Tripathy and Gupta 2005), and others have documented significant malnutrition (Dang *et al.* 2004). Of interest is the finding that maternal anemia is inversely proportional to birth weight at altitudes from 2220 to 4850 m (Nahum and Stanislaw 2004). The authors attributed this finding to the decreased oxygen delivery with increasing viscosity known to occur at high altitude, but it is not clear that the degree of polycythemia was high enough to decrease blood flow.

Infant mortality depends heavily on living standards and medical facilities and the very high infant mortality rates reported probably reflect these factors more than the effect of altitude per se. In Ethiopia, Harrison *et al.* (1969) reported a rate of 200 per 1000 live births at high altitude and 176 per 1000 at low altitude, whereas in the Andes a rate of 180 per 1000 was found in the rural area of Nunoa (4000 m) but only 73 per 1000 in urban La Paz (Baker 1978). In Himalayan Sherpas, Lang and Lang (1971) gave a figure of 51 per 1000 at 4300 m, and in North Bhutan the rate was 189 per 1000 (Jackson *et al.* 1966, p. 99). In experimental animals under controlled conditions, hypoxia increases neonatal mortality, so probably the high rates found in mountain peoples are at least partly due to the altitude. Apart from the direct effect of hypoxia an important indirect effect may be through the reduced amount of liver glycogen present at birth, an important energy store until suckling becomes established (Clegg 1978).

17.3.3 Growth through childhood

The high altitude baby starts life smaller than the average low altitude baby does, and its early growth is slower. Milestones such as sitting and walking are slightly later, but the differences between high and low altitude residents of the same race are less than those between different races or between urban and rural populations (Clegg 1978).

In Quechua Indians in Peru, throughout childhood the high altitude child lags behind his low altitude counterpart in height by about 2 years. The adolescent growth spurt is less pronounced in high altitude youths but their growth continues for about 2 years longer and their adult stature is not reached until 22 years of age (Frisancho 1978). In Ethiopia, there were no such differences. Indeed, high altitude males were taller and heavier for their age than lowlanders. In the Himalayas, a comparison of high altitude Sherpas (3075–5050 m) with Tibetans resident at 1400 m was made by Pawson (quoted by Frisancho 1978) who found no difference in the height of children in these populations, though other indices of maturation (skeletal and dental development and menarche) show the Sherpa children to lag behind the low altitude Tibetans. Recently, a study from Ecuador found very little difference in rates of body weight increase in children at high altitude compared with children from low altitude. There were some minor differences in rates of height increase but the authors conclude that hypoxia plays a relatively small role in shaping growth in the first 5 years after birth (Leonard *et al.* 1995).

On the other hand, investigations amongst the children of Kirghiz tribes of the Tien Shan mountains showed delayed growth in the high altitude children, equivalent to a lag of about 1 year. The altitude of residence was 2300–2800 m, but in the summer months they go up to 3500 m to graze their cattle (Frisancho 1978).

Menarche is a milestone well documented in studies from various high altitude regions; and, in girls living in the Andes, Himalayas and Tien Shan, it is 1–2 years later than in low altitude girls (Frisancho 1978, Jackson et al. 1966, pp. 40–4). The Ethiopian highlanders again are the exception as no difference was found (Harrison et al. 1969). Adrenarche, the increase in serum androgens, also occurs 1–2 years later in children at altitude compared with sea level in Peru (Goñez et al. 1993).

17.4 PHYSIOLOGY

17.4.1 Stature, lung development and function

Compared with Europeans and North Americans, most high altitude residents have a smaller stature and are lighter in weight, but when compared with people of similar race and living standards most of this difference disappears. The delayed growth (see above) is almost counteracted by the prolongation of active growth to beyond 20 years. The Han Chinese who have more recently migrated to high altitude regions do show some retardation of growth and stature but respiratory adaptations which are similar to high altitude populations (Weitz and Garruto 2004). It is important to note, however, that Tibetans who were second-generation lowlanders adapted more quickly to high altitude than lowland Caucasians (Marconi et al. 2004) which suggests an inherent characteristic to adaptation.

One of the most quoted aspects of lifelong adaptation to high altitude is the deep-chested development of the thorax in high altitude residents (Barcroft 1925). This has been documented by measurement of chest circumference and vital capacity in South American Indians living above 4500 m but is quite a small difference even in this population. Vital capacity was about 300 mL higher than predicted when corrected for body size (Velasquez 1976). However, at 3500 m these measurements were smaller and less than the values published in the USA. High altitude residents in the Himalayas do not have larger circumference chests or bigger vital capacities than lowlanders (Frisancho 1978) nor do younger white residents of Leadville (3100 m),

but those over 50 years of age did have significantly larger vital capacities, by 440 mL, than predicted (DeGraff et al. 1970). Sun et al. (1990) compared Tibetans and Han Chinese residents of Lhasa. Their mean ages, heights and weights were similar, but, whereas the Tibetans were lifelong residents, the Han have been resident for a mean time of 8 years. The Tibetans had vital capacities significantly greater than the Han did: 5080 mL compared with 4280 mL. High peak flows (>139%) were measured in both Tibetans and Ladakhis at 3300 m (Wood et al. 2003).

In Andean residents at 4540 m, the total lung capacity is about 500 mL greater than at sea level, most of the increase being due to increased residual volume (Velasquez 1976). Infants born at high altitude have greater thoracic compliance than infants of the same ethnic background born at low altitude (Mortola et al. 1990). In adults the thoracic blood volume is increased and the residual volume/total lung capacity ratio increases from 21 to 28% in high altitude compared with low altitude residents. There may be some benefit from this since it would have the effect of reducing the breath-by-breath oscillations of P_{CO_2} and, hence, pH. At altitude these oscillations would otherwise be increased due to the reduction in plasma bicarbonate as part of the acclimatization process (Chapter 5). However, these changes in lung volumes, even when found, are quite small and probably have little effect on performance. Vital capacity decreases with age at sea level but this reduction is much greater at altitude, at least in Andean residents (Monge et al. 1990), which may account in part for the increasing incidence of chronic mountain sickness with age (Chapter 21).

The increased lung capacity may allow for an increased area for gas diffusion which, together with the increased blood volume, results in increased lung diffusing capacity. Details of studies in Andean and Caucasian residents are given in section 6.4.2. This increase in gas transfer should give the altitude resident a distinct performance advantage over the newcomer to altitude. Work from Tibet by Chen et al. (1997) indicates that Tibetan highlanders also have higher lung diffusing capacities when compared with Han Chinese. The increase in pulmonary gas exchange can be induced after as little as 2 years in dogs brought up during maturation at 3800 m (McDonough et al. 2006). These findings suggest plasticity in this response if individuals are exposed to an hypoxic environment during important growth phases. Samaja *et al.* (1997), who studied Sherpas and Caucasian lowlanders at 3400 and 6450 m, found that the Sherpas were less alkalotic at the higher altitude due to a higher P_{CO_2}, although the P_{O_2} and S_{a,O_2} were the same as those of Caucasians. This indicates that their oxygen transport was more efficient.

17.4.2 Ventilatory control at rest and exercise

Newcomers to high altitude find, often to their surprise, that they have to hyperventilate on the slightest exertion. They may notice that high altitude residents seem to be relatively unaffected in this way. Reviews (Lahiri 2000, Moore 2000, Donnelly and Carroll 2005, Wilson 2005, Leon-Velarde and Richalet 2006) provide rich sources for the biochemical, genetic, cellular, and physiologic responses that are known to exist in high altitude populations.

Measurements of resting and exercise ventilation in high altitude residents confirmed that high altitude natives in the Andes do, in fact, hypoventilate compared to sojourners. Chiodi (1957) showed that resting ventilation was higher in newcomers to altitude than in residents. At 3990 m the values were 5.3 and 4.5 L min^{-1} m^{-2}, and at 4515 m, 5.6 and 4.9 L min^{-1} m^{-2} for newcomers and residents respectively. The P_{a,CO_2} values were in accordance with these differences. Santolaya *et al.* (1989) studied workers at the Aucanquilcha mine (5950 m) in Chile. Their mean P_{a,CO_2} was 27.5 mmHg whereas lowlanders at that altitude had a value about 5 mmHg lower, indicating ventilation 22% higher. They also showed no respiratory alkalosis (pH 7.4), which lowlanders would have at that altitude.

On exercise, Buskirk (1978) found a similar distinction in Andean high altitude residents as did Lahiri *et al.* (1967) in Sherpa subjects compared with lowlanders at altitude. It is likely that this lower ventilation in high altitude residents is due to their low hypoxic ventilatory response (HVR), especially the ventilatory response to prolonged hypoxia as opposed to acute hypoxia (Gamboa *et al.* 2003; and Chapter 5). HVR correlates with exercise hyperventilation (Schoene *et al.* 1984) and thus would be associated with both the objective and subjective response to exercise ventilation at high altitude. As discussed in

Chapter 5 this blunting of the HVR appears to take place over decades at altitude. Children resident at high altitude have normal HVR, and this blunting is seen in white subjects resident in Leadville (3100 m) in Colorado, so it does not seem to be genetically determined (Weil *et al.* 1971, Lahiri *et al.* 1976). There does, however, appear to be some differences in the ventilatory response to hypoxia between genders with women breathing more than men (Joseph *et al.* 2000).

Work by Zhuang *et al.* (1993) showed some interesting differences between lowland born Han Chinese and highland born Tibetans studied in Lhasa (3658 m). The Han had migrated to altitude in childhood, adolescence or adulthood. They showed the decline in HVR with length of residence at altitude as seen in Colorado altitude residents, but the Tibetans, who had a higher HVR than the Han, showed very little decline with age. However, Tibetans showed a paradoxical increase in ventilation on breathing 70% oxygen, a response not seen in Han subjects. Tibetan lifelong residents at 4400 m when studied at 3658 m and compared with Tibetans living there had blunted HVRs though their resting ventilation was similar (Curran *et al.* 1995). Recently the same team has looked at a group of men of mixed Han–Tibetan parentage. They found that HVR was decreased with time of residence at altitude, but that resting ventilation did not decrease, as is the case with Han subjects. They exhibited the same paradoxical response to oxygen breathing as did Tibetan subjects (Curran *et al.* 1997).

Beall and colleagues have compared Tibetan and South American Aymara highlanders. They found resting ventilation was roughly 1.5 times higher in the Tibetans and HVR about double that of the Aymara. They also found that the contribution of genetic differences to the variance in ventilation was 35% in the Tibetan population and nil in the Aymara. The figures for HVR were 31 and 21% respectively (Beall *et al.* 1997a; see also section 17.5.2).

17.4.3 Hemoglobin concentration

The increase in hemoglobin concentration at altitude is one of the best-known adaptations to altitude hypoxia. It is found in both acclimatized lowlanders and lifelong residents at altitude. This is discussed in detail in Chapter 8.

In the Andes, some workers have found very high hemoglobin concentration in residents (Talbott and Dill 1936, Dill *et al.* 1937, Merino 1950) and suggested that this is part of their long-term adaptation to altitude. However, subjects may have been included in these study populations who would now be considered to have chronic mountain sickness or Monge's disease (Chapter 21). Other studies have not found such high levels or a significant difference between residents and acclimatized lowlanders (Peñaloza *et al.* 1971). Frisancho (1988) reviewed the published data and showed that hemoglobin concentration values from mining areas in the Andes were higher than from nonmining areas, and that if studies from nonmining areas were compared with those from the Himalayas there was no significant difference. However, Beall *et al.* (1998) found Aymara Andean high altitude natives to have hemoglobin concentration significantly higher, by 3–4 g dL^{-1}, than Tibetans at a similar altitude. Normal values were established by Vasquez and Villena (2001) in natives to 4000 m in Potosi, Peru, and found to be 52.7 and 48.3% hematocrit and 17.3 and 15.8 g dL^{-1} hemoglobin for men and women respectively. Villafuerte *et al.* (2004) modeled optimal values in the Andean (hemoglobin 14.7 g dL−1) population and concluded that other factors have influenced the mean values which are higher and thus may not be optimal for oxygen delivery. Leon-Velarde *et al.* (2000) showed a gradual increase in erythrocytosis in both men and women which was felt to be excessive and thus not beneficially adaptive.

Much of the polycythemia persists in populations, both children and adults, who have low iron stores. This phenomenon has been studied in Bolivia (Cook *et al.* 2005), and nutritional intervention with weekly iron supplementation has been found to be beneficial (Berger *et al.* 1997), but intervention on a public health scale has not been universally undertaken.

In the Himalayas and on the Tibetan plateau, residents tend to have rather lower hemoglobin concentration than acclimatized lowlanders (Wu *et al.* 2005). As discussed in Chapter 8, it is thought that, although a modest rise in hemoglobin concentration (to perhaps 18.0 g dL^{-1}) is advantageous, values much above this level are probably detrimental. So the Tibetans' lower hemoglobin concentration values are considered to be evidence of better altitude adaptation.

17.4.4 The carotid body and chemodectoma

Chronic hypoxia causes an increase in the size and weight of the carotid body. This was first reported in high altitude Andean natives by Arias-Stella (1969). He found the weight of the two carotid bodies in residents of Lima to be just over 20 mg, whereas in altitude residents they totaled over 60 mg. Heath and co-workers found a similar increased weight of carotid bodies in patients with chronic hypoxic lung disease. They found a good correlation between carotid body and right ventricular weight, suggesting that a common correlation with hypoxia was the cause of the hyperplasia (Heath 1986).

The principal cell involved in this hyperplasia is the sustentacular (type II) cell with compression and obliteration of clusters of chief (type I) cells. This type of hyperplasia is similar to that seen in systemic hypertension (Heath 1986).

Chemodectoma, a tumor of the carotid body, is rare at sea level, but appears to be relatively common at high altitude. In 1973 Saldana *et al.* reported its occurrence in a higher proportion of Peruvian adults born and living at 4350 m than in those living at 3000 m. All were benign and the incidence was higher in women. An association between chemodectoma and thyroid carcinoma has been noted in two patients at 2380 m (Saldana *et al.* 1973). No cases of chemodectoma have yet been reported from the Tibetan plateau or the high Himalayan valleys.

17.4.5 Cardiovascular adaptations

Andean high altitude residents share with newcomers the raised pulmonary artery and right ventricular pressure due to the hypoxic pulmonary pressor response (Chapter 7), resulting in right ventricular hypertrophy (Recavarren and Arias-Stella 1964). Indeed, in Andean children at high altitude, the usual involution of the muscular coat of the pulmonary artery after birth does not take place, or does so only partially, so that the pulmonary arteries, both large and small, show far greater muscularization than is normal in sea level residents (Saldana and Arias-Stella 1963a,b,c, Huicho and Niermeyer 2006).

This finding of right ventricular hypertrophy, continued muscularization of the pulmonary arteries and raised pulmonary artery pressure in residents at high altitude should be regarded as a response to high altitude rather than an adaptation, since there is no evidence that it has any physiological benefit. Indeed, it merely throws more strain on the right heart.

The purpose of the hypoxic pressor response in humans at sea level, apart from its vital role in prenatal life, is presumably to redistribute blood away from areas of the lung that are hypoxic because of, for instance, atelectasis, and thus improve matching of ventilation and blood flow in various clinical situations. It would probably be beneficial to lose this response at altitude, and the altitude-adapted yak would seem to have done this (section 17.5).

Studies in Tibetan highlanders suggest that they have achieved a similar adaptation to the yak and do not have raised pulmonary artery pressures at altitude and little rise on exercise (Groves *et al.* 1993) though the numbers studied were small. Neither do they develop the structural changes in their pulmonary arterial tree that are found in Andean highlanders (Gupta *et al.* 1992). The incidence of right ventricular hypertrophic signs in the electrocardiograph (ECG) was found to be only 17% in Tibetans and 29% in Han Chinese at the same altitude (Halperin *et al.* 1998). Lifelong residents also have an increase in the number of branches to the main trunks of their coronary arteries (Arias-Stella and Topilsky 1971) and presumed adaptation by angiogenesis to optimize perfusion to tissues that are chronically more hypoxic (see Chapters 16 and 24).

Another adaptation of high altitude residents is that, on exercise at altitude, their maximum heart rate does not seem to be limited, as is the case for acclimatized lowlanders, and they maintained the presumably healthy heart rate variability both at low altitude and upon re-ascent to high altitude, also found in rats acclimatized to high altitude (Melin *et al.* 2003). This is discussed more fully in Chapter 7 and in relation to the adrenergic system in Chapter 15. A study by Passino *et al.* (1996) looked at the spectral analysis of ECGs of high altitude residents compared with lowlanders at altitude. The high altitude residents did not show the reduced vagal tone seen in lowlanders, which may indicate the mechanism which allows this higher maximum heart rate in highlanders. These high altitude natives maintained higher heart rate responses while running a marathon at 4220 m (Cornolo *et al.* 2005) as

well as after they had descended to low altitude (Gamboa *et al.* 2001), suggesting a maintained sympathetic tone after the hypoxic stress had been removed. Some genetic advantage must be conveyed to high altitude natives of uninterrupted lineage, as those high altitude inhabitants with Spanish admixture demonstrated a greater decrease in $V_{O_2,max}$ when exercised at 4228 m than did pure natives to these altitudes (Brutsaert *et al.* 2003).

One further curious finding is that Tibetans demonstrate improved work economy (Marconi *et al.* 2005). In other words, they have been shown to carry out workloads at a lower energy expenditure than low altitude controls (Ge 1994, Curran *et al.* 1998, Marconi *et al.* 2005, 2006). The reasons for such improvement is not fully understood but provide a fertile area for further investigation as understanding such adaptation may provide insight into more optimal functioning of patients with a variety of diseases with impairment of oxygen delivery.

17.4.6 Adaptation to cold

Cold is a feature of life at high altitude (section 3.8.1). Further aspects of cold adaptation are considered in Chapter 24.

17.5 ADAPTATION TO HYPOXIA OVER GENERATIONS

Most of the adaptations to hypoxia that have been shown in humans appear to develop during a lifetime of exposure. Even the blunting of the hypoxic ventilatory response has been shown to develop in people of lowland origin over a period of decades (Weil *et al.* 1971). The lower hemoglobin concentration in Sherpa and Tibetan subjects has been suggested as an example of adaptation over many generations in Tibetan stock, as is the blunted hypoxic pressor response (below).

17.5.1 The hypoxic pulmonary pressor response

Hypoxic pulmonary vasoconstriction to varying degrees is a response universal to most mammals which has sparked the curiosity of many physiologists (Moudgil 2005, Reeves and Grover 2005, Rhodes 2005). A better understanding of the cellular, biochemical and genetic aspects of this response has been unraveled over the last decade.

In animals, Harris (1986) has shown elegantly that in cattle the pulmonary pressor response, or lack of it, is genetically determined. The yak has little or no response, whereas the cow has a brisk response. The crossbred dzo has the blunted response of its yak parent, but the second cross of dzo and bull produces 50% brisk and 50% low response offspring. That is, the gene responsible for a low response is dominant and the characteristic is inherited in a Mendelian way. This vasomotor reactivity is mediated, in part, by the production of nitric oxide in Tibetan highlanders (Hoit et al. 2005), Tibetan sheep (Koizumi 2004), as well as in other animals, including the yak (Ishizaki 2005). Presumably, a low response is an advantage at altitude such that lower pulmonary vascular resistance results in better cardiac output and exercise capacity. A brisk response is a risk factor for brisket disease (named after the brisket, the loose skin at the animal's throat). Thus, we have a true adaptation achieved presumably by environmental pressure selecting for the low response gene. Similar adaptation has been found in the llama.

There is evidence that in populations of Tibetan origin a similar adaptation may have taken place. Jackson (1968) found little ECG evidence of pulmonary hypertension in Bhutanese and Sherpa subjects at altitude, in that their mean frontal QRS axis differed by only 10 from healthy Edinburgh adults, in contrast to both lowlanders and Andean residents at altitude, who have marked right axis deviation due to pulmonary hypertension (Chapter 7). Groves et al. (1993) found pulmonary artery pressures and resistance in five Tibetan subjects in Lhasa (3658 m) to be within normal sea level values at rest and exercise. This suggests that the Tibetan population demonstrates genuine altitude adaptation, presumably by natural selection over very many generations.

17.5.2 Arterial oxygen saturation

In 1994 Beall and her colleagues reported that the level of Sa,O_2 was influenced by a single gene in a population of Tibetan women they had studied at 4850–5450 m (Beall et al. 1994). They later studied

another Tibetan population in the Lhasa region (3800–4065 m) and calculated that this gene accounted for 21% of the variance in Sa,O_2 (Beall et al. 1997b). More recently the same group compared Tibetan with South American Aymara women. They found that the Tibetans had Sa,O_2 on average 2.6% higher than the Aymara, and also that whereas much of the variance of Sa,O_2 in the Tibetan women could be attributed to genetic factors, no significant proportion of the variance could be so attributed in the South American population (Beall et al. 1999). Therefore there is the potential for natural selection towards higher Sa,O_2 in the Tibetan but not in the Aymara population.

Beall et al. (2002) reported an unusual adaptation of Ethiopian highlanders at 3530 m who had a modest polycythemic response (15.9 and 15.0 g dL^{-1} in men and women, respectively) with surprisingly high Sa,O_2: approx. 95.3%. This is the first description of this form of adaptation in a population which, because of socio-political circumstances in the past, is just beginning to be studied. Understanding of this observation is yet to be unraveled.

17.6 DISEASES

It is clear from the biography of Yu-Thog the elder (786–911), the physician–saint and founder of traditional Tibetan medicine, that a number of medical conditions were known at high altitude from the earliest times. These included lung disease, leprosy, venereal disease, a 'swelling of the throat' (possibly diphtheria) and rabies, as well as urinary retention and stones in the urinary tract (Rinpoche 1973, p. 72).

Travelers to Lhasa in the eighteenth and nineteenth centuries, such as Huc and Gabet (Pelliot 1928, vol. 2 p. 250), reported epidemics of smallpox and in 1925 it was estimated that 7000 people died in and around Lhasa from this cause. Because of the prevalence of smallpox in Tibet, in the eighteenth century the Chinese placed a tablet in Lhasa giving instructions on how to curb the disease, and it was also reported in south Tibet and Bhutan by Saunders (1789) and in the Pamir (Forsyth 1875). The Tibetan cure for smallpox was the skin of the ox and rhinoceros (Rinpoche 1973, p. 72), though a form of inoculation was used, apparently borrowed from China and India (Das 1902). A kind of snuff prepared from the dried pustules of smallpox patients was inhaled, which induced a mild form of the disease, protecting the snuff taker from the severe form as described by the Pandit A-K (Walker 1885). These conditions (smallpox, rabies, leprosy, etc.) are not, of course, caused by altitude.

Gallstones, commonly perceived as a disease of the developed world, is also a common problem in high altitude populations. Commoner in women than men, increased alcohol consumption is associated with a lower risk (Moro *et al.* 1999).

17.6.1 Birth defects

Apart from congenital heart disease, considered in the next section, a high frequency of other birth defects has been noted by Castilla *et al.* (1999). In a collaborative study from three hospitals situated between 2600 and 3600 m in Bogota (Colombia), La Paz (Bolivia) and Quito (Ecuador) they found a high frequency of craniofacial defects, cleft lip, microtia, pre-auricular tag, brachial arch complex, constriction band complex and anal atresia; there was a low frequency of neural tube defects, anencephaly and spina bifida. The incidence of patent ductus arteriosus was not addressed.

17.6.2 Cardiovascular disease

CONGENITAL HEART DISEASE

Congenital cardiovascular malformations are common at altitude, with patent ductus arteriosus being 15 times commoner at Cerro de Pasco (4200 m) than at sea level in Lima (Peñaloza *et al.* 1964). Marticorena *et al.* (1959) reported an incidence of 0.72% of patent ductus arteriosus in children born around 4300 m, compared with an incidence of 0.8% for all congenital heart disease at sea level.

In Xizang (Tibet), among the resident Tibetan population the incidence of congenital heart disease has been shown to range from 0.51 to 2.25%, with patent ductus arteriosus being the most frequently encountered abnormality (Sun 1985). The greater the altitude the higher the prevalence; the highest documented incidence (2.5%) occurred in Chinese emigrants (Zhang 1985). Presumably the cause of these high rates is the lack of a sudden increase in oxygen levels in the few hours after birth which normally triggers the reduction in pulmonary vascular resistance and the closure of the ductus.

ATHEROSCLEROSIS

Studies of populations in the Andes suggest that both coronary artery disease and myocardial infarction are uncommon amongst high altitude residents. No cases were found in one series of 300 necropsies carried out at 4300 m, and epidemiological studies in South America have shown that both angina of effort and ECG evidence of myocardial ischemia are less at altitude than at sea level (Ramos *et al.* 1967). In the Tibetan ethnic population of North Bhutan no autopsy studies were available but angina seemed uncommon, and, as judged by ECG recordings, evidence of coronary artery disease was minimal. Studies from the Tien Shan and Pamir also suggest that degenerative cardiovascular disease is rare in these regions (Mirrakhimov 1978).

In autopsy studies of 385 Tibetan adults living in the Lhasa area, arteriosclerosis of the aorta and its main branches occurred in 81.8% and of the coronary artery in 65.5%. In Qinghai, coronary artery disease was common and autopsies on Tibetans showed the same incidence as in lowlanders, but the incidence of coronary infarction was low (Sun 1985). Serum cholesterol levels were low in Andean natives and in the Bhutanese high altitude group studied; in the latter there was no progressive increase with age (Jackson *et al.* 1966, p. 96).

Moderate altitude and presumably a more active lifestyle of physical activity conveys some protection against obesity. A modernization of lifestyle in some high altitude populations migrating to low altitude with decreased activity is associated with a higher prevalence of hypertension, obesity and cardiovascular disease (Smith 1999, Cabrera de Leon *et al.* 2004). Serum leptin levels, a marker as a risk for cardiovascular disease, is usually lower in the active, non-obese high altitude populations (Lindegarde *et al.* 2004). Even in the presence of relative obesity (BMI > 30), an active lifestyle in Aymara natives of Chile was associated with a low prevalence of type 2 diabetes mellitus (Santos *et al.* 2001). Obesity per se is also associated with pulmonary hypertension and respiratory disturbances during sleep (Valencia-Flores *et al.* 2004).

HYPERTENSION

Hypertension is uncommon in high altitude populations in South America. In a study of 300 high altitude natives in Peru no significant rise in either systolic or diastolic pressure occurred with age. Of individuals aged between 60 and 80 years in the same area, few had a systolic pressure above 165 mmHg or a diastolic pressure above 95 mmHg (Baker 1978). There was no significant hypertension in ethnic Tibetan populations of North Bhutan, and, of 70 individuals examined, levels of blood pressure above 165/90 mmHg were found in 4%. Hypertension was not found in a Sherpa population studied in northeast Nepal nor in populations studied in the Tien Shan or Pamir. In an Ethiopian group, a slightly higher systolic pressure was found in males. By contrast, Sun reports (1985, 1986) a relatively high incidence of hypertension among indigenous Tibetans. He also found an age-associated increase in blood pressure. There was no tendency for hypertension to decline at higher altitudes and the blood pressure was higher in women than in men. The incidence was greater in the urban population around Lhasa than in rural populations. Similar observations have been made in Tibetans living in high altitude areas of western Szechuan. However, Han (Chinese) immigrants to Tibet showed a lower incidence of hypertension than did the Tibetans. In Qinghai province (which contains the northeastern part of the Tibetan plateau) the incidence of hypertension appears to be lower than in Xizang.

The incidence of hypertension and lack of rise in blood pressure with age in the South American and Himalayan populations studied may be the product of diet and behavior associated with a traditional lifestyle. The cause of hypertension among Tibetans is not clear. On the plateau, obesity is uncommon and traditionally few smoke (though this is changing). However, they do have a very high intake of salt, estimated at up to 1 kg per month, much of it taken in their tea. They also add yak butter, which is often slightly rancid. In the Bhutanese and Sherpa varieties of 'Tibetan' tea neither the salt nor the butter content appears, by taste, to be as high. In all houses and nomad dwellings there is a continuous supply of this tea, which is offered to every visitor. Even when they have migrated to low levels, Tibetans still drink large quantities of it and may become very obese. The high salt and butter intake may be a factor in the high incidence of hypertension in Tibetans.

However, a 15-year survey of Tibetan native highlanders living on the Tibetan plateau showed a low incidence of systemic hypertension. A total of 7797 men and 8029 women were studied. Just over 2% of this group had hypertension compared with over 4% of Chinese immigrants to Tibet. The intake of salt varied. Tibetans in Zadou county (4068 m) had the highest intake with an average of 14.6 g day^{-1} and an incidence of hypertension of 3.48%. In Zhidou county (4179 m) the average salt intake was 2.2 g day^{-1} and hypertension was found in 2.62% (Wu 1994a). By contrast, in lowland Chinese the incidence of hypertension is 7.9% (Liu 1986).

17.6.3 Infection

Direct exposure to increased solar radiation inhibits the growth of some bacteria because of the ultraviolet component of sunlight. *Staphylococcus aureus* is greatly inhibited, but *Escherichia coli* is more resistant (Nusshag 1954). The number of bacteria in ambient air decreases with altitude, and a study on the Jungfraujoch (3400 m) in Switzerland showed that, despite a large number of tourists, few bacteria were present in the air.

High altitudes do not influence human bacterial flora *per se*. However, a lower incidence of many common infections of bacterial, viral and protozoal origin was observed in soldiers at altitudes up to 5538 m (Singh *et al.* 1977). Examination of nasal swabs in a high altitude population in north Bhutan showed that there was only a 4% carrier rate of coagulase positive staphylococci; normally the incidence is between 29 and 40% in Western communities. A high frequency of β-hemolytic streptococci, highly sensitive to penicillin, was found in throat cultures, whereas in Western communities sensitivity to penicillin would be minimal (Selkon and Gould 1966).

In the highlanders of Peru, Colombia and Ecuador, oroya fever is found, which is caused by *Bacillus bacilliformis* becoming parasitic in the red blood cells. Various hemorrhagic fevers are described in the highlands of Bolivia. These are considered to be viral in origin, the virus belonging to the same group as that which causes lassa fever. Hemorrhagic disorders have also been described in north-eastern Nepal.

Mosquitoes, which transmit malaria and yellow fever, are absent at high altitude, but typhus appears to be commoner than at lower levels. This may be because bathing is not usual at higher altitudes, because of the cold, and so lice are common.

Pulmonary disease also appears common at altitude and this in part may be related to the exposure of highlanders to the smoke from open fires inside their houses or tents. In Xizang (Tibet) the incidence of chronic bronchitis was 3.7% in a low altitude population and 22.9% in a population at 4500 m. This was complicated by emphysema in 5–12% of cases and by cor pulmonale in 0.98% (Sun 1985). In Qinghai province, chronic obstructive airway disease is relatively common but smoking is prevalent, particularly amongst immigrants to high altitude. In the Pamir too, respiratory infections were noted by Forsyth (1875), though they seem less common now.

In Nepal and throughout the subcontinent, pulmonary tuberculosis was relatively common, whereas in Ethiopia it was rare. In Ethiopia the major communicable diseases were measles, malaria, dysentery, scabies and syphilis, and the total incidence of communicable disease was greater in the low altitude population (Harrison *et al.* 1969).

In northern Bhutan, respiratory infections appeared to be commoner in the younger age groups but were rare in adults; antibodies to a number of common viral infections were found. A high proportion of the population had been exposed to influenza, mumps, measles, herpes simplex and the common cold (Jackson *et al.* 1966, p. 96); in Lhasa, other parts of Tibet and the Pamir, measles epidemics with a high mortality have been reported.

Leprosy occurs in Nepal and Bhutan (Ward and Jackson 1965) and was reported in Tibet in the nineteenth century (Das 1902) and in the western Himalayas (Moorcroft and Trebeck 1841, Vol. 1, p. 180). The incidence of venereal disease appears to have been high in Lhasa (Chapman 1938), south Tibet and Bhutan (Saunders 1789) and in the Pamir (Forsyth 1875). Where large flocks of sheep are found, as in Qinghai province, hydatid disease is common. European travelers in Central Asia (Deasy 1901, Grenard 1904, p. 249) have also mentioned plague.

Chronic eye infections are seen in the populations of the Pamir, Himalayas and Tibetan plateau; the smoke of yak dung fires exacerbates them. Instruments for the treatment of cataract were available to those who practiced traditional Tibetan medicine; in general, surgery was not commonly carried out.

In summary, where certain infections are common they are due to the low living standards of the people rather than to altitude per se.

17.6.4 Goiter

The frequency of goiter in mountainous areas has been recognized for centuries, but it is not confined to the mountains, and over 200 million people worldwide have goiter (Fig. 17.1). Iodine deficiency is due to low iodine content of the soil and therefore the water. Soils poor in iodine are found where the land remained longest under quaternary glaciers. When the ice thawed, the iodine-rich soil was swept away and replaced by new soil derived from iodine-poor crystalline rocks. Seaweed, which is rich in iodine, and other folk remedies have been used since ancient times for prophylaxis and treatment (Hetzel 1989).

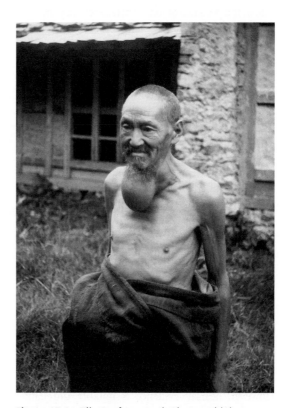

Figure 17.1 Tibetan from north Bhutan with large pendulous goiter.

Scientific proof that goiter was due to iodine deficiency was not available until Marine and Kimball (1920) published a controlled trial in high school children in Akron, Ohio. They showed a reduction in the size of goiters and prevention of their development in children treated with iodine. Iodine deficiency causes hyperplasia and retention of colloid in the thyroid, resulting in goiter and, eventually, hypothyroidism in adults. Children born to iodine-deficient mothers have a range of neurological and skeletal defects known collectively as cretinism, an association noted for centuries. This term covers a range of clinical conditions which seem to vary in frequency and importance from locality to locality and includes dwarfism, goiter, facial dysmorphism, deafness, deaf mutism and intellectual impairment. In populations with goiter, the overall work capacity of the population may be impaired, as, in addition to cretinism, there is a marked morbidity, infant mortality is raised and mental subnormality common.

Iodine deficiency may result from insufficient intake, goitrogenic substances and deficiency in intrathyroidal enzymes; an excess of calcium or fluoride in the presence of iodine deficiency may increase the incidence of goiter. McCarrison (1908 1913) carried out a classical study of goiter and endemic cretinism in the Gilgit Agency of Kashmir (Karakoram), and more recently Chapman et al. (1972) worked in the identical area. In 1906, McCarrison found a goiter incidence of 65%; in Chapman's study it was 74%. In the latter study 10 of 589 individuals examined were cretins, and hypothyroidism, excluding cretinism, was found in 24 subjects. Although the population as a whole appeared to be iodine deficient, the majority had adapted well. No evidence was found that goiter was caused by an infectious agent, a theory put forward by McCarrison.

The incidence of goiter may vary widely within a few miles; some 100 miles (160 km) north of Gilgit where goiter was endemic, it was not observed in the semi-nomadic Kirghiz tribesmen who inhabit the Pamir plateau of southern Xinjiang. Direct questioning of the nomads revealed that they knew about goiter but they were adamant that there was no history of its occurrence amongst them (Ward 1983), though Marco Polo noted a large population of people with goiter in Yarkand (Shache) as did Forsyth (1875). However, hearsay evidence is notably unreliable. Anecdotal evidence of goiter in other regions of the Himalayas, the Shimshall region of the Karakoram,

and west Bhutan, suggests also that the incidence may vary considerably within a few miles (Saunders 1789, Shipton 1938).

Moorcroft and Trebeck (1841, Vol. 2), while traveling in the western Himalayas and on the Tibetan border, comment on goiter that, 'scarcely a woman was free from it' (p. 25). Later they say, 'Goiter was here very common: the water was soft whilst at Gonh it was too hard to mix with soap: but so it was at Le where goiter does not prevail' (p. 30). Fraser (1820) alludes to surgical removal.

> We understand it [goiter] was sometimes cured when early means were taken, and these are said to consist in extirpation of the part by the knife. We saw some persons who had scars on their throat resulting from this mode of cure which had in these instances been completely successful.

Waddell (1899), in a village where goiter was prevalent, writes, 'I was surprised to see that several of the goats and the domestic fowls, as well as some of the ponies, had the same large swellings'.

According to Dr Sun Sin-Fu (personal communication), in Lhasa, about 60% of Tibetan indigenous inhabitants have goiter. Das (1902) commented too that Tibetan physicians recognized six varieties of goiter. Rockhill (1891, p. 265) also observed goiter, particularly in women in eastern Tibet, and other travelers noted the condition in northern Tibet (Bonvalot 1891, p. 116) and in the gorge country of south-east Tibet (Bailey 1957). The incidence of goiter in Himalayan valleys is high, and in the Tibetan ethnic population of north Bhutan it was the commonest clinical condition. In subjects less than 20 years old it was less marked, and younger individuals had a diffuse enlargement, whereas with age a nodular goiter was more common. No cases of cancer or thyrotoxicosis were seen, and two cretins were found in 349 individuals examined. The incidence of goiter was 60% in females and 19% in males (Jackson et al. 1966, pp. 40–4).

Ibbertson et al. (1972), in a survey of Sherpas (also of Tibetan ethnic origin) in the Sola Khumbu region of north-eastern Nepal, found that 92% had a palpable goiter, which was visibly enlarged in 63%; 75% had below normal protein-bound iodine levels in the blood and 30% were clinically hypothyroid. Classical myxedema was present in 5.9% of the population, deaf mutism in a further 4.7% and isolated deafness in a further 3.1%. Pitt (1970) describes Nepalese babies born with goiter. In many of these areas the incidence of goiter is much lower now after various projects for giving iodine by tablets or depot injections have been carried out. In a survey carried out in 1980–81 in Ethiopia, the gross goiter prevalence was found to be 30% among schoolchildren and 19% in household members (Wolde-Gebriel *et al.* 1993).

17.6.5 Sickle cell disease

Adzaku *et al.* (1993) reported on 136 patients resident at about 3000 m in Saudi Arabia and compared them with 185 patients living at sea level. Patients at both locations included those with homozygous disease (Hb SS), hemoglobin C (Hb SC) and sickle cell trait (Hb AS). The main finding was a marked increase in 2,3-diphosphoglycerate (2,3-DPG) in patients with sickle cell disease compared with normal controls at altitude and patients at sea level. Their hemoglobin concentration was not different

from sea level patients; they were anemic, with values around 8.0–9.0 g dL^{-1}. Sickle cell patients resident at low altitude have a high risk of crises on going to altitude (section 27.4.3). Adzaku *et al.* (1993) attribute the relative well being of their patients at altitude to their high 2,3-DPG, which, at this relatively modest altitude, would help tissue oxygenation, in contrast to the situation at extreme altitude (Chapter 12).

17.6.6 Dental conditions

There is no evidence that altitude has any direct effect on the teeth but the economic conditions, dictated in part by altitude, may well affect diet and hence dental condition. Generally, the diet of high altitude populations contains less refined sugars and more fiber, giving fewer caries than a more 'Western' diet. Green (1992) reported a much higher incidence of caries amongst Sherpa children along the popular trekking routes in Nepal (76%) than in villages off the routes (17%). The latter had not had the 'benefit' of cadging sweets from generous but misguided tourists.

18

Acute mountain sickness

SUMMARY

Acute mountain sickness (AMS) commonly afflicts otherwise healthy men and woman who go rapidly to altitude. Symptoms, which come on a few hours after arrival, include headache, anorexia, nausea, vomiting, lack of energy, malaise and disturbed sleep. Symptoms can occur as early as 8–24 h upon acute ascent to a new high altitude location but are usually worst on the second and third days at altitude and usually disappear by the fifth day. Symptoms may reappear on ascent to a higher altitude. This common self-limiting condition is termed AMS. Two other forms of AMS are high altitude pulmonary edema (HAPE) and high altitude cerebral edema (HACE) which are the subject of Chapters 19 and 20. These are potentially lethal.

The incidence of AMS depends upon the rate of ascent and the height reached. It is uncommon below 2000 m but is almost universal among those flying directly to altitudes above 3800 m. It occurs in both sexes and at all ages. Fitness confers no protection, and so far no physiological measurement gives reliable prediction of susceptibility for AMS. Strenuous exercise on arrival at altitude is a risk factor especially for HAPE. The mechanism underlying the symptoms is still debated, but cerebral edema is present in cases of AMS and causes most of the clinical symptoms. The edema is probably due to vasogenic mechanisms in which cerebral blood flow and permeability play a part. Abnormal fluid and sodium retention has been associated with AMS. Blunted ventilatory responses to hypoxia and the subsequent decrease in oxygen saturation have been found in some studies of AMS. Subclinical pulmonary edema and its subsequent effect on gas exchange may also play a greater or lesser role in the evolution of AMS.

Though there is debate about the mechanisms of AMS, there is a consensus about its management. AMS can be prevented or ameliorated by a slow rate of ascent which allows for normal acclimatization to occur and by drugs, of which acetazolamide is the best studied and most widely used while dexamethasone has also been shown to be quite effective in preventing and treating AMS. Treatment is hardly needed in the majority of cases, but ibuprofen and dexamethasone have been shown to be effective in the relief of headache; acetazolamide is also helpful as treatment and improves blood gases.

A scoring system for AMS has been devised, the Lake Louise system, which is recommended for research into AMS. It is described at the end of the chapter.

18.1 INTRODUCTION

It has been known for many years that travelers to high mountains experience a variety of symptoms, an early description of which was by de Acosta (Chapter 1.3). But the first modern account of acute mountain sickness (AMS) was by Ravenhill (1913). He pointed out that fatigue, cold and lack of food complicated previous descriptions by explorers and mountain climbers. He was serving as a medical officer of a mining company whose mines at 4700 m in Chile were served by a railway so that the patients he observed were suffering the uncomplicated effects of altitude alone. The local Bolivian name for AMS was *puna* or in Peru *soroche*. Tibetan names for AMS include *ladrak* (poison of the pass), *damgiri*, *duqri*, *yen chang* (from the Koko Nor region), *chang-chi* (from Szechuan) and *tuteck*. Ravenhill's description of simple AMS, which he calls *puna* of the 'normal' type, can hardly be bettered. He wrote:

> It is a curious fact that the symptoms of puna do not usually evince themselves at once. The majority of newcomers have expressed themselves as being quite well on first arrival. As a rule, towards the evening, the patient begins to feel rather slack and disinclined for exertion. He goes to bed but has a restless and troubled night and wakes up next morning with a severe frontal headache.

> There may be vomiting, frequently there is a sense of oppression in the chest but there is rarely any respiratory distress or alteration in the normal rate of breathing so long as the patient is at rest. The patient may feel slightly giddy on rising from bed and any attempt at exertion increases the headache, which is nearly always confined to the frontal region. (Ravenhill 1913)

To this description should be added the symptoms of irritability and occasionally photophobia. Sleep is often disturbed, probably because of periodic breathing. The patient may wake with a feeling of suffocation during the apneic phase. It should be noted, however, that periodic breathing is not a symptom of AMS. At altitudes above 5000 m, it continues in many subjects long after any symptoms of

AMS have resolved, and there is no correlation between its severity and AMS scores (Eichenberger *et al.* 1996). It is not a cause of AMS though its presence, by causing more severe intermittent hypoxia, may make matters worse. Ravenhill then goes on to describe *puna* of the cardiac and nervous types, corresponding in our present nomenclature to acute pulmonary edema and acute cerebral edema of high altitude (section 18.2).

After Ravenhill, although mountain sickness was well recognized, the distinction and importance of the two complicating forms seem to have been lost, at least in the English-speaking world until rediscovered by Houston (1960) and Hultgren and Spickard (1960) in the case of high altitude pulmonary edema and by Fitch (1964) for high altitude cerebral edema. However, high altitude pulmonary edema was well known to South American physicians with experience at altitude. Lizárraga (1955) gave the first detailed description of the condition after Ravenhill. A fuller account of the history of AMS is given in West (1998).

18.2 DEFINITIONS AND NOMENCLATURE

The terms *puna* and *soroche* are used loosely in South America, not only for the symptoms of acute mountain sickness but also for the dyspnea normal to exertion at high altitude (Ravenhill 1913). They are also used for chronic mountain sickness, a completely distinct clinical entity (Chapter 21). The term 'mountain sickness' needs to be qualified by the word 'acute' to distinguish it from this latter entity; the term 'acute mountain sickness' (AMS) is now well accepted for this condition or group of conditions. Finally, there is the recently described high altitude pulmonary hypertension affecting either infants or adults (Chapter 21).

Severe and potentially fatal altitude illnesses include high altitude pulmonary edema (HAPE, Chapter 20), and high altitude cerebral edema (HACE, Chapter 19).

18.2.1 Definition, signs and symptoms

AMS may be defined as a self-limiting condition affecting previously healthy individuals going rapidly to high altitude. After arrival there may be an asymptomatic period, but then within 6–24 h symptoms, including headache, anorexia, nausea, vomiting, fatigue, light-headedness and sleep disturbance can start gradually and peak usually on the second or third day. By the fourth or fifth day symptoms are usually gone and do not recur at that altitude. The Lake Louise scoring system (section 18.8) requires mild headache and at least one of the above symptoms to make the diagnosis as well as a score of three or more. There must be a history of recent height gain and (if altitude is reached abruptly as by air or cable car) several hours must elapse before the symptoms begin. The diagnosis is made on the history, and there may be no signs. However, physical examination may reveal crackles in the chest and peripheral edema. According to Hackett and Rennie (1979), the proportions of cases showing these signs were 23% and 18%, respectively. Mild fever may be present. Maggiorini et al. (1997) found a rise in body temperature of 0.5°C in mild cases (AMS score =3), 1.2°C in more severe cases of AMS (score >3) and 1.7°C in cases of HAPE; whereas, Loeppky et al. (2003) found a slight decrease in temperature with symptoms of AMS with no change in metabolic rate. Early speech impairment may also be an early sign of AMS (Cymerman et al. 2002.) With the advent of small portable pulse oximeters, $Sa_{,O_2}$ can be measured easily, and this value is often low in both patients with AMS and in subjects who will subsequently develop AMS (section 18.4.8).

Ascent to a higher altitude, even after acclimatization at a lower altitude, may precipitate a further attack. Descent and re-ascent after less than 7–10 days does not usually provoke symptoms, but descent for more than about 10 days renders the subject susceptible to AMS on re-ascent. The period of risk for AMS, therefore, corresponds with the period before acclimatization has taken place.

18.3 INCIDENCE OF AMS

The incidence of AMS depends upon the rate at which people ascend to altitude and the height reached as well as the exact definition of the condition. The lowest altitude at which some individuals can be affected is as low as 2000 m, the height of many ski resorts. Rapid ascent to 3100 m, for instance by the railway to the Gornergrat, in Switzerland or by road to Leadville, Colorado,

produces symptoms in a proportion of people by the next morning. Hackett and Rennie (1979) found an overall incidence of 43% in trekkers reaching the aid post at Pheriche (4343 m), though some affected trekkers would have dropped out before reaching this altitude. Among those who flew into the airstrip at Lukla (2800 m), the incidence was higher than among those who walked all the way (49% versus 31%). Maggiorini et al. (1990) found an incidence in climbers to European alpine huts of 9% at 2850 m, 13% at 3050 m and 34% at 3650 m. Pilgrims to 4300 m to a sacred lake in Nepal incurred a 68% incidence of AMS and 31% incidence of HACE (Basnyat et al. 2000). Frequent exposures to altitude reduce the risk of AMS and were found to increase the chance of reaching the summit on Aconcagua at 6962 m (Pesce et al. 2005). Similar data were generated at the Capanna Margherita Hut at 4559 m where individuals had a much lower risk of AMS with a history of previous exposures or slow ascent (Schneider et al. 2002). A study of a general tourist population arriving at resorts in Colorado at altitudes of 1900–2940 m found an incidence of 25% (Honigman et al. 1993). Among lowlanders who drive directly from Lima to Cerro de Pasco (4300 m) in Peru or who fly to La Paz in Bolivia (3700 m), there are very few who do not have at least mild symptoms on the morning after arrival. Murdoch (1995) reported an incidence of 85% in tourists flying into the airstrip at Shayangboche (3800 m) in Nepal. However, if the stay at altitude is only an hour or two, the incidence of AMS is negligible. This is the case, for instance, for the great majority of tourists who drive or take the train to the summit of Pike's Peak, Colorado (4300 m). It is important to note that over the last three decades increasing awareness of AMS from education has led to a lower incidence of AMS (Gaillard et al. 2004, Vardy et al. 2005).

18.4 ETIOLOGY OF AMS

18.4.1 Individual susceptibility

The etiology of AMS is multifactorial. The most important factors are the rate of ascent and the height reached. Symptoms can be induced in almost all subjects if ascent is made rapidly to a sufficient height, but for any given altitude/time profile there is great variation in individual susceptibility, but individuals with a previous history of AMS are more likely to experience it again.

18.4.2 AMS and fitness

There is no easy way to identify the susceptible individual as Ravenhill (1913) says:

> There is in my experience no type of man of whom one can say he will or will not suffer from puna. Most of the cases I have instanced were young men to all appearances perfectly sound. Young, strong and healthy men may be completely overcome. Stout, plethoric individuals of the chronic bronchitic type may not even have a headache. I have known several instances of this even when the persons have taken no care of themselves. (Ravenhill 1913)

Certainly athletic fitness provides no immunity. A superbly fit French paratrooper on a family trek to Everest Base Camp had to be evacuated to lower altitude with severe symptoms of AMS while his mother and aunt were unaffected. One study found no correlation between fitness as measured by $VO_{2,max}$ before an expedition to Mount Kenya and AMS symptom scores during the first days at altitude (Milledge et al. 1991a). Bircher et al. (1994) in a study of 41 mountaineers, who went to 4559 m in the Alps in 20–22 h, found no correlation between a measure of fitness (PWC_{170}) and AMS scores, and Savourey et al. (1995) similarly found no correlation between $VO_{2,max}$ and subsequent AMS on an Andean expedition. Thus, while common sense dictates that fitness may provide a margin of safety in any mountaineering situation, it won't convey protection from altitude illness.

18.4.3 Consistency in response to altitude

Individuals respond reasonably consistently, so that performance on one occasion is a guide to future performance. This clinical impression has been confirmed in a study by Forster (1984), who studied workers at Mauna Kea observatory in Hawaii, situated at 4200 m. These workers alternated 5 days

at the observatory with 5 days at sea level so that Forster was able to score the symptoms of AMS in 18 men on two altitude shifts. He showed that the rank order of scores correlated significantly on the two occasions. There is a tendency to acclimatize better on each subsequent trip to altitude.

However, there are numerous exceptions and case histories do show anomalies. For instance, someone who has had little trouble on the first two trips may develop AMS on a third. A respiratory or some other infection may be an added factor in such cases or may be mistaken for AMS (Bailey et al. 2003). Predictability of incurring altitude illness is greater in the case of individuals who have had HAPE than AMS.

18.4.4 AMS, gender, age and body build

Both men and women are at risk. One study (Kayser 1991) of trekkers going over the Thorong pass in Nepal (5400 m), found women to have a higher rate of sickness than men (69% versus 57%), but perhaps women are more ready to admit to symptoms than men. The young are probably at greater risk than the old (Hackett et al. 1976, Roach et al. 1995) and the risk among boys, at least of HAPE, seems especially high in South America (Hultgren and Marticorena 1978). However, Yaron et al. (1998) found a similar incidence of benign AMS in young children to that in adults. Subjects slimmer than average (body mass index <22) may be less susceptible to AMS than those who are standard or obese according to one study (Hirata et al. 1989); Kayser (1991) also found obesity to be a risk factor in men.

18.4.5 Smoking, diet and AMS

There has been an impression amongst mountaineers that smokers have less AMS than nonsmokers, perhaps because, being habituated to a modest level of carboxyhemoglobin they have, in effect, some pre-acclimatization. A recent chamber study (Yoneda and Watanabe 1997) seems to confirm that, at least for very acute, severe hypoxia, smokers had fewer symptoms, though their time of useful consciousness was not different from that of nonsmokers.

A high carbohydrate diet has some physiological benefit at altitude (section 14.8.1) and is preferred by many mountaineers, but does it reduce AMS? In a chamber study of 19 subjects given either a high (68%) or normal (45%) carbohydrate diet for 4 days before altitude exposure for 8 h, Swenson et al. (1997) found that there was no difference in the AMS scores between the two diets.

18.4.6 AMS and hypoxic ventilatory response (HVR)

There is some evidence that subjects with a low HVR (Chapter 5) measured at sea level are liable to develop AMS. The association has been shown by measurements of the response to acute hypoxia in the laboratory in studies of a few subjects (Lakshminarayan and Pierson 1975, Hu et al. 1982, Matsuzawa et al. 1989). In the last study, two of the 10 subjects had HVRs within the normal range. Richalet et al. (1988) studied a large group of climbers before they went on various expeditions to the great ranges. They found that a low ventilatory and cardiac response to hypoxia on exercise were risk factors for AMS. The same group recently reported a single case of high susceptibility in a subject who had had radiation to his neck as a child and had a very low HVR (presumably because of damage to his carotid bodies). He suffered severe AMS at only 3500 m (Rathat et al. 1993). However, a number of more recent studies in the field have failed to find a correlation. Two prospective studies found no correlation between HVR measured before going to altitude and symptom scores for AMS after arrival (Milledge et al. 1988, 1991b). Savourey et al. (1995) also reported no correlation with HVR measured before an Andean expedition and subsequent AMS. Interestingly, they did find that resting PO_2 at sea level or at simulated altitude was predictive for AMS. Selland et al. (1993) found that two of four subjects with a history of HAPE had HVRs greater than their control subjects' mean value. Hackett et al. (1987) in a study of 106 climbers on Mount McKinley found that, whilst a low Sa,O_2 predicted the likely development of AMS, there was no good correlation between HVR and Sa,O_2 on arrival at altitude. Hohenhaus et al. (1995) found that compared with control fit subjects, HVR was significantly lower in subjects who developed HAPE but not in subjects with AMS. Highlanders who generally have less AMS than lowlanders

have a blunted HVR (section 5.5.2). Interestingly, Hackett et al. (1988b) found low HVR values at altitude in patients with HAPE. Some had hypoxic depression of ventilation, which was relieved by oxygen breathing. On the other hand, Bartsch et al. (2002) did not note a relationship between HVR, measured at sea level, and subsequent AMS upon ascent to 4559 m but did document that those who did not raise their HVR on the first day had a higher incidence of AMS. After the initial increase in ventilation upon exposure to hypoxia, ventilation decreases back toward baseline within 20–30 min (hypoxic ventilatory depression, HVD). Burtscher et al. (2004) studied this poikilocapnic ventilatory response after 20–30 min of hypoxia in AMS-susceptible individuals and found that AMS was predicted in 86% subsequently exposed to high altitude. In conclusion it would seem that whilst susceptibility to HAPE is associated with a low HVR, susceptibility to AMS is not.

18.4.7 AMS and hypoxic vascular pressor responses

Hypoxia elicits complex vasomotor responses which result in improved blood flow and thus oxygen delivery to tissues while causing a vasoconstrictor response in the pulmonary vasculature.

So far as the pulmonary vasculature, a brisk increase in pressure in response to hypoxia is a risk factor for HAPE and is discussed in Chapter 19 (Hultgren et al. 1971, Kawashima et al. 1989). The finding that nifedipine which, by lowering the pulmonary artery pressure, is protective of HAPE does not protect from AMS (Hohenhaus et al. 1994) makes the relationship of HPVR and AMS unlikely.

On the other hand, using spectral analysis of the R–R interval and blood pressure (BP) variability the systemic vasculature and its autonomic regulation has been studied in 41 mountaineers at low altitude and 4559 m. AMS symptoms correlated consistently with a higher proportion of BP variability, suggestive of a marker for increased sympathetic tone and susceptibility to AMS. This finding may provide insight into subtle differences in inherent characteristics of AMS-susceptible individuals.

18.4.8 Oxygen saturation and AMS

Although hypoxia is not the immediate cause of the symptoms of AMS, the severity of hypoxia is important since the incidence increases with altitude. It is perhaps not surprising therefore, that a number of studies have shown a correlation between Sa,O_2 and AMS (Bircher *et al.* 1994, Roach *et al.* 1998). In the study by Bircher *et al.* (1994) subjects traveled to the Capanna Margherita (4559 m) by helicopter, and the saturations were measured on the second day when AMS symptoms were at their height. Some subjects had overt HAPE, and no doubt others had subclinical edema. In the study by Roach and colleagues (1998), 102 climbers on Mount Denali were studied at Base Camp (4200 m) and then questioned about AMS symptoms on their return from their summit bids. The Sa,O_2 measured before climbing from Base Camp correlated with subsequent AMS scores. Thus, a low Sa,O_2 on arrival at altitude is a good predictor for the later development of AMS. The authors comment that the reason for the low Sa,O_2 in these subjects could be either hypoventilation or impaired gas exchange. However, Bircher *et al.* (1994) did not find a difference in Pa,CO_2 between those with and without AMS and the collected results from over 90 subjects from a number of studies at this location by Bärtsch (personal communication) gave the same finding. However, other studies, mostly taking measurements earlier in altitude exposure, did find evidence of hypoventilation and higher PCO_2 in AMS subjects (section 18.5.2). Erba *et al.* (2004) studied subjects during sleep upon ascent to 4559 m and did not find a correlation between AMS and hypoventilation but did find one between the degree of nocturnal hypoxemia and AMS.

Another way of looking at the possible gas exchange abnormality was studied by Ge *et al.* (1997) who measured pulmonary diffusing capacity for carbon monoxide (DCO) in a group of 32 subjects at 2260 m and after ascent to 4700 m. In non-AMS subjects there was an increase in DCO at the higher altitude whilst in AMS patients the increase was insignificant. They also showed lower vital capacity, reduced expiratory flow in the middle of their forced vital capacity (FVC) and greater $(A-a)O_2$ gradient. These differences were thought to be due to subclinical pulmonary edema. Pollard *et al.* (1997) also found reduced FVC and forced expiratory volume in 1 s (FEV_1) at altitude and a correlation between these indices of lung function and arterial saturation. Probably a degree of subclinical pulmonary edema is common during the early days at altitude which is consistent with the findings of radiographic evidence of pulmonary edema in some well-trained cyclists after an endurance ride at moderate altitude (Anholm *et al.* 1996).

18.4.9 Exercise and AMS

AMS can and frequently does occur in the absence of any exercise as in chamber experiments or with only gentle walking short distances, as in helicopter transport to a mountain hut or a flight to La Paz, Bolivia. But until recently we could not answer the question of whether subjects climbing on foot to altitude would be more or less likely to have AMS than those who arrived there by air or motor transport given the same rate of ascent. Obviously, most people who fly to altitude have a more rapid height gain than those who walk and therefore more AMS. Again, the advice to people on arrival at altitude is to avoid exercise for some time but there are little hard data to support this. Bircher *et al.* (1994) did not find any difference in the incidence of AMS in relation to intensity of work (as assessed by heart rate) in groups of subjects who climbed to the Capanna Margherita. However, as the authors say, their study was not designed to look at this relationship, and the differences in exercise rates were not great. Roach *et al.* (2000) carried out a cross-over trial in which seven subjects were exposed to approximately 4800 m altitude equivalent in a chamber for 10 h on one occasion with, and on another without, four bouts of 30 min of 50% of altitude-specific exercise. The AMS scores were significantly higher during the exposure with exercise. This one study lends some credence to the time-honored advice to avoid strenuous exercise in getting to and on arrival at altitude, in order to avoid AMS. The same advice is probably even more pertinent in relation to HAPE where exercise raises pulmonary artery pressure and increases the risk of HAPE.

18.5 MECHANISMS OF AMS

18.5.1 Fluid balance and AMS

Clearly, hypoxia is a crucial starting mechanism for AMS but it is not the direct cause of symptoms.

Within a few minutes of exposure to high altitude Po_2 falls throughout the body but symptoms of acute mountain sickness are delayed for at least a few hours. This suggests that hypoxia initiates some process which requires a time course of 6–24 h before it, in turn, causes the symptoms. Some of this response appears to be secondary to the lowered barometric pressure, as opposed to just the hypoxia, per se, which also effects an increase in fluid retention secondary to an increase in aldosterone and anti-diuretic hormone (Loeppky *et al.* 2005b).

Current thinking favors the hypothesis that hypoxia causes some alteration of fluid or electrolyte homeostasis with either water retention or shifts of water from intracellular to extracellular compartments (Hansen *et al.* 1970, Hackett *et al.* 1981, Bartsch *et al.* 2002, Loeppky *et al.* 2005a).

In considering the possible role of disturbances in fluid balance in the mechanism of AMS we need to take into account two other variables apart from the rate of ascent:

- Whether or not the subject exercises upon arrival at high altitude
- Whether the subject has a physiological or a pathological response to altitude hypoxia, i.e. whether or not he or she gets AMS

EXERCISE AT LOW ALTITUDE

The effect of commencing daylong exercise (hill walking) continued for several days at low altitude was studied in the hills of North Wales. Full water and electrolyte balances were carried out before, during and after the exercise period. There was significant sodium retention, modest water retention, significant increases in plasma and interstitial fluid volumes at the expense of the intracellular compartment (Williams *et al.* 1979), later shown to be due to activation of the renin–aldosterone system during exercise (Milledge *et al.* 1982, see section 15.3.3). The increased interstitial fluid volume can cause overt pitting edema in a few subjects, but all were in a state of subclinical edema.

ALTITUDE WITHOUT EXERCISE OR AMS

It is surprisingly difficult to obtain reliable data on the effect of altitude on fluid and electrolyte balance in the absence of exercise and AMS. Papers usually indicate if exercise has been excluded (though not always) but seldom make it clear which if any subjects were free of AMS. Few papers quote strict balance studies, and those that do often give conflicting results. The usual physiological response to hypoxia is a diuresis. This seems to be the case in animals and is effected by stimulus of the peripheral chemoreceptors (Honig 1989) but is less easy to demonstrate in humans. Studies in the field have given conflicting results probably because of the difficulty in controlling factors such as temperature, sweating, sodium and water intake. However, Swenson *et al.* (1995), in a 6-h chamber study where these factors have all been controlled, have shown that there was an increase in urinary volume and sodium output with hypoxia. Further they found a good correlation between these two measurements and the subjects' hypoxic ventilatory response (HVR). There were only minimal symptoms of AMS in the 6h of the study. The diuresis and natriuresis did not correlate with changes in aldosterone, renin, ANP, vasopressin or digoxin-like immunoreactive substance.

There is a reduction of plasma, interstitial and intracellular volumes during the first few days at altitude (Frayzer *et al.* 1975, Jain *et al.* 1980). Similar changes were found in a study by Singh *et al.* (1990) and are shown in Fig. 18.1. Note that the changes, as a percentage of sea level values are quite small, the greatest being a 6–7% reduction in plasma and extracellular fluid volumes at two days. The changes in these compartments remained for up to 12 days whereas the reductions in total body water and intracellular fluid were restored by day 12 at altitude.

ALTITUDE WITH EXERCISE AND WITHOUT AMS

A study based on the Gonergrat (3100 m), Switzerland involved baseline studies at rest at low altitude followed by exercise in climbing to the Gornergrat on a daily basis while there (Milledge *et al.* 1983). Complete balance studies were continued throughout. The results were almost identical to those of exercise at low altitude. The plasma volume increased so that the hematocrit, instead of rising as is usual at altitude, actually fell as it did at sea level. Renin and aldosterone levels were high; whereas, subjects at rest at altitude have low aldosterone levels.

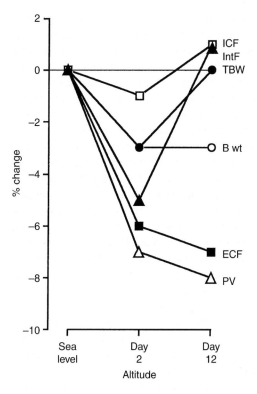

Figure 18.1   Changes in fluid compartments on going to altitude in the absence of exercise or acute mountain sickness (AMS). ICF, intracellular fluid volume; Int F, interstitial fluid volume; TBW, total body water; Bwt, Body weight; ECF, extracellular fluid volume; PV, plasma volume. Data from Singh *et al.* (1990).

The effect of exercise over-rides the effect of altitude in this situation.

ALTITUDE WITH EXERCISE AND AMS

There are no balance studies which have addressed exactly this question due to the formidable problems of carrying out balance studies on sufficiently large numbers of subjects to cover both good and poor acclimatizers. Studies measuring just 24-h sodium excretion have shown an inverse correlation between sodium excretion and AMS symptom scores and a direct correlation with aldosterone concentration. That is, those who develop AMS have higher aldosterone levels and retain more sodium. All subjects have a reduced urine volume with the AMS victims tending to have a greater anti-diuresis but this did not reach statistical significance (Bärtsch *et al.* 1988, Milledge *et al.* 1989).

SODIUM AND WATER BALANCE IN AMS

Table 18.1 attempts to bring together these changes showing that the subject with AMS is in a similar state of expanded plasma and extracellular fluid volume as a subject starting day-long exercise at low altitude. They are both in a state of subclinical edema.

These effects are shown in Fig. 18.2. It is suggested that this increase in extracellular fluid in turn results in the dependent and periorbital edema often seen in patients with acute mountain sickness (Hackett and Rennie 1979). It also causes mild cerebral edema, resulting in the symptoms of AMS. More severe cerebral edema causes the full blown condition of HACE and pulmonary edema causes HAPE.

Some evidence of fluid retention is provided by the clinical observation of lower urine output in soldiers with AMS than in soldiers free of symptoms (Singh *et al.* 1969) and by the finding that trekkers with AMS gained weight, while trekkers without AMS had lost weight by the time they reached 4243 m (Hackett *et al.* 1982). The 'normal' response to altitude seems to be a mild diuresis; whereas, subjects destined to get AMS have an anti-diuresis.

Because of this anti-diuresis the anti-diuretic hormone (vasopressin) might be thought to underlie this mechanism, but that seems not to be the case (see section 15.2.3). The effect of altitude on the renin–aldosterone system is reviewed in section 15.3. Briefly, ascent to altitude alone has a variable effect

Table 18.1   Changes in sodium and water control with exercise at low altitude and in response to altitude in subjects with and without acute mountain sickness (AMS)

Parameter	Exercise Low altitude	No AMS High altitude	With AMS High altitude
Urine volume	↓	↑	↓
Water balance	? Positive	? Negative	? Positive
Na excretion	↓	↑	↓
Plasma volume	↑	↓	? ↑
Extracellular volume	↑	↓	? ↑
Plasma aldosterone	↑	↓	↑

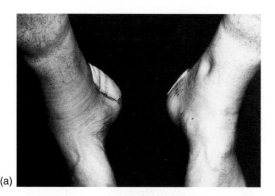

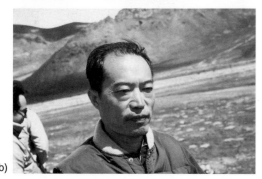

Figure 18.2   (a) Pitting edema of the ankle after hill walking at low altitude. (b) Periorbital edema at high altitude.

on plasma renin activity but results in lower than normal aldosterone levels at rest. Exercise stimulates the release of renin which in turn, via angiotensin, stimulates aldosterone release and if continued long enough causes salt and hence water retention (Williams *et al.* 1979, Milledge *et al.* 1982). This may be important especially in HAPE, in which a history of exercise is often a prominent feature (Chapter 19). AMS symptom scores were found to correlate with aldosterone levels and with reduced 24-h urine sodium output on the first day at altitude in subjects who had ascended to 4300 m on foot on Mount Kenya (Milledge *et al.* 1989). A similar result was reported from a study in the European Alps (Bärtsch *et al.* 1988) although Hogan *et al.* (1973), in a chamber experiment, found that subjects with AMS had lower aldosterone concentrations than did asymptomatic subjects.

Atrial natriuretic peptide (ANP), which increases urinary sodium excretion and hence fluid excretion, is elevated by hypoxia in rats (Winter *et al.* 1987) and man (Bärtsch *et al.* 1988, Cosby *et al.* 1988, Milledge *et al.* 1989). The relationship between ANP levels and AMS is variable. One study found a tendency to higher levels in subjects more resistant to AMS (Milledge *et al.* 1989); whereas, two other studies found the opposite (Bärtsch *et al.* 1988, Cosby *et al.* 1988). It seems that despite its name ANP is not a very powerful natriuretic hormone. Subjects, hill walking at low altitude, have raised ANP levels while retaining sodium vigorously (Milledge *et al.* 1991b). ANP may have an effect by increasing capillary permeability, but its significance in the aetiology of AMS remains to be established (Bärtsch *et al.* 1988).

Although the favored hypothesis is that fluid is retained and somehow causes AMS, it has proved very hard to substantiate this. Measurements of urine output have usually not shown a clear difference between those with and without AMS (Milledge *et al.* 1989) though this negative finding often goes unreported. Westerterp *et al.* (1996) applied the technique of labeled water and bromide to the problem. A group of 10 subjects were transported by helicopter to the Obervatoire Vallot (4350 m) and studied for 4 days. Fluid intake correlated closely with food intake and both were reduced in those with AMS. There was reduced evaporative water loss at altitude which resulted in increased urine output in the case of subjects without AMS but not in AMS sufferers. The change in total body water was small and not significantly different between those with and without AMS. However, those with AMS showed a fluid shift greater than 1 L between intra- and extracellular compartments. The shift could be in either direction making it difficult to understand the mechanism. However, only one AMS subject had a reduction in extracellular volume while three showed the expected increase. On the other hand, Cumbo *et al.* (2002) found a correlation between markers of dehydration and AMS. Recently, Loeppky *et al.* (2005a) demonstrated that anti-diuretic hormone rose within 90 min of exposure to approx. 4900 m in subjects who developed AMS and continued to do so. Thus, most of the evidence supports a response in AMS victims that favors fluid retention.

18.5.2 Role of P_{CO_2} in AMS and cerebral blood flow

The symptoms of AMS are largely related edema of the brain (Krasney 1994), and much debate has been generated about the regulation of cerebral blood flow (CBF) at high altitude and the development of edema. On going to high altitude the subject experiences not only hypoxia but also hypocapnia, both of which have potent effects on CBF.

The possibility that hypocapnia over a number of hours might be a factor in the genesis of AMS was tested by Maher *et al.* (1975). They exposed two groups of subjects to simulated altitude in a hypobaric chamber. One group had CO_2 added to the atmosphere to maintain their P_{CO_2} at control levels; the other group breathed air and became hypocapnic. Hypoxia was similar in the two groups, though to achieve this the group with CO_2 added was taken to a lower barometric pressure. Far from alleviating symptoms of AMS the added CO_2 increased their severity.

Sutton *et al.* (1976) found that in a group of subjects air lifted to a camp at 5360 m on Mount Logan, the severity of AMS correlated best with the P_{CO_2}. Forwand *et al.* (1968) found AMS symptom scores correlated well with P_{CO_2} but not with pH or P_{O_2}. In a study of 42 trekkers, Hackett *et al.* (1982) found that those who gained weight on ascent to 4300 m had the highest incidence of AMS and reduced their $Pa_{,CO_2}$ very little, whereas those who lost weight (presumably mainly fluid) had less frequent AMS and a low $PA_{,CO_2}$. Two studies of men in decompression chambers also found a correlation between AMS and hypoventilation (King and Robinson 1972, Moore *et al.* 1986). Maher *et al.* (1975) suggested that the mechanism connecting P_{CO_2} and AMS was the well-known effect of CO_2 in increasing the cerebral blood flow.

Hypoxia also causes an increase in cerebral blood flow. In subjects with a brisk ventilatory response and low P_{CO_2} these two effects are, to a degree, counterbalanced. Whereas, in subjects at high altitude with little increase in ventilation and P_{CO_2} close to sea-level values, cerebral vessels will be dilated and may contribute to cerebral edema and a rise in intracranial pressure. This in turn causes the symptoms of AMS and is shown in Fig. 18.3 on the right of the diagram. Another possibility, referred to above, is that the higher P_{CO_2} and lower P_{O_2} would cause peripheral vasodilatation which, by lowering central venous pressure, would lower the level of ANP and result in an anti-diuresis.

Acclimatization to high altitude attempts to maintain oxygen delivery to tissue beds. The brain is no exception and requires a finely regulated mechanism

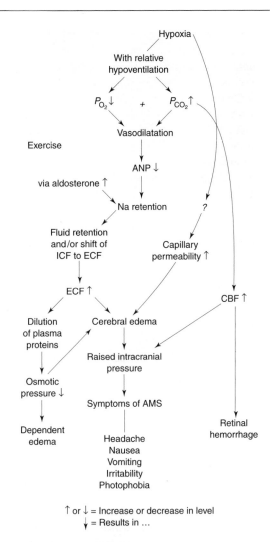

Figure 18.3 Possible mechanisms underlying acute mountain sickness (AMS). ICF, intracellular fluid; ECF, extracellular fluid; CBF, cerebral blood flow; ANP, atrial natriuretic peptide.

of increase in blood flow and an increase in oxygen content in the blood provided by erythropoietic response over a number of days. This balance was demonstrated by Severinghaus *et al.* (1966) who showed that cerebral blood flow was increased on going to altitude and then fell toward sea level values with acclimatization. One study, which confirmed this general pattern, found no difference in cerebral blood flow between subjects with and without AMS (Jensen *et al.* 1990); however, two more recent studies (Baumgartner *et al.* 1994, Jansen *et al.* 1999), using velocity in the middle cerebral artery measured by

Doppler ultrasound, have shown greater increase on going to altitude in subjects with AMS than in non-symptomatic controls. The Sa,O_2 was lower in AMS subjects and accounted for much of the difference in flow. On the other hand, Jansen *et al.* (1999) showed that AMS subjects had greater response in flow to changes in PCO_2 (voluntary hyperventilation) than controls, suggesting brisker vasomotor response in these susceptible individuals.

These same investigators demonstrated a loss of CBF autoregulation during hypoxia and phenyl-ephrine infusion in high altitude natives (Sherpas) and sojourners to altitude as compared to subjects at sea level (Jansen *et al.* 2000.) Manipulation of systemic blood pressure with phenylephrine nor-mally results in a concomitant adjustment in CBF which did not occur consistently at high altitude. These investigators did not look at symptoms of AMS. Insight into the importance of CBF autoreg-ulation may be gleaned from a study by Van Osta *et al.* (2005) where they found that symptoms of AMS correlated with loss of this precise mechanism.

The correlations between CBF, altitude and AMS are not consistent. Another study looked at the cere-bral blood flow response to a 15-min hypoxic and hyperoxic challenge in one group of subjects who had suffered HAPE, another who had been to alti-tude with no AMS and a third unselected control group. The study showed no predictive value of alti-tude tolerance (Berre *et al.* 1999).

Another important factor has to do with the effect of exercise at high altitude on CBF. Imray *et al.* (2005) studied nine subjects acclimatized to 5260 m. At low altitude cerebral oxygenation increased during maxi-mum exercise; whereas, at high altitude maximum cerebral oxygenation occurred at 30% of maximum exercise and then fell slowly as exercise progressed to higher levels. All of these factors may play a role in the effect of CBF on vasogenic edema and thus AMS.

18.5.3 Intracranial pressure and AMS

There is a striking similarity of symptoms between AMS and the effects of high intracranial pressure due to cerebral tumors etc. The evidence for raised intracranial pressure in AMS is:

- The CSF pressure was found to be elevated by 60–210 mmH$_2$O during AMS compared with that after recovery (Singh *et al.* 1969).

- In cases of malignant cerebral AMS, papilledema has been noted (Dickinson 1979).
- In those dying with cerebral AMS, cerebral edema with flattening of the cerebral convolutions has been found (Dickinson *et al.* 1983, Singh *et al.* 1969).
- Computerized tomographic examination of the brain in patients with HAPE showed diffuse low density areas in the cerebrum representing edema (Fukushima *et al.* 1983).
- Direct measurement has been made in one unreported study (B.H. Cummings, personal communication). One of three subjects, with pressure transducers implanted in their skulls before a Himalayan expedition, was mountain sick on return from 5700 m to Base Camp at 4750 m. His intracranial pressure was normal at rest but elevated on the slightest exertion. Other subjects without AMS had normal pressures even on exercise.
- Using an indirect measure of intracranial pressure (tympanic membrane displacement) exposure to acute hypoxia at 3440 m was associated with a rise in pressure. However, on going to 4120 m and 5200 m the pressure returned to sea level values. There was no correlation between intracranial pressure and AMS scores (Wright *et al.*1995).

Despite the lack of good direct evidence and some dissenting data (Fischer *et al.* 2004), the con-sensus view seems to be that the symptoms of AMS are best explained as being due to cerebral edema and raised intracranial pressure (Hackett 1999). A magnetic resonance imaging (MRI) technique described by Morocz *et al.* (2001) can track changes in cerebral edema in a non-invasive manner and may provide a valuable tool for investigation in the future. Other mechanisms of cerebral edema are considered in Chapter 19.

18.5.4 Derangement of clotting mechanism

In reports on necropsy material, the presence of thromboses in lungs and brain figures prominently. No doubt parts of the pathological picture, such as the development of hyaline membrane in the alve-oli and possibly some thrombi, are secondary to the autopsy conditions, but there is evidence of alterations in coagulation associated with altitude (Singh and Chohan 1972). It has been suggested that thrombosis may form a basis for the development of both pulmonary hypertension and edema (Dickinson *et al.* 1983). However, Hyers *et al.* (1979) were unable to show differences in activated coagulation between those who are susceptible to pulmonary edema and more normal individuals at altitude.

Bärtsch *et al.* (1987) studied a range of clotting factors in 66 subjects presenting at the Capanna Margherita (4559 m) with varying degrees of AMS. They found that coagulation time, euglobulin lysis time and fibrin(ogen) fragment E were normal in all subject groups. Fibrinopeptide A (FPA), a molecular marker of *in vivo* fibrin formation, was elevated in patients with HAPE. However, FPA was not elevated in subjects with simple AMS, even with widened $(A–a)O_2$ suggesting early HAPE. They conclude that the fibrin formation which takes place in HAPE is an epiphenomenon and not causative and thus probably not related to the pathogenesis of AMS.

18.5.5 Microvascular permeability and AMS

Hypoxia may increase microvascular permeability directly or via mediators. Numerous animal studies have shown that hypoxia increases lymph flow with variable results on the lymph/plasma ratio for protein. The problem is to separate hemodynamic effects from permeability itself. Staub (1986) has reviewed the effect of hypoxia on microvascular permeability and concludes that, 'On best analysis ... the change in permeability is slight, albeit statistically significant'.

However, there is no really good animal model and the failure to show an important change in an animal which does not get HAPE in no way excludes the importance of permeability changes in humans. Findings have served to strengthen the evidence for some effect of hypoxia on microvascular permeability:

- Larsen *et al.* (1985) have shown in rabbits that neither hypoxia alone nor the infusion of cobra venom (which activates the complement system) alone caused pulmonary edema.

However, the two insults together did cause permeability-type pulmonary edema. This suggests the possibility that hypoxia, with some other factor, may increase microvascular permeability.

- Schoene *et al.* (1986, 1988) and Hackett *et al.* (1986), by analysing bronchoalveolar lavage and pulmonary edema fluid, respectively, have shown conclusively that in HAPE the edema is of the high protein permeability type rather than hemodynamic. They also found significant levels of leukotriene B_4 and factors chemotactic for monocytes in the lavage fluid, suggesting that the release of these and other mediators of inflammation may be involved in the mechanism of HAPE.

- Richalet *et al.* (1991) found a rise in plasma levels of most of the six eicosanoids measured in subjects taken abruptly to the Vallot observatory on Mount Blanc (4350 m). All subjects had AMS. The levels of these vasoactive mediators affecting permeability had a time course parallel to that of AMS symptoms.

- Roach *et al.* (1996) measured urinary leukotriene E_4 in subjects taken to 4300 m with a 4-day stop-over at 1830 m. There was a significant increase in levels of urinary leukotriene though the correlation with AMS did not reach significance. The authors conclude that leukotrienes may be involved in the genesis of AMS. On the other hand, leukotriene blockade did not prevent AMS upon rapid exposure to 4300 m (Muza *et al.* 2004). In fact, lower urinary leukotriene E_4 levels were measured on Denali where leukotriene blockade also did not have an effect on AMS (Grissom *et al.* 2005).

- Bauer *et al.* (2006) demonstrated fluid shifts from the intra- to extravascular space with exercise at high altitude that was decreased with acclimatization, suggesting some adaptation of the endothelium with adaptation. The mechanism of the response may be related to endothelial adaptation to hypoxia as demonstrated by Gonzalez and Wood (2001) who documented the effect of hypoxia on adherence of leukocytes to the vascular endothelium and subsequent inflammation marked by reactive oxygen species (ROS) which abated with time for acclimatization, a process thought to be mediated by an upregulation of inducible nitric oxide synthase and not unique to the pulmonary vasculature.

- Choucker *et al.* (2005) demonstrated that hypoxia alone stimulated granulocyte function, but that exercise inhibited the inflammatory response.

Most of these studies have concentrated on the pulmonary microvascular permeability, but the same mechanism could affect microvascular permeability generally, including cerebral microvessels and thus contribute to cerebral edema as shown in Fig. 18.3 (center). Hypoxia has been shown to increase permeability of endothelial monolayers to a range of proteins *in vitro,* though quite severe hypoxia (12–19 mmHg) and incubation for 48–72 h was needed to show the effect (Gerlach *et al.* 1992). The mechanism of this permeability is open to question, but the seminal question is how much permeability in the cerebral vasculature is caused by increased pressure and how much by inflammatory mediators?

As a reflection of generalized microvascular endothelial leak, proteinuria is also common during the first few days at altitude, especially in subjects with AMS (Chapter 15) and this may be due to increased microvascular permeability in the kidneys (Winterborn *et al.* 1986). If increased permeability has a role in AMS there is the question of whether it initiates or continues the process. Kleger *et al.* (1996) investigated this by measuring the escape rate of ^{125}I-labeled albumin as well as various cytokines in the plasma of 24 subjects taken rapidly to 4559 m altitude. Ten subjects developed AMS and four HAPE. They found no significant increase in albumin escape in any group of subjects. The only significant increase in cytokine levels was in the HAPE patients and that was of IL-6 on the second and third days at altitude when HAPE was established. Swenson *et al.* (1997) measured a number of cytokines in the plasma of 19 subjects exposed to 10% oxygen for 8 h. They found no change in the concentration of the measured cytokines by the end of the exposure time. These findings suggest that if cytokines do play a role in AMS it is probably in the development of the illness towards HAPE or HACE. In Chapter 19 there is further consideration of

mechanisms in relation to HAPE, some of which may also apply to benign AMS.

Vascular endothelial growth factor (VEGF) is a permeability factor that is inducible by hypoxia. Walter *et al.* (2001) documented an increase in VEGF upon ascent to 4559 m, but there was no difference between subjects with and without AMS or HAPE. On the other hand, Schoch *et al.* (2002) showed in mice that hypoxia induced an increase in VEGF, as well as evidence (documented by fluorescein marker) of cerebral edema which was prevented by inhibition of VEGF by a neutralizing antibody. Tissot van Patot *et al.* (2005) studied free plasma VEGF and found higher levels in subjects at 4300 m who had AMS.

Several investigative teams have looked the effect of hypoxia on reactive oxidant species and their role in clinical AMS. Bailey *et al.* (2001) documented free radical mediated vascular permeability in male volunteers ascending to high altitude, especially in the muscle vascular bed, which they contended may be related to the cerebral leak in AMS. In a subsequent study, rapid ascent to 4559 m induced an increase in cytokines, markers of muscle damage, neuronal damage, and ROS which suggested tissue damage, but no correlation with AMS could be substantiated (Bailey *et al.* 2003). Thus, the role of oxidative stress as a causative one or merely an epiphenomenon is debatable. Magalhaes *et al.* (2003) exposed mice to an equivalent altitude of 7000 m and looked at the effect of the exposure on oxidative stress and the blocking of this stress. Hypoxia increased the stress but blockade resulted in a lower glutathione concentration (a marker of ROS). This same group (Magalhaes *et al.* 2004b) confirmed the increase in markers of oxidative stress with hypoxia in humans but found no additional changes with rapid reoxygenation. In another study (Bailey *et al.* 2005), ROS were induced in humans by hypoxia (12% for 18 h). Lumbar punctures, brain MRI, AMS and ROS were all performed. Although 50% of the subjects developed AMS, there was no correlation between mild evidence of cerebral edema, clinical symptoms of AMS, or increase of intracranial pressures.

At this point, the pathophysiology of brain edema in AMS remains a puzzle, but important clues about the roles of increased mechanical factors on the endothelium as well as humoral factors which induce endothelial permeability leak are being pieced together.

18.5.6 Anorexia, leptin and AMS

Leptin, a hormone, produces the sensation of satiety and is thought to be important in body weight regulation. Tschop *et al.* (1998) measured its level in subjects in two field studies at the Capanna Margherita (4559 m). They found it to be elevated at altitude compared with sea level and to be higher in subjects with AMS than in those without. The neuropeptide cholecystokinin (CCK) also suppresses the appetite. Bailey *et al.* (2000) found it to be increased in plasma from subjects with AMS compared with subjects free of symptoms on the Kangchenjunga Medical Expedition 1998, but further work is necessary to understand the mechanism of AMS.

18.6 PROPHYLAXIS OF AMS

AMS only occurs during the first few days at a given altitude. It seems therefore that acclimatization confers protection in some way from AMS. Allowing time for acclimatization is therefore the best way to prevent AMS. There is an impression that there are limits to acclimatization which vary for different individuals. At altitudes above this limit a person is therefore at risk of AMS, HAPE and HACE even after acclimatization to lower altitudes has been achieved.

18.6.1 Rate of ascent

A slow rate of ascent will prevent AMS, but due to the great variation in susceptibility to AMS, it is not possible to be dogmatic in advice on rate of ascent. A suggested rule of thumb is that, above 3000 m, each night should be spent not more than 300 m above the last, with a rest day – that is two nights at the same altitude – every 2–3 days. In addition, anyone who experiences symptoms of AMS should go no higher until they improve. It is not certain where the rule originated, possibly from the epidemiological study of trekkers on the route to Everest Base Camp (Hackett *et al.* 1976). Recently, Murdoch (1999) has looked for evidence of its efficiency in preventing AMS in the same area. He surveyed 283 trekkers asking about AMS symptoms and speed of ascent. There are two clear messages from this study.

First, that there is huge individual variation in susceptibility. Half the trekkers ascending at the very low mean rate of 100–200 m day^{-1} became sick while almost half the trekkers ascending at 500–600 m day^{-1} remained free of AMS. Obviously there was a process of self-selection, with those feeling fine going fast and those feeling less well going slowly. Second, that overall, the incidence of AMS was higher the faster trekkers ascended. His conclusion is that, while the rule for many, if not most trekkers, is slower than is really necessary, the rule should continue to be the guideline, in the interest of a substantial minority. Basnyat *et al.* (1999) also found evidence from their questionnaire survey of the same trekking route that rate of ascent was an important risk factor. AMS risk decreased by 19% for each additional day spent between the airstrip at Lukla (2804 m) and the place of survey, Pheriche (4243 m).

18.6.2 Fluid intake

Trek leaders often urge their clients to drink plenty as they gain altitude in order to avoid AMS. There seems no good scientific reason for this advice. Providing enough fluid is taken to avoid dehydration, further intake will only be excreted and if all taken as water, could lead to symptomatic hyponatremia. However, there is a recent epidemiological study that appears to lend some support for this practice. Basnyat *et al.* (1999) gave questionnaires to Everest Base Camp Trekkers at Pheriche (4243 m) and found that 30% of them had AMS. They asked about daily fluid intake and found that the higher the intake (up to 5 L day^{-1}) the lower the incidence of AMS (odds ratio 1.54). But in the only controlled trial to address this issue, Aoki and Robinson (1971) found that there was no effect of hydration on AMS incidence. They achieved dehydration by treatment of one group with furosemide, hyperhydration in another with vasopressin and a third group was given a placebo. All groups were decompressed at the same rate in a chamber. Clearly, more work is needed to answer this question.

18.6.3 Drugs for prophylaxis

ACETAZOLAMIDE (DIAMOX®)

Cain and Dunn (1965) were the first to show that acetazolamide increases ventilation and Pa,o_2, and decreases $Pa,_{CO_2}$. It has been shown to reduce the incidence and severity of AMS in a number of double-blind controlled trials in the field (Forward *et al.* 1968, Birmingham Medical Research Group 1981, Larsen *et al.* 1982). All symptoms are improved, as well as general performance, as judged by peer review. Sleep was improved and the profound desaturation associated with periodic breathing (Chapter 13) was relieved (Sutton *et al.* 1979). It has been shown to prevent patients with asthma from developing AMS (Mirrakhimov *et al.* 1993). In these trials, the dose was 250 mg, orally, every 8 h, started 1 day before ascent, except in the Birmingham trial where the dose was one 500 mg slow release tablet daily. This dose, or 250 mg normal release twice daily (which is cheaper), used to be the recommended regimen. More recently many are recommending half that dose morning and evening since it is believed that protection is adequate and side effects are fewer (Basnyat *et al.* 2003, 2006), but a higher dose 250 mg b.i.d. was found to be more efficacious in tourists ascending to 3630 m (Carlsten *et al.* 2004). Whatever the dose decided upon, medications can be started upon arrival at altitude.

The duration of treatment depends upon the circumstance and situation. In many treks, the exposure to conditions when AMS may be a problem is limited to a few days, and obviously treatment can be discontinued when the party has descended from altitude. In situations where subjects go to altitude and stay there, the risk of AMS is limited to the first four or five days so that treatment could reasonably be stopped after that.

However, a study by the Birmingham group (Bradwell *et al.* 1986) has shown that taking acetazolamide for three weeks at 4846 m conferred a benefit in that the group on treatment lost less weight, lost less muscle bulk and had superior exercise performance than those on placebo. Here the drug was being used not so much to prevent AMS as to reduce altitude deterioration.

The side effects of acetazolamide consist of a mild diuresis and paraesthesiae in the hands and feet, which tend to diminish with continued use of the drug. A few people find this tingling very disturbing, and some are troubled by gastric side effects. Also, carbonated beverages (soft drinks, beer, wine, sparkling wine) taste flat; this is due to the inhibition of carbonic anhydrase in the tongue so that the conversion of CO_2 to carbonic acid fails to take place in the time available as the drink passes over the tongue, and the acid sensing buds are not stimulated. The safety of acetazolamide is assured by its widespread use in glaucoma where it is used for years at doses similar to that recommended for AMS prophylaxis.

The ethics of the use of acetazolamide (or that of any drug) especially if used throughout an expedition needs consideration but in the end it is for the individual or team to decide.

The mechanism of action of acetazolamide is thought to be due to its inhibition of carbonic anhydrase rather than its diuretic action. It is quite a mild diuretic and more powerful diuretics are said to be less effective though no direct comparisons have been made in controlled trials. Interference with CO_2 transport is thought to result in intracellular acidosis, including the cells of the medullary chemoreceptor. In this way it acts as a respiratory stimulant. It has recently been shown to shift the ventilatory CO_2 response curve to the left, as happens with acclimatization (section 5.12) although it does not affect the slope. The acute effect after a single dose results in a reduction in the hypoxic ventilatory response, though with a few hours' administration this is restored (Swenson and Hughes 1993).

Acetazolamide also acts as a respiratory stimulant by promoting the excretion of bicarbonate by the kidneys, thus correcting the respiratory alkalosis due to hypoxic induced hyperventilation. In effect the subject is given an artificial respiratory acclimatization. The importance of this renal effect is suggested by Swenson *et al.* (1991) in a study in which the drug benzolamide, a selective inhibitor of renal carbonic anhydrase, reduced high altitude periodic breathing, a feature of acetazolamide use. A trial of benzolamide as a prophylactic for AMS (Collier *et al.* 1996) showed it to be beneficial compared with placebo suggesting that inhibition of cerebral carbonic anhydrase may not be the important action of acetazolamide.

Another possible mechanism is via its effect on cerebral blood flow (Vorstrup *et al.* 1984). Acetazolamide increases cerebral blood flow, which would increase cerebral PO_2. However, increased PCO_2, which has the same effect on cerebral blood flow, seems to increase the symptoms of AMS at the same level of hypoxia (section 18.5.2). Additionally, the dosage used in this study (1 g i.v.) was very large compared with that used in AMS prophylaxis.

Jensen et al. (1990) found that, although 1.5 g aceta-zolamide caused a 22% increase in cerebral blood flow after 2 h, there was no change in AMS symptoms. Also, Hackett et al. (1988a) found no change in CBF (as measured by trans-cranial Doppler ultrasound) in subjects with or without AMS after 0.25 g acetazolamide intravenously.

SPIRONOLACTONE

Jain et al. (1986) compared spironolactone with acetazolamide and placebo. They found both drugs to be effective in ameliorating AMS, with spironolactone being possibly superior. This confirms a previous uncontrolled report (Currie et al. 1976).

DEXAMETHASONE AND ASPIRIN

Dexamethasone (4 mg, every 6 h) has been tried on the grounds that it is effective in cerebral edema. In a double-blind cross-over chamber study it was found to be an effective prophylactic (Johnson et al. 1984) and was found to be superior when compared with acetazolamide (Ellsworth et al. 1991). Rock et al. (1989) carried out a dose ranging chamber experiment and concluded that 4 mg every 12 h was the minimum effective dose. The same group had previously found that, if dexamethasone was given for only 48 h after arrival at altitude, it was effective in reducing symptoms, but that after stopping the drug, symptoms of AMS began (Rock et al. 1989). The combination of acetazolamide and dexamethasone has been shown to be more effective than acetazolamide alone, especially in preventing the cerebral symptoms of AMS (Bernhard et al. 1998). Aspirin has been shown to be similarly effective as a prophylactic (Brutscher et al. 1998) but, like dexamethasone, does not affect oxygen saturation. In a later study Burtscher et al. (1999) found that aspirin alone was not very effective in preventing the headache of AMS in subjects skiing to a mountain hut, whereas aspirin in combination with dexamethasone was. There was no placebo arm in this trial.

Dexamethasone remains an excellent drug to prevent or treat AMS or early cerebral edema but, unlike acetazolamide, does not facilitate acclimatization and thus may mask symptoms of AMS or HACE. It is an important adjunctive therapy for individuals ascending rapidly to altitudes higher than 3000 m for a rescue but should never be taken as a means to mask symptoms of moderate or severe AMS or HACE while the climber continues to ascend. Dexamethasone can produce rapid resolution of symptoms, improve cognitive function (Lafleur et al. 2003) and keep patients ambulatory so that they help in their own descent and/or rescue.

OTHER DRUGS

Theophylline (300 mg) has been shown to be beneficial as a prophylactic in a placebo-controlled, double-blind trial by Kuepper et al. (1999). Fischer et al., on the other hand, in studying acetazolamide, theophylline and placebo did not find a decrease in CSF volumes with theophylline. A decrease in CSF volume was found with the other drugs which correlated with a decrease in symptoms of AMS. This drug also reduces sleep disturbance and periodic breathing, but little data are available to recommend it as an important adjunct to medications to prevent or treat AMS.

Herbal extracts have been advocated both as preventative and curative for AMS. As is usual in herbal medicine there are few good trials to guide us. However, some remedies have now been tested. An extract of *Gingko biloba* (EGb 761) was studied by Roncin et al. (1996) in a placebo-controlled trial and found to be effective as a prophylactic. Based on its anti-oxidant, rheologic effects, and stimulatory effect on NO production (Jowers et al. 2004) other studies of ginkgo biloba were spawned. One-day treatment with ginkgo prior to ascent to 4205 m showed marginal benefit of ginkgo in preventing AMS. In a head-to-head study, ginkgo was not as effective in preventing AMS as acetazolamide (Gertsch et al. 2004). Thus the initial enthusiasm for ginkgo has waned.

Coca, from the coca leaf, is very commonly taken in South America either infused as a tea or chewed. Many people are convinced of its efficacy in preventing AMS, but there seem to be no trials to confirm this.

18.7 TREATMENT OF AMS

Most cases of AMS will get better in 24–48 h with no treatment. If there is progression of symptoms to those of acute pulmonary edema, or serious cerebral edema, action is vital since these two disorders are frequently fatal in a matter of hours. Their treatment is discussed in Chapters 19 and 20, respectively.

18.7.1 Rest, acetazolamide

Rest alone often relieves the symptoms of AMS (Bärtsch et al. 1993), and this fact needs to be borne in mind in trials of therapy in AMS. Acetazolamide had been shown to be an effective treatment of AMS as well as a prophylactic (Bradwell et al. 1988, Grissom et al. 1992). The earlier study used a single large dose (1.5 g) whereas the later study used the more conventional 250 mg every 8 h. Pa,O_2 as well as symptoms were improved.

Dexamethasone was shown, in a double-blind trial, to be effective as an emergency treatment for acute AMS (Ferrazzini et al. 1987). The dosage used was 8 mg initially followed by 4 mg every 6 h. Levine et al. (1989) also found it to be effective in relieving AMS symptoms compared with placebo but it had no effect on fluid shifts, oxygenation, sleep apnea, urinary catecholamine levels, chest radiographs or perfusion scans. These findings emphasize the dictum that, in the event of HAPE or HACE, patients should be taken to lower altitude as soon as possible.

18.7.2 Aspirin, paracetamol, nonsteroidal anti-inflammatory agents, dexamethasone

For the headache of AMS, aspirin, nonsteroidal anti-inflammatory drugs, or paracetamol is often used, but there are no controlled trials, and they are often ineffective. A double-blind, placebo-controlled trial of ibuprofen (400 mg) showed it to be more effective than placebo in relieving headache (Broom et al. 1994). Keller et al. (1995) carried out a trial comparing dexamethasone with hyperbaria (in a Certec bag) for 1 h. Assessment 1 h after treatment found hyperbaria to be better, but at 11 h dexamethasone was more effective.

18.7.3 Other drugs

The possibility that the headache in AMS and in migraine might have a common mechanism stimulated a group from Heidelberg to carry out a placebo-controlled trial of sumatriptan, a 5-HT antagonist effective in migraine. Although the pooled results failed to show significant benefit, analysis of male and female subjects separately showed significant benefit in men (Utiger et al. 1999).

18.7.4 Oxygen

Oxygen may help, but frequently does not, and its use, besides being impractical in most cases, would impede acclimatization. Voluntary hyperventilation often helps and probably does promote acclimatization. Inhalation of 3% CO_2 in air has been claimed to alleviate symptoms in one study (Harvey et al. 1988) but not in another (Bärtsch et al. 1990). Both found a rise in Pa,O_2, due presumably to hyperventilation. In the latter study most subjects given air to breathe had a reduction in symptoms, indicating the importance of the placebo effect or perhaps the beneficial effect of rest.

The place of portable inflatable pressure chambers (the Gamow bag) is considered in Chapter 19.

18.8 SCORING AMS SYMPTOMS

In studies on AMS there is obviously a need to score the symptoms in some way and it is preferable for all researchers to use the same system so that results of different studies can be compared. The most complicated scoring system is the Environmental Symptom Questionnaire (ESQ) (Sampson et al. 1983). This consists of 67 questions in its ESQ-III version, many of which are overlapping and of uncertain relevance to AMS. Most workers have used more simple formats, scoring only three to five symptoms often on a scale of 0 to 3, with 0 for no symptoms and 1, 2 and 3 for mild, moderate and severe symptoms. Either an observer can administer the questionnaire to all subjects or self-assessment by each subject can be used; the two methods give similar results. A document was produced at the Lake Louise Hypoxia Symposium in 1991, which, after defining AMS, suggested a simple method of scoring along these lines. This was modified at the next Hypoxia Symposium in 1993 and is shown in Table 18.2 (Roach et al. 1993). It is important to note that one of the modifications introduced was the caveat that headache must be present for the

Table 18.2 Lake Louise consensus: scoring of AMS (From Roach *et al.* 1993)

(a) AMS self assessment. The sum of the responses is the AMS Self-report score. Headache and at least one other symptom must be present for the diagnosis of AMS. A score of 3 or more is taken as AMS. It is suggested that this part of the scoring system be always used and reported separately. The question relating to sleep will not always be relevant, eg. in short one day studies or in evening assessment when twice daily scoring is used.

Symptom	Scoring	
1. Headache	0	None at all
	1	Mild headache
	2	Moderate headache
	3	Severe headache, incapacitating
2. Gastrointestinal symptoms	0	Good appetite
	1	Poor appetite or nausea
	2	Moderate nausea or vomiting
	3	Severe, incapacitating nausea and vomiting
3. Fatigue and/or weakness	0	Not tired or weak
	1	Mild fatigue/weakness
	2	Moderate fatigue/weakness
	3	Severe fatigue/weakness
4. Dizziness/light-headedness	0	None
	1	Mild
	2	Moderate
	3	Severe, incapacitating
5. Difficulty sleeping	0	Slept as well as usual
	1	Did not sleep as well as usual
	2	Woke many times, poor night's sleep
	3	Could not sleep at all

(b) Clinical assessment. This portion of the scoring system contains information gained by examination. The Clinical Assessment score is the sum of scores in the following three questions.

Sign	Scoring	
Change in mental status	0	No change
	1	Lethargy/lassitude
	2	Disorientated/confused
	3	Stupor/semiconscious
	4	Coma
Ataxia (heel/toe walking)	0	None
	1	Balancing manoeuvres
	2	Steps off the line
	3	Falls down
	4	Unable to stand
Peripheral edema	0	None
	1	One location
	2	Two or more locations

(c) Functional score. The functional consequences of the AMS Self-reported score should be further evaluated by one optional question asked after the AMS self-report questionnaire. Alternatively, this question may be asked by the examiner if clinical assessment is performed.

Overall, if you had any of these symptoms, how did they affect your activities?	0	Not at all
	1	Mild reduction
	2	Moderate reduction
	3	Severe reduction (e.g. bedrest)

diagnosis, as well as at least one other of the symptoms listed. The importance of insisting that headache is present for the diagnosis is illustrated by a paper comparing a previous system (Hackett's) with the Lake Louise system (Roeggla *et al.* 1996). It was found that the Lake Louise system gave a spuriously high incidence, 25%, compared with 8% using the Hackett system, at the moderate altitude of 2940 m. Unfortunately, the authors used the earlier 1991 version. Only 9% of their subjects had headache. Had they excluded from the diagnosis subjects without headache the two systems would have given almost identical results.

There have been a number of studies comparing the ESQ with the Lake Louise system. Bärtsch *et al.* (1993) did just this and found the percentages of subjects diagnosed as having AMS in Alpine huts at four altitudes was comparable whichever system was used. Maggiorini *et al.* (1998) applied questionnaires to 490 climbers in alpine huts up to 4559 m. Using a Lake Louise score of 4 or more as the cut-off, they found a sensitivity of 78% and specificity of 93% compared with the ESQ AMS-C. Ellsworth *et al.* (1991) found similar results in 400 climbers on Mount Rainier. The Lake Louise system being much simpler is, therefore, to be preferred.

There remains the question of the score at which AMS is said to be present. On the self-report section,

five questions yield a possible top score of 15. The consensus report suggests a score of 3 or more (with headache) be deemed AMS, though from the study quoted above a score of 4 or more seemed to give better sensitivity and specificity. It is not clear what is to be done with the other two parts of the assessment, the clinical and functional scores, if they are used. Clearly, if these scores are added to the self-reported scores a greater cut of value would be appropriate. In the paper by Bärtsch *et al.* (1993) a figure of >5 for the total Lake Louise score was suggested. Until more data are available on the other parts of the assessment, reliance should be placed mainly on the self-reported score, which has been well validated.

These systems have all addressed the situation in adults. The diagnosis of AMS in children presents especial problems. Children too young to express their symptoms verbally may be irritable, miserable, tearful and refuse food. This behavior is even more nonspecific than symptoms in adults. The only safe course is to assume that this behavior in a child who has gained altitude in the previous hours or days indicates AMS until proved otherwise. Yaron *et al.* (1998) have addressed the problem of scoring AMS in pre-verbal children. They devised a 'fussiness' scale derived from the Lake Louise system. For more details of this see Chapter 28.

High altitude cerebral edema

SUMMARY

High altitude cerebral edema (HACE) is a severe form of acute mountain sickness (AMS) characterized by the same symptoms, headache, malaise and fatigue which can progress to ataxia, altered consciousness, hallucinations, coma and death. Signs include papilledema, extensor plantar responses and other neurological signs. There may be mild fever, cyanosis, increased pulse and respiratory rates. Computerized tomography (CT) and post-mortem appearance indicate cerebral edema, and magnetic resonance imaging (MRI) scans show lesions in the splenium and corpus callosum. In untreated cases remaining at altitude, death can occur in a few hours or days.

The incidence of HACE is less than for HAPE, usually occurs at a higher altitude, but many patients have a mixed picture with signs and symptoms of both conditions.

Prevention of HACE is the same as for AMS; that is, to make a slow ascent to altitude and to descend if symptoms do not improve. The diagnosis is made on the history and clinical examination. In a patient with symptoms of AMS, if any neurological signs appear or if there is any clouding of consciousness or hallucinations, then HACE is the likely diagnosis. Often the earliest sign is ataxia, which is easily missed in a patient lying in a tent with a headache especially as he may be irritable, and insist that he is all right.

The most important action in treatment, as in HAPE, is to get the patient down. If this is impossible or while awaiting evacuation, oxygen, if available, will help. Dexamethasone 4–8 mg initially, followed by 4 mg every 6 h often relieves the neurological symptoms and signs, and treatment in a portable compression bag (Gamow or Certec) is also beneficial, at least for a few hours. Recovery is often rapid on descent, but a number of cases have been described in which recovery was delayed by days or weeks, and, of course, some victims die regardless of descent or medication.

The mechanism of development of cerebral edema is not understood. It is probably the same as in AMS at first, but instead of being self-limited, it progresses to an advanced stage giving rise to the signs and symptoms described and eventually to death. The consensus at present is that the edema is vasogenic in origin with an increase in the permeability of the blood–brain barrier. Various hypotheses have been advanced to account for this and are discussed.

19.1 INTRODUCTION

The symptoms of acute mountain sickness (AMS) are probably due to mild cerebral edema, which, though unpleasant, are not serious. In a small minority of cases, usually at altitudes higher than 3500 m, the condition progresses to more severe symptoms. Unmistakable signs of cerebral edema and increased intracranial pressure become manifest and progress to coma. Death can occur if the patient is not treated and has been reported even if descent or other interventions have been initiated. This severe form of AMS is called high altitude cerebral edema (HACE).

Ravenhill (1913) called the condition '*puna* of a nervous type'. He describes three cases who recovered on being sent down to low altitude. As with acute pulmonary edema of high altitude, his work was forgotten, and it was only during the 1960s that description of this serious form of acute cerebral edema of high altitude emerged (e.g. Singh *et al.* 1969).

19.2 CLINICAL PRESENTATION

19.2.1 Epidemiology

Symptoms of AMS usually precede HACE (Chapter 18). HACE can occur in unacclimatized individuals usually at 3000 m or higher. Because of difficulty in knowing the number of people exposed, its incidence has never been accurately determined, but HACE certainly is much less common than AMS or HAPE. A 1% incidence in trekkers in Nepal between 4200 and 5500 m was reported by Hackett *et al.* (1976). An extraordinarily high incidence of 31% was reported by Basynat *et al.* (2000) in a group of pilgrims who ascended rapidly in Nepal. Often HACE and HAPE may co-exist (Yarnell *et al.* 2000). Symptoms of stupor and coma were described in 13% of 52 patients with HAPE (Gabry *et al.* 2003) which is similar to the findings of Hultgren *et al.* (1996) in the Canadian Rockies. Sometimes in HAPE, the severity of hypoxemia is so great that it is difficult to know whether the symptoms are secondary to cerebral edema or the effects of hypoxemia.

The age and sex distribution, like that for AMS, shows no group to be immune. Possibly the younger male is rather more at risk, perhaps because he is more likely to push on to higher altitude with symptoms, a feature of many histories in fatal cases. People native to high altitude can become victims of HACE. The impression is that the incidence in them is lower but there are no good published data.

19.2.2 Symptoms and signs

Symptoms of AMS usually precede those of HACE by 24–36 h, but the presence of milder cerebral edema before the progression to HACE has not been confirmed (Fischer *et al.* 2004.) Headache, loss of appetite, nausea, vomiting and photophobia are common. Climbing performance decreases dramatically, and in fact, patients may just stop any activity and become irritable and withdrawn and wish only to be left alone. Behavior may become bizarre and irrational, and survival instincts cease. The clinical transition from AMS to HACE is often difficult to ascertain, but the appearance of ataxia, irrationality, hallucinations or clouding of consciousness should alert one to the likelihood that the patient now has HACE. The patient may report blurring of vision which may be due to retinal hemorrhages or to papilledema. Deep-tendon reflexes may be brisk, and later the plantar reflexes may become extensor. There may be ocular muscle paralysis with diplopia. The pulse is often rapid, and cyanosis usual.

As the condition progresses, all symptoms and signs become more evident. The headache becomes worse, and ataxia intensifies so that the patient can no longer sit up (truncal ataxia) or walk in a coordinated manner. If coma ensues, breathing becomes irregular. Death may come in a few hours or in a day or two in untreated cases. Residual and permanent neurologic impairment, including dementia (Usui *et al.* 2004), have been reported.

Although with a recent ascent to high altitudes greater than 3000 m and the symptoms described above, good clinical evaluation must be made, as many of the symptoms are nonspecific and may be secondary to many other conditions including structural (tumors), psychiatric (psychosis), metabolic (hypoglycemia, ketoacidosis, hyponatremia), toxic (ingestions), epileptic (Firth and Bolay 2004, Daleau *et al.* 2006), or cerebro-vascular (stroke, hemorrhage, migraine) abnormalities.

19.2.3 Case histories

CASE 1 (HOUSTON AND DICKINSON 1975)

A 39-year-old Japanese female flew from 1500 m to 2750 m, and during the next 2 days, climbed to 3500 m, where she developed a severe headache.

On day 4, at 3800 m, she began to vomit. On day 5, at 3 960 m, she became breathless and weak, was vomiting and needed assistance to walk. On day 6 she lost consciousness and was carried down to 3 350 m where she was found to be deeply unconscious and cyanosed, with a temperature of 40.6°C and a pulse of 140 beats min^{-1}. Crackles filled the chest. Reflexes were brisk and plantars flexor. Slight papilledema was present. She was treated with oxygen, furosemide and penicillin. On day 8 she was flown to a hospital at 1500 m where she was found to be in the same condition but with extensor plantar reflexes. Lumbar puncture showed a pressure of 270 mm H_2O, but examination of the CSF was normal. She slowly improved over 2 weeks and eventually recovered completely.

Comment. The symptoms of HACE are dominant in this case but the patient also had signs of HAPE.

CASE 2 (DICKINSON *ET AL.* 1983)

A 46-year-old man trekked from 1500 m to 3650 in 2 days. On the way he began to feel unwell, was tired, anorexic and later began to vomit. At 3650 m he became unconscious and was evacuated to a hospital at 1500 m. On examination he was deeply unconscious, responding only to pain. He was cyanosed and hyperventilating. There were crackles and wheezes in the lungs; papilledema and retinal haemorrhage were present. Respirations were 40 breaths min^{-1}, the pulse was 120 beats min^{-1}, and the temperature 40°C. He remained unconsciousness and died after 4 days in the hospital.

Comment. This is a typical case of HACE, which seemed to have reached an irreversible stage before descent.

CASE 3 (HOUSTON AND DICKINSON 1975)

A 42-year-old fit man reached 3600 m from sea level in a few days. He spent 2 days at this altitude and on day 3 climbed to 4940 m, returning to sleep at 3960 m. On day 4, after carrying about 25 kg to 4940 m, he complained of severe headache, and went to sleep on arrival at the camp. Next morning he was confused and unable to talk coherently. He could not coordinate hand and foot movements and was disorientated in time and space. He was carried down to 3600 m where he became coherent

and was able to walk without assistance. He was given an intramuscular steroid and by late afternoon seemed normal. The next day he was taken down to 2130 m where he was completely normal.

Comment. A typical case of HACE where prompt action in bringing the patient down saved his life.

CASE 4 (ABRIDGED FROM HOWARTH 1999)

A 42-year-old member of a scientific expedition had trekked to Kangchenjunga Base Camp (5100 m) and spent a week at this altitude including climbing twice to about 5400 m on day outings. He had had no sickness during all this time. With three companions he set out to climb a 6200 m peak on the return trek. On the first day from Base Camp their porters took the wrong route to their intended camp at 5500 m necessitating some climbing over very rough ground. During the early part of the day the patient had been going strongly, but later he was slow and reached camp at 2.45 p.m., cold and exhausted. He complained of a bad headache but took some hot soup and painkillers. AMS was diagnosed, and it was hoped he would improve with rest. However, over the next 2 h he deteriorated and became ataxic. He was given acetazolamide and dexamethasone but vomited most of the tablets. Evacuation was started, but it required a man on each side to support him and over the boulder-strewn ground, going was very slow. He continued to deteriorate, and they had to stop for rest every 20 yards or so. The party was benighted but fortunately was able to radio other members of the expedition for help. The rescue party met them with oxygen and injectable dexamethasone after which the patient improved though descent over now steepening scree was still very slow. A temporary camp at about 4900 m was reached at 11.30 p.m. By next morning the patient was much better, and during the day was able to walk slowly back to Base Camp.

Comment. This case illustrates the unpredictability of AMS in that typical HACE developed in a climber who would seem to have acclimatized well. In some subjects who have no problems up to a certain point there seems to be a critical altitude above which they quite abruptly start having symptoms. It also emphasizes the importance of making an early diagnosis and getting the patient down as soon as possible, easier with hindsight of course.

19.2.4 Investigations

Unless the case of presumed HACE is, in fact, another condition, such as mentioned in section 20.2.2, blood counts and biochemistries are usually normal, but white counts may be high. Chest radiographs may show evidence of concomitant pulmonary edema. Although normally not necessary to perform except to rule out a CNS infection or hemorrhage, lumbar punctures show raised pressures, 44–220 mmH$_2$O, (Singh *et al.* 1969, Houston and Dickinson 1975), but normal CSF chemistries and cell counts. Computerized tomographic scanning of the brain in 12 patients with HAPE and HACE (Koyama *et al.* 1984) showed evidence of cerebral edema with diffuse low density of the entire cerebrum and compression of the ventricles. Recovery to normal CT findings occurred within a week in three cases, but abnormal findings persisted for 1–2 weeks in two cases; one case took over a month to clear.

Hackett *et al.* (1998) reported MRI scans in nine patients with HACE compared with three with HAPE and three who had been to altitude with no illness. They found intense T$_2$ signals in white matter, especially in the splenium and corpus callosum in the subjects with HACE. There were no lesions in the grey matter (Fig. 19.1). With this one study, there was no correlation between the severity of edema on imaging and the subsequent clinical course.

19.2.5 Treatment

The treatment for HACE is very similar to that for HAPE. Get the patient down to lower altitude as soon as possible, especially before their condition renders them unable to care for themselves. Recognizing the symptoms early while the victim is still ambulatory may mean the difference between a successful descent, with recovery, and death on the mountain. Whilst awaiting evacuation, oxygen therapy is advised but often is only of marginal benefit. Dexamethasone has been shown to be of benefit in a double-blind, randomized, placebo-controlled trial in AMS (Ferrazzini *et al.* 1987). It is particularly the cerebral symptoms which seem to be helped by this drug, so it is a critical drug to have available and use in this situation. The dose utilized in the trial was 8 mg initially, followed by 4 mg every 6 h. Enthusiasm for dexamethasone should be tempered by the finding that, although symptoms are relieved, the physiological abnormalities (fluid shifts, oxygenation, sleep apnea, urinary catecholamine levels, chest radiograph, perfusion scans and the results of psychomotor tests) are not improved (Levine *et al.* 1989). The drug is no substitute for descent.

Some authors have recommended diuretics, but the delicate balance between cerebral perfusion and pre-existing hypovolemia in the mountains accentuated by diuresis is a risk not worth taking in the field setting. Once in the hospital setting where monitoring is possible, the usual measures taken to decrease intracerebral edema (mannitol, hypertonic saline, etc.) are reasonable.

Portable hyperbaric bags (Gamow bags) are now available, and their use in HAPE is discussed in Chapter 20. In HACE, their use is less well documented (Freeman *et al.* 2004); but, if available

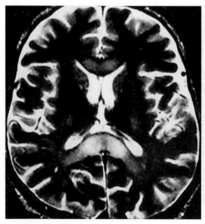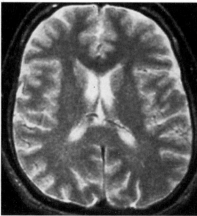

Figure 19.1 Left, Axial T2-weighted magnetic resonance image of patient showing markedly increased signal in corpus callosum (arrows), including both the genu and the splenium, as well as increased signal of periventricular and subcortical white matter.

and if descent is necessarily delayed, a hyperbaric bag should be tried. Their use may have therapeutic benefit and make it possible for a patient to descend unaided, instead of having to be carried. Recovery after descent may not be as rapid as is usually the recovery from HAPE (Dickinson 1979, and Cases 1 and 2). Some reports detail recoveries from 2 to 14 days or even longer (6 weeks; Hackett *et al.* 1998) with some reports of persistent neurologic impairment. Better education about altitude maladies (Vardy *et al.* 2005) and the increasing availability of helicopter rescue in remote areas of the Himalaya (Graham and Basynat 2001) are improving the outcomes of HACE and other altitude illnesses.

19.2.6 Post-mortem appearance

There have been a few reports of post-mortems in HACE (Singh *et al.* 1969, Houston and Dickinson 1975, Dickinson *et al.* 1983). The usual findings in the brain are of cerebral edema with swollen, flattened gyri, and compression of the sulci. There may be herniation of the cerebellar tonsils and unci. Spongiosis, especially in the white matter, may be marked. In many cases there are widespread petechial hemorrhages; in some there are ante-mortem thrombi in the venous sinuses, or there may be subarachnoid hemorrhages. There seems to be considerable variation in the findings. It must always be remembered that the few cases that reach autopsy are highly selected and may be unrepresentative of the condition as seen clinically in the field.

19.3 MECHANISMS OF HACE

19.3.1 Cytotoxic versus vasogenic edema

The mechanism for the development of cerebral edema at altitude is reviewed in Chapter 18, and there may be many responses of edema formation which AMS and HACE have in common. There is agreement that hypoxia induces an increase in extracellular fluid. It may also cause increased microvascular permeability. The images on MRI suggest that the leak is vasogenic in origin, i.e. an increase in permeability of the vascular endothelium, but these findings do not differentiate between a leak caused by increased pressures or factors such as inflammation that increase the vulnerability of the endothelial lining.

Cytotoxic edema results from hypoxic-induced failure of cellular ion pumps with a rise in intracellular sodium and osmolarity and consequent cellular swelling from an influx of water (Fishman 1975). Membrane failure from cytotoxic causes was, for some time, touted as a possible cause of HACE, but the degree of hypoxia and/or ischemia to cause such membrane dysfunction is much greater than one would see in most altitude settings. Thus, the hypothesis that failure of the membrane pumps leads to cellular permeability has, for many years, not been felt to be the initiating mechanism of HACE.

19.3.2 Cerebral blood flow

An inordinate increase in cerebral blood flow would seem a likely culprit, leading to cerebro-vascular damage and subsequent leak of fluid from the intra- to extravascular space. Hypoxia increases cerebral blood flow (Severinghaus *et al.* 1966), particularly when there is no marked reduction in P_{CO_2}. The usual increase in alveolar ventilation upon ascent to altitude and the resulting hypocapnia lead to cerebral vasoconstriction. The body's response upon rapid ascent, though, is to optimize blood flow and oxygen delivery such that the increase in cerebral blood flow from hypoxia over-rides the vasoconstriction from the hypocapnia.

Attempts to find a correlation between AMS and HACE and cerebral blood flow have not been consistent. While Baumgartner *et al.* (1994) found a correlation between CBF and AMS, Jensen *et al.* (1990) found none. Furthermore, a doubling of CBF by hypercapnia in sheep did not cause brain edema (Yang *et al.* 1994). These same factors may become more pronounced to cause the symptoms of HACE, but that theory is mere speculation.

In an attempt to find a relationship between autoregulation of CBF with hypoxia and systemic blood pressure, Jansen *et al.* (2000) studied subjects at low altitude and Sherpas who had not experienced HACE and sojourners at high altitude and found an inconsistent decrease or maintenance of autoregulation of CBF in response to hypoxia and an increase in SBP raised by phenylephrine in all groups. Thus it does not seem likely that one could

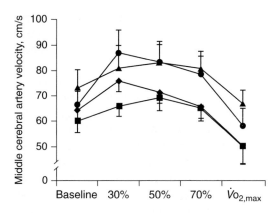

Figure 19.2 Changes in middle cerebral artery blood velocity during exercise at different altitudes (■, 150 m; ◆, 3610 m; ●, 4750 m; ▲, 5260 m). Values are means and SE. Velocity at rest increased with increasing altitude ($P < 0.05$). At all altitudes, velocity increased during submaximal exercise ($P < 0.05$–0.0001) but fell at maximal oxygen uptake ($\dot{V}_{O_2,max}$; $P < 0.01$–0.0001).

base an etiology for the mechanism of HACE on normal autoregulation of CBF. On the other hand, a subsequent study in subjects rapidly ascending to 4559 m showed a correlation between CBF, Sa_{O_2}, and AMS scores (Van Osta *et al.* 2005).

Imray *et al.* (2005) found intriguing results when they measured cerebral perfusion and oxygenation in unacclimatized subjects at 150 and 5260 m during progressive exercise. Whereas cerebral oxygenation was maintained throughout exercise at low altitude, at high altitude it increased up to 30% of maximal exercise and then fell progressively as the exercise intensity increased (Fig. 19.2). The authors speculate that this phenomenon may contribute not only to performance at high altitude but also to the brain's vulnerability to edema. There clearly needs to be more work done in this area.

19.3.3 Cranial vault capacity

The question of why certain individuals are susceptible while others are not is as puzzling in HACE as in other forms of AMS. One possible factor might be the relative sizes of the brain and cranial cavity. In a recent review of etiology, Hackett (1999) discusses this 'tight fit' hypothesis. Those with a tight fit brain in the box of their cranial cavity will have a greater rise in pressure for a given increase in fluid volume in the brain. Those with looser brains

are less susceptible. As we get older our brains shrink which may be why older people are less susceptible to AMS and HACE. More data are necessary to make this hypothesis stronger.

19.3.4 Venous thrombosis

Venous thrombosis has been found on CT scan in one patient (Asaji *et al.* 1984) and in some postmortem studies of HACE. It may develop late in the condition as a consequence of intracranial hypertension. It will certainly exacerbate the condition.

19.3.5 Vascular endothelial growth factor

Severinghaus (1995) suggested that vascular permeability, operating in situations of angiogenesis and induced by vascular endothelial growth factor (VEGF), may be involved in HACE. Hypoxia stimulates the release of transforming growth factor which attracts macrophages. These, in turn, release VEGF and other factors which eventually give rise to growth of new capillaries. The more immediate effect is to increase capillary permeability as capillary basement membranes are broken down. He suggests that even earlier than these events, hypoxia may case osmotic brain swelling. Dexamethasone is very effective in preventing angiogenesis, and it may be this action which explains its effectiveness in HACE. This theory received support from the finding of VEGF mRNA in rat brains after only 3 h of hypoxia (Figure 19.3). The level reached a peak of three times control at 12–24 h (Xu and Severinghaus 1998). This could explain the increased permeability of the blood–brain barrier and the vasogenic edema.

Two studies lend credence to this theory. Schoch *et al.* (2002) found increased VEGF expression and increased vascular permeability, as measured with a fluorescein marker in mice brains, which correlated with the degree of hypoxic exposure which was prevented by inhibition of VEGF activity (Fig. 19.4). By measuring free VEGF upon acute ascent to 4300 m, investigators found a correlation between free VEGF and AMS symptoms (Tissot van Patot *et al.* 2005). These studies are strongly suggestive of induction of vascular permeability by VEGF in its response and attempt to initiate angiogenesis secondary to an hypoxic stimulus.

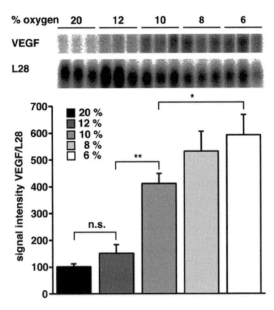

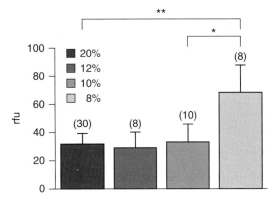

Figure 19.3 Increased expression of VEGF mRNA in mouse brain after hypoxic stimulation. Total RNA was extracted from brains of normal mice and mice exposed to 6–12% oxygen for 24 h. (*Upper panel*) Northern blots of total RNA sequentially hybridized with a ^{32}P-labelled probe for murine VEGF and the ribosomal protein L28. (*Lower panel*) Mean and standard deviation ($n = 3$) of VEGF mRNA pixel densities as quantified with a Phosphoimager and corrected for L28. Normoxic control was set to 100%. **$P < 0.001$; *$P < 0.05$; n.s., not significant.

Figure 19.4 Two-fold increase in vascular permeability after exposure to 8% oxygen. Sodium fluorescein injected intravenously in controls or hypoxic mice was quantified following homogenization of brain hemispheres. Results are expressed as relative fluorescence units (r.f.u.). Values are mean and standard deviation. **$P < 0.0001$; *$P < 0.001$; $n = 8$–30 as indicated.

19.3.6 Nitric oxide and cerebral edema

Clark (1999) suggested that the mechanism of cerebral edema in HACE may be via the induction of inducible nitric oxide synthase (iNOS) in the brain by hypoxia. This gives rise to increased levels of nitric oxide (NO) which by increasing vascular permeability causes edema. In most cases this is quite mild and self-limiting giving rise to the symptoms of benign AMS. However, if there are even low levels of cytokines as well, due to a mild infection for instance, there will be a synergistic effect on iNOS induction and permeability. This results in HACE.

20

High altitude pulmonary edema

SUMMARY

High altitude pulmonary edema (HAPE) is a potentially lethal form of mountain sickness which, like acute mountain sickness (AMS), affects previously healthy persons who go rapidly to high altitude. A few hours after arrival patients suffer the usual symptoms of AMS but then become more breathless than their companions. Over the next few hours the breathlessness increases, a cough develops which is first dry but later productive of frothy white sputum. The sputum may become blood-tinged. The signs of obvious pulmonary edema are found and cyanosis may be detected. Some patients literally drown in their own secretions and become comatose and can die if no action is taken. Patients have tachycardia and tachypnea with mild pyrexia and leucocytosis and a characteristic X-ray appearance. The pathology, in fatal cases, is of patchy edema of the lungs.

The most important management is to get the patient down; if there is unavoidable delay, oxygen, if available, and drugs which vasodilate the pulmonary vasculature are helpful. If descent is not feasible, hyperbaric treatment in a Gamow (or Certec) bag gives temporary relief and may be useful in enabling a patient to improve and walk down rather than having to be carried.

The mechanism of the edema formation is not left ventricular failure since wedge pressures on cardiac catheterization are normal. However, there is severe pulmonary hypertension. There are a number of hypotheses about how this results in edema. The most favored mechanism is that the hypoxic vaso-constriction is uneven. Vessels which are not downstream from the constricted vessels are exposed to higher pressures which suffer stress failure of these vessels allowing proteins and later blood cells to leak out into the interstitial space and then alveolar spaces. Later, there is evidence of inflammation, as cytokines and arachidonic acid metabolites are found in the edema fluid, and these contribute to the vascular leakage. Exercise seems to be a risk factor presumably by raising the pulmonary artery pressure.

Many patients who suffer HAPE show susceptibility to the condition on subsequent altitude exposure. These subjects are found to have a brisk hypoxic pressor response in their pulmonary circulation and it is thought that this susceptibility may have a genetic origin.

20.1 INTRODUCTION

There are a number of accounts in the early climbing literature of climbers dying of 'pneumonia'. In retrospect many, if not most, of these fatalities were probably due to high altitude pulmonary edema (HAPE). One of the best known was the death of Dr Jacottet on Mont Blanc in 1891. He died in the

Vallot hut (4300 m) after taking part in a rescue on the mountain. Refusing to go down, he spent a further two nights in the hut with obvious symptoms of acute mountain sickness (AMS). He died during the second night. The post-mortem showed 'acute edema of the lung' (*oedéme considerable*) (Mosso 1898).

In 1913, Ravenhill described what he called *puna* of the cardiac type as a lethal form or development of AMS. Though he was wrong in attributing the condition to cardiac failure, his description of three cases fits well with HAPE. However, his work was forgotten.

For the first half of the twentieth century the condition would not be at all common in the European Alps, because few unacclimatized people spent nights above 2500 m or in the Himalaya where approach marches to the mountains were long enough for acclimatization to take place. But in South America, as Ravenhill's experience showed, railways and later roads had been built to altitude up to 3000 or 4000 m, thus putting large numbers of people at risk. However, even in these countries the condition does not seem to have been recognized for many years after Ravenhill. West (1998) has unearthed a description of a case reported by Alberto Hurtado in 1937 in an obscure booklet. But the case is atypical in a number of ways and Hurtado says (in translation from the Spanish),

> this is undoubtedly a type of Soroche (mountain sickness) which is quite rare and infrequent and is characterized by intense congestion and edema of the lung. Possibly there is in these cases a prior cardiac condition....

This case also had further long-term problems suggestive of a cardiac condition. Although this could be considered as the first case report of HAPE after Ravenhill, there was mention of some cases of soroche who had cough with frothy pink sputum and who made a rapid recovery on descent to low altitude. This was in an article by Harold Crane, the chief surgeon of a hospital at the mining town of Oroya (3750 m) in Peru. The article was published in the *Annals of the Faculty of Medicine*, Lima in 1927. The first series of cases (seven) to be published was by Leoncio Lizárraga Morla in 1955 in the same journal. He mentioned that the condition

was recognized by Carlos Monge M. as early as 1927. The cases described were typical of HAPE and included chest X-rays and ECGs typical of HAPE. This paper was followed by others, including Bardáles, from Peru in the later 1950s. The first reference in English to the condition we now call HAPE was in a letter to the *Journal of the American Medical Association* by Bardáles in 1956. In it he describes the condition briefly in high altitude residents returning to altitude, saying it is particularly common in young people. For a fuller description of these papers and the full references, see West (1998).

An interesting side light showing the situation in the English-speaking world in the mid 1950s is given by a letter to Dr Griffith Pugh which he published with a comment in *The Practitioner* (Pugh 1955). Dr Pugh was the leading authority on altitude medicine and physiology in UK at the time. The letter gave an excellent account of a fatal case of HAPE and asked whether acute pulmonary edema is a common symptom of high altitude sickness. Pugh, in his response, indicates that he knew of no such case from his experience or from the literature. The original letter and response together with a commentary are to be found in West (1999).

Herbert Hultgren visited Peru in 1959 and saw cases of HAPE. He and his companion Spickard wrote up their experiences in the *Stanford Medical Bulletin* published in May 1960 under the title, 'Medical Experiences in Peru'. In it they mention 41 cases of acute pulmonary edema in residents returning to altitude after a stay of 5–21 days at low altitude. They correctly suggested that the mechanism was not left ventricular failure but related to pulmonary hypertension. Not surprisingly, this important observation was not recognized at the time and so the condition was brought to the notice of the English-speaking medical world by Houston (1960) who published his landmark paper on 'acute pulmonary edema of high altitude' later in the same year in the *New England Journal of Medicine*. Houston said 'this single case is presented in the hope of stimulating further reports' and 'pulmonary edema of high altitude deserves further study'. Both hope and declaration have been amply fulfilled in the succeeding years by the description of hundreds of cases from all the major mountainous areas and hundreds of studies aimed at elucidating the mechanism of the condition have been conducted, some of which will be reviewed in this chapter.

20.2 CLINICAL PRESENTATION

HAPE, like AMS, affects previously healthy individuals on ascent to altitude and often presents in the absence of AMS. There is a wide range of altitude of presentation from 2000 to 7000 m (Lobenhoffer *et al.* 1982). A typical history is that the subject ascends rapidly to altitude and is very active getting there or on arrival. The subject suffers the symptoms of AMS after arrival, though not necessarily very severely, and then becomes more short of breath and lethargic. The patient may experience chest pain. Physical signs are of tachycardia, tachypnea and crackles at the lung bases. A dry cough develops which later progresses to one productive of frothy white and eventually blood-tinged sputum. Over a few hours the condition progresses with increasing respiratory distress, orthopnoea, cyanosis, bubbling respirations, coma and death.

20.2.1 Case histories

CASE 1 (HOUSTON 1960)

A male patient left sea level, reaching 5090 m by car and on foot 5 days later. He had no symptoms until 1 day later when he noted dyspnea progressing to severe orthopnea. Within a few hours his breathing became progressively more congested and labored. He sounded as though he was literally drowning in his own fluid with an almost continuous loud bubbling sound as if breathing through liquid. A white froth resembling cotton candy had appeared to well up out of his mouth, which was open. This was even though he was sitting up with his head tilted back. The patient died within 8 h of the onset of symptoms.

CASE 2

A Sherpa on a large expedition had carried a load from 6400 m to 7000 m and returned. The following morning he complained of severe headache and malaise. He was anorexic and remained in his sleeping bag. On examination at mid-morning he was found to be cyanosed and breathless on the slightest exertion, and he had a dry cough. His pulse and respiratory rate were increased. Fine crackles were heard at the lung bases. At noon he started down for a lower camp at 5800 m accompanied by two expedition members. It was at once apparent that he could not carry even a light load. Every 100–200 m he had to stop even though the route was over an easy downhill glacier. He began coughing frothy white sputum, which later became blood-tinged. At about 100 m above the camp he was given oxygen and was able to complete the journey without stopping. After breathing oxygen for about 3 h at the camp he declared himself well and refused any more oxygen. He descended unaided to a lower camp next day, carrying a load.

CASE 3

A 20-year-old college student from Chicago flew in the morning to Denver, Colorado, and drove that afternoon from the airport to the Keystone Ski resort in Summit County (3000 m) where he was going to spend the week skiing. By mid-afternoon, he was skiing at 3700 m. That night he developed a headache which progressed to malaise, dyspnea and a dry cough which by morning had progressed to one with frothy sputum. He could not sleep and went to the resort clinic where he was found by pulse oximeter to have an oxygen saturation of 70%. His examination revealed crackles, a tachycardia, cyanosis and tachypnea. Application of $3 \, L \, min^{-1}$ flow of oxygen by nasal prongs resulted in a rise in his oxygen saturation to 91%. He was sent to his hotel room with oxygen therapy with his family. Emergency medical help was available 24 h each day. He was seen daily in the clinic and had improved by the fourth day such that he was able to ski the last 3 days of his vacation.

20.2.2 Incidence

Because of the problem of knowing the number of people at risk, it is difficult to obtain data on the incidence of HAPE. As with AMS, its incidence will depend upon the rate of ascent and the height reached. Hackett and Rennie (1976) saw seven cases in 278 trekkers who passed through Pheriche (4243 m) on their way to Everest Base Camp, giving an incidence of 2.5%. The incidence of AMS in the same group was 53%. Menon (1965) found an incidence of 0.57% in Indian troops flown to the modest altitude of Leh (3500 m). Hultgren and Marticorena (1978) gave an incidence of 0.6% in adults going to La Oroya, 3750 m. In these series a diagnosis was only made in clear, overt cases. If the chests of all new-comers to altitude are auscultated, crackles will be heard in many who would not be otherwise diagnosed as HAPE, and radiographic signs are also found on chest X-ray in many subjects after intense exercise (Anholm *et al.* 1999, Cremona *et al.* 2002). Hence, we now believe that a degree of subclinical edema is probably present in subjects with and without simple AMS which contributes to the reduced Sa,O_2 (section 18.4.8). However, in simple AMS or in subjects without any symptoms of altitude illness, the edema is self-limiting; whereas in HAPE it is progressive.

The incidence will be affected by health education of people going to altitude. It is the impression of health workers at the aid post at Pheriche (4243 m) that the incidence is less following some years of publicity about the dangers of HAPE amongst trekkers and the trekking agencies.

20.2.3 Symptoms of HAPE

Table 20.1 shows the symptoms from the largest series managed by a single physician (Menon 1965) who reported 101 cases. The frequency of chest pain, second only to breathlessness is unusually high. Only 21% of patients complained of chest pain in a German series (Lobenhoffer *et al.* 1982). Hallucinations are not uncommon and, with confusion and irrational behavior, may make management difficult. Nocturnal dyspnea and the symptoms of AMS – headache, nausea and insomnia – are all common, and almost all patients have marked limitation in their exercise capabilities.

Table 20.1 High-altitude pulmonary edema: symptoms in 101 cases (Menon 1965)

Symptom	No. of cases
Breathlessness	84
Chest pain	66
Headache	63
Nocturnal dyspnea	59
Dry cough	51
Hemoptysis	39
Nausea	26
Insomnia	23
Dizziness	18

20.2.4 Signs

These depend upon the stage of the condition. Probably the earliest signs are crackles at the lung bases and tachycardia although the former is not always reliable. Crackles may be heard in subjects who have no other signs of HAPE and who do not progress to the full blown condition (Maggiorini 2006). The presence of early edema may be the cause of dry cough on exertion and of the shift to the left of the pressure/volume curve of the lung (Mansell *et al.* 1980, Gautier *et al.* 1982), the reduction in forced vital capacity (Welsh *et al.* 1993, Fischer *et al.* 2005), and the increase in closing volumes (Cremona *et al.* 2002). The pulse rate increases early and was over 120 in 70 of 101 patients in Menon's series (1965). The respiratory rate was over 30 in 69 cases; cyanosis was detected in 52 subjects.

The pulmonary artery pressure is high in this condition (section 20.2.7) giving the signs of right ventricular heave and accentuated pulmonary second sound in about half the patients. Signs of right ventricular failure are not prominent but 15 of Menon's patients had raised jugular venous pressure and dependent edema is found in a number of cases. The temperature is normal in at least 25% of cases but was found to be mildly elevated (37–39°C) in 70% of Menon's cases. In only two cases was it above 39°C. Maggiorini *et al.* (1997) found temperature to be elevated by a mean of 0.8°C compared with climbers without HAPE. The systemic blood pressure is either normal or mildly elevated (systolic 130–140 mmHg) as is found in some subjects on ascent to altitude who do not have HAPE.

Some subjects (15 in Menon's series) have mental confusion and amnesia following recovery. This may be due to hypoxia or cerebral edema (Chapter 19).

20.2.5 Radiology

A number of studies have reported patchy infiltrates (Hultgrem and Spickard 1960, Menon 1965, Vock *et al.* 1989, Vock *et al.* 1991, Koizumi *et al.* 1994).

Figure 20.1 shows a chest radiograph of a patient with HAPE and a second radiograph 4 days later after treatment. The typical features are of cotton wool blotches irregularly positioned in both lung fields, best seen by computerized tomography (Fig. 20.2). They are frequently asymmetrical; possibly being denser on the side which has been dependent.

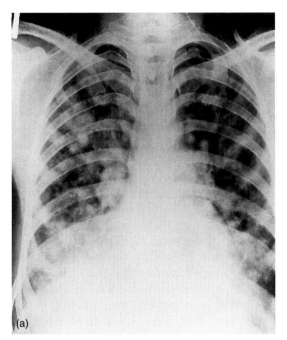
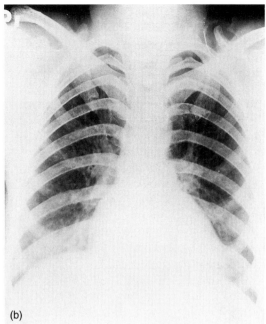

Figure 20.1   Radiograph of a patient with high altitude pulmonary edema: (a) on admission and (b) 4 days later. (Reproduced with permission of Dr T. Norboo of Leh, Jammu and Kashmir, India.)

Very often, the right side is more densely shadowed (Menon 1965). Quite frequently, the lower zones, especially the costo-phrenic angles, are spared as well as the apices. The pulmonary vessels may be seen to be engorged (Marticorena *et al.* 1964). The radiographic appearance in early cases shows more pathology than would be expected from clinical examination (Menon 1965). In patients with a second attack of HAPE there is no consistent pattern in the areas of lung involved. In treated cases the radiographic lesions clear rapidly (see Fig. 20.1), often within 2 days (Houston 1960), though usually lagging behind the improvement in symptoms.

20.2.6 Investigations

THE ELECTROCARDIOGRAPH

The ECG shows tachycardia. The P waves are often peaked (P pulmonale), and there is right axis deviation of the AQRS (mean, +123°). Some patients show elevation of the S–T segment (Marticorena *et al.* 1964). T-waves may be inverted in the precordial leads but this may be seen in asymptomatic subjects at altitude (Milledge 1963). The ECG appearances can be attributed to the very high pulmonary artery pressure and the consequent increase in right ventricular work.

HEMATOLOGY

Menon (1965) found that haemoglobin concentration was 14.0–16.0 g dL^{-1} and the sedimentation rate was normal. The white cell count was raised in 75 of 95 cases. This elevation was due to an increase in neutrophil count.

BLOOD GASES

P_{O_2} and arterial oxygen saturation are low compared with normal values for altitude. P_{CO_2} is very variable and is not significantly different from controls (Antezana *et al.* 1982, Schoene *et al.* 1985).

URINE

Proteinuria was present in four of 101 cases (Menon 1965), but using more sensitive tests there was an increase in urine protein in all subjects during the first few days at altitude, the degree of proteinuria correlating with the severity of AMS (Pines 1978; Chapter 15).

20.2.7 Cardiac catheter studies

There have been a number of catheter studies carried out on patients with HAPE before treatment (Penaloza and Sime 1969, Antezana *et al.* 1982) or

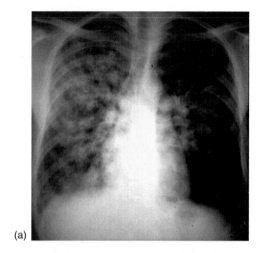

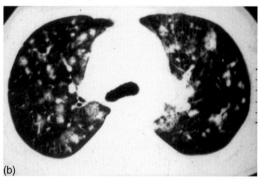

Figure 20.2   (a) Radiograph of a 37-year-old male mountaineer with HAPE which shows a patchy to confluent distribution of edema, predominantly on the right side. (b) Computerized tomography scan of 27-year-old mountaineer with recurrent HAPE showing patchy distribution of edema. (From Bartsch *et al.* 2005.)

soon after starting treatment (Fred *et al.* 1962, Hultgren *et al.* 1964, Roy *et al.* 1969). In all these studies there was found to be a high pulmonary artery pressure compared with healthy subjects at the same altitude (Table 20.2). The wedge pressures were normal. The pulmonary artery pressure ranged up to 144 mmHg systolic at the high end (Hultgren *et al.* 1964) but were still quite high at 60–80 mmHg systolic (Table 20.2). The normal wedge pressure implies normal pulmonary venous and left atrial pressures; in one subject direct measurement of left atrial pressure was made via a patent foramen ovale and was normal (Fred *et al.* 1962). The cardiac output was within the normal range so the calculated pulmonary resistance was markedly raised. There was no evidence of left ventricular failure. Breathing 100% oxygen resulted in a fall of pulmonary artery pressure to normal values within 3 min in two of five subjects. However, in the other three, pressures fell but plateaued out at 40–50 mmHg pulmonary artery pressure, well above the upper limit of normal at that altitude (Antezana *et al.* 1982).

Non-invasive echocardiography has afforded investigators the opportunity to evaluate patients during and after their bouts of HAPE (Kawashima *et al.* 1989, Yagi *et al.* 1990, Hackett *et al.* 1992, Vachiery *et al.* 1995, Busch *et al.* 2001, Berger *et al.* 2005). Similar responses were found during hypoxic exercise (Fig 20.3). These findings have confirmed the earlier catheterization studies (Table 20.2).

20.2.8 Population at risk

The etiology of HAPE is similar to that of AMS (section 18.4), all ages and both sexes being susceptible. There is an impression that children and young adults are more prone to HAPE than older people. Individual susceptibility for HAPE is more clear-cut

Table 20.2   Cardiac catheter studies in HAPE at 3700 m (Data from Antezana *et al.* 1982)

Group	Pulmonary artery pressure (mmHg)		Wedge pressure (mmHg)	Cardiac output (L min^{-1})
	Systolic	Diastolic		
HAPE (*n* = 5)	81	49	5	5.8
Controls (*n* = 50)	29	13	9	6.4

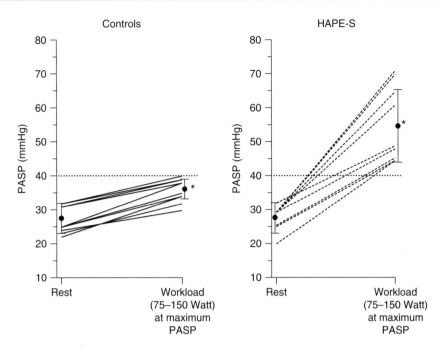

Figure 20.3   PASP response to exercise. Discrimination between controls and HAPE-S subjects by their PASP response to exercise estimated by Doppler echocardiography. HAPE-S, subjects susceptible to high-altitude pulmonary edema ($n = 9$), CONTROLS, control subjects ($n = 11$). No significant differences at rest between both groups ($p = 0.28$). *Mean maximal PASP in controls (36 ± 3 mmHg) vs. HAPE-S (55 ± 11 mmHg) subjects, $p < 0.002$.

than for AMS in that subjects (HAPE-S) who have suffered HAPE on one occasion are very likely to have problems on subsequent altitude trips. HAPE has been described in both South (Hultgren and Spickard 1960) and North America (Scoggin *et al.* 1977) in permanent high altitude residents, mostly children, who have made brief forays to low altitude (1–14 days) and have subsequently developed HAPE. The role of smooth muscle remodeling and vasoconstrictive reactivity has been speculated as an etiology of this sporadic and unpredictable clinical presentation. Finally, individuals with congenital absence of a pulmonary artery are predisposed to developing HAPE (Hackett *et al.* 1980).

20.2.9 Physiologic characteristics

LUNG VOLUMES

One possibility is that HAPE-susceptible individuals have a restricted lung vasculature or just smaller lungs. Surface area of the pulmonary vascular bed may influence vascular resistance encountered when HPVR and augmented blood flow merge to stress the microvasculature. A study by Steinacker *et al.* (1998) tested this idea by comparing eight such subjects with controls at rest and on exercise in normoxia and hypoxia. The HAPE-prone group had 35% smaller functional residual capacity, 7–10% smaller vital and total lung capacities and did not increase their diffusing capacities as much on exercise under hypoxia. This lends support to the hypothesis of smaller lungs in HAPE-susceptible individuals. A similar conclusion had been reached by Podolsky *et al.* (1996) who studied the pulmonary response to exercise in HAPE-susceptible subjects at sea level and 3810 m. They found greater vascular reactivity in HAPE subjects. The reactivity was not affected by altitude or oxygenation so was due to either flow-dependent pulmonary vasoconstriction or a reduced vascular cross-sectional area.

VENTILATION

Susceptible subjects have characteristics which appear to accentuate the effects of hypoxia on acute ascent to high altitude. For instance, the primary defense against hypoxemia is the hypoxic ventilatory response (HVR). Several studies have demonstrated that HAPE-S subjects have relatively blunted HVR responses (Hyers *et al.* 1979, Hackett *et al.* 1988, Matsuzawa *et al.* 1989, Selland *et al.* 1993, Schirlo *et al.* 2002). A more blunted HVR results in less alveolar hypoxia, the effect of which can be especially strong in individuals with brisk hypoxic pulmonary vasoconstrictive responses (HPVR).

PULMONARY HEMODYNAMICS

As mentioned previously (section 20.2.7), susceptible subjects have a greater HPVR than control subjects who had been to altitude previously without problems (Hultgren *et al.* 1971, Vachiery *et al.* 1995, Eldridge *et al.* 1996, Scherrer *et al.* 1996). Hohenhaus *et al.* (1995) studied both the pulmonary pressor and hypoxic ventilatory responses in HAPE-susceptible subjects and concluded that they had lower HVR than controls but not significantly different from subjects who had simple AMS. The latter had a wide range of HVR. Some HAPE-susceptible subjects had very brisk pressor responses but not all subjects could be separated from controls by this test.

PULMONARY VASOACTIVE MEDIATORS

An imbalance of vasoactive mediators may be responsible for an accentuated HPVR, and there

may be genetic predisposition to such disarray. An increased concentration of thromboxane B_2 was found in broncho-alveolar lavage fluid of HAPE victims compared to controls (Schoene *et al.* 1986, 1988), but more recently attention has shifted to the opposing influences of nitric oxide (NO) and endothelin-1 (ET-1). NO is an evanescent, endothelially derived molecule that is a potent pulmonary vasodilator. During the development of edema in HAPE-S at 4559 m, exhaled NO was 30% lower than in control subjects which also showed an inverse relationship with pulmonary artery pressure (PAP) (Duplain *et al.* 2000, Fig. 20.4a). It was hypothesized that a defect in NO synthesis predisposed HAPE-S individuals to accentuated PAP and thus HAPE. A subsequent study (Busch *et al.* 2001; Fig. 20.4b) noted that when HAPE-S subjects were exposed to 2 h of acute hypoxia, exhalation of NO decreased, whereas control subjects had no change in NO exhalation. These findings also correlated with an increase in PAP as NO fell. Hypoxia per se may induce systemic endothelial dysfunction in HAPE-S subjects compared to controls (Berger *et al.* 2005). This response is not isolated to the pulmonary vasculature and results in decreased NO production which correlated with an increase in PAP in this study. HAPE-S subjects have also been found to have impaired release of NO when exposed to hypoxia (Berger *et al.* 2005).

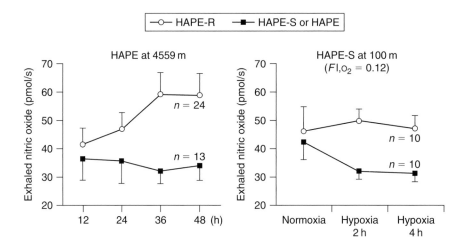

Figure 20.4 *Left*: exhaled nitric oxide (NO) after 40 h at 4559 m in individuals developing HAPE and in individuals not developing HAPE (HAPE-R) despite identical exposure to high altitude (Duplain *et al.* 2000). *Right*: exhaled NO in HAPE-susceptible subjects (HAPE-S) and HAPE-R individuals after 4 h of exposure to hypoxia ($FI_{,O_2} = 0.12$) at low altitude (elevation 100 m) (Busch *et al.* 2001). *n*, No. of subjects.

Endothelin-1 is a potent vasoconstrictor, and plasma levels were found to be 33% higher in HAPE-S subjects compared to controls at 4559 m (Sartori *et al.* 1999b). PAP values were higher in HAPE-S subjects, and these levels correlated with the increase in ET-1. It is not clear though whether these higher values are secondary to increased ET-1 production or decreased clearance.

Inherent sympathetic activity may play an important role in HAPE-susceptibility. Duplain *et al.* (1999a) measured sympathetic activity directly from postganglionic nerve discharge in HAPE susceptible subjects in response to a short hypoxic test. They found at both high and low altitude that the test subjects had two to three times the response compared with controls suggesting that sympathetic over-activation may be a part of the susceptibility.

ALVEOLAR FLUID CLEARANCE (AFC)

Most of the early studies of HAPE focused on leak from the microvasculature, but fluid flux in the lung also involves clearance of fluid from the alveolar and interstitial spaces to the lymphatic drainage. This process of active water and sodium transport across the alveolar epithelial cells is mediated by a Na^+–K^+-ATPase pump which is inhibited by hypoxia (Planes *et al.* 1997, Pham *et al.* 2002) (Fig. 20.5). It was hypothesized that individuals with impaired AFC would be HAPE-susceptible.

Similar sodium and water transport mechanisms exist in the nasal epithelium and are thought to be reflective of the alveolar epithelium (Mairbaurl *et al.* 2003, Sartori *et al.* 2004). Scherrer and colleagues have reinforced the proposition that pulmonary hypertension by itself does not cause pulmonary edema (section 20.7.3 and Sartori *et al.* 1999b). However, in transgenic mice with disruption of the gene for the α sub-unit of the amiloride-sensitive epithelial sodium channel, hypoxia did induce pulmonary edema. The same group has found a similar defect in epithelial ion transport in HAPE-susceptible human subjects (Lepori *et al.* 1999).

Taking advantage of the fact that one of the effects of beta-2 receptor agonists is to facilitate AFC, Sartori *et al.* (2002) used high doses of inhaled salmeterol in 37 HAPE-susceptible climbers taken to 4559 m and reduced the incidence of HAPE by 50%. Compared to controls, the HAPE-S subjects also had trans-nasal epithelial sodium transport that

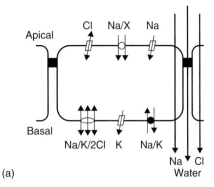

(a)

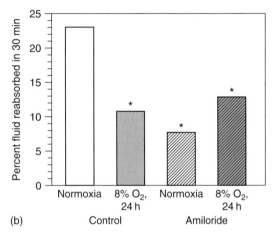

(b)

Figure 20.5 Alveolar fluid balance. (a) Removal of alveolar fluid is driven by the active reabsorption of Na^+ that enters the cell via Na channels and Na-coupled transport (Na/X) and is extruded by Na^+–K^+-ATPases. Thus active Na reabsorption generates the osmotic gradient for the reabsorption of water. (b) Hypoxia inhibits the reabsorption of fluid instilled into lungs of hypoxia-exposed rats, which is fully explained by inhibition of amiloride-sensitive pathways (mostly Na channels). *$p < 0.05$ vs. control values in normoxia. Modified from Vivona *et al.* (2001).

was 30% lower than non-HAPE controls. Beta-agonists lower PAP and decrease inflammation so that beneficial effect in decreasing HAPE may not be totally attributable to the facilitation of AFC. Mason *et al.* (2003) tracked the association of AFC by use of nasal transmembrane potentials and lung volumes (vital capacity) befores, during and after an ascent to 3800 m. The findings suggested that an altered respiratory epithelial transport may play a role in the accumulation of extra-vascular water.

GENETIC MARKERS

With an increasing array of genetic markers at the disposal of investigators, HAPE has come within the sights of researchers who are studying genes and disease states. Hanoka *et al.* (1998) found an association of certain HLA complexes (HLA-DR6 and HLA-DQ4) in patients with a history of HAPE. Hypothetically, there could be an association of angiotensin converting enzyme (ACE) insertion/deletion (I/D) gene polymorphism and vasoconstriction and fluid retention and thus potentially related to HAPE susceptibility. Morrell *et al.* (1999) reported that Kyrghyz highlanders with pulmonary hypertension had a high incidence of the D allele of the ACE gene compared with subjects suspected but found not to have pulmonary hypertension, but two more recent studies in a large number of subjects at altitudes from 3000 to 4559 m (Dehnert *et al.* 2002, Kumar *et al.* 2004) demonstrated no relationship between ACE I/D gene polymorphisms and HAPE. In 49 HAPE-susceptible and 55 healthy climbers, Hotta *et al.* (2004) also found no relationship between ACE-I/D genes and HAPE susceptibility, but in a subset of HAPE subjects the D allele of the ACE-I/D polymorphism was associated with pulmonary vascular hyper-responsiveness in patients who were catheterized and challenged with hypoxia.

As mentioned earlier, an impairment of NO synthesis can lead to less pulmonary vasodilatation with hypoxic stress which may be a permissive factor in the development of HAPE. Gene polymorphisms for endothelial-derived NO synthase (e-NOS) were studied in HAPE-susceptible subjects, and two variants of the e-NOS gene were present in 25.6 and 23.2% versus 9.8 and 6.9% in HAPE-S versus controls. These results suggest a genetic etiology to e-NOS related pulmonary vascular reactivity and HAPE susceptibility.

In another line of genetic investigation, Saxena *et al.* (2005) studied polymorphisms of the pulmonary surfactant protein A1 and A2 genes (SP-A1 and SP-A2). SP-A is a potent anti-oxidant which protects against inflammatory reactions and oxidative damage and thus lung injury. The polymorphisms have been associated with respiratory distress syndrome, chronic obstructive pulmonary disease, and pulmonary infection. In this study, HAPE subjects homozygous for SP-A1 and SP-A2 had a higher degree of oxidative damage. HAPE subjects heterozygous for the polymorphisms had a lower degree of oxidative damage while control subjects without a history of HAPE and no gene polymorphisms had little to no oxidative damage.

These studies are just the beginning of what will become a plethora of genetic studies in the future which will further unravel the fascinating mechanism of HAPE.

20.2.10 Summary of HAPE susceptibility

A number of physiologic, cellular and genetic markers have provided investigators with important insight into the underlying mechanisms of HAPE:

- Smaller lung volumes and presumed vascular bed
- Blunted ventilatory responses to hypoxia
- Accentuated hypoxic pulmonary vasoconstriction
- Imbalance of vasoactive mediators that enhance (endothelin-1) and relax hypoxic pulmonary vascular tone
- Impaired trans-alveolar epithelial sodium and water clearance
- Gene polymorphisms which mediate e-NOS and surfactant

20.3 PREVENTION AND TREATMENT

20.3.1 Slow ascent

It is thought that HAPE occurs in individuals who have not yet acclimatized with special disposition in those who have characteristics which make them susceptible. It can occur in individuals with AMS; therefore, if a sufficiently slow ascent is undertaken both AMS and HAPE may be avoided (section 18.6.1). However, because of the rush of modern-day life, people often ascend at a rate that puts them at risk of AMS and HAPE.

20.3.2 Exercise

Many case histories from Houston (1960) onwards emphasize the point that patients have been very energetic while getting to high altitude or on arrival there. Ravenhill (1913) was of the opinion that physical exertion rendered a man more susceptible to

AMS in general. The Indian Army, with great experience of HAPE since the war with China in the Himalayas in 1962, advises all inductees to altitude to take no unnecessary exertion for the first 72 h. Exercise, by increasing cardiac output, raises the pulmonary artery pressure, especially in subjects susceptible to HAPE and it is believed that the higher the PA pressure, the greater the risk of HAPE. In healthy subjects at altitude, Eldridge *et al.* (1998) have shown that strenuous exercise results in the appearance of RBCs, WBCs and gdT cells in the lavage fluid. The latter cells indicate damage to the endothelium and play a role in inflammation. Anholm *et al.* (1999) found radiographic evidence of pulmonary edema in a group of cyclists at the end of a run a modest altitude. However, HAPE can occur in the absence of hard physical exertion; 66 of Menon's 101 cases had taken no exercise more strenuous than office work, travelling as passengers in a truck or walking about on level ground (Menon 1965). Nevertheless, the anecdotal evidence is strong enough to advise people who have to make a rapid ascent to altitude to avoid hard physical exertion for 2 days or more.

20.3.3 Drugs

Some of the emerging suggestions for therapy to prevent HAPE have evolved from important physiologic observations which, as mentioned previously, are associated with susceptibility to HAPE. This section will address a number of pharmacologic interventions which are potentially effective for both prevention and treatment.

ACETAZOLAMIDE

Acetazolamide (section 18.6.2), by preventing or at least reducing AMS, probably also reduces the risk of HAPE, but no studies have directly addressed this issue. On the other hand, acetazolamide, not by carbonic anhydrase inhibition or NO release, has been shown to reduce HPVR (Höhne *et al.* 2004, Swenson 2006, Höhne *et al.* 2006) and may by its effect on calcium channels reduce HPVR and subsequent susceptibility to HAPE.

CALCIUM CHANNEL BLOCKERS

Oelz *et al.* (1989) showed that nifedipine was of value in the treatment of HAPE. Six subjects with clinical physiological and radiographic evidence of HAPE

were treated with 10 mg of nifedipine sublingually and 20 mg slow release orally every 6 h thereafter. Despite continued exercise at 4559 m this treatment without oxygen resulted in clinical improvement, better oxygenation, reduced $(A–a)Po_2$ gradient and pulmonary artery pressure, and clearing of alveolar edema. The sublingual preparation is very rapidly absorbed and occasionally results in systemic hypotension. Therefore most physicians now do not use it.

Bartsch *et al.* (1991) took advantage of the strong relationship between an accentuated HPVR and HAPE, used a calcium-channel blocker, nifedipine, in a group of HAPE-susceptible individuals in a controlled trial upon ascent to the Margherita Hut at 4559 m and essentially prevented HAPE while also mitigating the expected rise in PAP in these subjects.

NITRIC OXIDE

Nitric oxide (NO) produced by endothelial cells is a naturally occurring potent vasodilator. It was first used in the treatment of HAPE by Scherrer *et al.* (1996) who took 18 HAPE-susceptible subjects to 4559 m. Their pulmonary artery pressures were higher and Pa,o_2 lower than control, non-susceptible subjects. NO lowered their PA pressure and raised their Pa,o_2 whereas in control subjects Pa,o_2 fell. The latter was thought to be due to increasing V/Q mismatching. In HAPE subjects, NO goes preferentially to ventilated, non-edematous areas dilating the vessels there. This shifts blood flow from edematous to non-edematous areas with improvement in V/Q matching. The beneficial effects of NO were confirmed by Anand *et al.* (1998) in 14 patients with established HAPE. They compared NO treatment with 50% O_2 and NO plus O_2 50%. Both NO and O_2 were effective in reducing PA pressure and improving Pa,o_2 but the combination had an additive effect. Omura *et al.* (2000) exposed rats to normobaric hypoxia ($FI,o_2 = 0.10$) with one group on 83 ppm NO and the other controls. Mortality was reduced from 39.5 to 6.2% on NO with heavier lung weight in the controls suggesting that NO was beneficial in minimizing pulmonary edema in this rat model of HAPE. These studies are of great interest in understanding the mechanisms of HAPE, but NO is not suitable for use in the field; and if the patient reaches a hospital, the descent, calcium channel blockers and oxygen are almost always effective in relieving the condition.

PHOSPHODIESTERASE-5 (PDE-5) INHIBITION

Other interventions may affect e-NOS which result in pulmonary vasodilatation. There has been recent interest in PDE-5 inhibitors (sildenafil, tadalafil) which inhibits cGMP in the lungs, lower PAP and increase exercise performance at high altitude (Ghofrani *et al.* 2004, Richalet *et al.* 2005a) and prevent HAPE (Maggiorini 2006). This line of drugs may provide prophylactic as well as therapeutic benefits in HAPE.

GLUCOCORTICOIDS

Maggiorini *et al.* (2006) also noted that high dose dexamethasone prevented the increase in PAP as much as tadalafil which initially seemed surprising. Dexamethasone may promote eNOS synthase by inhibiting hypoxia-induced endothelial dysfunction (Murata *et al.* 2004) which would have some of the same salutary effects as other vasodilators in preventing HAPE. Other effects of glucocorticoids, however, make dissecting this beneficial mechanism difficult. For instance, dexamethasone increases the Na^+–K^+ ATPase pump at the epithelial layer (Noda *et al.* 2003), and pulmonary vascular permeability was reduced in rats treated with hypoxia (Stelzner *et al.* 1988).

OTHER VASODILATORS

Hackett *et al.* (1992) have shown that several vasodilators are beneficial in HAPE as indicated by a reduction in pulmonary artery pressure, pulmonary vascular resistance and improved gas exchange (Fig. 20.6). Nifedipine and hydralazine were of equal benefit but rather less effective than oxygen. Phentolamine, an alpha-blocker, was more effective than oxygen and, when combined with oxygen, was even more effective.

20.3.4 Field treatment

In mild to moderate cases of HAPE in an environment where medical help is available, e.g. a ski resort, and when Sa,O_2 can be improved to greater than 90% on low-flow oxygen, patients can be treated

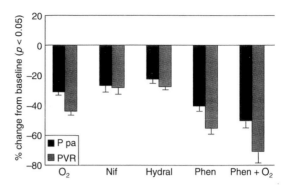

Figure 20.6   Percentage change in mean pulmonary artery pressure (Ppa) and pulmonary vascular resistance (PVR) with five different interventions in subjects with HAPE. Nif, nifedipine; Hydral, hydralazine; Phen, phentolamine. (Reproduced with permission from Hackett *et al.* 1992.)

with oxygen and close observation without going down unless the clinical situation worsens (Zafren *et al.* 1996). In other situations when the patient is more severely ill and where medical care is not available, the single most important maneuver in treating HAPE is to get the patient down as fast and as far as possible. Even a descent of as little as 300 m may improve a patient's condition dramatically (report of Case 2, in section 19.2). However, there are often unavoidable delays while awaiting evacuation and there are a number of therapeutic possibilities.

OXYGEN

Breathing air enriched with oxygen, if available, is an obvious and invaluable treatment. It relieves hypoxia and reduces pulmonary artery pressure (section 19.2.6), but, while most patients benefit, in some, the relief is only partial, and in a few, deterioration may continue. The dosage of oxygen is usually dictated by its supply. If there is sufficient, a flow of 6–10 L min^{-1} is indicated for the first few hours, reducing to 2–4 L min^{-1} when there is improvement.

DIURETICS

Since the patient has edema, diuretics have been used in the treatment of HAPE (Singh *et al.* 1965); however, since subjects at high altitude are often volume depleted to begin with, any presumed benefit of diuretics is outweighed by the risk of further volume depletion and the dangers in the field setting thereof.

ANTIBIOTICS

Many cases of HAPE have mild fever and leucocytosis suggesting that infection may play a part; however, there has never been any evidence that pneumonia initiates or perpetuates HAPE. Menon (1965) discontinued the use of antibiotics in his last 44 cases of HAPE with no apparent disadvantage to the outcome. Unless there is evidence of a concurrent infection, antibiotics should not be used in HAPE.

OTHER DRUGS

Digoxin has been used in cases of HAPE in its early clinical history. Menon (1965) observed the effect of an intravenous dose of 0.5–1.5 mg in 66 patients and claimed that the response was uniformly good within a few hours, even in patients given only 1 L min^{-1} of added oxygen. However, there was no evidence of myocardial failure nor was there atrial fibrillation, the current indications for digoxin therapy, and its use is no longer advised.

Morphine (15–30 mg i.v.) has been used, again with the clinical impression that this resulted in a reduction in pulmonary edema. As it does in acute left ventricular failure, it also makes the patient more comfortable, possibly by causing peripheral vasodilatation and a decrease in pre-load on the right ventricle and thus a shift of blood from central to peripheral circulations. However, its respiratory depressant effects should make for caution in its use, especially in the field setting.

EXPIRATORY POSITIVE AIRWAYS PRESSURE

Feldman and Herndon (1977) suggested that expiratory positive airways pressure might be beneficial in HAPE by analogy with its use in other forms of pulmonary edema. They proposed a simple device in which the subject exhaled through an underwater tube to achieve the desired positive pressure whilst inspiration was direct from atmosphere.

Schoene et al. (1985) used a commercial expiratory positive pressure mask on four patients with HAPE on Mount McKinley. They showed that, using the mask, arterial saturation was increased with increasing positive pressure (up to 10 cm water). There was a concomitant rise in P_{CO_2} but not of heart rate. The intrathoracic pressure would be negative during inspiration so the cardiac output would probably not be reduced. A similar effect can be achieved by pursed lips expiration as used by patients with severe emphysema; mountain guides advise this, presumably because they have found it to be beneficial.

PORTABLE HYPERBARIC CHAMBER: THE GAMOW OR CERTEC BAGS

A lightweight rubberized canvas bag has been developed into which a patient can be zipped and the bag pressurized using a foot pump. There is a pressure relief valve set to 2 psi. This pressure gives the equivalent altitude reduction of almost 2000 m from a typical base camp altitude of 4000–5000 m. There are currently two commercially available bags: the Gamow from the USA and Certec from France. There have been numerous accounts of their use in HAPE and HACE, with good results (Robertson and Shlim 1991). One report draws attention to the considerable placebo effect of the procedure. Roach and Hackett (1992) have reviewed the efficacy of hyperbaric treatment. They conclude that both oxygen and hyperbaria are effective. There may be a rebound effect some hours after treatment (typically 1–2 h duration). A recent controlled trial in benign AMS has shown that 1 h in the bag at pressure (193 mbar) was significantly more effective in reducing symptoms than control (1 h at the trivial pressure of 20 mbar) (Bärtsch et al. 1993). The effort of maintaining the necessary pumping for even 1 h is considerable, especially at altitude where the number of rescuers might be limited. Duff (1999b), reporting a case, makes the useful point that some patients with severe HAPE or HACE may be orthoponeic when made to lie flat in a compression bag and in their confused state may become belligerent. Their condition may be confused with claustrophobia. The solution is to position the bag at a 30° head-up angle.

20.3.5 Summary of prevention and treatment

Prevention of HAPE should be undertaken in individuals with a previous history of HAPE, especially if they are undergoing an unavoidably rapid ascent. These measures are:

- Encourage slow ascent, if at all possible, to allow for acclimatization
- Use of nifedipine or other pulmonary vasodilators (PDE-5 inhibitors, maybe acetazolamide or dexamethasone) if rapid ascent is unavoidable, especially in HAPE-S subjects
- Use of drugs which increase alveolar fluid clearance (inhaled beta-agonists, dexamethasone) upon ascent

The treatment of HAPE should consist of:

- Mild to moderate HAPE patients where medical help is available can be treated with oxygen and observation unless the clinical situation deteriorates.
- With more severe HAPE or in areas where medical help is not available, getting the patient down in altitude as fast and as low as possible is the most prudent approach.
- While awaiting evacuation, or if evacuation is not possible, give oxygen or hyperbaria. Nifedipine 20 mg slow release should be given and a broad-spectrum antibiotic should be considered. Sildenafil or tadalafil may also be beneficial.
- The use of expiratory positive airway pressure, with a respiratory valve device, or failing that, by pursed lips breathing, will give some temporary improvement.

20.4 OUTCOME

In fully established cases, where evacuation to lower altitude is impossible and no intervention is undertaken, death within a few hours is usual. If cases are recognized early and taken down, patients usually recover completely in 1 or 2 days, but occasionally they continue to deteriorate and die even after being brought down to lower altitude, especially if there are symptoms of cerebral edema (Dickinson et al. 1983). Only one case has been reported as progressing to adult respiratory distress syndrome (Zimmerman and Crapo 1980). Usually, the

pulmonary hypertension reduces rapidly on going to low altitude and the inverted T waves on the ECG return to normal (Singh et al. 1965, Fig. 3). But Menon (1965) mentions two soldiers (out of 101 cases) who having recovered from HAPE had to be evacuated later because of breathlessness, precordial pain and inverted T waves in their EGC, and Fiorenzano et al. (1997) reported one case with prolonged T-wave inversion in the precordial leads suggesting prolonged pulmonary hypertension. Even patients who have apparently fully recovered have been shown to have significant hypoxaemia and widened (A–a)Po_2 gradients for up to 12 weeks (Guleria et al. 1969). However, after recovery at lower altitudes, many climbers have returned within a few days to climb their peaks without further trouble (Schoene et al. 1986, 1988).

20.5 PATHOLOGY

20.5.1 Post-mortem examination

There have been a number of post-mortem studies which have shown a similar pathology in the heart and lungs (Hultgren et al. 1962, Arias-Stella and Kruger 1963, Marticorena et al. 1964, Nayak et al. 1964, Singh et al. 1965, Dickinson et al. 1983, Hultgren et al. 1997). The lungs are heavy and feel solid. The cut surface weeps edema fluid, usually blood stained, but a striking feature is the non-uniform nature of the edema. Areas of hemorrhagic edema alternate with clear edema and with areas which are virtually normal (or over-inflated). Pulmonary arterial thrombi are commonly found.

On microscopy, alveoli are filled with fluid containing red blood cells, polymorphs and macrophages, though not in great numbers. Hyaline membranes are found in the alveoli, identical with those seen in respiratory distress syndrome of the new-born. The pulmonary capillaries are congested with small arteries and veins containing thrombi and fibrin clot. Perivascular edema and hemorrhage are found. In post-mortem studies of high altitude natives from South America the pulmonary arteries are very muscular and the right ventricle is hypertrophied. In lowlanders the pulmonary vessels have normal musculature (Dickinson et al. 1983).

20.5.2 The edema fluid

The hyaline membranes are probably formed by coalescence of proteins, suggesting a high protein edema. It has been shown in life that the edema fluid is rich in protein. Hackett *et al.* (1986) sampled pure edema fluid by bronchoscopy in one case and showed it to have a plasma/fluid ratio of 0.8:1.1 for total protein. Schoene *et al.* (1986) took bronchoalveolar lavage fluid from three cases of HAPE and compared it with lavage fluid from three controls at the same altitude (4400 m). The fluid from patients was rich in high molecular weight protein, red blood cells and macrophages. These findings suggest a 'large pore' leak type of edema. In further studies the same group (Schoene *et al.* 1988) also found that the fluid was rich in alveolar macrophages and a high concentration of high molecular weight proteins. There was evidence of activation of complement (C5a) and release of thromboxane B_2 and leukotriene B_4. Tsukimoto *et al.* (1994) also showed under tightly controlled laboratory conditions in the rat, that elevation of the capillary pressure alone resulted in the appearance of leukotriene B_4 in the BAL fluid. Recently, a Japanese group (Kubo *et al.* 1998) has carried out BAL in seven patients with early HAPE and found increased cell counts of macrophages, lymphocytes and neutrophils plus markedly elevated concentrations of proteins, lactate dehydrogenase, IL-1β, IL-6, IL-8, and TNFα. IL-6 and TNFα were shown to correlate with the Pa,O_2 and pulmonary artery driving pressure ($P_{PA} - P_{wedge}$). Swenson *et al.* (2002) carried out bronchoalveolar lavage (BAL) in HAPE-S subjects as soon as they arrived at the Margherita Hut and developed signs of HAPE. The BAL fluid showed a high protein concentration but no signs of inflammation. This important study determined that an inflammatory response does not play a role in the initiation of HAPE.

20.6 MECHANISMS OF HAPE

There is evidence suggesting that a degree of subclinical pulmonary edema is common during the second and third days at altitude. There is a reduction in vital capacity, a shift of the pressure/volume curve of the lung (Mansell *et al.* 1980, Gautier *et al.* 1982), and an increase in alveolar arterial oxygen difference (Sutton *et al.* 1976). This might simply be part of a generalized increase in extracellular fluid volume which shows itself as subcutaneous edema in the face on rising in the morning and in the ankles later in the day. In the skull, the same edema raises the intracellular pressure and may give rise to the symptoms of AMS, but the progression from this mild edema to clinical pulmonary edema requires a further mechanism or mechanisms.

20.6.1 Facts that require explanation

Any hypothesis that seeks to explain the mechanism of HAPE must take into account the following facts:

- The edema is of the high protein type
- The patchy distribution of the edema seen on post-mortem and radiology (Fig. 20.1)
- The very high pulmonary artery pressure and normal wedge (and left atrial) pressures (Table 20.2); the improvement which follows treatment with different drugs which reduce the pulmonary artery pressure indicates the importance of this factor in the mechanism of HAPE
- The presence of vascular thrombi and fibrin clots in pulmonary vessels (section 20.4.1)
- The individual susceptibility which is associated with an increased hypoxic pulmonary pressor response (Hultgren *et al.* 1971) and response to exercise (Kawashima *et al.* 1989)
- The increased risk of HAPE with exercise on arrival at altitude

20.6.2 Left ventricular failure

Although HAPE resembles left ventricular failure (LVF) clinically, which is why Ravenhill (1913) called it *puna* of the cardiac type, it is not now thought to be due to left ventricular failure per se. Most catheter studies have shown normal wedge pressures and the edema fluid is of the high protein permeability type. On the other hand, Maggiorini *et al.* (2001) found elevated pulmonary capillary wedge pressures, consistent with pulmonary venoconstriction, but the chest radiograph and pathology are not typical of LVF.

20.6.3 Pulmonary hypertension

The extraordinarily high pulmonary artery pressure found in HAPE must play a role in the mechanism of the condition. High pulmonary artery pressure by itself does not cause edema, as for instance in primary pulmonary hypertension, or in a group of men studied by Sartori and colleagues (1999b). These individuals had suffered a period of hypoxia in the neonatal period and as a result had exaggerated pulmonary hypoxic pressor responses. When taken up to high altitude, they had high PA pressures but did not develop HAPE. This is perhaps not surprising since the resistance vessels, the arterioles, are upstream of capillaries and therefore capillary pressure should be normal. One must therefore postulate some further mechanism as well as, but related to, the pulmonary hypertension. The following have been proposed.

20.6.4 Uneven pulmonary vasoconstriction and perfusion

Hultgren (1969) suggested that the edema is caused by a very powerful, but uneven, vasoconstriction so that there is reduced blood flow in some parts of the lung and torrential blood flow in others. He showed (Hultgren et al. 1966) that if one progressively ties off more and more of the pulmonary arterial tree in a dog, thus forcing the total cardiac output through only a portion of the lung, pulmonary edema results in that part of the lung that remains perfused.

A case report by Dombret et al. (1987) provides confirmation in humans of Hultgren's experimental findings. The reported patient had a massive pulmonary embolus resulting in perfusion being reduced to only the left upper and middle lobes. She developed symptoms and signs of pulmonary edema, which on radiograph were shown to be confined to those same perfused lobes.

Evidence in favor of this mechanism as being the cause of HAPE is provided by Viswanathan et al. (1979) who, at sea level, studied 12 subjects who had recovered from HAPE. They showed that, on being given 10% oxygen to breathe, they had a greater pulmonary pressor response than controls and on lung scanning their perfusion was more uneven.

This hypothesis accounts well for the patchy distribution of the condition. High flow through less severely constricted areas might well produce edema by capillary stress failure (section 20.6.5). Added support for this hypothesis came from a paper by Hackett et al. (1980), who collected four cases of HAPE occurring at very modest altitudes (2000–3000 m) in subjects who had a congenital absence of the right pulmonary artery. The edema developed in the left lung, which received the total cardiac output. That four cases of HAPE developed in such an uncommon condition (only 50 cases have been described in the world literature) strongly suggests a causative rather than a coincidental association. Pulmonary blood flow was re-distributed in rats when exposed to severe hypoxia (Kuwahira et al. 2001), while Hanaoka et al. (2000) demonstrated a more marked cephalad distribution of blood flow in HAPE-susceptible subjects when exposed to hypoxia. Using magnetic resonance imaging in HAPE-susceptible subjects and controls, Hopkins et al. (2005) found marked heterogeneity of blood flow in the HAPE-susceptible subjects when exposed to hypoxia.

20.6.5 Stress failure of pulmonary capillaries

It has been proposed that HAPE is caused by damage to the walls of pulmonary capillaries as a result of very high wall stresses associated with increased capillary transmural pressure (West et al. 1991, West and Mathieu-Costello 1992a). These high capillary pressures are the result of uneven hypoxic pulmonary vasoconstriction as originally proposed by Hultgren (1969). Extensive laboratory studies have now shown that raising capillary transmural pressure causes ultrastructural damage to the capillary walls, including disruption of the capillary endothelial layer, alveolar epithelial layer, and sometimes, all layers of the wall (Tsukimoto et al. 1991, West et al. 1991, Costello et al. 1992, Elliott et al. 1992, Fu et al. 1992). The result is a high permeability form of pulmonary edema (Tsukimoto et al. 1994). Figure 20.7 is an electron micrograph showing rupture of a pulmonary capillary wall in a rat exposed to a barometric pressure of 294 mmHg for 4 h. Note the red blood cell in the process of moving

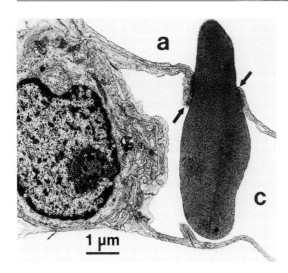

Figure 20.7 Electron micrograph of a pulmonary capillary in a rat exposed to a barometric pressure of 294 mmHg for 4 h. Note rupture of the capillary wall with a red cell moving out of the capillary lumen (c) into an alveolus (a). (From West *et al.* 1995.)

from the capillary lumen to the alveolar space (West *et al.* 1995).

The work on stress failure began because of two key observations about HAPE. The first is that, as described above, there is a very strong relationship between the occurrence of HAPE and the height of the pulmonary arterial pressure. This suggests that HAPE is caused in some way by high vascular pressures in the pulmonary circulation. The second observation was that samples of alveolar fluid obtained by bronchoalveolar lavage in patients with HAPE show that the fluid is of the high permeability type with a large concentration of high molecular weight proteins and many cells. This observation strongly suggests that HAPE is associated with damage to the walls of the pulmonary capillaries by some mechanism. The problem therefore was to reconcile a hydrostatic pressure basis for the disease with the development of abnormalities in the capillary walls. As a result, extensive studies of the effects of raising pulmonary capillary pressure on the ultrastructure of pulmonary capillaries were carried out. These showed that stress failure is common in rabbit lung when the capillary transmural pressure rises to 40 mmHg and that when it occurs it causes a high permeability type of pulmonary edema.

It is not at all surprising that pulmonary capillaries break under these conditions because the calculated wall stress of the capillary is extremely high (West *et al.* 1991, West and Matthieu-Costello 1992b). The surprising thing is not that the capillaries fail, but that they do not fail more often. Stress failure is now believed to play a role in a number of lung diseases (West and Mathieu-Costello 1992c) and is also the cause of bleeding into the lungs of racehorses, which is extremely common (West *et al.* 1993).

Bronchoalveolar lavage studies in patients with HAPE show the presence of inflammatory markers including leukotriene B_4, other lipoxygenase products of arachidonic acid metabolism, and C5a complement in the lavage fluid (Schoene *et al.* 1988). These lavage studies were not done in early stages of HAPE as was the study of Swenson *et al.* (2002) where no inflammatory markers were found. At first sight these findings might seem to argue against stress failure of pulmonary capillaries as a mechanism. However, an important feature of the ultrastructural changes in stress failure is that the basement membranes of capillary endothelial cells are frequently exposed (Tsukimoto *et al.* 1991). The exposed basement membrane is electrically charged and highly reactive, and can be expected to activate leucocytes and platelets. In bronchoalveolar studies of the rabbit preparation, leukotriene B_4 is seen in the lavage fluid (Tsukimoto *et al.* 1994). Platelet activation will result in the formation of fibrin thrombi, which are a feature of the pathology of HAPE (Arias-Stella and Kruger 1963). As mentioned above, the study of Swenson *et al.* (2002) put to rest the role of inflammation in the initiation of HAPE as they found no evidence of inflammation in BAL fluid in HAPE-S subjects in the early stages of the development of HAPE.

A striking feature of stress failure of pulmonary capillaries is that some of the breaks are rapidly reversible when the pressure is reduced. In one study carried out in rabbit lung, it was found that about 70% of both the epithelial and endothelial breaks closed within a few minutes of the pressure being reduced (Elliott *et al.* 1992). This rapid reversibility of most of the disruptions may explain why patients with HAPE often rapidly improve when they descend to a lower altitude.

Stress failure of pulmonary capillaries had not previously been suggested as the mechanism of

HAPE. However, Mooi and co-workers (1978) studied the ultrastructural changes that occurred in rat lungs when the animals were exposed to acute decompression in a hyperbaric chamber. The appearances that they described are consistent with the findings seen in stress failure.

The mechanism of stress failure has clear implications for therapy. The main objective should be to reduce the pulmonary artery pressure. The pressure is high because of hypoxic pulmonary vasoconstriction, and the best way to reduce it is by rapid descent to a lower altitude, which reduces the alveolar P_{O_2}. In addition, oxygen should be given if this is available. Calcium channel blockers such as nifedipine are also effective because they reduce pulmonary artery pressure (Oelz *et al.* 1989).

A recent case report by Grissom *et al.* (2000) indicates that alveolar hemorrhage occurs early in HAPE. They report a case of HAPE in a climber who made a rapid ascent of Denali, Alaska and on whom they carried out BAL. The fluid yielded an abundance of hemosiderin-laden macrophages. These have been reported at necropsy and indicate bleeding into the alveoli. They appear from 48 h after bleeding. Bronchoscopy was performed in this case less than 48 h after symptoms started so the timing of this result indicates bleeding occurred well before the onset of symptoms. This finding is consistent with capillary stress failure early in the course of the condition due to high pulmonary artery pressure.

20.6.6 Venular constriction

Since patients with HAPE have such a powerful arteriolar constriction in response to hypoxia, perhaps they have some degree of venular constriction as well. There is some pathological evidence for this from Wagenvoort and Wagenvoort (1976). This would not give high wedge pressures because when the catheter is wedged the blood in that segment runs off even through constricted venules and the wedge pressure reflects only the large vein and left atrial pressures, not the pressure in capillaries when the blood is flowing. To explain the patchy nature of the condition one must further postulate that the venular constriction is uneven.

20.6.7 Arterial leakage

Severinghaus (1977), impressed with the extraordinarily high pulmonary artery pressure in these patients, suggested that perhaps the fluid leak was upstream of the resistance vessels (i.e. in the arteries). He pointed out that when there was generalized arterial vasoconstriction, Laplace's law would mean reduction in diameter of small vessels but distension of large vessels (even though their wall tension was as great or greater). Radiography frequently shows distended hilar vessels (Marticorena *et al.* 1964). These larger vessels, not designed for such high pressure, suffer minor ruptures or fenestrations, which then leak high protein fluid and eventually red blood cells. The leakage is into the perivascular spaces which, when full, 'back up' to eventually cause alveolar flooding. This sequence occurs wherever the initial leak takes place since the perivascular space is the low pressure region of the lung.

Some evidence for such a mechanism was provided by two studies in animals (Milledge *et al.* 1968, Whayne and Severinghaus 1968) and in excised dog lungs (Iliff 1971). This evidence was reviewed by Severinghaus (1977) who quoted Hultgren's report on two horses which died suddenly after running at altitude. Both were found to have a ruptured pulmonary artery. Both this and the preceding hypothesis would account for exercise being a risk factor since it increases both flow and pressure in the pulmonary artery.

20.6.8 Multiple pulmonary emboli

Multiple scattered pulmonary emboli, even of inert substances, such as glass beads, cause a rapid profuse pulmonary edema in animals (Saldeen 1976) and this has been shown to be of the protein rich increased permeability type (Ohkuda *et al.* 1978). The finding in post-mortem studies of frequent vascular thrombi and fibrin clots has led to the microembolization hypothesis for HAPE on the premise that there is a derangement of the clotting system. The effect of hypoxia on coagulation has been studied by a number of workers (section 18.5.4). It seems that most clotting factors are unaffected by hypoxia; they are not disturbed in AMS. Some evidence of *in vivo* fibrin formation was found by Bärtsch *et al.* (1987) in patients with

HAPE but this was considered to be an epiphenomenon and not causative. If it does occur it will cause further deterioration in the patient. It is possible that changes in the red blood cells with hypoxia might alter their rheological properties and be a factor in AMS and HAPE. However, Reinhart et al. (1991) found no difference between subjects with and without AMS with respect to a number of rheological parameters. Platelets are clearly activated at high altitude and show signs of clumping as the day progresses (Lehmann et al. 2006), but there is no difference in the groups in terms of developing HAPE.

It has even been suggested that rapid ascent may cause bubble formation by decompression and thus air microembolization (Gray 1983). If this were the case, HAPE should be much more common in chamber studies than in the mountains, but this is not so.

20.6.9 Hypoxia, vascular permeability and inflammation

Hypoxia may increase vascular permeability, either directly, or more likely, via the release of chemical mediators. Against this suggestion is evidence that, in dogs, hypoxia does not alter the threshold for edema formation at a given microvascular pressure (Homik et al. 1988). However, it may require some other agent acting with hypoxia to produce the effect, as suggested by the work of Larsen et al. (1985). They showed in rabbits that neither hypoxia alone nor activation of the complement system (by infusion of cobra venom) alone caused pulmonary edema, but the two insults together did. Such a mechanism may well produce secondary intravascular coagulation, which would result in further pulmonary edema. On the other hand Duplain et al. (1999b) found in a group of HAPE-susceptible individuals, some of whom developed HAPE at altitude, that there was no tendency for the exhaled nitric oxide to increase with HAPE. Exhaled NO is a marker for inflammation, so this is evidence against inflammation being a factor in the genesis of HAPE. In a well-designed study, after baseline studies at low altitude, Swenson and colleagues (2002) took HAPE-susceptible subjects to 4559 m. At the first sign of HAPE, subjects underwent bronchoscopy and BAL. The fluid was high in protein,

but there were no markers of inflammation in the BAL fluid of their HAPE subjects. This study complemented the earlier field studies (Schoene et al. 1986, 1988). In those studies, the investigators could not control the stage of the illness in which the subjects were studied. These studies were the first to use BAL which demonstrated high proteins and inflammatory mediators in severe cases of HAPE. Thus, the speculation that inflammation played a role in the permeability leak was put to rest with Swenson's research which supports the mechanism of the leak being primarily secondary to high pressures.

20.6.10 Hypoventilation

Grover (1980) has pointed out that hypoventilation has two disadvantages for a subject in relation to HAPE. It will mean that the subject is more hypoxic at a given altitude than a subject with the normal altitude hyperventilation and also has a higher $P\text{CO}_2$. The higher $P\text{CO}_2$ means that there is no peripheral vasoconstriction and reduction in plasma volume on going to altitude; hence the plasma osmotic pressure is not raised. The subject is, therefore, more susceptible to pulmonary edema. A number of studies have found subjects with a history of HAPE to have low hypoxic ventilatory responses (Hackett et al. 1988, Matsuzawa et al. 1989). This might lead to relative hypoventilation at altitude, although Hackett et al. concluded that the low HVR played a permissive rather than a causative role in the pathogenesis of HAPE, allowing hypoxia to cause depression of ventilation. They found oxygen breathing increased ventilation in some of their subjects at altitude.

20.6.11 Neurogenic pulmonary edema

In some cases of head injury, a form of acute pulmonary edema is found which can be mimicked in experimental animals by creating lesions in the fourth ventricle. High levels of catecholamines are found, and the edema can be prevented by pretreatment with α-adrenergic blocking drugs; therefore, it is assumed that the edema is caused by a surge of sympathetic activity. During the first few days at altitude there is increased sympathetic activity and possibly a similar mechanism is at work. The effectiveness of the alpha-blocker, phentolamine, in HAPE (Hackett *et al.* 1992) suggests that this may be the case, findings also supported by the study of Duplain *et al.* (1999a).

20.6.12 Infection

Before 1960, many cases of HAPE were attributed to pneumonia. While in some cases, infection plays no part in HAPE, in others it may be a factor, especially in those where individuals who are not normally susceptible to AMS but develop a secondary infection and succumb. Carpenter *et al.* (1998) showed that rats given a mild respiratory infection and allowed to recover had greater lung edema and higher cell counts and protein concentration in BAL fluid when exposed to 10% O_2 a week later than

control rats. This gives support to the clinical impression that a concomitant or even previous respiratory infection is an important risk factor for HAPE.

20.6.13 Mechanisms: conclusions

It is now agreed that the genesis of HAPE is from high pressures in the fragile pulmonary microvasculature. The mechanism of abnormally powerful pulmonary hypoxic vasoconstriction, which is uneven and leads on to capillary stress failure, seems to have the most evidence in its favor. Other inherent characteristics, above and beyond the brisk hypoxic pulmonary vasoconstriction, include slower alveolar fluid clearance, and blunted hypoxic ventilatory response, and others, all play additive roles in the clinical spectrum of the disease.

21

Chronic mountain sickness and high altitude pulmonary hypertension

SUMMARY

Chronic mountain sickness (CMS) was first recognized by Carlos Monge M. in Peru and is also known as Monge's disease. It is found in all populations who remain at altitude for a number of years. The incidence is increased with altitude and with age; it is higher in males than females. In Tibet at least, it is more common in immigrant Han Chinese than in native Tibetans. It is characterized by excessive erythrocytosis with hematocrit values greater than 80%, hypoxemia and in some cases pulmonary hypertension. The condition improves after descent to low altitude.

In cases without overt lung disease various factors which cause relative hypoventilation, such as a reduced hypoxic ventilatory drive or disturbed breathing patterns during sleep, may be involved in the mechanism. Patients with underlying conditions such as chronic obstructive lung disease (chronic bronchitis, emphysema), kyphoscoliosis and other lung diseases may also have excessive erythrocytosis and in the past were sometimes diagnosed as 'CMS (or Monge's disease) with lung disease' but are now generally excluded from the diagnosis of CMS (León-Velarde *et al.* 2005).

The symptoms that result from this excessive erythrocytosis are rather vague and include headache, dizziness, physical and mental fatigue, anorexia and breathlessness. There may be symptoms of burning hands or feet. Signs are few and include cyanosis and a florid complexion.

Prevention, apart from remaining at low altitude, can only be directed at secondary risk factors such as smoking and occupational dust air pollution. Relocation to low altitude cures the condition but many patients are not able to take this option. The removal of 1–3 units of blood is beneficial but needs to be repeated as the hemoglobin concentration rises again. Respiratory stimulants have been used with reported success, including, recently, acetazolamide.

High altitude pulmonary hypertension (HAPH), previously termed sub-acute mountain sickness or high altitude heart disease, is a condition affecting either infants born or brought up to altitude within their first year, or adults resident or coming and remaining at altitude for months or years. In Tibet, the infants are usually the children of lowland Han Chinese; the highland Tibetan infants are relatively less susceptible. As the condition develops the infants become breathless, irritable and edematous. The pathology is of pulmonary hypertension and right heart failure. In adults, it has been reported in Han Chinese and, less often, in the Tibetan population, in Kyrgyz highlanders and in Indian soldiers stationed

Table 21.1 Nomenclature for chronic high altitude diseases and previous terms or synonyms and essential features

Suggested name	Synonyms	Features
Chronic mountain sickness	Monge's disease	Excessive erythrocytosis
	HA excessive polycythemia	Hypoxemia
	Excessive erythrocytosis	Pulmonary hypertension in some cases
		Rt heart failure
	HA pathologic erythrocytosis	Headache, dizziness, fatigue
		Recovery on descent to low altitude
High altitude pulmonary hypertension	CMS of the vascular type	Pulmonary hypertension
	High altitude heart disease	Right ventricle hypertrophy
	Hypoxic cor pulmonale	Right heart failure
	Infant sub-acute mountain sickness	Moderate hypoxemia
	Pediatric high altitude heart disease	No excessive erythrocytosis
	Adult sub-acute mountain sickness	

Abstracted from the ISMM Consensus statement (León-Velarde *et al.* 2005).

at about 6000 m for long periods. When symptoms develop they are those of right heart failure with signs of that condition. Descent results in reversal of signs and symptoms. Short-term trials of drugs such as nifedipine and sildenafil have shown them to be effective in lowering pulmonary artery pressure whilst remaining at altitude, but there have been no long-term trials to observe the effects on disease progression.

21.1 INTRODUCTION

There are two chronic conditions which affect people resident at high altitudes for months or years or infants born at altitude. There are numerous terms used in the literature for these conditions. Two consensus statements have been published on this topic which include an attempt to rationalize these terms. (León-Velarde 1998 and 2005) Table 21.1 sets out a schema of terms and synonyms abstracted from the latest statement (2005).

Following the consensus statement we shall use the terms chronic mountain sickness (CMS), for the condition of excessive erythrocytosis, and high altitude pulmonary hypertension (HAPH), for the condition where pulmonary hypertension predominates. There is considerable overlap in the two conditions. Most patients with CMS are also found to have pulmonary hypertension and may go on to

develop right heart failure whilst some patients with HAPH have a degree of excessive erythrocytosis. However, in most patients one or other response to chronic altitude hypoxia dominates so the consensus group decided to keep the two diagnoses though recognizing that some patients had both conditions. The situation is, perhaps, analogous to that of HAPE and HACE. It is interesting that excessive erythrocytosis (CMS) is the common pathology in the Andes whilst HAPH is more common in the high altitude areas of Asia.

Chronic mountain sickness (CMS) has been well known for many years. The other condition, HAPH, has only been recognized as a chronic condition in adults in the Andes since 1971 (Penalosa and Sime) and in China reported in the Chinese literature by Chen *et al.* in 1982. A more acute condition was reported by Anand in Indian soldiers stationed at between 5800 m and 6700 m for several months (mean 1.8 years). The condition was recognized rather earlier in children born or brought up to altitude at an early age (Khoury and Hawes 1963).

21.2 CHRONIC MOUNTAIN SICKNESS

21.2.1 Historical

In 1925 Carlos Monge M. reported a case of polycythemia in a patient from Cerro de Pasco (4300 m) in Peru to the Peruvian Academy of Medicine (Monge 1925). In 1928 he reported a series of such patients with red cell counts significantly higher than normally found at altitude (Monge C. and Whittembury 1976). (*Note.* Carlos Monge M. is the father and Carlos Monge C. the son: the M and C are the initial letters of the mothers' names, as is Spanish custom.) This condition has come to be known also as Monge's disease. The 1935 international expedition, led by Bruce Dill, reported one case of CMS in the English literature (Talbott and Dill 1936). In 1942 Hurtado published detailed observations of eight cases, outlining the symptomatology and hematological changes at altitude and the effect of descent to sea level and return to altitude (Hurtado 1942).

Outside South America, CMS was observed in Leadville (3100 m), a mining town in Colorado, USA, by Monge M. in the late 1940s (Winslow and Monge 1987, p. 15) and from the 1960s the condition has been studied there by Weil and colleagues (1971) from Denver (section 21.2.3). Reports of CMS from the Himalayas indicate the condition to be prevalent in immigrant Han Chinese in Lhasa (3658 m) but less common in the indigenous Tibetan population (Pei *et al.* 1989).

21.2.2 Clinical aspects of CMS

DEFINITION OF CHRONIC MOUNTAIN SICKNESS

The latest consensus statement defines CMS as

> A clinical syndrome that occurs in natives or long-life residents above 2500 m. It is characterized by excessive erythrocytosis ([Hb] $\geqslant$ 19 dL^{-1} for females and $\geqslant$ 21 dL^{-1} for males), severe hypoxemia and in some cases moderate or severe pulmonary hypertension, which may evolve into cor pulmonale, leading to congestive heart failure. The clinical picture of CMS gradually disappears after descending to low altitude and reappears after returning to high altitude. (León-Velarde *et al.* 2005)

The consensus statement also excludes from the definition of CMS patients with any chronic pulmonary disease or any other chronic condition which worsens the hypoxemia of altitude, though it does allow a diagnosis of secondary CMS in such cases.

SYMPTOMS

Patients typically have rather vague neuropsychological complaints including headache, dizziness, paresthesia, somnolence, fatigue, difficulty in concentration and loss of mental acuity. There may also be irritability, depression and even hallucinations. Dyspnea on exertion is not commonly complained of, but poor exercise tolerance is common and patients may gain weight. The characteristic feature of the disease is that the symptoms disappear on going down to sea level, only to reappear on return to altitude.

A symptom more recently reported in CMS is that of burning feet or hands. This was first described by León-Velarde and Arregui in 1994 (quoted by Thomas *et al.* 2000). In a study by Thomas *et al.* (2000) this symptom was present in all 10 unselected CMS patients but also four out of five control subjects, resident at the same altitude, and free of CMS. They complained of intermittent burning usually confined to the feet. The symptoms subsided in patients who went down to low altitudes and reappeared on return to high altitude.

SIGNS

Although normal people are mildly cyanotic at an altitude of 4000 m, patients with CMS stand out since, with a high hemoglobin concentration and lower oxygen saturation, they have a far higher concentration of reduced hemoglobin. In Andean Indians, the population with the greatest number of patients, the signs may be florid:

> The combination of virtually black lips and wine red mucosal surfaces against the olive green pigmentation of the Indian skin gives the patient with Monge's disease a striking appearance. (Heath and Williams 1995, p. 193)

The conjunctivae are congested and the fingers may be clubbed. In Caucasians and at lower altitudes such as Leadville (3100 m), the appearances are rather less striking, resembling patients with polycythemia secondary to hypoxic lung disease at sea level. Some patients show very little in the way of signs.

INVESTIGATIONS

The red cell count, hemoglobin concentration and packed cell volume are raised; values as high as $28.0\,g\,dL^{-1}$ hemoglobin and a hematocrits of over 80% have been recorded (Hurtado 1942). Like secondary polycythemia at sea level and unlike polycythemia rubra vera there is no increase in white cell numbers. Blood gases, compared with healthy controls at the same altitude, show a higher Pa,CO_2 and lower Pa,O_2 and oxygen saturation (Peñaloza and Sime 1971, Kryger et al. 1978a). The lower Pa,O_2 is partly due to hypoventilation as shown by the increased Pa,CO_2 and partly (in many cases) by an increased alveolar–arterial oxygen pressure, $((A–a)O_2$ gradient).

Manier et al. (1988) found a mean of 10.5 mmHg in CMS patients at La Paz (3600 m) compared with the normal $(A–a)O_2$ of 2.9 mmHg at this altitude. Using the multiple inert gas technique, they attributed most of this to increased blood flow to poorly ventilated areas of lung rather than to true shunting. Tewari et al. (1991) found a reduced diffusing capacity (DLCO) in lowland soldiers with excessive polycythemia on return to low altitude. The DLCO improved with time at low altitude and return to a normal hematocrit. The DLCO was lower in smokers than nonsmokers though both were well below predicted values. In some cases of CMS standard pulmonary function tests show abnormalities indicating obstructive and/or restrictive defects, suggesting that patients have coexisting chronic lung disease.

Thomas et al. (2000) investigated the pathology underlying the burning feet and hands symptom by taking peripheral nerve biopsies (sural nerve) in 10 CMS patients who all had this symptom. They found a neuropathy consisting of a thinning of the basal laminal layer of endoneural micro-vessels. This is the opposite of that seen in diabetic neuropathy but has been reported in severe chronic hypoxia due to COPD (Malik et al. 1990).

HEMODYNAMICS AND PATHOLOGY

The very high hematocrit increases the viscosity of the blood. The systemic blood pressure may be moderately elevated and the pulmonary artery pressure is significantly higher than that of healthy high altitude residents. Peñaloza et al. (1971) found a mean pulmonary artery pressure of 64/33 mmHg in 10 cases of CMS compared with 34/23 mmHg in controls. Cardiac output was not significantly different, so that calculated resistance was just over twice that of controls. As well as the effect of increased viscosity there would also be pulmonary vasoconstriction due to hypoxia. In present terminology we would say patients who have high pulmonary artery pressure have both CMS and HAPH.

As might be expected these hemodynamic changes lead to increased right ventricular hypertrophy and associated electrocardiogram (ECG) changes. Halperin et al. (1998) found that 90% of cases of CMS had ECG evidence of right ventricular hypertrophy. There is also thickening of the pulmonary arteries to a greater degree than in normal residents at high altitude (Arias-Stella et al. 1973).

PREVENTION

Descent to low altitude without return is a sure preventative but not an option for many altitude residents whose livelihood depends upon their work at altitude. Attention to any secondary risk factors such as smoking is obvious. Since many patients are miners, efforts can also be made to avoid occupational health risks such as dust and air pollution, but these are frequently difficult to eliminate. In this respect pollution of drinking water by cobalt may be important in some cases (see section in 22.2.5).

TREATMENT

As already mentioned, symptoms and signs classically clear up on going down to sea level. However, many patients want to remain at altitude for family or economic reasons. In these cases, venesection is beneficial. Venesection not only lowers the raised hematocrit but also improves many of the neuropsychological symptoms. It also improves pulmonary gas exchange (Cruz et al. 1979) and exercise performance in some subjects (Winslow and Monge 1987, p. 212). In Leadville, Colorado, with about 60 patients being regularly bled for therapeutic purposes, the blood bank has no need of any other donors (Kryger et al. 1978a)!

An alternative to venesection for residents at high altitude is the long-term use of respiratory stimulants. Kryger *et al.* (1978b) have reported success with medroxyprogesterone acetate. They showed a fall in hemoglobin concentration after 10 weeks' treatment in 17 patients. The drug stimulated ventilation and P_{O_2} and reduced P_{CO_2} by a modest amount. Although the changes in blood gases were small, they suggest that the main benefit may have been in oxygenation at night since hypoxemia may be much greater then. The only side effect reported was of loss of libido in four patients. In all but one, this could be overcome by lowering the dose to a level that still kept the hemoglobin concentration down. In one patient the dose had to be reduced to a point which did not hold down the hemoglobin concentration.

In previous editions we reported that there had been no trials of acetazolamide in CMS. There has now been a double-blind controlled trial of acetazolamide in CMS (Richalet *et al.* 2005b). Three groups of patients ($n = 10$ in each group) were treated with either acetazolamide 250 or 500 mg daily or placebo for 3 weeks. There was significant decrease in haematocrit, serum erythropoietin, and soluble transferrin and an increase in nocturnal S_{a,O_2} of 5%. The results for the 250 mg group were as good as for the 500 mg. This simple low cost therapy would seem to offer benefit to the large number of patients with this condition.

21.2.3 Epidemiology of CMS

ANDES

CMS is found most commonly in the Andes, where it was first described mainly affecting the local Amerindians, especially the Quechuan population living on the altiplano at altitudes about 3300–4500 m. Men are affected far more commonly than women. The average age is 40 years with a range from 22 to 51 years in one reported series (Peñaloza *et al.* 1971). Occasional cases are seen in expatriate mining company staff. It used to be thought that CMS was virtually confined to the Andes but this is not the case, as is discussed below.

HIMALAYAS AND TIBET

Until recently there have been few reported cases of CMS in the Himalayas. Winslow noted one Sherpa on the American Medical Research Expedition to

Everest to have a hematocrit of 72% (Winslow and Monge 1987, p. 17). Pei *et al.* (1989) describe their experience of CMS in Lhasa (3658 m). The condition is not uncommon among male cigarette-smoking Han Chinese. These subjects had immigrated some years before becoming polycythemic and then displayed the usual signs and symptoms of CMS. In a 12-month period there were 24 patients admitted to their hospital with CMS. All were male, 23 were Han and only one Tibetan. Six were nonsmokers, the rest, including the one Tibetan, were smokers. The mean duration of altitude exposure in the lowlanders was 26 years (range, 9–43 years). However, though the incidence in Tibetans may be less than in Han immigrants, CMS is now being reported in this population. Wu *et al.* (1992) reported a series of 26 cases in native-born Tibetans living at between 3680 m and 4179 m with typical symptoms of CMS and hemoglobin concentration of 22.2 g dL^{-1} mean compared with 16.6 g dL^{-1} in healthy controls at the same altitude.

In Himalayan residents, hemoglobin concentration tends to be lower than the values from the Peruvian Andes, although much of this difference disappears if results from mining towns are excluded (Frisancho 1988). It is speculated that this may be because the geography allows residents to move to lower altitudes more easily than from the altiplano of the Andes, and the way of life of the Sherpas, with seasonal migration, contributes to this movement in altitude. Like the inhabitants of the Andes, Tibetans live on a high altitude plain and cannot easily move up and down.

Although more evidence is needed it would seem that people of Tibetan stock are less at risk of CMS than Andean highlanders, and certainly than lowland Han subjects long resident at altitude. This may be due to genuine genetic adaptation to altitude over very many generations.

A review comparing incidence of CMS in the Andes with that in Tibet seems to bear out this earlier speculation (Moore *et al.* 1998b). This review also presents more evidence on incidence at various altitudes, men versus women, and Tibetan versus Han Chinese.

NORTH AMERICA

The condition is well recognized in Leadville, Colorado (3100 m). Kryger *et al.* (1978a) described

20 cases, all male, and mentioned that, of about 60 cases known to physicians there, only two were female. One case of apparently classical CMS in a 67-year-old woman has been reported from as low as 2000 m in California (Gronbeck 1984).

21.2.4 Scoring of chronic mountain sickness

A symptom/sign scoring system for CMS was proposed at the 6th World Congress of Mountain Medicine in Qinghai in August 2004 and included in the consensus statement (León-Velarde *et al.* 2005). The purpose was to provide a means of comparing cases from one study to another. Symptoms/signs are scored as 0 to 3 indicating: 0, no symptom; 1, mild; 2 moderate; and 3 severe symptom/sign. The list of symptoms/signs are as follows: breathlessness/palpitations, sleep disturbance, cyanosis, dilatation of veins, paresthesia, headache, tinnitus. Hemoglobin level: males >18 but $<21\,dL^{-1} = 0$; $\geqslant 21\,dL^{-1} = 3$; females >16 but $<19\,dL^{-1} = 0$, $\geqslant 19\,dL^{-1} = 3$.

21.2.5 Mechanisms of CMS

CMS WITH NORMAL LUNGS

Patients with CMS have lower Pa,O_2 and Sa,O_2 and higher Pa,CO_2 values than healthy subjects at the same altitude. The greater hypoxemia results in higher erthropoietin levels and thus greater erthrocytosis. So what is the cause of this more severe hypoxia? The raised Pa,CO_2 points to a degree of hypoventilation but there may also be some gas transfer defect as well. As mentioned above, a widened $P(A-a)O_2$ gradient has been shown in CMS patients (Manier *et al.* 1988).

Severinghaus *et al.* (1966a) found that CMS patients have an extremely blunted HVR compared with healthy resident controls of the same age. Maybe people at the low end of the spectrum for HVR in the population are destined to get CMS if they remain for years at altitude. The HVR decreases with age (Kronenberg and Drage 1973) and with duration of stay at altitude (Wiel *et al.* 1971); perhaps patients with CMS are those in whom the process is faster than average (Fig. 21.1).

Kryger *et al.* (1978a), however, found no difference in HVR between patients and age-matched

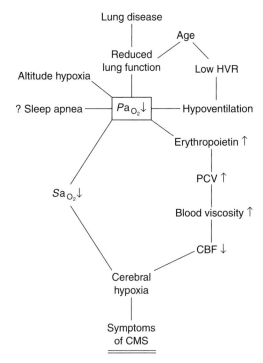

Figure 21.1   Possible mechanisms in the development of chronic mountain sickness (CMS). HVR, hypoxic ventilatory response; CBF, cerebral blood flow; PCV, packed cell volume.

controls in Leadville, Colorado. They did find that their patients had a greater dead-space/tidal volume ratio and that their ventilation increased on breathing 100% oxygen; they therefore appeared to have hypoxic ventilatory depression. They concluded that blunted chemical drive to breathing is not the cause of CMS.

SLEEP

During sleep, even in normal subjects, the ventilation is depressed. If there are frequent periods of apnea, either central or obstructive, Sa,O_2 will be further reduced and could contribute to the etiology. A study by Sun *et al.* (1996) found that CMS patients had more disordered breathing and lower mean Sa,O_2 values when asleep than a group free of CMS. In periods of disordered breathing non CMS controls increased their cerebral blood flow whereas the CMS group did not. Therefore the latter had a reduction in their calculated brain oxygen delivery. Recently Spicuzza *et al.* (2004) in a study of CMS patients and controls at 4300 m confirmed the greater hypoxemia in CMS patients when awake and showed that they were also more hypoxic when asleep. In particular the total time spent with $Sa,O_2 < 80\%$ was significantly greater in the CMS patients. This level of desaturation would be expected to trigger a greater erythropoietin release. Reeves and Weil (2001) in their review of over 900 patients with CMS studied over the years emphasize the profound hypoxia in these patients, when asleep.

GENDER

Women (at least before the menopause) seem to be protected from CMS as from the hypoventilation syndrome (the Pickwickian syndrome) at sea level, possibly by the stimulating effect of progesterone on ventilation. León-Velarde et al. (1997) compared pre-menopausal and postmenopausal women at Cerro de Pasco (4300 m) in Peru and found significantly higher hematocrit and lower Sa,O_2, and peak expiratory flows in the postmenopausal group, supporting the protective role of female sex hormones.

AGE

Age has effects on lung function as well as its effect on HVR. The Pa,O_2 declines with age and, although this has little effect on oxygen saturation at sea level, it has much more effect at altitude because subjects are already on the steep part of the oxygen dissociation curve. A study by León-Velarde et al. (1993) at 4300 m in Peru found an increasing incidence of CMS with age. Taking a hemoglobin concentration of above 21.3 g dL^{-1} as 'excessive erythrocytosis', the incidence at 20–29 years was 6.8% which increased to 33.7% at age 60–69 years. This study also found a decreasing vital capacity with age at altitude, in both those with and without CMS, but the reduction was significantly more marked in the CMS group. Sea level subjects showed no reduction in vital capacity between 20–29 years and 60–69 years.

COBALT

Cobalt is a known stimulant of erythropoiesis. In a review of their experience over many years, Reeves and Weil (2001) collected details of more than 750 men and 200 women with CMS. They noted that one of the contributing factors to the variation in the erythropoietic response to altitude was ingested toxins and minerals such as cobalt. Jefferson et al. (2002) in a study from Cerro de Pasco (4300 m) found that 11 of their 21 subjects with CMS had detectable cobalt levels in their serum compared with none in their controls. However, Bernardi et al. (2003) in their study also in Cerro do Pasco found normal cobalt levels in CMS patients. Cerro de Pasco is a mining town and cobalt is one of the many minerals in the rocks. It was not found in samples of drinking water tested by Jefferson et al. but perhaps leaches in at times. It may, therefore, act as a risk factor in some cases of CMS in some localities.

CEREBRAL BLOOD FLOW IN CMS

Polycythemia (rubra vera) results in reduced cerebral blood flow (CBF) (Thomas et al. 1977) due to increased viscosity. However, the few studies of CBF, (measuring blood velocity by Doppler ultrasound) in CMS have either shown no significant differences between subjects with and without CMS when awake breathing air (Sun S et al. 1996), or the expected reduced flow in CMS patients compared with controls (Claydon et al. 2005).

GENETICS AND CMS

There seems to be a difference in response to long-term, chronic hypoxia in different populations and only a proportion of any population is susceptible to CMS. These considerations lead to the question of whether there is a genetic component to susceptibility. Mejia et al. (2005) in a case–control study looked at a variety of candidate genes including: erythropoietin, erythropoietin-receptor, HIF-1α (von Hippel-Lindau and others). They found no association between the polymorphisms linked to the candidate genes and severe polycythemia.

EXCESSIVE ERYTHROCYTOSIS WITH LUNG DISEASE

In cases of excessive erythrocytosis with definite lung disease, it is easy to understand that the combination of altitude with fairly mild lung disease precipitates polycythemia and cor pulmonale (Fig. 21.1). Removal of altitude hypoxia by descent to sea level is sufficient to reverse the process. At altitude, these patients are more hypoxic than normal people because of their lung disease, hence their stimulus to erythrocytosis via erythropoietin secretion is greater and they become abnormally polycythemic. The importance of lower respiratory tract disease is emphasized in a study by León-Velarde *et al.* (1994) which shows that subjects with chronic lower respiratory disease had higher hemoglobin concentration, lower $Sa_{,O_2}$ and higher CMS symptom scores than healthy controls or subjects with chronic upper respiratory disease.

SUMMARY

Figure 21.1 shows the interaction of factors involved in CMS. Altitude hypoxia and hypoventilation will result in a low $Pa_{,O_2}$. This hypoventilatory response may be due to a low HVR, to hypoxic depression of ventilation or some unknown cause. If lung function is also reduced by lung or chest wall disease, this will reduce $Pa_{,O_2}$ still further. Aging results in both reduced lung function and reduced HVR, especially in a life spent at high altitude, thus further lowering the $Pa_{,O_2}$. The low $Pa_{,O_2}$ results in a low $Sa_{,O_2}$. It also stimulates secretion of erythropoietin and hence an increase in hematocrit. However, it should be noted that a study of erythropoietin levels in subjects at Cerro de Pasco (4300 m), although showing the expected higher mean values at altitude than at sea level, did not demonstrate any difference between subjects with and without CMS (León-Velarde *et al.* 1991). The rise in hematocrit causes a rise in blood viscosity and probably, a fall in cerebral blood flow, which, with a low $Sa_{,O_2}$, results in chronic severe cerebral hypoxia and symptoms of CMS.

21.3 HIGH ALTITUDE PULMONARY HYPERTENSION

21.3.1 Introduction and history

It has been known for 60 years that hypoxia results in pulmonary hypertension. This was first demonstrated by von Euler and Liljestrand (1946) in cats and shortly afterwards by Motley *et al.* (1947) in man. This hypoxic pressor response is important in the fetus since blood must be diverted away from the nonfunctioning lung through the ductus arteriosis to the rest of the body. Its effect in life after birth may be to improve ventilation/perfusion ratios in the lung when parts of the lung are unventilated, for instance by bronchiolar occlusion in asthma or lobar consolidation in pneumonia. In these situations, the areas underventilated become hypoxic and it is clearly beneficial for vasoconstriction in these areas to reduce the blood flow and divert it to other, ventilated parts of the lung. But at altitude, with global hypoxia there is vasoconstriction throughout the lung and the pulmonary artery pressure rises with no benefit to gas transfer apart from possibly some slight improvement in the upright lung due to rather more even perfusion. It is of note that animals adapted to high altitude, such as the yak (Harris 1986) or pika (Ge, L.R. *et al.* 1998) do not have this pressor response and Tibetans have a greatly diminished response (Groves *et al.* 1993.)

As early as 1956 Rotta *et al.* found pulmonary hypertension in acclimatized lowlanders and residents at altitude. In 1962 Penaloza *et al.* and Arias-Stella *et al.* presented their data on pulmonary hypertension and pulmonary artery pathology respectively showing hypertension and muscularization of the pulmonary arterioles in healthy people resident at altitude in the Andes. This remodeling results in sustained hypertension even when hypoxia is relieved by oxygen breathing (see section 7.5.1) or descent to low altitude, although after some months or years at low altitude hypertension does remit.

Patients with CMS often also had pulmonary hypertension (section 21.2.2) and sometimes developed right heart failure, but the severe erythrocytosis had been described earlier and, since blood counts were so much easier to carry out than cardiac catheterization, the hypertension tended to be dismissed and attributed mainly to the increased viscosity due to high hematocrit rather than to hypoxic vasoconstriction followed by remodeling. This early work in Peru has been thoughtfully reviewed by Reeves and Grover (2005).

In 1988 Sui *et al.* published their experience with infants born at low altitude and taken to high altitude in Tibet. They called the condition sub-acute infantile mountain sickness. Shortly afterwards Anand *et al.* (1990) reported a similar condition in adults, soldiers stationed for some months or more at extreme altitude and called it adult sub-acute mountain sickness. Both conditions were essentially right heart failure due to chronic pulmonary hypertension and would be called HAPH in the nomenclature suggested by the consensus statement

(Table 21.1). Since then there have been numerous reports of this condition from high altitude regions of Asia (Ge and Helun 2001, Aldeshev *et al.* 2002, Wu 2005).

21.3.2 High altitude pulmonary hypertension in infants

The Spaniards who first colonized the Andes became well aware that their infants did not thrive if born at high altitude. They made it their practice to arrange delivery at low altitude and not to bring their babies to high altitude before 1 year of age.

The lowland Han Chinese colonists of Tibet face the same environmental problem. Wu and Liu (1995) described a Chinese infant of 11 months born in Lhasa (3658 m) who presented with dyspnea, cyanosis and congestive heart failure. At postmortem, marked right ventricular hypertrophy and muscular thickening of the peripheral pulmonary artery tree were found. There was no other pathology such as congenital heart disease and the authors called the condition high altitude heart disease. Sui *et al.* (1988) had reported the postmortem findings on 15 infants who died in Lhasa of a syndrome they called infantile sub-acute mountain sickness. The presenting symptoms were commonly dyspnea and cough, with often sleeplessness, irritability and signs of cyanosis, edema of the face, oliguria, tachycardia, liver enlargement, rales in the lungs and fever. The majority of infants had been born at low altitude but two were born at high altitude, one of Han and one of Tibetan parents. The condition was usually fatal in a matter of weeks or months. The post-mortem findings were of extreme medial hypertrophy of muscular pulmonary arteries and muscularization of pulmonary arterioles. There was massive hypertrophy and dilatation of the right ventricle and of the pulmonary trunk.

21.3.3 High altitude pulmonary hypertension in adults

Anand *et al.* (1990) described a condition in 21 soldiers who, after a full acclimatization period, had been posted to between 5800 m and 6700 m for several months (mean, 1.8 years). They called the condition adult sub-acute mountain sickness. The patients presented with dyspnea, cough and effort angina. The signs were of dependent edema. They were treated at high altitude with diuretics with improvement. When they were evacuated to low altitude by aircraft they were found to have cardiomegaly with right ventricular enlargement and, in most cases, pericardial effusion. The pulmonary artery pressure was elevated (26 mmHg) and rose significantly on mild exercise to 40 mmHg. Recovery was rapid after descent from high altitude. Investigations showed a generalized increase in the volume of the fluid compartments of the body and total body sodium, even in subjects without overt disease at these altitudes for this length of time (Anand *et al.* 1993). The increase in central blood volume is the probable cause of the decrease in forced vital capacity, and the radiographically engorged pulmonary vessels found in the subjects of Operation Everest II (Welsh *et al.* 1993). A similar condition was described by Wu (2005) in his review of CMS on the Qinghai–Tibetan plateau. It would seem that this HAPH with right heart failure is the human form of a similar condition affecting cattle taken to high altitude, and known as brisket disease (Hecht *et al.* 1959). The brisket is the loose skin area of the cow's neck, which is dependent and becomes swollen with edema fluid in this condition.

Pei *et al.* (1989) reviewed their experience of CMS in Lhasa based on 17 cases. Sixteen were Han Chinese men whilst the 17th was a Tibetan woman. The men had all moved from lowland China to Tibet to an altitude of 3600 an average of 15 years before admission to hospital. Their symptoms and signs were cough, dyspnea, dependent edema, liver enlargement and raised jugular venous pressure. The mean hematocrit was 70% and in the five patients who were catheterized the pulmonary artery pressure was 57/28 mean. Reviewing the natural history of the disease, they suggested that the earlier stage of the disease was dominated by polycythemia while cardiopulmonary involvement increases with the duration of the disease.

CLINICAL FEATURES

Mild or moderate pulmonary hypertension does not give rise to symptoms. There may be signs, an accentuated second heart sound and ECG and echo-cardiographic evidence of hypertension but

Table 21.2   Prevalence (percentage of population) of high altitude heart disease (HAPH) at various altitudes of residence in Han and Tibetan children and adults

Altitude (m)	Han		Tibetan	
	Children	Adults	Children	Adults
<3000	0.47	0.07	0.2	0
3000–4000	1.47	0.71	0.37	0.24
4000–5000	3.64	1.72	1.04	0.46

Children are more susceptible than adults and Han Chinese than Tibetans. The prevalence increases with altitude. Data of Wu and Ge quoted in Ge and Helun 2001.

symptoms only develop when the right heart begins to fail. The symptoms are of headache, dyspnea, cough, irritability, sleeplessness and sometimes angina on exertion. Clinical signs include cyanosis, tachycardia, tachypnoea, edema of face, liver enlargement and crackles in the chest (Ge and Helun 2001). On going down to low altitude all these symptoms and signs typically disappear in a few days or weeks although occasionally the hypertension may be detectable for a year or more.

EPIDEMIOLOGY AND PREVALENCE

Some populations are more susceptible than others. In Qinghai and Tibet the Han Chinese immigrants are more susceptible than Tibetans (by a factor of 3–4). Children are more susceptible than adults (by a factor of about 3). These data are shown in Table 21.2.

Men are more susceptible than women. Aldeshev and colleagues have reported on their studies of HAPH in the high altitude population in Kyrgyzstan (Aldeshev *et al.* 2002). A health survey, including ECG, was carried out in three villages between 2800 and 3100 m. ECG recordings on 741 subjects (347 males, 394 females) were analyzed. Fourteen percent had one or more criteria for cor pulmonale, 23% of males and only 6% of females, a highly significant difference.

NATURAL HISTORY OF HAPH

Aldeshev *et al.* (2002) carried out right heart catheterization in Bishkek (760 m) on a group of 136 male highlanders resident between 2800 and 3600. Three groups were identified: (1) a group

with normal pulmonary artery pressures, (2) those with normal pressures but who had a greater than two-fold increase in pressure on breathing a hypoxic gas mixture, and (3) a group with frank pulmonary hypertension. The percentages for these groups were: 59, 21 and 20%. They were able to follow up 25 subjects 10 years later. Of the normotensive group, there was no increase in pressure. All 10 of the subjects followed up in the hyper-responsiveness group showed increase in pressures as did the seven subjects followed up in the hypertension group.

GENETIC CONTRIBUTION TO HAPH

It has been well established that brisket disease in cattle affects only certain breeds and that the pulmonary hypertensive trait in susceptible breeds is genetically determined (Cruz *et al.* 1980). HAPH is the human equivalent of this condition. Fagan and Weil (2001) have reviewed the evidence of the genetic contribution to the control of pulmonary artery pressure at altitude. They conclude that the differences among diverse altitude populations (such as indicated above) suggest an evolutionary, genetic influence on the response of the pulmonary circulation to the hypoxia of altitude. Tucker and Rhodes (2001) reviewed the role of pulmonary vascular smooth muscle in the development of HAPH in various animals and humans. There was good evidence for the hypothesis that the amount of smooth muscle predicted the degree of response. Cattle and pigs are high responders and have thick muscle layers; sheep, dogs and a variety of animals native to high altitude are low responders and have thin muscle walls to their pulmonary arteries. Humans, rats and mice are intermediate. That these differences are genetically determined is supported by studies in cross breeds between yak and cattle (Anand *et al.* (1986).

Aldeshev *et al.* (2002) reported their results of ACE genotyping in 78 male highlanders who had undergone cardiac catheterization. There was a three-fold higher frequency of the I/I allele in highlanders with HAPH, compared with normal highlanders and the mean pulmonary artery pressure was significantly higher in subjects with I/I than with I/D or D/D. A comparison of the frequency of these alleles between lowlanders resident in Bishkek and high altitude residents showed a significantly lower frequency of I/I and higher D/D in the highlanders, suggesting possibly evolutionary selection of D/D alleles in the high altitude population.

TREATMENT OF HAPH

The whole process of pulmonary arterial vasoconstriction and remodeling is reversed by descent to low altitude and the relief of hypoxia. However, the option of emigration from their high altitude homes and relocating to low altitude is not open to many patients with HAPH. For these patients the possibility of drug treatment may be considered. However, such trials as have been reported are all short-term, so we do not know the long-term result of drug treatment on disease progression.

Antezana *et al.* (1998) showed that nifedipine reduced the pulmonary artery pressure (*P*pa) in patients with AHPH by 20% in two-thirds of patients. The effect was greatest in those with the highest pressures and was not correlated with [Hb]. The phosphodiesterase inhibitor, sildenafil, has been shown to be effective in lowering *P*pa (and improving gas exchange) in healthy subjects taken to altitude for 6 days (Richalet *et al.* 2005a). Aldashev *et al.* (2005) studied 22 patients with HAPH in a controlled trial of two doses of sildenafil (25 mg and 100 mg, every 8 h) or placebo, for 3 months. The two doses were equally effective in lowering *P*pa and in increasing the length of the 6 min walking test. Sildenafil was said to be well tolerated. There do not seem to have been any trials of acetazolamide in HAPH.

22

Other altitude-related conditions: neurovascular disorders, eye conditions, altitude cough, anesthesia at altitude

SUMMARY

A cluster of neurovascular signs and symptoms has been reported in mountaineers for many years. These vary from transient ischemic attacks (TIAs), often with symptoms of dysphasia or transient visual disturbance or even blindness, to longer lasting strokes with hemiplegia, etc. The problems usually occur after some time at altitude and so are not considered part of acute mountain sickness (AMS). The condition usually resolves rapidly and recurrence is unusual. However, few patients expose themselves to altitude risk again. Also reviewed in this chapter is the effect of altitude on factors involved in clotting, which in general seem little disturbed at altitude. Risk factors for thrombosis and mechanisms are discussed.

Eye problems at altitude include retinal hemorrhage, transient visual disturbance or blindness, which may be neurovascular or migrainous in origin, and problems following corneal surgery. Retinal hemorrhages are quite common at altitude but are normally a symptomless, benign condition diagnosed only if the retina is inspected. Small hemorrhages are seen which clear in a few days. The incidence is variable, often being over 50% when looked for. It is usually seen early in altitude exposure. Only in rare cases, when the hemorrhage affects the macula, is vision disturbed. Problems after corneal surgery are confined to patients who have had radial keratotomy for myopia. In these patients the hypoxia of altitude results in a change in the refractive properties of the operated eye, making for long-sightedness. At extreme altitude this can render the patient almost blind. The problem resolves after descent.

Altitude cough, though known for many years, has only recently been scientifically investigated. It afflicts most climbers who remain at altitude for more than a few days and in severe cases can cause sleep disturbance, fatigue and even fracture of ribs.

Although hyperventilation of the cold dry air at altitude may be a factor, it seems that hypoxia itself is important. The cough threshold for citric acid is lowered by stay at altitude and this can be prevented by therapy with anti-asthma inhalers. Altitude also affects mucociliary function in the nose and this can be prevented by regular moistening of the nasal mucosa with saline.

General anesthesia at altitude is dangerous because of the respiratory depressant effects of anesthetics. They abolish the hypoxic ventilatory response (HVR) so that ventilation is reduced and with the low inspired P_{O_2} the risk of severe hypoxia is considerable. This risk of hypoxia extends into the post-operative period because even small concentrations of anesthetic gases depress the HVR. It is therefore advised that general anesthetic be avoided at altitude. Either local anesthetic should be used or the patient brought down to low altitude. If general anesthetic must be given at altitude, ketamine is probably the agent of choice; oxygen should be added at high concentrations.

22.1 NEUROVASCULAR DISORDERS

22.1.1 Historical background

Increasingly, cases with neurological signs, some transient and others permanent, are being reported from expeditions at altitude in both lowlanders and highlanders. These are not associated with AMS, or high altitude cerebral or pulmonary edema (HACE, HAPE). It is likely that some have a vascular origin, such as spasm, thrombosis, embolus or hemorrhage. Others may be focal neurological disorders or are of unknown etiology.

Sporadic cases of vascular disorders have been described in the mountain and geographical literature over the last century (Table 22.1).

Table 22.1   Cerebrovascular accidents at altitude*

Date	Altitude (m)	Time at altitude	Signs	Outcome	Source
1895	4300	?	Right hemiparesis	Recovered	Roborovsky (1896)
1924	6000	?	Hemiparesis	Died	Norton (1925)
1938	6400	?	Right hemiparesis	Recovered	Tilman (1948)
1943	6400	6 weeks	Dysphasia	Recovered	Shipton (1943)
1954	6000+	?	Hemiparesis	Died	Evans (1956)
1961	6400	7–8 weeks	Right hemiparesis	Recovered	Ward (1968)
1978	6400	?	Hemiparesis	?	Messner (1979, p. 137)
1982	8200	7 weeks	Left hemiparesis	Recovered	Clarke (1983)
1983	6100	?	Semi-conscious	Recovered	Asaji et al. (1984)
1986	4900	Several days	Headache, visual disturbance		
			Numb right hand, ?migraine	Recovered	Jenzer and Bärtsch (1993)
1990	4800	9 days	Right hemiparesis	Recovered	Sharma et al. (1990)
1990	5300	Several days	Headache, weak right hand and right leg, ?migraine	Recovered	Jenzer and Bärtsch (1993)
1994	3867	4 days	Right lat. rectus palsy	Recovered	Murdoch (1994)
1994	4242	12 days	Right lat. rectus palsy	Recovered	Murdoch (1994)
1995	3660	100 mile race	Diplopia	Recovered	Murdoch (1994)
1997	7600	Several days	Right hemiparesis, CT scan edema, left parietal lobe	Recovered	Basnyat (1997)

* All subjects were male adults. The two patients who died were Sherpas; the remainder were climbers from low altitude.

In 1895, while exploring the Amne Machin range in eastern Tibet, Roborovsky, a Russian traveler, suffered a 'stroke' in crossing the Mangur Pass (4270 m). He described

a stroke of paralysis which attacked the right part of my body from head to the toes of my right foot; my tongue hardly obeyed my will. I lay in a disgusting and unbearable state for eight days.

Over the next few weeks he gradually recovered and continued his journey (Roborovsky 1896).

Cases of hemiplegia also occurred on Everest expeditions in 1924 and 1936. One, a Gurkha soldier, died, and the other, a Sherpa porter, recovered (Norton 1925, p. 68, Tilman 1948). Evans (1956, p. 169) on Kangchenjunga recorded a further fatal case of hemiplegia in a Sherpa. Each of these three cases was in a fit young man who had spent a considerable period above 6000 m.

In 1954, a young American mountaineer, stormbound in a tent at 7465 m on K2, developed thrombophlebitis in the calf and, after a further 2 days, had a hemoptysis. A provisional diagnosis of pulmonary embolus was made and he was evacuated; however, during the descent he was swept away in an avalanche (Houston and Bates 1979).

Shipton (1943), after climbing to 8865 m on Everest, described an episode of transient aphasia with severe headache. This was possibly due to a migraine attack. Apart from severe headache he had no other symptoms and was fully recovered by the next morning.

22.1.2 Varieties of neurovascular disorders

Basnyat et al. (2004) have reviewed neurological conditions at altitude that fall outside the definition of AMS. These they list as:

- Transient ischemic attacks (TIAs) and strokes or cerebro-vascular accidents (CVAs)
- Migraine
- Cerebral venous thrombosis
- Subarachnoid hemorrhage
- Seizures, epileptic fits
- High altitude syncope
- Space occupying lesions
- Transient global amnesia
- Delirium at high altitude
- Cranial nerve palsies
- Possible coagulation problems
- Ophthalmological problems

The cases of Roborovsky and of Shipton mentioned above could be considered as examples of TIAs. Wohns (1986) reported two cases of TIA on Everest north-east ridge and a third patient who suffered TIAs on three separate high altitude climbs. Jenzer and Bärtsch (1993) reported a case of a climber with transient aphasia, right sided sensory and motor impairment with headache. He had similar symptoms on a subsequent expedition. In Operation Everest III (Comex), a 40-day chamber study of eight subjects, there were three cases of TIA towards the end of the study at an altitude equivalent to above 8000 m. They all recovered rapidly (Richalet et al. 1999). Murdoch (1996) reported cases with various focal neurological defects at altitude with, again, rapid recovery. The distinction between TIA and stroke is somewhat arbitrary. A number of cases typical of stroke (hemiparesis, aphasia) have been reported (Table 22.1) but in contra-distinction to stroke seen in hospital practice, almost all cases seen at altitude make complete recovery within 24 h.

22.1.3 Migraine

Migraine is very common at sea level so its occurrence at altitude may be coincidental. However, anecdotal reports suggest that altitude may well be a trigger for attacks. Engel et al., as early as 1944, reported that migraine developed repeatedly in patients taken to high altitude in a chamber (quoted by Basnyat et al. 2004). The severity of attacks may be worse at altitude (Murdoch 1995) and may be attended by various transient, focal neurological defects. A case report by Jenzer and Bärtsch (1993) illustrates this. A healthy 25-year-old mountaineer suffered mild migraine at low altitude but after a climb to over 8000 m he experienced very severe headache together with some aphasia and sensory impairment of his tongue and right hand. Four years later he had another episode, similar in many ways to the first. Both episodes lasted a number of hours and subsequent neurological examination including computed tomography (CT) scans were all negative. The headache may not be the typical one-sided headache of migraine and may be hard to distinguish from that due to AMS.

22.1.4 Cerebral venous thrombosis

Dickenson *et al.* (1983) noted cerebral venous thrombosis in autopsies of patients evacuated to Kathmandu after death at altitude. Song *et al.* (1986) made the same finding in his patients all of whom had been at altitudes of greater than 5000 m for more than 3 weeks. Patients usually present with hemiparesis. They suggested that plasma volume depletion due to dehydration and polycythemia may be a factor in the genesis of the condition.

Jha *et al.* (2002) reported their experience of stroke in Indian Army personnel admitted to their hospital from high altitude. Of the 30 stroke patients, the majority had ischemic strokes but two patients had cerebral venous thromboses. Superior sagittal sinus thrombosis was diagnosed in a case of a climber in the French alps who developed right sided weakness and dysphasia with seizures (Boulos *et al.* (2000). He was found to have a low protein C level and the same deficiency was found in one family member. The patient gradually improved on anticoagulant treatment. From Israel a case of sagittal and transverse sinus thrombosis was reported by Torgovicky *et al.* (2005) in a chamber instructor who presented with severe frontal headaches persisting for a month following routine high altitude chamber training. She also made a slow recovery on anti-coagulant therapy. Complete coagulation screening failed to find any defect. The patient had been taking oral contraceptives.

22.1.5 Subarachnoid hemorrhage

This condition, which affects otherwise healthy young individuals, may strike while the patient is at high altitude and could be misdiagnosed as AMS especially in cases where the vascular malformation leaks rather than ruptures. Hackett (2001) mentions three patients he looked after at altitude with neurological defects, two of whom were subsequently shown to have cerebral arteriovenous malformations and the third, an aneurism. Whether ascent to altitude is a risk factor for subarachnoid hemorrhage is debatable. The vasodilatation that occurs then with increased cerebral blood flow might be a trigger.

22.1.6 Seizures

Although seizures are a feature of acute, very severe hypoxia such as used in the selection of Everest climbers by the Russian 1982 expedition (Gazenco *et al.* 1987), they are not normally seen in AMS or HACE and are not a response to the sort of chronic hypoxia experienced by people going to high altitude. Whether altitude hypoxia is a trigger for seizures in an individual with susceptibility is still an open question. There is some anecdotal evidence that it might be so (Hackett 2001). A recent case report of a mountaineer in the Andes is very suggestive. This 35-year-old man had no previous history of epilepsy but suffered two epilepiform seizures after a night at 5200 m. He had no symptoms of AMS or HAPE. He was later shown to have the typical spike and wave pattern on his EEG on hyperventilation and his father had a similar EEG (Daleau *et al.* 2006). (For further discussion see Chapter 24.)

22.1.7 Space occupying lesions

Shlim *et al.* (1991) reported three cases of patients asymptomatic at low altitude who developed symptoms at altitude found to be due to brain tumors and Hackett (2000) reported a case of a man who suffered diplopia and ataxia on two occasions when he ascended from sea level to 4000 m. He was later diagnosed as having a subarachnoid cyst in the left frontal region. There is slight swelling of the brain on going to altitude even in subjects without AMS (Hackett 1999). Presumably in these patients with a space occupying lesion, the extra pressure from this swelling is enough to cause the lesion to become symptomatic.

22.1.8 Transient global amnesia

The term high altitude global amnesia (HAGA) has been used by Litch and Bishop (2000) to describe a variety of neurological features associated with transient loss of memory and confusion but not associated with any motor or sensory disturbance or obvious HACE or HAPE. As the cerebral cortex is vulnerable to hypoxia, local hypoxia of the limbic cortex may be implicated.

22.1.9 Cranial nerve palsies

Lateral rectus (6th nerve) palsy has been widely reported at altitude (Virmani and Swamy 1993, Shlim *et al.* 1995, Murdoch 1994). In most cases these palsies are not associated with AMS or HACE and the condition is rarely seen in cases of HACE. The resulting diplopia and palsy may last for weeks or months but, in the absence of HAPE is usually benign (Murdoch 1994). Other cranial nerves can be affected, e.g. facial and hypoglossal (Basnyat 2001).

22.1.10 Cortical blindness and transient visual defects

Transient blindness has been reported in otherwise healthy individuals at altitude. Six cases at an altitude of 4300 m were reported by Hackett *et al.* (1987c), four on Denali in Alaska and two at Pheriche near Everest. These individuals were not suffering from pulmonary edema or severe AMS. They did not have retinal hemorrhage. The blindness lasted from 20 min to 24 h, with intermittent periods of normal vision. Oxygen breathing relieved it and recovery was complete. It was thought to be due to hypoxia or ischemia of the visual cortex. Houston (1987) also reported various visual disturbances on acute exposure to altitude in chambers. There is some suggestion that subjects with a history of migraine are more susceptible.

22.2 PLATELETS AND CLOTTING

There has been considerable interest in factors in the blood associated with clotting, and the effect of hypoxia, with and without symptoms of AMS, on these systems. This is because of the frequent finding of thrombi in various organs at post-mortem in cases of AMS and its complications (Dickinson *et al.* 1983), and the frequency of cases of cerebrovascular accidents at altitude.

22.2.1 Platelet counts

In mice, there is a profound fall in platelet count on exposure to hypoxia. Counts are down to 36% of control by day 12 (Birks *et al.* 1975). In humans, no such fall has been found. It has been reported that in the first few days there is either no change (Maher *et al.* 1976, Sharma 1982), or a small fall of 3% in subjects with AMS and a rise of 3% in asymptomatic subjects (Sharma 1980). Chatterji *et al.* (1982) found a 12–26% reduction in platelet count on day 2 or 3 at altitude in two studies at 3200 m and 3700 m. Counts increased towards control values over the next 10 days. These small changes may simply reflect hemoconcentration or dilution. With more prolonged exposure Sharma (1981) found a 14% increase by 21–31 days followed by a fall to sea level values at 180 days. At 4300 m, a rise of between 50 and 100% has been found, both on arrival and 2 weeks later, after climbs to higher altitude (Simon-Schnass and Korniszewski 1990). Hudson *et al.* (1999) also found a significant increase in platelet count in 28 subjects on going up from 600 m to 3600 m in Bolivia with a slight further rise after one week. They also found that residents of El Alto (4200 m) had higher counts than residents of Santa Cruz (600 m).

22.2.2 Platelet adhesiveness

Under a variety of conditions platelets become more sticky, and this property may be important in initiating platelet thrombi. Sharma (1982) has also studied the effect of altitude on platelet adhesiveness. On acute exposure to altitude he reported an increase in platelet adhesiveness in subjects with AMS, compared with their sea level results. However, this was only on days 2 and 10 of altitude exposure and not on days 1 and 4. Also, the sea level values for symptomatic subjects were markedly less than for the asymptomatic group. Actual values at altitude were the same for both groups. He also reported (with others) that high altitude residents had significantly higher platelet adhesiveness than lowlanders at sea level (Sharma *et al.* 1980).

22.2.3 Coagulation

Singh and Chohan (1972a) found an increase in fibrinogen level and fibrinolytic activity in 38 subjects at altitudes between 3670 m and 5470 m, but, in six subjects thought to have pulmonary hypertension on clinical grounds, the fibrinogen levels were lower, suggesting consumption coagulopathy. In these patients, factors V and VIII were increased, as was platelet factor III. Maher *et al.* (1976) also found a fall in fibrinogen level in eight subjects in a simulated altitude of 4400 m but no change in thrombin or prothrombin times; platelet factor III was normal. Partial thromboplastin time was shortened and factor VIII activity was reduced. Hyers *et al.* (1979) found accelerated fibrinolytic activity in subjects with and without susceptibility to AMS but no change in fibrinogen, partial prothrombin time, platelet lysis time or fibrinopeptide A. In patients with HAPE, fibrinogen levels and venous clot lysis time have been reported to be increased (Singh *et al.* 1969a, Singh and Chohan 1972a).

Bärtsch *et al.* (1982) showed, in 20 subjects taken rapidly to 3700 m, that there were no changes in coagulation tests 1 h after arrival. After strenuous exercise there was shortening of clotting time, euglobulin lysis time, and increase in factor VIII activity – changes that are all found on exercise at sea level. There was no change in fibrinopeptide A and no rise in fibrin degradation products or fibrin fragment E (i.e. no evidence of intravascular clotting). In a later study the contact phase of blood coagulation was studied in subjects who had ascended to 4559 m in 3 days. There was no evidence of activation of this system even in subjects who developed acute HAPE (Bärtsch *et al.* 1989).

An extensive study of the clotting cascade during a 40-day chamber experiment, Operation Everest II, when subjects were taken in stages up to the simulated equivalent altitude of Mount Everest, showed no significant changes in clotting factors, though thrombosis round the sites of Swan–Ganz catheters was common (Andrew *et al.* 1987).

In summary, it seems that the physiological response to hypoxia has not been shown to involve any important changes in platelet count or adhesiveness or in other clotting factors. However, there may be changes associated with AMS and especially HAPE (Singh and Chohan 1972b). These may include changes suggesting disseminated intravascular coagulation but this is still not proved. The changes so far demonstrated seem to appear rather too late in the course of altitude exposure to be considered causative, so, even if present, they may represent an effect or a complication of AMS rather than being essential in its genesis.

22.3 SPLINTER HEMORRHAGES

Splinter hemorrhages may occur under the fingernails of high altitude natives, and are more pronounced in those with CMS and in climbers at extreme altitude (English 1987). In South American high altitude dwellers, the incidence appears to increase with altitude, rising from 34.9% at 150 m to 57.9% at 4200 m (Heath and Williams 1995, pp. 311–13). In over 1000 healthy Chinese children born at altitude, examination of the nails showed an increase in number of capillary loops and abnormal loops (Han *et al.* 1985). The cause of these hemorrhages may be associated with increased capillary fragility or it may be embolic or traumatic in origin.

22.4 RISK FACTORS FOR THROMBOSIS

The risk factors for thrombosis include decreased physical activity, dehydration, increased hematocrit and cold.

Physical activity may be greatly decreased at altitude. Individuals may spend several days recumbent in a sleeping bag in bad weather and, even in good weather, activity can be restricted by fatigue to a shorter working period each day than at lower levels.

Dehydration is common, with increased respiratory water loss owing to cold and a high respiratory rate. A diminished sensation of thirst, together with the practical difficulties of melting snow to produce water, results in an inadequate fluid intake.

A hematocrit of 45–60% is normal for sea level visitors to altitude and some high altitude residents. When the hematocrit exceeds 50% the apparent viscosity increases steeply. Vasoconstriction further increases viscosity and thus cold will contribute (Whittaker and Winton 1933, Pappenheimer and Maes 1942).

22.5 MECHANISMS OF VASCULAR ACCIDENTS

The mechanism of vascular accidents is debatable. Short-lived attacks may be due to spasm, or possibly a manifestation of migraine. Thrombosis is another possibility, due to a high hematocrit and dehydration (Ward 1975, pp. 289–92), and disturbances of coagulation and platelet function may also occur. In some cases hemorrhage cannot be ruled out. As with 'stroke' at lower altitudes, there may be different causes.

22.6 CASE HISTORIES

22.6.1 Patient A

A man, aged 32, while climbing at 8400 m, suddenly experienced a severe pain in the right side of his chest and collapsed. He was unable to move for 30 min and then started to cough up dark red blood. After a night at 8200 m he crawled down to a lower camp at 7800 m, continuing to complain of severe pain and coughing up blood.

Three days later, that is, 5 days after the initial incident, he reached camp at 7400 m. He was barely conscious and his feet and hands were gray–white in color and had the consistency of wood. He was evacuated to a camp at 6400 m where his general condition was poor and he was still coughing up blood. On examination, air entry at the base of the right lung was found to be greatly diminished, and there was deep frostbite to both legs below the knees, but both popliteal and femoral arteries were palpable. Deep frostbite was also present in the distal parts of all fingers and both thumbs.

In the next 2 days he was evacuated to 4600 m and then flown to hospital at 1100 m. Here a chest radiograph showed shadowing in the right lower zone, presumably an infarct. Later he developed a lung abscess in this part of the lung and then an empyema with bronchopleural fistula. After a rib resection and drainage this resolved (Figs 22.1–22.3).

Eventually, bilateral below-knee amputation was carried out and all fingertips on both hands were removed after mummification. There remained some scarring of the right hand with restriction of finger and thumb movement (Ward 1968).

22.6.2 Patient B

A man climbed from 7850 m to 8750 m in 13 h using supplementary oxygen and then spent 35 min on the summit. He bivouacked for the night a few hundred meters lower. The night temperature was estimated

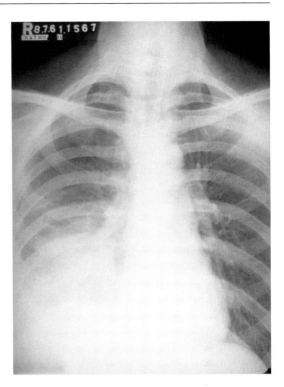

Figure 22.1   Patient A: thrombosis of the right lower lobe, which occurred at 8350 m.

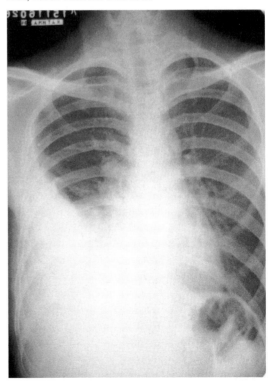

Figure 22.2   Patient A: after the development of a right pleural effusion.

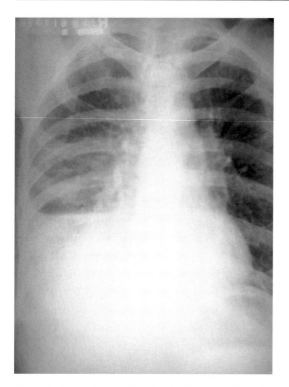

Figure 22.3 Patient A: after the development of a right pyopneumothorax and bronchopleural fistula.

at −30°C with winds gusting to 80–95 km h⁻¹ (50–60 mph). During the night his supply of oxygen ran out and he shivered continuously. Later he estimated that he had had nothing to drink for 30 h while above 7900 m.

Next day he descended and developed a persistent cough. A day later he complained of pain in the left side of his chest and, when examined, was told that he had pneumonia and pleurisy. He continued to have chest pain and then 4–5 days later began coughing up blood. Eleven days after he had reached the summit, chest radiograph showed a left pleural effusion. Three days later he was admitted to hospital in the USA. Six weeks after the initial incident, at operation, a fibrous tissue mass occupying 50% of the lower half of the left thorax was excised. He made an uneventful recovery and post-operatively reached an altitude of 5800 m. His stamina has in no way been impaired (Wickwire 1982).

22.6.3 Patient C

A man, aged 40, complained of severe headache at 6400 m. This continued for 3 days and was relieved

by codeine tablets. By the evening of the third day he noticed that he could not speak properly. On examination he had nominal aphasia but could understand the spoken word. There was some evidence of right facial weakness with involuntary movements confined to the right side of the face. Both carotid arteries were palpable. There was loss of power in the right arm, but no loss of sensation. The lower limbs could not be examined as the patient was in a sleeping bag.

After sedation and continuous oxygen by mask for 8 h, he was able to descend to 5000 m, with some difficulty due to weakness of the arms and legs. For a further 3 days speech remained slurred, he was often at a loss for a word and individuals' names were mixed. After 15 days there were no residual signs; a note written at this time contained lucid statements and logical arguments and his writing was normal. There appeared to be no permanent after-effects (Ward 1968).

22.7 MANAGEMENT

22.7.1 Prevention

Adequate hydration is extremely important and, as the majority of mountaineers at extreme altitudes appear to be dehydrated, the danger of thrombosis occurring probably increases with length of stay.

Posture too may be significant, particularly while bivouacking, when a fetal position is assumed to prevent too much heat loss. As the knees, hips and arms are kept flexed there is an increased risk of thrombosis, so arm and leg stretching should be carried out regularly. Lying in a sleeping bag, particularly if the calves are constricted, may lead to the formation of 'silent' calf thrombosis. Regular movement is therefore important. In subjects with an abnormally high hematocrit (e.g. over 0.65), after adequate hydration, venesection should be considered if the subject plans to remain at altitude. Hemodilution has been used for treating polycythemia in mountaineers; it is considered to be a potentially hazardous maneuver (Sarnquist *et al.* 1986).

22.7.2 Treatment

Treatment will depend upon the diagnosis but all patients will benefit from descent and hydration.

Oxygen may improve those who are severely shocked. Anticoagulants are potentially dangerous and adequate laboratory facilities should be available before they are used. However, in exceptional circumstances in cases of thrombosis and if the physician is experienced, small doses of a short-acting anticoagulant may be given. Return to altitude after a vascular episode should be considered with caution, but some have returned with future expeditions to climb at high altitude without recurrence of symptoms.

22.8 RETINAL HEMORRHAGE

22.8.1 Clinical features

In 1970 Frayser *et al.* reported retinal hemorrhages in 35% of subjects flown to 5330 m. Since then retinal hemorrhages have been found in a proportion of climbers on a number of expeditions (Rennie and Morrissey 1975, Clarke and Duff 1976). The condition is almost always symptomless and self-limiting. The hemorrhages are usually multiple, often flame shaped and adjacent to a vessel. If near the disc there may be some blurring of vision. A case has been reported in a skier, who also had HAPE, at an altitude of only 2930 m in Colorado, though he had been briefly up to 3470 m (Honigman *et al.* 2001).

Besides hemorrhages, 'cotton wool' spots have been reported in one case (Hackett and Rennie 1982) and some mild papilledema may be present as well. There is usually engorgement of both arteries and veins (Fig. 22.4).

The hemorrhages are usually found during the first few days after ascent to altitude (the 'at risk' time for AMS) and subjects are often suffering from AMS, though the correlation with severity of AMS is not strong (Rennie and Morrissey 1975). A study by Wiedman and Tabin (1999) did find a significant correlation between retinopathy and HACE ($p = 0.02$).

22.8.2 Incidence of retinal hemorrhage

The incidence varies from zero on one 10-member expedition to Mount Kongur (7719 m) in Xinjiang, to 15 of 16 members on an expedition to Peak Communism (7495 m) in Russia (Nakashima 1983). It seems that people going to altitude for the first time

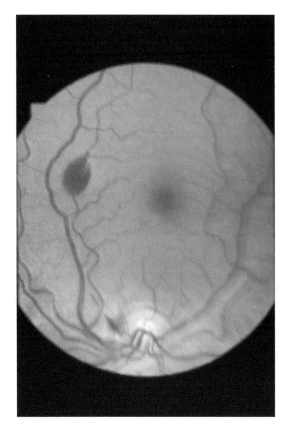

Figure 22.4   Retinal hemorrhage at altitude.

are especially liable to show this phenomenon (Clarke and Duff 1976) whereas experienced high altitude climbers and Sherpa residents are relatively immune. Wiedman and Tabin (1999) found retinopathy in 19 of 21 climbers who went to over 7500 m and in 14 of 19 who ascended to between 5000 and 7500 m.

22.8.3 Mechanism of retinal hemorrhage

At the time when retinal hemorrhage appears, the cerebral blood flow is increased (Severinghaus *et al.* 1966a). The blood flow through the retinal vessels is increased by 105% (Frayser *et al.* 1970). Rennie and Morrissey (1975) found arterial diameter to be increased by 24% and venous diameter by 19%. They suggest that, in the presence of these dilated vessels, the sudden rise in vascular pressure associated with coughing and straining may cause a microvessel to rupture; cough is common and severe at altitude (see section 22.10). However, Sakaguchi and Yurugi (1983) have produced retinal hemorrhage in monkeys in a chamber when presumably cough was absent. In 16 exposures five monkeys showed retinal hemorrhage, whereas no retinal hemorrhage was produced in 46 rabbits. The authors point out that rabbits, unlike monkeys or humans, have arteriolar–venular anastomotic vessels in their retina, which may protect them.

22.9 ALTITUDE AND THE CORNEA

22.9.1 Hypoxia and the cornea

The cornea relies on the direct diffusion of oxygen from the air for its oxygen supply. At altitude it therefore suffers from hypoxia but, unlike other tissues in the body, there can be no compensatory mechanisms of acclimatization such as increased ventilation and hemoglobin concentration. The effect of hypoxia on the cornea is to increase its hydration, causing it to swell. Shutting the eyes as in sleep results in lowering the Po_2 further so that any swelling will be worse after a night's sleep. Normally this swelling is not noticed and causes no change in the refraction of the eye in either normal eyes or myopia (short sight).

22.9.2 Dry eye syndrome

Dry eye syndrome is a common condition and may be present in climbers and trekkers. It is due to reduced production of tears. The condition may is exacerbated by dry air, windy conditions and glare – all common at altitude. Symptoms include irritation of the eyes, burning sensation, light sensitivity and blurred vision (Mader and Tabin 2003). In all but the most severe cases tear substitute eye drops are adequate to avoid symptoms. However, in the mountains there is the practical problem of which preparation to use. Artificial tear preparations can contain preservatives, in which case they can be reused after opening but the preservatives themselves can cause irritation. If the drops are preservative free they are liable to bacterial contamination and, after opening, can only be used for 24 h. Climbers can benefit from wrap-around goggles that protect the eye from wind, dust and UV light. Such goggles may also increase the humidity around the cornea, thus providing additional comfort (Mader and Tabin 2003).

22.9.3 Refractive errors, glasses and contact lenses

Altitude hypoxia has no effect on corneal refraction (unless there has been surgery on the cornea, see below) but subjects with refractive errors who rely on glasses or contact lenses need to consider the effect of the wilderness environment on their ability to maintain ocular hygiene. The problem with glasses are obvious and most mountaineers will have found their own solutions including prescription glacier glasses or will have tried contact lenses. There are a number of types of lenses available each with its own advantages and disadvantages. For a discussion of this topic the reader is referred to Mader and Tabin's review (2003).

22.9.4 Surgery for myopia

A number of operations have been devised to change the refraction of the cornea in myopia, one of the most successful and frequently performed being radial keratotomy (RK). Millions of young people have now benefited from this operation which consists of making four to eight radial incisions in the cornea from the edge of the central area to the periphery. The effect of this maneuver is to cause a flattening of the cornea as the incisions heal and contract, reducing the power of the cornea/lens system and thus correcting much or all of the refractive error of the eye. Originally, the incisions were made by a diamond scalpel but now a laser is usually used. Another operation is photorefractive keratectomy (PRK). Here a laser is used to ablate and remodel the anterior surface of the cornea, reducing its curvature.

22.9.5 Hypoxia and the post-surgical myopic patient

Mader and White (1995) and Mader et al. (1996) have studied the effect of hypoxia on subjects following surgery. In the first study four normal corneas were compared with four which had undergone RK.

Patients were studied at 12 000 ft (3658 m) and 17 000 ft (5182 m) and remained for 24 h at each altitude. They found that from sea level to 12 000 ft there was a change in refraction of the operated eyes of −0.59 diopter and at 17 000 ft of −1.75 diopters. There was no change in the normal eyes. In the second study at 14 100 ft (5182 m), six subjects with RK, six with PRK and nine with myopia were studied daily for 3 days. There was no change in refraction in the subjects with myopia or PRK, whereas the RK subjects had significantly changed refraction.

The mechanism of this change is probably due to the swelling of the cornea because of hypoxia causing further flattening of the RK cornea (Winkle et al. 1998). The effect is to make the subject far-sighted. These changes are all reversible after return to sea level. However, although the changes at moderate altitude are probably only of nuisance value, at extreme altitude they can result in near blindness which in turn can lead to catastrophe as in the case of an American climber on Everest in 1996 (Krakauer 1997). If subjects who have had RK wish to climb high they should be advised to take a selection of cheap positive lens glasses to correct the change in refraction that can be expected. It is not possible to predict this change accurately.

22.10 HIGH ALTITUDE COUGH

22.10.1 Background

It has been common knowledge amongst mountaineers that cough is a problem at high altitude, especially after some time spent at extreme altitude. Tasker writes in his account of the winter expedition on Everest's west ridge:

> Alan (Rouse) . . . was still racked by frequent coughs and periodically, as if by autosuggestion I found that I too was succumbing to a bout. Once started, there was no escape. The cold dry air compounded the irritation in the throat and the victim's body would be shaken by the hacking cough until randomly flung free of its spell. The nights at Base Camp as well as on the mountain were often punctuated by staccato bursts of noise disturbing the sleep of the sufferer and all those around.
>
> (Tasker 1981)

Apart from disturbing the sleep of climbers, cough is quite debilitating and can even cause rib fracture (Steele 1971).

Although well known to climbers, altitude cough attracted no scientific study until Barry and colleagues carried out their work on the British Mount Everest Medical Expedition (BMEME) in 1994. They first documented the reality of increasing cough frequency with altitude and length of stay. They did this by using voice-activated tape recorders and showed that the number of coughs at night increased from zero at sea level to a mean of 60 per night at 7000 m (Barry et al. 1997a).

22.10.2 Mechanism

It has been generally assumed that the cause of altitude cough is the cooling and drying of the upper airway due to hyperventilating cold, dry air at altitude. However, anecdotal reports of cough in long-term chamber studies such as Operation Everest II, where the temperature and humidity were controlled at comfortable levels, gave pause for thought as to whether this was the whole story. In Operation Everest III (COMEX '97) cough frequency was monitored, again with voice-activated tape recorders, and shown to increase with altitude (Mason et al. 1999).

In 1994 Barry and his team also measured the cough threshold to citric acid. In this test the subject is given a nebulizer of increasing concentrations of citric acid and the concentration which first provokes cough is noted. This threshold was reduced at altitude (Barry et al. 1997a). In the Operation Everest III study the cough threshold for citric acid also was shown to decrease at 8000 m even though the temperature was kept at 18–24°C and relative humidity at 30–60%

Barry et al. (1997b) also documented a decrease in mucociliary clearance by the saccharin time test and found that the sensation of nasal blockage was increased at Everest Base Camp. In a double-blind, placebo-controlled trial at Kangchenjunga Base Camp in Nepal in 1998, the same team showed that salmeterol or nedocromil could prevent the reduction in cough threshold, though the effect on cough frequency was not significant (Bakewell et al. 1999). Also it was shown, in a controlled trial, that moistening the nasal mucosa by saline spray four times a day prevented the increase in saccharin times seen in the control group.

It is probably too early to make a coherent hypothesis taking into account the results of all these studies. It is apparent that altitude cough is not simply an effect of cold dry air and hyperventilation, though these may be factors. Results from chamber studies suggest that hypoxia per se is at least a factor. The importance of the changes in the nasal mucosa is also not clear. Finally, combining results of two separate studies from BMEME '94 showed that those individuals who had the greatest change in cough threshold also had the greatest increase in dynamic carbon dioxide ventilatory response (see section 5.16) (Barry *et al.* 1997c). This is in line with an earlier finding by Banner (1988) of a correlation between cough induced with hypotonic aerosol and the ventilatory response to carbon dioxide. This raises the possibility that central mechanisms may be involved.

22.11 ANESTHESIA

22.11.1 Summary

A considerable number of major medical centers are at altitudes of 1500–2000 m. General anesthetics are administered there safely, and with only minor modifications of techniques. Above 2000 m, increasing attention must be paid to the effects of decreased barometric pressure. Anesthetics are not normally administered above 4000 m, and the response to general anesthesia in this situation has not been systematically studied. Anesthesia above this altitude might, however, be required in an emergency and is potentially very dangerous. This is because anesthesia abolishes the peripheral chemoreceptor response to hypoxia. This, together with the low PI,O_2, means that the patient is at serious risk of severe hypoxia. The use of intravenous ketamine with oxygen enrichment may be the technique of choice but local anesthetic is considered safer at altitude (Stoneham 1995). Patients requiring general anesthetic should, wherever possible, be evacuated to lower altitude.

22.11.2 Avoidance of hypoxia

During anesthesia with spontaneous ventilation, breathing is almost always depressed and alveolar ventilation may be reduced to half the value appropriate to the metabolic rate. Whether breathing is spontaneous or artificial, there is usually an increase in the alveolar/arterial PO_2 gradient, equivalent to a

shunt of about 10% of pulmonary arterial blood flow. For these reasons maintenance of a normal arterial PO_2 requires, at sea level, an increase in the inspired oxygen concentration to 35–40%. The inspired PO_2 is thus about 300 mmHg and this should be maintained regardless of barometric pressure. The concentration of oxygen breathed by the anesthetized patient should therefore be increased in accordance with altitude, as shown in Table 22.2.

Nitrous oxide is an effective anesthetic at an alveolar partial pressure of about 750 mmHg (70% nitrous oxide at sea level is only a partial anesthetic). It will be clear from Table 22.2 that it cannot make a very effective contribution to anesthesia above 2000 m, at which altitude only 46% of the inspired gas is available for nitrous oxide. It is contraindicated at any higher level and general anesthesia must then be based on potent volatile anesthetic agents vaporized in oxygen-enriched mixtures. Intravenous anesthetics should only be used with oxygen enrichment of the inspired gas according to Table 22.2.

22.11.3 Hypoxic ventilatory drive

Survival at altitudes much in excess of 5000 m depends upon hyperventilation in response to hypoxic drive, although this is counteracted by negative feedback, resulting from reduction of the PCO_2. It is now established that anesthesia (and even sub-anesthetic concentrations of anesthetics) will totally abolish the peripheral chemoreceptor response to hypoxia (Knill and Celb 1978). It is therefore possible to envisage a situation in which a patient at 6000 m, who would normally have an arterial PO_2 of 45 mmHg and a PCO_2 of 23 mmHg, might perhaps be anesthetized with halothane and air. There would be rapid inactivation of peripheral chemoreceptors with decrease of PO_2 to about 23 mmHg, which would threaten life. An increased oxygen concentration is therefore essential, not only during anesthesia, but in the postoperative period, because the peripheral chemoreceptors are severely depressed by as little as one-tenth of the anesthetic concentration of volatile anesthetic agents.

22.11.4 Performance of vaporizers

Calibrated vaporizers depend upon known dilution of saturation concentrations of volatile anesthetics.

Table 22.2   Minimal concentrations of oxygen in the inspired gas required to maintain a normal arterial Po_2 in the anesthetized patient

Altitude (m)	P_B (mmHg)	Oxygen concentration (%)	PI,o_2 (mmHg)
Sea level	760	40	285
2000	596	54	296
4000	462	72	298
6000	354	100	307

P_B, atmospheric pressure; PI,o_2, partial pressure of inspired oxygen.

The saturation concentration equals the vapor pressure divided by the barometric pressure. Vapor pressure depends only on temperature. Thus, if the barometric pressure is halved, the saturation concentration is doubled. If the dilution ratio of the vaporizer is unaffected by the reduction in barometric pressure (a reasonable assumption), it may be expected that the vaporizer will then deliver twice the concentration shown on the dial. However, the pharmacological effect depends on partial pressure. Twice the concentration at half the barometric pressure gives the same partial pressure as at sea level. Therefore, as a first approximation, probably adequate for clinical purposes, a temperature controlled calibrated vaporizer may be expected to produce the same effect for the same dial setting at altitude as at sea level.

These concepts have never been tested at altitude. However, Ward, Nunn and Woolmer anesthetized one another in a chamber at a pressure of 375 mmHg in 1961, in preparation for the Himalayan Scientific and Mountaineering Expedition (Silver Hut) 1960–61. The apparatus was based on equipment designed for use in Antarctica (Nunn 1961). With a carrier gas of 60% oxygen in nitrogen, obtained with oxygen flow through an injector, and a standard halothane vaporizer (Fluotec Mark 2), uneventful anesthesia was easily obtained in all three subjects and recovery was rapid and uneventful. In view of the subsequent discovery of the effect of anesthetics on the peripheral chemoreceptors, we would now favor 100% oxygen at this simulated altitude of nearly 6000 m.

22.11.5 Practical considerations

The greater the altitude the lower is the possibility of a trained anesthetist and appropriate equipment being available. Dangers are multiplied by anesthesia being attempted in this very hostile environment by someone who is untrained. The first rule must be to avoid anesthesia above 4000 m if at all possible and to evacuate rather than attempt surgical intervention on the spot.

If anesthesia is essential, then oxygen enrichment of the inspired gas is essential for both patient and anesthetist throughout the perioperative period. The safest technique is probably a nonirritant volatile anesthetic (halothane, enflurane or isoflurane) vaporized in oxygen-enriched air according to Table 22.2. It was demonstrated that this technique could be accomplished at sea level by medical officers without special training in anesthesia who were destined for the Antarctic (Nunn 1961). Transport of sufficient oxygen, the vaporizer and the gas delivery system would clearly present logistic difficulties. Use of the open mask is not recommended because of the difficulty in controlling the inspired oxygen concentration. Ruttledge (1934) described a near disaster when chloroform was administered on an open mask at 4300 m on the Tibetan plateau during the march in on the 1933 Everest expedition. This would be expected on present understanding.

Intravenous anesthesia should not be attempted at altitude by those without experience because of the dangers of respiratory obstruction and depression. However, ketamine ($2–4\,mg\,kg^{-1}$) might well be satisfactory because the patient's airway and respiratory drive are well maintained with this drug. This is logistically very attractive for major disasters, mass casualties and warfare. There is good analgesia, and duration is sufficient for any procedure likely to be considered. Hallucinations may occur but would be the least of the patient's problems. Ketamine should only be administered with oxygen enrichment. A study of the use of ketamine anesthesia at 1850 m without supplementary oxygen found that saturation values fell below 90% in significant numbers of patients, particularly in adults. However, the authors conclude that ketamine was acceptable provided that supplementary oxygen and staff experienced in airway management were readily available (Pederson and Benumof 1993).

A report from Khunde Hospital (3900 m) in Nepal describes the successful use of ketamine in 11 cases. A low dose ($2.0 \, mg \, kg^{-1}$) was used and premedication with midazolam prevented the nightmares commonly encountered with ketamine. Oxygen saturation was maintained either with supplemental oxygen or by encouraging the patient to breathe faster and deeper (Bishop et al. 2000).

A recent paper from Leh, India (3454 m) reports the results in a series of 11 local children who underwent surgery for ligation of patent ductus arteriosis under general anesthesia. Under controlled hypotension (systolic pressure between 70 and 90 mmHg), general anaesthesia (GA) was induced with sodium thiopentone and suxamethonium and used to facilitate intubation. GA was maintained with oxygen: nitrous nxide, 40:60, supplemented with vecuronium as muscle relaxant and tramadol for analgesia. Halothane was used for controlled hypotension during ligation of the PDA. All children were extubated on the table as there was no facility for elective ventilation. Supplemental oxygen by nasal catheter was given for a short period following transfer to the recovery room. Their systemic oxygen saturation remained 90% on room air, 2 h after discontinuing oxygen. All children survived the operation and were discharged within 5–6 days (Kumar et al. 2005). The PI,O_2 would have been about 177 mmHg, a lower figure than most anesthetists would like but in this situation, with a light anesthetic and high altitude resident children, there seems to have been no problem.

22.11.6 Post-anesthetic period

In the post-anesthetic period, after a general anesthetic, the hazard of hypoxia due to respiratory depression discussed above is still very real. Indeed, in the hours after the operation, the danger may be greater since the patient may not be so closely watched as during anesthesia.

It should be remembered that, even at sea level, patients are normally mildly hypoxic during this stage. Hypoxia may cause restlessness, irritability and confusion, which may be misinterpreted as being due to pain. Additional analgesics may then be administered which further depress respiration and the patient may die from hypoxic cardiac arrest. This was probably the sequence of events in a Sherpa operated upon for debridement of frost-bitten fingers at an altitude of 3900 m. Clearly, supplementary oxygen must be given during the post-anesthetic period if available. The patient must be closely watched and stimulated to breathe either by verbal encouragement or, possibly, by the use of a respiratory stimulant such as doxapram.

The physiology and pathology of heat and cold

SUMMARY

This chapter deals briefly with the physiology and pathology of heat and cold. Thermal balance, the difference between heat gain and heat loss, determines our body temperature. The various components of this balance are discussed and the ways that the body defends itself in hot and cold conditions, and the processes of acclimatization and adaptation to either heat or cold are considered.

The pathology of heat includes the effect on the whole body, heat lassitude and hyperthermia and locally, sunburn, snow blindness and prickly heat.

The body's response to cold is discussed and the pathology of cold affecting the whole body, hypothermia and locally, frostbite and nonfreezing cold injury (trench foot); their diagnosis and management.

23.1 HEAT: INTRODUCTION

The traveler, if from a cool climate, is at risk of medical problems when he or she goes to a hot climate. In these days of rapid transport, the change from cool to hot climate can be very abrupt with no time for heat acclimatization and this situation increases the risk for the newly arrived traveler. There is a variety of illnesses associated with heat from the relatively trivial, prickly heat and mild sunburn to the lethal, heat stroke. One might suppose that the mountaineer or visitor to high altitude would not be at risk of heat problems but apart from the fact that the approach to mountains is often through tropical or subtropical lowlands, the mountain environment can be hot. The great ranges are mainly at low latitudes with the sun high in the sky. At altitude there is less air to filter out the solar radiation and snow reflects this back on a climber, further increasing the heat load. Finally, having started out in the cold early morning dressed in high insulating clothes and exercising quite hard, the climber is at real risk of suffering from over-heating, dehydration and salt depletion.

The effects of sunlight in causing sunburn and snow blindness are obviously of importance to mountaineers and travelers to altitude.

23.2 HEAT: THERMAL BALANCE

Humans, like all warm-blooded animals, maintain a constant internal temperature unless the limits of their thermo-regulatory systems are exceeded. These mechanisms are both physiological and technical. The technical include clothing, shelter and heating or cooling of our environment. The physiological mechanisms include regulation of blood flow to the skin, sweating and shivering. In considering the problem for subjects in a hot environment we need to consider, on the one hand, the factors tending to make for a rise in temperature, the heat gain; and, on the other, the ways in which the body can reduce the temperature: the heat loss. The balance of heat gain and heat loss determines the temperature of the body.

23.2.1 Heat gain

Heat gain is from either external or internal sources. Externally, heat is gained via convection, conduction and radiation. The important factors are the ambient temperature and solar radiation. Internally, heat is gained as a by-product of metabolism. At rest between 272 and 355 kJ h^{-1} (65 and 85 kcal h^{-1}) are gained from this source but even moderate exercise raises this to 1.25–2.5 MJ h^{-1} (300–600 kcal h^{-1}). Solar radiation can add up to about 630 kJ h^{-1} (150 kcal h^{-1}).

23.2.2 Heat loss

Heat is lost to the environment also by convection, conduction, radiation and evaporation of sweat. Normally about 65% (170–210 kJ h^{-1} (40–50 kcal h^{-1})) of heat loss is by radiation from the body to air. This depends upon the air temperature and when the air temperature reaches 37°C no heat lose takes place by this mechanism. Evaporative heat loss is very important in hot climates. For every liter of sweat evaporated, 2.5 MJ (600 kcal) of heat are lost (though not all comes from the subject). But the efficiency of sweating depends upon the humidity of the air, becoming less efficient as the humidity and temperature rise, until at 37°C and 100% humidity no evaporation can take place. At more normal humidity levels, air movement increases the rate of evaporation, hence the beneficial effect of

fans in hot climates. Note that sweat that drips off the body rather than evaporating is wasted from the point of view of heat loss. The effect of sweating is to lose water and salt leading to dehydration and salt depletion if not replaced.

23.3 HEAT ACCLIMATIZATION

The human body can acclimatize to heat to some degree. Most of the research has been carried out in fit young subjects in whom a program of increasing exercise has been prescribed after an abrupt change from a cool to a hot climate. Under these conditions it has been possible to demonstrate changes in a number of physiological systems which together mitigate the effects of high ambient temperature on physical performance. These changes take place over the first 2 weeks and are enhanced by exercise. The changes include:

- Increase in aldosterone levels leading to conservation of salt
- The reduction in the salt content of sweat
- Lowering of the temperature at which sweating starts
- Increase in sweat rates up to twice the unacclimatized rate
- Increase in the plasma volume and cardiac output

This last adaptation allows a greater increase in skin blood flow, which increases heat transfer to the skin and increased heat loss (Armstrong and Maresh 1991).

These changes help to dissipate heat when the subject is under a heat load and reduce the risk of illnesses due to heat stress. The converse is that before acclimatization has occurred, during the first few days in a hot climate, travelers are rightly advised to avoid exercise, especially in the heat of the middle of the day.

23.4 HEAT ILLNESSES

Heat illness occurs when heat gain is greater than the subject is accustomed to. The onset is in the setting of high environmental temperature for some hours; often the patient has recently arrived in a hot country. High humidity, direct sunshine and especially exercise are aggravating factors.

There are three degrees or stages of heat illness:

- Lassitude, heat cramps, syncope
- Heat exhaustion
- Heat stroke

23.4.1 Lassitude, heat cramps or syncope

The subject feels lethargic and may have muscle cramps, often in the calves or thighs. Part of the mechanism is probably dehydration and/or salt depletion. The body temperature is normal. The treatment is the same as for heat exhaustion (see below).

23.4.2 Heat exhaustion

This is a further stage of heat illness. The setting is the same as above; often the patient has been exercising in the heat. He/she complains of weakness, faintness, anorexia, nausea, vomiting and muscle cramps. There may be flu-like symptoms. The skin is often pale and moist or frankly sweaty. The body temperature is normal and there are no central nervous system (CNS) signs. In cases which have developed in a short time, hours or a day, dehydration is likely to be dominant whereas in cases developing over a number of days, especially if water has been taken but little salt, salt depletion is likely to be more important. Often both are present and require correction.

Management consists of rest, reducing the heat gain, getting the patient out of the sun and into as cool a place as possible, then to replace salt and water as appropriate. One teaspoonful of salt to a liter of water is a reasonable domestic remedy. Both these stages of heat illness normally recover quickly and completely, though the patient may have a headache for a day or two.

23.4.3 Heat stroke, hyperthermia

Heat stroke is a true life-threatening medical emergency. The setting is the same as for heat exhaustion but with continued, more severe heat stress. The crucial difference from heat exhaustion is that the body

temperature is elevated to 40°C or above. If the rise is to above 42°C for more than 45 min there is danger of permanent brain damage or death (Bouchama and Knochel 2002). This explains the urgency of making the diagnosis and starting treatment.

The progression of the condition is due to the breakdown of the body's thermo-regulation and the cessation of sweating. It is this cessation of sweating that triggers the rapid rise in temperature if the heat stress continues and is a very serious clinical sign. Mustafa *et al.* (2003) have recently shown that rabbit carotid artery responded to being heated above 37°C by vasoconstriction, which might lead to cerebral ischemia and may be part of the mechanism for heat stroke.

The clinical picture is of a patient in the setting of a high heat load who has stopped sweating. The skin, instead of being pale, cool and sweaty becomes red, hot and dry. The patient becomes confused, uncoordinated, and drowsy and then loses consciousness. The body temperature will be found to be between 40 and 47°C. Seizures may occur during cooling. There is tachycardia and hyperventilation with $Pa,_{CO_2}$ often less than 20 mmHg. A quarter of patients have hypotension.

23.4.4 Primary treatment of heat stroke

The essential of treatment is to reduce the heat stress and institute cooling by whatever means are available as quickly as possible. If the patient is conscious, fluid and salt may be given by mouth. Cooling is best effected by wetting the skin and evaporating it by air movement. Water can be sprayed and fans played on the patient or the patient can be placed in an ice-cold bath of water if available. Circumstances will dictate the method used but speed is more important than sophistication. Ice packs, if available, can be used placed over superficial arteries, e.g. in the groin and axilla but, compared with evaporative heat loss, are relatively inefficient. After initial treatment, it is important to admit the patient to hospital in order to be able to deal with possible complications.

23.4.5 Secondary care

On investigation in hospital, there will usually be found both respiratory alkalosis and lactic acidosis (Bouchama and De Vol 2001). Hypercalcemia and hyperproteinemia are common and reflect hemoconcentration. Hypophosphatemia and hypokalemia are also common though hypoglycemia is rare. Rhabdomyolysis and hyperkalemia may be a problem after cooling (Knochel 1989). The most serious complications after initial treatment are those of multi-organ failure including encephalopathy, kidney or liver failure, myocardial infarction, intestinal ischemia and disseminated intravascular clotting (Bouchama and Knochel 2002).

23.5 LOCAL EFFECTS OF A HOT CLIMATE

23.5.1 Sunburn

Sunburn is caused by ultra-violet radiation, mainly by the shorter wave UV-B, 290–320 nm (Diffey 1991). It is an acute inflammatory reaction after excessive exposure to the sun. The reason that many patients are taken unawares by sunburn is that, by the time the skin reddens, the damage has been done and the burn will develop over the next few hours. There is great variation in susceptibility to sunburn depending upon the type of skin the individual has, mainly the degree of pigmentation. Blond, blue-eyed subjects or red heads are many times more susceptible than well-pigmented black individuals. The former can burn after as little as 15 min in the tropical midday sun. Acquiring a tan provides some protection from sunburn but it only increases tolerance by a factor of 2 or 3. More important in light-skinned people is the thickening of the statum corneum of skin by sunlight exposure (Diffey 1991). Both tanning and thickening regress over a month or so of no exposure. Factors that influence the radiation load include:

- The height of the sun, time of day (75% of radiation arrives between 9 a.m. and 3 p.m.) (Diffey 1991).
- The latitude and time of year.
- Cloud cover or haze, athough this can be deceptive since ultra-violet radiation is filtered less by cloud than is visible light so one can become sunburnt under light cloud cover.
- Type of terrain, which determines the reflected solar load. Snow and ice, for instance, reflect 80% of the radiation compared with 20% from sand.

- Altitude. Roughly there is a 6% increase in radiation for every 1000m gain in altitude (Diffey 1991).

CLINICAL PICTURE

In the setting of recent exposure to the sun, an erythema develops after 2–6 h and reaches a maximum at 12–24 h. There is a burning pain in the affected part, possibly fever, malaise and even nausea and vomiting in severe cases. The skin may go on to blister formation. The condition resolves in 4–7 days usually with peeling.

The possibility of photosensitizing drugs needs to be borne in mind. Drugs can cause either photoallergic dermatitis or just an increase in sensitivity to sunburn. There is a long list of drugs that have been reported as causing photosensitivity but the ones most likely to be encountered in the mountain or wilderness settings are probably the tetracyclines, especially demeclocycline and doxycycline (travelers may be on this for malaria prophylaxis); quinine, topical nonsteroidal anti-inflammatory drugs (NSAIDs), diuretics such as bendroflurazide, oral hypoglycemic agents and antidepressants. Sulfonamides can cause photosensitivity but are rarely used now apart from acetazolamide. Photosensitivity is listed as a rare side effect of this drug.

TREATMENT

Most cases do not require any active treatment. Simple pain relief (paracetamol or NSAIDs) can be given. There has been debate about the efficacy of topical steroids in relieving the pain and inflammation of sunburn but a recent controlled trial has shown two commonly used ointments to be effective (Duteil *et al.* 2002). So it would seem reasonable to use a topical steroid in cases of significant sunburn.

More severe cases may require rehydration and salt replacement and may indeed have heat exhaustion as well (see section 23.4.2). If blistering is extensive the danger of secondary infection needs to be considered.

PREVENTION

Prevention is achieved by avoiding excessive solar radiation. The danger is particularly during midday.

Travelers should either keep out of the sun or cover up with clothes, hats etc. or apply adequate sunscreens to exposed skin areas. The latter should be of sufficient 'factor' e.g. 30, and applied liberally. If swimming, the screen should be waterproof.

LATE EFFECTS

The late effects of sunburn should not be ignored. They include an increased risk of developing skin cancers, including melanomas.

23.5.2 Snow blindness (photophthalmia)

Snow blindness is an inflammation of the cornea and conjunctiva due to ultra-violet light of wavelength 200–400 nm. At altitude this makes up 5–6% of solar radiation, compared with 1–2% at sea level. Snow reflects 80% of light waves and the eyes are particularly vulnerable.

ACUTE

Within a few hours the epithelial cells of the cornea die. There is loss of surface adhesion and the cells are brushed off the cornea by the mechanical act of blinking. The corneal nerve endings are then exposed. Within about 4 h, symptoms are felt that range from a feeling of 'grit in the eye' to excruciating pain and sensitivity to light. The slightest eye movement causes spasm of the eyelids, pupillary vasoconstriction, eye pain and headache. There is conjunctival inflammation, the eyelids are swollen and the secretion of tears profuse. The condition lasts 6–8 h and disappears in 48 h.

Treatment includes cold compresses, hydrocortisone eye ointment, an eye patch to exclude light, and the avoidance of light. The pupils should be dilated with atropine and an ocular antibiotic used in case corneal ulceration occurs. Analgesics may be necessary.

CHRONIC

Chronic snow blindness occurs in those inhabitants of mountainous and snowy regions over a long period. Visual disturbances, with sensitivity to

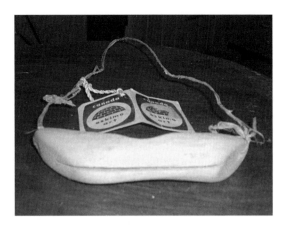

Figure 23.1   Traditional Inuit goggles made from bone used to prevent snow blindness.

light and chronic conjunctival inflammation, are reported.

PREVENTION

Inhabitants of mountainous and Arctic regions have used primitive prevention methods for centuries. These include yak wool and hair pulled forward over the eyes, slits in wood, or cardboard strapped to the head. The Inuit of northern Canada have used goggles made from bone as shown in Fig. 23.1.

Glasses or goggles with lenses that cut out radiation of wavelength 250–400 nm are normally used for protection. The quality of the lens is important, and it can be made of plastic or glass. The main advantage of plastic is that it is lightweight and unbreakable, but it does not filter out all the ultra-violet light; glass is heavier, but filters out most of the ultra-violet light. Ideally, the external surface is mirror finished to reflect light, and the internal surface should not reflect light onto the cornea. Frames should have side and nasal shields for protection against sun, and a safety cord may attached. A spare pair of glasses or goggles should always be carried. Goggles should have adequate ventilation to stop them steaming up (Lomax *et al.* 1991, Petetin 1991).

23.5.3 Prickly heat (miliaria rubra)

Prickly heat is a condition in which the sweat glands become blocked due to a hot humid climate.

Clinically the sufferer has an acute papulo-visicular eruption, usually on the trunk and in the skin flexures, groin, axilla, under pendulous breasts etc. There is a prickling sensation, hence the name, there may be itching and the patient feels the need to scratch. This may lead to secondary infection. It especially affects children, though all ages and both sexes can be susceptible.

Treatment is palliative since the condition is eventually self-limiting. Calamine lotion is traditional and gives some relief. Frequent cool showers if available are helpful, loose cotton clothes are advised.

23.6 COLD: INTRODUCTION

The situations where cold may become a serious problem are either on an adventure holiday, trekking or expedition in very cold climates or in the mountains; or when there is an emergency in the course of a normal journey that results in unexpected cold exposure especially if there is injury or severe illness.

23.7 COLD: THERMAL BALANCE

The same underlying considerations apply as in a hot environment. The body temperature is determined by the balance of heat gain and heat loss. Heat gain is from metabolism especially during exercise. There may be some gain from solar radiation but probably not much and none from the air. Heat loss will be by convection, conduction and radiation. The maintenance of body temperature in a cold environment depends upon reducing heat loss by technical means (clothing and footwear) and physiological mechanisms.

23.8 PHYSIOLOGICAL RESPONSE TO COLD

The body responds to cold by vasoconstriction of the skin, especially in the extremities. This conserves heat in the core of the body, the trunk and brain. The body is prepared, in effect, to sacrifice the extremities for the sake of preserving the core of the body. The other response is by shivering which increases metabolic heat production. In subjects exposed frequently to cold, cold tolerance develops to a degree but significant cold acclimatization is difficult to achieve. Modern cold weather clothing is so efficient that the cold weather adventurer can maintain the microclimate near his skin at a comfortable temperature in almost any weather condition. However, the effect of wind is considerable. Wind chill, as is now well known, has the cooling effect of a much lower temperature than still air on exposed skin. Wind also has the effect of reducing the insulation of clothing by causing increased exchange of air within and under clothing layers.

23.9 COLD PATHOLOGY: HYPOTHERMIA

Cold can affect the body either generally to cause hypothermia or locally to cause local cold injury, frostbite or trench foot. There are broadly three settings that produce hypothermia:

- Immersion in cold or freezing water
- 'Exposure' on hills or wilderness in cold, wet, windy weather
- Chronic cold due to insufficient heating especially elderly people with other illnesses

The onset of hypothermia, in immersion cases, is in a matter of minutes, in 'exposure', in hours and in the chronic situation in days. Risk factors include lack of food and exhaustion, which in the hills, leads to stopping walking and thus losing the metabolic heat of exercise. Children are at greater risk because their smaller body to surface area ratio means they lose heat faster, as are the elderly because of their lower metabolic rate. Occult hypothyroidism is a not uncommon added factor in the elderly. Alcohol is also a risk factor. It has a vasodilator effect on the peripheral circulation but more importantly its effect on the brain is to befuddle the victims so that they make stupid mistakes in the cold situation or just collapse, sleep in the open and drift into hypothermia.

Table 23.1 shows the stages of hypothermia and the relation of core temperature to neurological responses, signs and symptoms but it should be appreciated that there is considerable individual variation in this relationship.

Table 23.1 Stages of hypothermia

Core temperature (°C)	Responses	Signs and symptoms	Classification
37 to 35	Normal	Cold sensation, shivering	Normal
35 to 32	Normal	Physical, mental impairment	Mild
32 to 28	Attenuated	Shivering stops	Moderate
		Loss of consciousness	
<28	Absent	Rigid, risk of VF, appears dead	Severe

VF, Ventricular fibrillation. Note there is considerable individual variation in the relation of core temperature to signs, symptoms and neurological responses.

23.9.1 Clinical features: mild hypothermia

Individuals suffering from mild hypothermia complain of feeling cold and lose interest in any activity except getting warmer. They also develop a negative attitude towards the aims of the party and, as cooling continues into moderate hypothermia the patient becomes uncoordinated, unable to keep up and then starts to stumble. There may be attacks of violent shivering.

23.9.2 Severe hypothermia

At core temperatures below 32°C there is altered mental function and the patient becomes careless about self-protection from the cold.

Thinking becomes slow, decision making difficult and often wrong, and memory deteriorates. There may be a strong desire for sleep and eventually the will to survive collapses with the individual becoming progressively unresponsive and lapsing into coma. Slurred speech and ataxia may suggest a stroke. Gastrointestinal mobility may slow or cease, and gastric dilatation and ileus are common (Paton 1983).

Individuals show a great range of response to cold and loss of consciousness may occur with a core temperature as high as 33°C or as low as 27°C, depending on the rate of cooling. Consciousness is usually lost at around 30°C but patients have been reported to be conscious though confused at lower temperatures than this (Lloyd 1972, Paton 1983). As the temperature drops heart rate slows and breathing becomes slower and shallower. These may be a physiological response to the reduced metabolic rate.

Though shivering usually stops as the temperature drops below 30°C, it has been observed at a core temperature of 24°C (Alexander 1945). Some cases have been reported to cool without shivering (Marcus 1979).

When the temperature drops to below 30°C, ventricular fibrillation may supervene. Survival depends on sufficient cardiac function to maintain output adequate for brain and heart perfusion. Cardiac function is more relevant to survival than brain temperature.

The patient with profound hypothermia may be indistinguishable from one who is dead. The skin is ice cold to touch and the muscles and joints are stiff and simulate rigor mortis. Respiration may be difficult or impossible to register; the peripheral pulses may be absent and blood pressure unmeasurable. In profound hypothermia pupils do not react to light and other reflexes are absent.

The electrocardiogram (ECG) shows a slow rhythm with multifocal extra systoles, broad complexes and atrial flutter (Jessen and Hagelstein 1978). There may also be J waves present (Osborne 1953).

Both hemoglobin and white cell count will be raised because of a shift of fluid from plasma to the interstitial space. Thrombocytopenia has been reported (Vella *et al.* 1988).

Even when there is evidence of a total stoppage of cardiorespiratory function, survival is possible (Siebhke *et al.* 1975). A flat electroencephalogram (EEG) is not a certain indicator of death in hypothermia. The only certain diagnostic factor is failure to recover on re-warming (Golden 1973, Lilja 1983). Before brain death can be diagnosed the core temperature must be normal (NHS 1974); however, brain death can be the cause of hypothermia.

23.9.3 Management of hypothermia

The management of hypothermia in the field is 'the art of the possible'. Hamilton and Paton (1996) carried out a survey and concluded that most rescue groups attempting to measure temperature did so by the oral method. A low-reading thermometer was carried by a majority of teams. For reheating, commercial heating pads were used by most groups. The incidence of hypothermia was, surprisingly, the same for summer and winter. Cardiorespiratory resuscitation in the field was started in 76% of cases and the criteria for starting were the absence of a pulse, cardiac arrest and the likelihood of rapid evacuation.

MILD HYPOTHERMIA

Individuals should be stopped from walking and placed in shelter out of the wind, rain or snow. Any available warm or windproof clothing should be put on. They should be protected from further cooling and warmed by any method available.

To avoid further loss by evaporation, wet clothing should be replaced by dry, but if dry clothing is not available wet clothing should be wrung out and put back on. If wet clothing, which has some insulating value, is left on, it should be covered with an impermeable material to prevent further heat loss. As large amounts of heat may be lost from the head, it should be covered. Warm fluids should be given, but never alcohol.

A patient with mild hypothermia can recover with these simple procedures, but recovery will be hastened if external heat is added (e.g. getting into a sleeping bag with another person). Central re-warming methods have been described (Lloyd 1973, Foray and Salon 1985) using warmed inhaled air which can be applied in the field with suitable apparatus.

SEVERE HYPOTHERMIA

The management of severe hypothermia in the field will depend upon the local situation, possibilities for evacuation and access to specialist medical facilities. Where these are good, as in the mountains

of Europe and North America, patients should be evacuated as soon as possible with the minimum of treatment in the field. However, active treatment in the field has been successful (Fischer *et al.* 1991). When bad weather delays evacuation the patient should be re-warmed slowly and treated as gently as possible to avoid ventricular fibrillation.

If cardiac arrest occurs in a hypothermic patient this produces a dilemma for rescuers because it may be due to some other cause and because the heart may be beating even if clinically undetectable. Mechanical irritation of chest compression may trigger ventricular fibrillation with total loss of cardiac function. However, a consensus seems to be:

- If breathing is absent, becomes obstructed or stops, then standard airway management should be started including mouth-to-mouth resuscitation.
- Chest compression should be started if no carotid pulse is detected for 60 s, if the pulse disappears, or if cardiac arrest occurred within the last 2 h.
- Resuscitation should be started only if there is a reasonable expectation that it can be continued effectively with only brief interruption until the patient can be brought to a hospital where full advanced life support is available (Lloyd 1996). Cardiac resuscitation has been continued for 6.5 h with ultimate success (Lexow 1991).
- Misguided attempts at cardiac massage may precipitate ventricular fibrillation (Mills 1983a). The mortality rate from hypothermia in the field is of the order of 50% but with increasing expertise in management this figure should improve.
- The diagnosis of death in hypothermia should be made with caution because profound hypothermia can simulate death. Strictly, the diagnosis of death can only be made when the patient fails to revive after the core temperature has been brought to normal.

23.9.4 Prevention of hypothermia

The prevention of hypothermia in the mountains is mainly a matter of application of good mountaineering principles: good planning, adequate equipment and anticipation of possible weather conditions, accidents etc. Also an appreciation of the risk of hypothermia in other members of the party and taking action in time to avert it. Modern clothing has reduced the risk of hypothermia but it needs to be used intelligently. The concept of layering of clothing – inner thermal layers with an outer breathable, windproof and water resistant shell – needs to be understood. Common sense and experience will inform many measures which help to prevent hypothermia. For instance, clothes should be removed before over-heating, to avoid sweating and added before cooling becomes severe. When resting, get out of the wind somehow and, on a glacier, sit on a pack or rope, not directly on the ice.

23.10 COLD PATHOLOGY: FROSTBITE

Frostbite is caused by freezing of the tissues, usually skin but in severe cases deeper tissues as well. The affected parts are usually the fingers, toes, nose and ear tips. The setting is usually in the mountains, Arctic or Antarctic wilderness and the victims, mountaineers, skiers or explorers. However, in northern Canada, Alaska and Siberia victims can be ordinary residents caught out in the winter. In some cases alcohol is an added factor in the situation. Victims of severe injury or illness in the mountains or wilderness are at particular risk (as in the case of Patient A, Chapter 22).

23.10.1 Recognition and immediate management of frostbite

Frostbite often comes on insidiously. Under cold conditions, fingers and toes often become numb and this usually does not lead to frostbite. However, if there is further sufficient cooling the tissues actually freeze and frostbite is produced without the victim realizing it. Cold fingers and toes may be pale but are soft to the touch. The frost-bitten digit appears waxy white and is hard to the touch; it is in fact, frozen. The immediate management is to get the patient to a place of warmth and safety, being as gentle with the frost-bitten part as possible. It is important to avoid a sequence of freeze–thaw–freeze which results in much more damage than just freeze–thaw.

Having reached a safe base the affected part should be re-warmed as rapidly as possible. This best done in a stirred water bath at 40°C. Thereafter clean dressings and measures to avoid infection are the key to management until the patient is admitted to hospital, if the damage is any more than superficial.

23.10.2 Secondary management of frostbite

Full management in hospital is beyond the scope of this chapter. Two points, only, will be made:

- In severe cases where there is a question of amputation, management should be conservative. In frostbite, the early appearance of blackened skin is worse than the actuality. The underlying tissue is probably viable. This is unlike gangrene from vascular occlusion where the appearance underestimates the real extent of trouble. The difference is shown in Fig. 23.2.

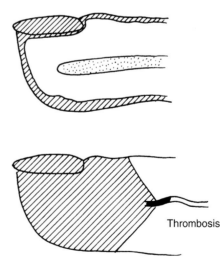

Figure 23.2   The difference between gangrene due to frostbite and due to digital artery occlusion. *Upper*: superficial frostbite: gangrene (shaded area) is limited to the superficial 2–3 mm of tissue. Tissue damage is less than it appears. *Lower*: Arterial thrombosis: gangrene extends through all tissues. Tissue damage is more than it appears.

Table 23.2 Classification scheme for severity of frostbite injuries; after Cauchy *et al.* 2001

Grade	Extent of initial lesion, day 0	Bone scan, day 2	Blisters at day 2	Prognosis at day 2
1	No lesion	Unnecessary	No blisters	No amputation
2	Lesion distal phalanx only	Reduced radiotracer uptake	Clear blister fluid	Tissue excision
3	Lesion dist., inter. and proximal phalanx	No radiotracer uptake on digit	Hemorrhagic blister fluid	Bone amputation of digit
4	Lesion in carpal/tarsal	No tracer uptake in carpal/tarsal	Hemorrhagic blisters carpal/tarsal	Bone amputation of limb

The initial assessment on arrival in hospital, day 0, is made after rapid re-warming.

- A new grading (Table 23.2) of frostbite has been proposed by Cauchy *et al.* (2001). This has a strong bearing on prognosis and helps guide the timing and need for amputation.

This classification is based on a series of 70 cases of severe frostbite seen and treated at the hospital in Chamonix, France. From the bone scan on day 2 it is possible to make a prognosis as to the outcome and decide on the need and extent of amputation.

23.11 COLD PATHOLOGY: NONFREEZING COLD INJURY

Prolonged exposure of tissue in wet, cold conditions in temperatures below 15°C will result in nonfreezing cold injury, often with lasting damage to muscles and nerves.

'Trench foot' is the commonest form of this condition and is a significant cause of injury in military operations when, for combat reasons, long periods have to be spent with feet in water or in deep snow. Water both increases and accelerates the risk of injury, as does any factor that impedes circulation to the extremities, such as a cramped position, immobility, tight clothing, tight boots and tight socks. Mountaineers are at risk when powder snow gets into their boots by the ankle or is melted by foot warmth; damp socks will increase cooling.

Exactly the same sequence occurs with the hands in mittens or gloves made sodden by water or snow. However, because the hands are easier to inspect and keep dry and warm, 'trench hand' is uncommon.

Nonfreezing cold injury, though initially reversible, becomes irreversible if cooling is prolonged. It often occurs in tissues immediately proximal to frostbite.

23.11.1 Clinical features

When first seen, the affected part will be pale and sensation and movement poor. The pulse may be absent, but freezing has not occurred. If these features do not improve on warming, nonfreezing cold injury is present.

After a few hours the part becomes swollen, numb, blotchy pink-purple and heavy. After 24–36 h a vigorous hyperemia develops with a bounding pulse and burning pain proximally but not distally. Edema with 'blood blisters' appears and, if the skin is poorly perfused, it will become gangrenous and slough. At night a pain like an electric shock makes sleep difficult.

In severe cases there is a progressive reduction in sensation. The joints become stiff and muscles cease to function. To maintain balance the legs are kept apart and the sensation of movement has been likened to walking on cotton wool (Ungley *et al.* 1945). Hyperemia appears to be due to vasomotor paralysis with paleness on elevation and redness when the part is dependent. This phase may last from days to weeks, as may changes in sensation. Persistent anesthesia suggests neurone degeneration with the prospect of long-term symptoms (Burr 1993).

23.11.2 Prevention and treatment

With modern outdoor clothing and footwear this condition is seen much less frequently. Nevertheless, it does still occur. In 1988 the incidence in one USA marine unit of 355 soldiers was 11%. Tobacco smoking (but not race) was associated with a higher incidence of trench foot though the difference did not reach significance (Tek and Mackey 1993). In situations where it may arise, i.e. prolonged exposure to cold, wet conditions, vigilance is required to check the condition of the feet frequently.

The patient should be removed from the cold; whole-body warming should be started (Lahti 1982) and dehydration corrected. Rapid warming of the part has been advocated but not universally adopted. Because of pain, analgesics should be given, the patient rested and the part raised. Blisters that develop should be left unless infected, when drainage should be carried out. Sympathectomy does not appear to be very effective as hyperemia occurs naturally.

Gangrene may occur later, and this may be more widespread and affect deeper tissues more extensively than freezing cold injury. Conservative management should be adopted and surgical procedures kept to the minimum. In the long term, nonfreezing cold injury may be more serious than freezing cold injury because of the unrecognized cooling effect on deeper and more proximal structures.

24

Pre-existing medical conditions at altitude

SUMMARY

Very little information exists to assist medical practitioners in advising their patients with medical problems who are traveling to high altitude for recreation or work. The deficiency in guidelines is largely secondary to the dearth of clinical studies which have been carried out to provide assistance to both physicians and patients. This area of clinical research is a fertile one for investigators in the future who should be able to provide physicians with data from which sound advice and protocols for adventuring patients to follow can be drawn.

The purpose of this chapter is to review the studies on a number of common clinical problems which adventuresome patients might have and thus provide advice as best as possible for practitioners to give their patients. It will also be emphasized that physicians should advise patients that they are at greater risk for exacerbation of their disease or occurrence of related incidents when they go not only to high altitude but also to places that are remote from medical care. If physicians are better informed, then their patients who decide to go to high altitude will do so knowing that they are undertaking the trip with an accepted and informed risk.

24.1 INTRODUCTION

With more and more people going to altitude for adventure holidays, expeditions and skiing, doctors are more frequently being asked to counsel patients on the advisability of their trip. People are also continuing these pursuits into later life (including the authors of this book) and thus are increasingly likely to be suffering from chronic diseases which may prompt questions as to their fitness for altitude. The lack of good clinical studies on the effect of sojourning to high altitude in many human maladies makes this area a fertile arena for future investigation. An excellent earlier review (Hackett 2001) will be updated in this chapter.

Apart from the effect of altitude itself, the mountain environment poses other hazards. The great ranges are situated mostly in under-developed countries and in wilderness areas where gastro-intestinal problems are common and medical help uncertain. Altitude holidays usually involve quite strenuous exercise and put a strain on the joints, especially knees, hips and backs. Finally, the different culture and lifestyle of such a holiday may impose psychological stresses which may be too much for some people unused to the difficulties and privations of such a trip.

There is also the consideration that on an expedition or trek the aphorism, 'No man is an island' applies with greater force than in normal urban life. One member's illness affects the whole team and may even imperil the safety of other members; therefore, it is ethically imperative that if a person knows he/she has some pre-existing condition which might affect performance, it should be made known, at least to the leader or medical officer if there is one. As a general rule, individuals should be as fit as possible before they leave for a holiday at altitude though fitness does not protect against altitude illnesses but does add an element of safety as the fitter one is the better one can cope with long days, arduous rescues, or escapes from impending bad weather. Every individual on a trek, climb or expedition owes it to their companions to be as fit, mentally and physically, as possible to deal with the unexpected or very strenuous.

Those who have problems with their health should find out as much as possible about their condition before setting out. They may have to pursue other sources of information since many primary care physicians are ill-informed about altitude or foreign travel. The action of specific medicines they use must be understood and an adequate supply taken, particularly when regular doses are necessary as with diabetes mellitus or asthma (Rennie and Wilson 1982).

Finally, there is always an element of increased risk with high altitude travel, especially in individuals with pre-existing medical conditions, and the advisability of going on such a trip must be weighed between the traveler and his/her physician. Most travelers are rather keen to go on trips no matter what, but each individual must undertake these adventures with informed and assumed risk and take full responsibility for the consequences.

24.2 CARDIOVASCULAR DISORDERS

The initial response upon ascent to high altitude is mediated by an increase in sympathetic tone which may bring out the manifestations of occult cardiovascular disease. Over the first week, however, heart rate, blood pressure and myocardial stress return close to sea-level values as acclimatization proceeds,

oxygen delivery to the tissues is improved and sympathetic tone decreases (Chapter 7). Evaluation of cardiac disease should, therefore, be taken in the context of this response.

24.2.1 Coronary artery disease

Coronary artery disease is one of the major causes of death in men and women over 40. If angina of effort is present at sea level it is likely that ascent to altitude will increase symptoms especially in the first few days before acclimatization has occurred. If exercise is limited by pain and the exercise capacity reduced, it is likely that symptoms will occur at altitude, and the risk of cardiac irregularities and infarction may be increased. Clearly, such patients with unstable or exercise-induced angina should not consider an active holiday at high altitude, and even non-strenuous trips for business or pleasure should be avoided. Visits to moderate altitude by asymptomatic patients with coronary artery disease are probably safe. Roach et al. (1995) surveyed 97 older people visiting Vail, Colorado (2500 m): 20% had coronary artery disease. They reported that no adverse signs or symptoms occurred. Erdmann et al. (1998) studied a group of cardiac patients, with impaired left ventricular function but no residual ischemia, up to an altitude of 2500 m. They were compared with a group of controls. In both groups exercise capacity was reduced by altitude, but there were no complications or sign of ischemia. Elderly subjects, even those with coronary artery disease, acclimatize well at altitude (Levine et al. 1997). So it would be prudent for patients with such disease to limit their activities during the first few days at altitude to allow time for acclimatization.

Recent data in isolated animal hearts (Xie 2004), intact rats (Asemu et al. 1999, Neckar et al. 2002, Zhu et al. 2006), and humans (Schmid et al. 2006, del Pilar Valle 2006) suggest that exposure to intermittent hypoxia may be cardio-protective by minimizing ischemia–reperfusion injury and vulnerability to dysrhythmias. The mechanism of these observations is thought to be secondary to alterations in the potassium and calcium channels induced by intermittent periods of hypoxic exposures. This area of research provides important direction for future investigations in heart disease and high altitude.

MYOCARDIAL INFARCTION

A recent cardiac infarction is a contraindication to ascent; but after a mild infarct providing the patient has been symptom-free for several months, there is probably little risk in going to altitude (Halhuber *et al.* 1986). The exercise of hill walking at low altitude (470–1220 m) has been shown to be well tolerated in patients with a history of myocardial infarction and stable disease (Huonker *et al.* 1997). There was no evidence of coronary insufficiency on continuous ECG and echocardiography. Schmid *et al.* (2006) exercised patients to exhaustion about a month after a documented infarction and revascularization both at low and high (3454 m) altitude and found no adverse events.

Patients with poorly controlled heart failure due to coronary artery disease should obviously be advised not to go to high altitude. Those with well-controlled disease who can manage a high level of exercise such as hill walking at low altitude may well be able to cope with the added strain of altitude. Agostoni *et al.* (2000) found in patients with controlled congestive heart failure that the limitation found at altitude was proportional to that degree of limitation at low altitude, but no patient was limited in their exercise test by cardiac-related symptoms.

As an aside, however, it must be remembered that cold tends to make the platelets stickier and theoretically could increase the possibility of infarction. Cold also is thought to predispose to coronary artery spasm.

CORONARY BYPASS SURGERY AND ANGIOPLASTY

Patients who have had successful coronary bypass surgery before any myocardial infarction and have a good exercise tolerance can certainly enjoy an altitude holiday. One such patient was the subject of correspondence in the *Journal of the American Medical Association* and a subsequent editorial (Berner *et al.* 1988, Rennie 1989). He enjoyed a trek to 5760 m with no adverse effect. Another was a 67-year-old climber who enjoyed two Himalayan expeditions after his operation although on the second expedition his altitude ceiling was limited to 4700 m. However, ambulatory monitoring of his ECG when climbing and asleep at 4700 m did not show any evidence of ischemia. Patients can be warned that their condition may limit their performance and accept that but their fear, and that of their companions, centers on the risk of sudden death due to cardiac causes. Clearly, there is a risk that the graft may block at any time but there is no evidence that altitude may precipitate this event. The same considerations apply to patients who have had coronary angioplasty (Schmid *et al.* 2006).

RISK IN CARDIAC PATIENTS

In the wider context of cardiac disease, Halhuber *et al.* (1985) found in 1273 'cardiac patients' who ascended to 1500–3000 m a negligible morbidity. These patients included 434 with coronary artery disease of whom 141 had had myocardial infarction. Only one of these had a new infarct at altitude. Additionally, patients with controlled dysrhythmias appear to have no increase in events although the increased sympathetic tone upon acute ascent does increase myocardial irritability even in normal individuals (Alexander 1995).

A larger question is that of occult coronary artery disease especially in those with known risk factors such as a family or smoking history, obesity, a sedentary lifestyle, etc. Risk factors which can be modified obviously should be, although there will be little benefit in the short term. The patients' primary care physicians must make a reasonable assessment of such risk and evaluate the patients accordingly.

MEDICAL CHECK-UP

Should doctors carry out 'check-ups' and tests to identify any patients at risk? Is altitude a significant risk factor for sudden cardiac death? Shlim and Houston (1989) reviewed deaths amongst trekkers in Nepal. By obtaining the number of trekking permits issued, they were able to give a number for the denominator as well. Out of 148 000 trekkers in 3.5 years there were eight deaths, none of which were known to be cardiac in origin although two were of unknown cause. There were six helicopter evacuations for cardiac reasons out of a total of 111 evacuations. Two were men in their late 50s with severe known cardiac disease; one was a young man with persistent ectopic beats and three had chest pain thought eventually to be noncardiac. These reports suggest that if altitude is a risk factor for sudden cardiac death, it is a minor one.

So should a symptomless subject be advised an exercise ECG test before undertaking an altitude trip? In view of the apparent low risk and the known poor sensitivity of the test (50%) the answer should be 'No'. Rennie (1989) argues that the predictive value of such a test might be 0.001%, i.e. it would identify only one patient with silent disease who would have a fatal event during a trip, for every 100 000 tests carried out! Further, the specificity of the test being only 90%, the great majority of positive tests will be false positives.

So what should the general practitioner do when asked for advice from someone proposing to go on an adventure holiday to altitude? He should take a history including coronary disease risk factors, advise on these and the advisability of getting fit. He should check weight and blood pressure. In the absence of any evidence of disease no further tests are indicated. He should point out that 'getting away from it all' also involves getting away from easy access to medical treatment and that people going on such holidays must take a greater responsibility for their own health than on a standard package holiday.

24.2.2 Hypertension

Acute hypoxia has a variable effect on blood pressure in hypertensive subjects but there is a tendency to elevation both at rest and at exercise at 3460 m (Savonitto *et al.* 1992). However, Halhuber *et al.* (1985) found that mild hypertensives who ascended and lived at up to 3000 m had few symptoms and both systolic and diastolic pressure fell. No cases of cerebrovascular accident or cardiac failure were noted in 593 patients. This improvement was continued for 4–8 months after returning to lower levels. Those with well-controlled hypertension may go to altitude. In two treated hypertensives, a 6-week stay at altitudes between 3500 and 5000 m produced little change in either systolic or diastolic pressure. Subjects with borderline hypertension may well have higher pressures on going to altitude but at present there is no evidence that this means greater risk of vascular incidents (though no evidence of risk does not mean evidence of no risk). Ledderhos *et al.* (2002) demonstrated an accentuated reno-vascular response in young men with borderline hypertension

in that eight of 18 subjects showed an anti-diuresis and symptoms of AMS but no other adverse events.

There is variability in the blood pressure response in patients with hypertension, and very little systematic data are available to predict what individual's response will be. Given the large number of patients who go to altitude for recreation and the known physiology of an increased sympathetic response in the first few days, it seems prudent that patients with difficult to control hypertension should stay on their low altitude medications and monitor their blood pressure upon ascent. In collaboration with their physicians, they should be given guidelines to follow, and if their pressure is beyond those, then medical advice should be sought.

24.2.3 Other cardiac conditions

Patients who have had valve replacements should, in general, not take hard physical exercise. Poor lung function is more often associated with mitral than aortic valve replacement. The risks of going to moderate altitude, provided anticoagulants are taken and hard exercise avoided, are probably acceptable, but the usual risks of activity and anticoagulation should be respected.

After repair of a ventricular septal defect, residual pulmonary hypertension is not uncommon, and patients who have had a correction of Fallot's tetralogy may often have some residual strain on the right ventricle due to obstruction of the pulmonary outflow tract. Ascent to altitude in both will increase pulmonary artery pressure and may put the individual at risk of HAPE.

Following operation for coarctation of the aorta some residual cerebral hypertension may be present and in theory cerebral edema may be more common. Providing cardiac pressures are normal, the ascent to altitude following repair of patent ductus arteriosus and atrial septal defect is probably acceptable.

24.3 LUNG DISEASE

As the first defense between the body and high altitude, the lung has potentially many interactions which may be worsened by sojourns to high altitude (Hackett 2001, Cogo *et al.* 2004). Appropriate advice to patients who wish to travel to high altitude relies on a careful evaluation of the type of lung disease, its severity, the patient's itinerary, and co-morbid conditions which may make venturing more hazardous.

24.3.1 Asthma

Asthma sufferers are often young and active, so the question of the advisability of an asthmatic individual undertaking an altitude trip is a common one. An attack of asthma may be provoked by cold air and exercise (Kaminsky et al. 1995), but in fact many asthmatic patients have less trouble at altitude than at home, possibly because the freedom from inhaled allergens is of greater importance than the effect of hyperventilation in cold air (Simon et al. 1994, Boner et al. 1995). Of interest are the observations that various levels of hypoxic exposure actually decrease methacholine reactivity (Denjean et al. 1988, Dagg et al. 1997) although these findings are not universal (Saito et al. 1999). On the other hand, the resultant hypocapnia from the hyperventilation at high altitude may increase airway resistance to an important clinical degree (Newhouse et al. 1964, van den Elshout et al. 1991). Thus, there are many confounding factors which make the effect of ascent to high altitude on airway reactivity difficult to predict.

It has been known for a long time that the house-dust mite is a pesky provocateur of asthma, and the lower level of dust mites at high altitude may result in improved symptoms of asthma, particularly in children living there (Grootendorst et al. 2001). Decreased eosinophil counts, decreased peripheral T-lymphocyte activation and house-dust mite specific IgE (Boner et al. 1993, Peroni et al. 1994, Simon et al. 1994) may be involved in the mechanism of this improvement. Also, the increased sympathetic and adreno-cortical activity will counter the broncho-constriction of asthma in the first few days at altitude. In fact, some recommend treatment of steroid-dependent asthma with sojourns at high altitude (Allegra et al. 1995, Karagiannidis et al. 2006, Schultze-Werninghaus 2006). Some investigators suggest that avoidance of allergens at high altitude is essential to the management of more severe asthmatics (van Velzen et al. 1997, Grootendorst et al. 2001).

In one study (Louie and Pare 2004), asthmatics, trekking in the Himalaya, demonstrated a 76 ± 23 L min^{-1} decrease in peak flow measurements while Cogo et al. (1997) showed a decrease in bronchial responsivity to methacholine and hypertonic saline in known asthmatics ascending from low to high altitude. These results are similar to those of Allegra et al. (1995).

Heavy exercise at high altitude can elicit a decrease in airflow even in those athletes who are not aware of their airway reactivity (Durand et al. 2005), and simple measurements of peak flow may be an easy way to monitor patients (Valletta et al. 1997). The airway hyper-reactivity found with exercise in athletes at high altitude may be blocked in part by nifedipine (Henderson et al. 1983), acetazolamide (O'Donnell et al. 1992), and cromolyn sodium (Juniper et al. 1986).

RECOMMENDATIONS

Consulting physicians must advise their patients carefully. Mild to moderate asthmatics should be advised to go to high altitude with all the caveats of increased risk, location, logistics and availability of healthcare stressed. The importance of taking a sufficient supply of medication, using it regularly, and the risk of an asthma attack in a remote environment are all important points that the patient must understand. The patient must have a ample supply of bronchodilators and steroids and be instructed on how to use them properly to prevent or abort an attack of asthma. The patient must understand his/her signs and symptoms, such that he/she can begin or intensify therapy and get down if symptoms worsen. Patients with severe asthma must be warned carefully about being in a high altitude environment where they cannot receive medical care since their margin of safety is much less than the mild to moderate asthmatics. There is no evidence that asthmatics are at greater risk of acute mountain sickness than non-asthmatics though it must be presumed that poorly controlled patients must be at some risk, and acetazolamide prevents acute mountain sickness in asthmatic patients (Mirrakhimov et al. 1993).

24.3.2 Chronic obstructive lung disease

Chronic bronchitis and emphysema (COPD), primarily in patients from sea level ascending to high altitude, will be discussed in this section. Depending on the severity of the obstructive disease in these patients, all the stresses of high altitude with its increased ventilatory demand and stimulation of hypoxic pulmonary vascular response may be accentuated by their impairment of gas exchange and decreased respiratory muscle strength. Consequently, ventilatory capacity is reduced and oxygen uptake impaired. If patients are short of breath on exercise at sea level, they will certainly be worse at altitude. Even mild cases will find their performance markedly diminished at altitude.

The physician of patients with COPD must try to make a reasonable estimate of what effect an ascent to high altitude will have on his/her patient which should be based on the severity of the patient's disease in terms of gas exchange and ventilatory reserve, the altitude and location where the patient is going, access to medical care, and urgency of the trip. Very few studies have been done to help the practitioner design specific guidelines. Graham and Houston (1978) took eight patients with severe COPD (FEV_1 of 1.27 L) to the modest altitude of 1920 m and documented a drop in Pa,O_2 at sea level from 66 mmHg to 54 mmHg with no adverse clinical events. Ascent to modestly higher altitudes, both simulated and actual (~2348 m), in similarly impaired patients with COPD can result in marked hypoxemia with Pa,O_2 below 50 mm Hg at rest (Dillard *et al.* 1989, Christensen *et al.* 2000, Berg *et al.* 1992, Secombe *et al.* 2004) and exercise.

Short-term exposure to these altitudes in patients with mild to moderate COPD is probably safe, but the clinician must assess the severity of the disease, the potential downsides to the period of accentuated hypoxemia, and the duration of the sojourn. The advisability of supplemental oxygen at rest, exercise, and sleep must be determined since low-flow oxygen should take patients out of the danger zone, i.e. Pa,O_2 greater than approx. 60 mmHg or Sa,O_2 greater than approx. 88%, values based on physiology and the guidelines for patients with hypoxemic lung or heart disease at low altitude (Standards for the diagnosis and care of patients with COPD 1995).

Prediction of patients who would fall below these values can be determined on sound clinical evaluation or precise testing in the laboratory (Gong *et al.* 1984, Dillard *et al.* 1991, 1993, 1998, 2005). For air-flight or travel to moderate altitude in patients with $Sa,O_2 \leq 93\%$ at low altitude with moderate to severe COPD, empiric low-flow oxygen

is probably adequately prescribed without formal testing, but an arterial blood gas would be important to draw to insure that the patients are not CO_2 retainers since those patients usually have enough respiratory mechanical limitation such that they cannot invoke an increase in ventilation and thus are in danger at high altitude in spite of the modestly decreased air density encountered there. The physician should advise these patients not to go to altitude.

Another consideration concerns patients with bullous disease who upon ascent theoretically could experience expansion of the bullous and thus predisposition to pneumothorax. Since even with rapid ascent there is equilibration of atmospheric pressure across tissue planes, this risk is more theoretic than real. Small clinical studies in which patients with bullous lung disease were taken to moderate altitude (up to 5488 m) did not find a clinically significant incidence of bullous expansion and no cases of pneumothorax (Yanda and Herschensohn 1964, Tomashefski *et al.* 1966).

RECOMMENDATIONS

Clinicians must make an over-all assessment of their patients, both from the aspect the severity of their pulmonary disease and co-morbid conditions. Only then can the risk–benefit balance be determined. A careful history about anticipated altitude of the trip, duration of sojourn, and availability of medical care are all important factors. From a pulmonary standpoint, adults with $FEV_1 < 1.5$ L should be more formally evaluated to determine whether they need supplemental oxygen. Arterial blood gases are important to determine their gas exchange impairment as well as the presence or not of CO_2 retention. Since testing of patients in a simulated hypoxic environment is impractical, Dillard *et al.* (1989) suggest an equation to determine if the Pa,O_2 would become <55 mmHg during airflight. The predicted Pa,O_2 at altitude is

$$0.519 \times Pa,O_2 \text{at sea level})$$
$$+ (11.85 \times FEV_1) - 1.76$$

Of course, this equation is only good for the altitude of the cabin of a commercial flight (≈ 2400 m), and if the patient anticipates higher altitudes, one must remember that the Sa,O_2 will fall more rapidly the higher one goes as one falls onto the steeper portion of the oxygen–hemoglobin dissociation curve. Medications must be optimized. Treatment of upper and lower respiratory infections must be anticipated and treated. Access to medical care in the area of travel should be investigated, and assumed risk by the patient must be understood.

24.3.3 Interstitial lung disease

This section will deal with a number of diseases which affect function at altitude. Examples of these conditions include interstitial pulmonary fibrosis, sarcoidosis, cystic fibrosis, silicosis and many more. These conditions affect both gas exchange and lung mechanics in a way that exposure to high altitude may strongly influence both physiology and function in an adverse way. Gas exchange is characterized by a widened $(A–a)PO_2$ which only widens more with exposure to hypoxia, so in the same way as patients with COPD these individuals must be evaluated to ascertain whether exposure to high altitude is going to result in a degree of hypoxemia that is dangerous. Furthermore, these patients have reduced lung compliance and at high altitude increased ventilatory demand. With a lower tidal volume and a higher respiratory rate pattern of breathing, the work of breathing is higher, and a high level of dyspnea is incurred. Thus, activity and function are impaired.

More and more patients with cystic fibrosis live into adulthood and try to live a more normal life which might include recreation at high altitude. These patients have problems of both airway obstruction and gas exchange. Several studies found that Pa,O_2 fell to a precarious level with acute exposure to modest altitude (2000–3000 m) which was worsened by exercise (Rose et al. 2000, Ryujin et al. 2001, Thews et al. 2004, Fischer et al. 2005). One paper describes two cases where an altitude holiday appeared to tip the patients into cor pulmonale (Speechley-Dick et al. 1992). Cystic fibrosis patients with stable disease who are proposing to go to altitude or indeed to fly in commercial aircraft can be tested in the laboratory by breathing a hypoxic gas mixture (15% oxygen in nitrogen) for 10 min. The arterial oxygen saturation measured by a pulse oximeter gives a good indication of how they will fare at altitude (Oades et al. 1994).

One must also consider the clinical course in cystic fibrosis of unpredictable recurrent infections which at altitude may be even more precarious than usual. Thus, advising patients with cystic fibrosis can be quite a gamble, and it is probably prudent for patients with all but mild disease to forgo a high altitude venture.

24.3.4 Pulmonary vascular disease

The hypoxia of high altitude accentuates any form of pre-existing pulmonary vascular disease, whether it be primary pulmonary hypertension (PPH) or pulmonary thrombo-embolic disease PTE). As detailed in Chapter 19, individuals who may have normal or slightly elevated resting pulmonary artery pressure (PAP) at low altitude but accentuated PAP with exercise or ascent to high altitude are predisposed to the development of HAPE. Furthermore, individuals with congenital absence of one pulmonary artery have been reported to be predisposed to the development of HAPE. These findings emphasize the delicate balance of high pressures in the pulmonary vasculature and the fragile blood-gas barrier of the alveolar–capillary interface.

There have been no studies of patients with PPH ascending to altitude. Anecdotal experience tells us that these patients do not do well at even modest altitudes. In fact, sometimes early in the disease when patients may be asymptomatic at low altitude, they may present after a sojourn to modest altitude with symptoms of dyspnea with little or light exercise. For some reason probably related to parenchymal mechanoreceptors, an increase in PAP with exposure to altitude results in marked dyspnea even before the accentuated hypoxemia becomes a factor. Most patients do, however, have hypoxemia eventually at low altitude which can be markedly worse at moderate altitude. Thus, the acute and chronic manifestations of severe PHT leads to remodeling of the pulmonary vasculature, fixed PHT, right-heart failure and cor pulmonale. The prognosis for PPH is poor to begin with such that forays to high altitude should be strongly discouraged.

The pre-existence of thrombo-embolic disease (PTE) presents a difficult clinical dilemma. Although there have been cases of PTE at high altitude who have had pro-thrombotic conditions (Boulos et al. 1999, Folsom et al. 2002), there is little consistent evidence that travel to high altitude predisposes people to hypercoagulability or PTE. Only Anand *et al.* (2001) who studied over 20000 patients found that 44 with venous and two with arterial embolism were from high altitude while seventeen were from low altitude, but these patients were high altitude residents and thus not applicable to short-term exposure.

It seems reasonable to evaluate patients with pre-existing TE disease and PTE carefully. Those with uncomplicated TE or PTE events with no known predisposing conditions should have no contraindications from going to high altitude for recreation. Following guidelines of continuing their anticoagulant therapy, if still indicated, and staying well hydrated and active seems reasonable. Those with ongoing TE disease should be conservative in their approach to travel to high altitude. Patients with chronic TE and PTE with or without PHT should avoid exposure to high altitude.

24.3.5 Diseases of ventilatory control and ventilation

The physiology of ventilation should lead to common sense evaluation of patients with abnormalities in the control of ventilation, awake and asleep. The most common clinical abnormality of respiratory control is obesity–hypoventilation syndrome. Although no studies have been done in this population at high altitude, obesity is associated with a higher incidence of AMS, compared to non-obese individuals (Ri-Li *et al.* 2003), but while the underlying mechanism remains unstudied, the presumed cause should be more accentuated hypoxemia from hypoventilation. At low altitude, these patients often evolve into patients with pulmonary hypertension and cor pulmonale (Alpert 2001, Kessler 2001), and thus it is reasonable to surmise that these conditions would only worsen at high altitude, acutely and especially chronically. Furthermore, obese patients living at moderate altitude have a high prevalence of PHT (Lupi-Herrera *et al.* 1980) and systemic hypertension (Valencia-Flores 2004). It is, therefore, prudent to advise these patients whose condition has not been helped with intervention with respiratory stimulants, such as progesterone or acetazolamide, not to go to high altitude in order to avoid the complications of right-heart deterioration.

Patients with obstructive (OSA) and central (CSA) sleep apnea usually have profound oxygen desaturation during the hypopneic and apneic phases of their respiratory cycle during sleep. Their response to going to high altitude is unpredictable. This author (R.B.S.) by observation and Burgess *et al.* (2004) has actually observed a decrease in apneic index during sleep in patients with OSA ascending to high altitude. It was thought that the hypoxic stimulus from high altitude actually stimulated respiration in a way that minimized the upper airway relaxation and/or stimulated respiratory drive in a way that overcame the conditions leading to obstruction. On the other hand, in a small field study Netzer and Strohl (1999) found an increase in obstructive apneas and hypopneas in people ascending to 4200 m on Aconcaqua.

Patients with known OSA who insist on going to high altitude should continue their use of nasal CPAP and perhaps with supplemental oxygen if oxygen desaturation persists in spite of the resolution of the apneas.

24.4 BLOOD DISORDERS

24.4.1 Anemia

The cause of anemias should be diagnosed and treated prior to ascent. The impaired oxygen-carrying capacity from the anemia could lead to poorer performance and if severe enough, high-output heart failure. Pre-menopausal women may have inadequate iron stores (Richalet *et al.* 1993) and might benefit from iron therapy before or during an excursion to altitude when the erythropoietic stimulus is greatest.

24.4.2 Patients on anti-coagulants

Patients with recurrent clotting or bleeding problems may be taking unnecessary risks, whilst for those on anti-coagulants, if well controlled, there is no increased risk from altitude per se other than the fact that their being remote from medical help will be a risk.

24.4.3 Sickle cell trait

Hypoxia and sickle cell disease are not a good combination (Green *et al.* 1971), and even aeroplane flights in pressurized cabins or driving over mountain passes as low as 2500 m can induce a vaso-occlusive crisis and may be the first hint of underlying disease (Mahoney and Githens 1979). Reports in the literature indicate that there is a 20–30% risk that altitude travel over 2000 m may precipitate a crisis in patients with either homozygous sickle cell disease (Hb SS), sickle cell/hemoglobin C disease (Hb SC) or sickle cell trait (Hb AS) (Adzaku *et al.* 1993). These crises are either vaso-occlusive (mainly in Hb SS patients) or abdominal, splenic infarcts (mainly in Hb SC patients). Thus, sickle cell trait or disease should be considered in patients presenting with abdominal pain, and patients with known disease should be advised to venture to high altitude with care.

24.5 DIABETES MELLITUS

Glucose tolerance is normal at altitude when energy expenditure and food intake balance one another. Exercise at altitude may improve sugar uptake; and for well-controlled diabetics, there appears to be no contra-indication to mountaineering.

Those taking insulin should appreciate not only the considerable energy output that may be demanded over a few days, up to 25 MJ day^{-1} (6000 kcal day^{-1}) or more, but also the variation from day to day and within the day. During severe exercise they may need less insulin than on rest days because of increased glucose uptake by muscle metabolism. During rest days at altitude, insulin requirement will be similar to that at sea level. Because of these great variations diabetics should be encouraged to use quick acting insulin, have three to four injections each day, with monitoring of their blood sugar. Ready access to glucose in the form of sugar or chocolate is necessary and for emergencies i.v. glucose should be available, as hypoglycemia can be produced very rapidly by severe activity.

As insulin freezes at 0°C it should be kept warm close to the body. Frozen insulin may be thawed out without loss of potency, but care should be taken to prevent breakage and spare ampoules carried. Accidents to diabetics may be complicated by diabetic coma. Thus, the companions of diabetic trekkers or mountaineers should be carefully instructed in the problems that diabetics face, should be able to recognize hypoglycemia and diabetic coma and know what to do in emergencies. Hypothermia can produce hypoglycemia, and

exhausted diabetic mountaineers are at considerable risk. Extra easily assimilated carbohydrates must be taken for bivouacs. Clearly, insulin-dependent diabetes does present the patients, their companions and trip leaders with problems. Many will consider the risks of serious mountaineering at altitude to be unjustifiable. However, many diabetics on well controlled insulin treatment have made successful, rather more modest trips to altitude. It is essential to discuss the situation with the expedition/trek leader and doctor (if there is one) at an early stage in planning.

24.6 GASTROINTESTINAL DISORDERS

Intestinal colic and diarrhea are frequently encountered in mountainous areas, but altitude per se is not a factor. Simple traveler's diarrhea can be treated by Imodium® unless there is evidence of parasitic infection when specific medicine should be given.

The incidence of peptic ulcer appears to be less at altitude (Singh *et al.* 1977). However, patients with known peptic ulcer should be well controlled prior to the expedition as complications in the field can be fatal. Drugs taken because of joint problems, non-steroidal anti-inflammatory agents, or aspirin for headache, may cause gastric hemorrhage which should be considered as a cause of unexpected weakness. These drugs should not be taken on an empty stomach.

Those with inflammatory disorders of the bowel, such as Crohn's disease or ulcerative colitis in an active phase, should not go on expeditions. An expedition, which lasts weeks or months, should be considered very carefully for an individual in the quiescent phase and medication and diet planned to ensure that the condition gets no worse. Adequate treatment for an acute exacerbation must be available and evacuation should be easy.

Hemorrhoids, perianal hematoma and fissure-in-ano are often considered trivial conditions except by sufferers. They are not, and pre-expedition treatment must be undertaken. On an expedition a prolapsed pile should be replaced as soon as possible. Peri-anal hematoma is classically a self-limiting condition lasting 5 days before resolution. The clot, however, may be evacuated under local anesthetic. Acute fissure-in-ano may be exquisitely painful. Anesthetic ointment should always be available, and if necessary, under local anesthetic, a fissurotomy may be carried out. Any recurrent perineal or ischiorectal abscess must be dealt with prior to an expedition, as must fistulae and pruritus ani. Abscesses can be drained in the field. Even when an adequate anesthetic is available this is painful postoperatively.

Patients with hernias must have these repaired prior to an expedition. Any hernia occurring in the field should be reduced and kept reduced by a home-made truss. Irreducible and strangulated hernias can and have been operated on under local anesthetic, and the simplest operation consistent with the operator's skill and the patient's condition should be carried out.

Patients with recurrent appendicitis should consider an appendicectomy prior to an expedition. In the past, prophylactic appendicectomy has been advised before very long periods away from good medical cover, but this is not necessary. If appendicitis occurs during an expedition, it should be treated conservatively with antibiotics, i.v. fluids and nothing by mouth. Often it resolves, but if an abscess or appendix mass forms this may resolve or it will point on the abdominal wall or rectum and can be drained. Ruptured appendicitis and peritonitis should be drained under local anesthetic.

24.7 ORTHOPEDIC CONDITIONS

Those with arthritis, particularly of the joints of the lower limb should carefully consider the degree and amount of exercise that has to be taken on a mountain trek. Nonsteroidal anti-inflammatory drugs can be very beneficial and should be started early rather than being heroic about the pain. Treatment of painful joints particularly of the hip whether by replacement prosthesis, arthrodesis or some other method may make a short trek possible. One member of the successful Everest 1953 expedition who climbed to 8500 m had a fixed, flexed elbow, the result of an accident as a child.

24.8 ENT CONDITIONS AND DENTAL PROBLEMS

Nasal polyps or a deflected nasal septum which interferes with breathing should be treated prior to ascent. Patients with perennial rhinitis and sinusitis should ensure supplies of their usual medication.

Dental problems theoretically are not made worse by altitude, but anecdotally dental abscesses seem to be quite common. Anyone planning a holiday or expedition out of range of dental help on the mountains or anywhere else, is well advised to have a through dental check-up and any suspect teeth dealt with before setting out.

24.9 OBESITY

Obesity has been reported as being a risk factor for acute mountain sickness (Chapter 18) and the overweight will have an increased oxygen uptake for a given task. At night obese individuals may suffer from a greater fall in arterial P_{O_2} as the weight of the abdomen interferes with normal lung expansion. The repeated episodes of hypoxemia lead to increased pulmonary hypertension. In addition, they are more likely to have sleep disorders with, in particular, obstructive sleep apnea during which the arterial P_{O_2} can fall precipitously. In residents at altitude this may cause an undue increase in red blood cells and may be implicated as a cause of chronic mountain sickness (Chapter 21).

24.10 NEUROLOGICAL PROBLEMS

24.10.1 Headache

Headaches are common on ascent to altitude, probably because of mild cerebral edema. These are features of acute mountain sickness and resolve spontaneously in a few days. There is anecdotal evidence that altitude tends to trigger migraine attacks which can be severe. One sufferer had an attack of transient nominal aphasia at 5500 m. A history of migraine is a risk factor for acute mountain sickness (Chapter 18).

24.10.2 Epilepsy

There is no evidence that epileptics are worse off or that seizures are more frequent at altitude; however, the consequences of an epileptic attack need to be considered both on the affected individual and his companions. Understanding this, it is probably reasonable for patients with well-controlled epilepsy, who have not had a seizure for 6 months, to go on a trek but not to rock or ice climb. Some anti-epileptic preparations may affect breathing adversely during sleep, whilst others in high doses may affect coordination.

24.10.3 Sleep

Nightmares and vivid dreams are not unusual at altitude, and sleep may be very disturbed. Those who take drugs at sea level to induce sleep should remember that these often depress respiration and can lead to severe transient hypoxia. In any event, sleep at altitude is usually lighter and often less refreshing than at sea level (Chapter 13).

24.11 MENTAL OUTLOOK

Mountaineering is a potentially dangerous sport with an appreciable mortality. It requires time and patience to master all the skills necessary to move safely in mountain country, which is no place for the danger-mystic with or without religious overtones.

Mental agility, emotional stability, and patience are important, and the gregarious extrovert who can only be effective with constant activity and an impressionable audience is not so likely to function effectively as the more self-sufficient. Those who are obliged to live harmoniously in close proximity for long periods should be stable, loyal and have both a social and intellectual tolerance for their companions. Above all, a sense of humor and the ability to control and sublimate hostile and aggressive impulses are of great importance.

Considerable attention has been paid to the possible effects of emotional deprivation with reference to sexual abstinence, in isolated male communities. Most agree that sexual deprivation is usually of minor significance and, as a subject of conversation, ranks rather lower than food, drink or the task in hand. At high altitude reduction in libido has been reported in some lowlanders. High altitude residents do not appear to be affected. Instructions on the frequency of sexual intercourse are included in a work on traditional Tibetan medicine:

> During winter one can indulge in intercourse twice or thrice daily, since sperm increases in winter. In the autumn and spring there must be an interval of two days, and during the summer an interval of 15 days. Excessive intercourse affects the five sense organs. (Rinpoche 1973)

Elderly, enfeebled Tibetans drank the urine of young boys to increase their sexual vigor (MacDonald 1929).

For the majority of people, venturing into the high mountains is a wonderful experience even if, at times, the conditions are harsh and uncomfortable. Most have graduated via family trips into the hills, short camping trips near home, hill walking, etc. But some suddenly get the idea that they want to make some big trek or expedition with no previous experience and have quite unrealistic ideas of their own performance. Sometimes all works out well, and they adapt to what is a very different life-style with no problem, but others are clearly psychologically quite unsuited to it and become psychiatric casualties, to the distress of themselves and their companions.

Another element, which is important to emphasize, is risk. As mentioned above, venturing into any high altitude environment involves increased risk. The team and the individual must be self-sufficient and not depend on outside help to rescue them. No one is really responsible for their welfare but themselves. Team members on a trek, a climb or an expedition must accept the individual and collective risk and responsibility. Doing so as a team reduces the individual risk, as sharing in the 'fellowship of the rope' is one of the finest experiences of the mountain life.

25

Women at altitude

SUMMARY

Women respond to altitude in very much the same way as men. They acclimatize in a similar way and are as likely to get acute mountain sickness (AMS). Their exercise performance is similarly affected by altitude. Recent studies into the effect of the menstrual cycle have failed to find significant differences in performance or susceptibility to AMS in different phases of the cycle. Women seem to have an advantage over men in that they lose less weight at altitude probably because they suffer less loss of appetite. The risk of altitude in pregnancy is not known, but in the present state of knowledge women in the early stages of pregnancy are advised not to go beyond moderate altitudes. This is because of the possible risk of hypoxia on organogenesis in the fetus and likely discomfort for the mother in later pregnancy. Oral contraceptives (the pill) are widely used for both contraception and for menstrual regulation by women at altitude. Although there is the theoretical risk that altitude and increased hematocrit may lead to thrombosis, there is no direct evidence that this is the case.

25.1 INTRODUCTION

Until recently, studies of the effect of altitude on humans have used fit young men as their subjects, but the record of increasing success by women at very high altitudes has stimulated a modicum of studies either involving or including women. Both older (Braun 1997, Butterfield 1997, Moore 1997, Sandoval 1997, Zamudio 1997) and more recent studies are reviewed in this chapter, but in trying to provide answers to frequently asked questions, we discover that there is still room for more studies to elucidate the age-old queries about the differences in adaptation and performance between men and women going to and living in high, thin air.

25.2 CLIMBING PERFORMANCE

In 1970 Setuko Wanatabe, a Japanese climber, was the first woman to climb Everest, and since then more than 75 women from many nationalities, levels of education, and walks of life have also made the ascent, some without the use of supplementary oxygen.

Women, without supplemental oxygen, have climbed other 8000 m peaks including K2 and Kangchenjunga, and it will probably not be long before someone claims the record of the first woman to climb all fourteen 8000 m peaks.

Clearly, women can acclimatize and perform and train (Purkayasta *et al.* 2000) at altitude as well as men, even if there are fewer women participating in high altitude climbing, especially in the elite category. In this section the differences in physiology between women and men will be discussed though, as women's achievements demonstrate, similarities are probably greater than differences. Additionally, this chapter will deal primarily with women going to altitude while Chapter 17 focuses more on women native to high altitude.

25.3 ACCLIMATIZATION

Women acclimatize in a similar way to men. With respect to respiratory acclimatization their increase in ventilation in response to chronic hypoxia was documented as long ago as 1911 by Mabel FitzGerald (FitzGerald 1913). She measured the alveolar P_{CO_2} of acclimatized men and women, over a range of altitudes and showed that the $PA,_{CO_2}$ is about 2 mmHg lower in women than men. Their P_{O_2}, which was calculated from an assumed R, was presumably slightly higher. Others, including Hannon (1978) have confirmed this finding, and using arterialized capillary blood, Barry et al. (1995) found that P_{CO_2} fell more in women than men during acclimatization as did their bicarbonate. Loeppky et al. (2001) also found a consistently lower $Pa,_{CO_2}$ and higher $Pa,_{O_2}$ in women when compared to men which was accompanied by a higher respiratory rate and thus higher dead-space ventilation. Women's greater ventilation at all altitudes is assumed to be due to the stimulatory effect of sex hormones and disappears after the menopause.

Women increase their hemoglobin concentration, [Hb], hematocrit and red cell mass in the same way as men in general, though some women fail to do so due to low iron stores as a consequence of their menstrual blood loss. Richalet et al. (1994) reported two such cases in their study on Samaja and documented these women's low iron stores. It was also shown that their erythropoietin response was good. In an early study on Pikes Peak (4300 m) (Hannon et al. 1966) it was shown that women on iron supplements had similar rises in [Hb] to men, whereas women not taking iron had a slower increase in [Hb].

If susceptibility to acute mountain sickness (AMS) is seen as slow acclimatization then, again, there is probably no significant difference between men and women, as was documented by Hackett

et al. (1976), Maggiorini et al. (1990) and Honigman et al. (1993). Furthermore, the presumed association between AMS and fluid retention (Hackett and Rennie 1979, Hackett et al. 1982) has not been documented to occur at a greater rate in women when some increase in fluid retention is thought to occur during the luteal phase of the menstrual cycle, although there are contradictory results in this area of research.

25.4 PERFORMANCE AND THE MENSTRUAL CYCLE

Women in the luteal phase of the menstrual cycle have higher respiratory drives to hypoxia and hypercapnia and thus greater exercise ventilation (Schoene et al. 1981), and men at extreme altitudes with higher hypoxic respiratory drives have greater ventilatory responses and thus arterial oxygenation and extreme altitude performances (Schoene 1982, Schoene et al. 1984). Beidleman and colleagues (1999) tested the possibility that this greater respiratory response may be affected by the stimulation of progestational hormones in the midluteal phase of the menstrual cycle. They hypothesized that this ventilatory stimulation might improve oxygen transport especially at altitude. They undertook a chamber study at sea level and 4300 m equivalent in eight female subjects testing them in their early follicular and midluteal phases. They found that there was no difference between the phases for peak and submaximal exercise ventilation. $Sa,_{O_2}$ was 3% higher at altitude during the midluteal phase but $V_{O_2,max}$ and time to exhaustion were no different between phases at sea level or altitude.

25.5 WEIGHT LOSS

Women seem better able to maintain their weight on going to altitude than men do. In a group of women studied on Pikes Peak (4300 m) Hannon et al. (1976) found that they lost only 1.49% of their body weight compared with 4.86% in a group of men. This was attributed to the fact that the women seemed to regain their appetites sooner than men do. Collier et al. (1997) also found less weight loss in a group of women trekkers to Everest Base Camp (5340 m). The women had no significant weight loss during their stay at this altitude, while the men lost an average of $0.11\,kg\,m^{-2}\,day^{-1}$. In seven men who climbed to altitudes of 7100–8848 m the weight loss averaged $0.15\,kg\,m^{-2}\,day^{-1}$ whilst the one woman who climbed to above 8000 m lost no weight.

25.6 CATECHOLAMINES AND CARBOHYDRATE METABOLISM

In a 12-day study on Pike's Peak (4200 m) Mazzeo *et al.* (1998) found no difference in catecholamine response between men and women nor between the follicular and luteal phases of the menstrual cycle. However, for a given noradrenaline urinary excretion the heart rate and blood pressure response was lower in the follicular than in the luteal phase.

As mentioned in section 15.8, sensitivity to insulin appears to be increased at altitude in men. Braun *et al.* (1998) found that after nine days at altitude (4300 m) the blood glucose response to a standard meal was reduced in women possibly due to increased stimulation of peripheral glucose uptake or suppression of hepatic glucose production. They found that the glucose response was lower in the estrogen than in the estrogen plus progesterone phase of the menstrual cycle.

Mawson *et al.* (2000) found that the total energy requirements of women at 4300 m were 6% above sea-level values. Although there was a transient rise in BMR this did not explain all the increase. Unlike men, blood glucose utilization rates in young women after 10 days at 4300 m were lower at rest and no different during submaximal exercise from those observed at sea level. There was no correlation with circulating estrogens or progesterone (Braun *et al.* 2000).

25.7 PREGNANCY AND ORAL CONTRACEPTIVES

The risk to a pregnancy of going to altitude is not known with confidence, but it would seem wise to advise pregnant women against ascent to more than a modest altitude. In the early months of pregnancy, during organogenesis, there is the risk that hypoxia might result in fetal abnormalities. Later in pregnancy the increased bulk of the uterus and raised diaphragm will make for discomfort in the mother and interfere with her breathing.

There are no data on the risk of using oral contraceptives at altitude, but it is well known that they increase the risk of thrombosis at sea level. However the risk is less in current formulations and is even smaller in nonsmokers. The increased hematocrit at altitude and dehydration, should it occur, may increases this risk. After some weeks at altitude vascular episodes, some thrombotic in nature, have been reported though not in women. A survey by Miller (1999) of 926 trekkers on the Everest Base Camp route found that of 316 women, 30% were using an oral contraceptive mostly for control of menstruation. A significant number did report irregularities of menstruation especially if pills were not taken regularly, but there were no medical complications. However, though reassuring, the numbers were too small to draw firm conclusions regarding safety. A discussion of this question can be found in the *International Society of Mountain Medicine Newsletter* (1998). In earlier editions we advised against the use of the pill. Clearly women are using it and the advice now should be that if used it should be taken regularly.

25.8 WOMEN AND COLD

Cold injury, hypothermia, frostbite and immersion injury are seldom reported in women at altitude. A factor may be the relatively thicker layer of subcutaneous fat found in women. Also, it is possible that women are more meticulous in their preparation for cold conditions and so avoid cold injury through negligence.

26

Extremes of age at altitude: Children and the elderly

SUMMARY

Children respond to altitude in a similar way to adults with the physiological changes of acclimatization. However, infants in the first few months of life have hypoxic responses that are in transition from the fetal to childhood settings. This may result in quite severe hypoxia which has been documented recently.

Children are at risk at altitude if they are too young to be able to voice their symptoms of acute mountain sickness (AMS) which then may not be diagnosed promptly. Any child who has recently ascended to altitude and becomes unwell must be assumed to be suffering from AMS unless there are clear signs of an alternative diagnosis. Children are as likely to get AMS, high altitude pulmonary edema (HAPE) and high altitude cerebral edema (HACE) as adults are. The management of all forms of AMS is similar to that in adults with appropriate adjustment of dosage of drugs. Children are more at risk of hypothermia and cold injury because of their larger surface to weight ratio and especially if they are being carried and not exercising. Infants are at risk of high altitude pulmonary hypertension (HAPH) if they remain at altitude for months. The justification for taking young children to altitude is questionable and is discussed.

Increasing numbers of elderly people are going on holidays to the mountains. If they are otherwise fit, age is no bar to enjoying such holidays. Their exercise capacity will be less than that of younger mountaineers and their goals must be adjusted accordingly. With age comes the likelihood of various medical conditions, especially heart, lung disease, and locomotor defects, which may interfere with performance at altitude. However, the risk from occult disease, specifically asymptomatic coronary artery disease, is very small. The elderly are no more likely to get AMS than young people, indeed in practice they seem to suffer less, perhaps because they are likely to gain altitude more slowly or they may be less susceptible.

26.1 INTRODUCTION

Studies of the effect of altitude on humans have usually used fit young men as their subjects. There have been few studies addressing the question of the effect of altitude specifically on children or elderly people. Such studies as have been published are reviewed in this chapter but in trying to provide answers to frequently asked questions we still have to rely often on anecdote or extrapolation from young adult data. This chapter deals mainly with lowland children and

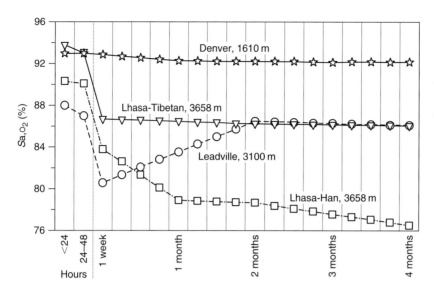

Figure 26.1 Arterial oxygen saturation in quietly sleeping infants at various altitudes and in various populations. (From Niermeyer 2003, with permission.)

elderly people going to altitude, highland populations being the subject of Chapter 17.

26.2 CHILDREN

26.2.1 Introduction

The increased accessibility of the high altitude regions of the world to adults means that more children are now being taken on adventure holidays to these places. Even infants have been carried over 6000 m peaks in Nepal (Pollard *et al.* 1998). Many lowland Han Chinese children are taken to high altitude in Tibet and Qinghai. Many school parties are venturing to high altitude. Are these children at risk from the effects of altitude? What advice should a doctor give to parents considering taking children to altitude? The International Society of Mountain Medicine set up an *ad hoc* committee (24 members from 10 countries) who produced a consensus statement, 'Children at altitude' to try and answer these questions (Pollard *et al.* 2001). This provides an excellent summary of knowledge in this field up to 2001.

26.2.2 Infants at altitude

There are some special considerations that apply to infants at altitude relating to the immaturity of their respiratory control mechanisms and the fact

that their pulmonary arteries are undergoing involution of the thick muscular layers at this time.

In the neonate, hypoxia has a depressant effect on ventilation. Normally this reverses to the adult pattern of stimulation in the first few weeks of life, but a study by Parkins *et al.* (1998) found that even at 3 months infants responded to 15% oxygen breathing by frequent periods of isolated and periodic apnea. The mean saturation on 15% oxygen was 92% in these infants. The responses were very variable, but some infants had saturations which fell to less than 80% for up to a minute (at which time the intervention was stopped).

Niermeyer (2003) has reviewed her own and others' work on infants at high altitude. There are remarkable differences in arterial saturations in the first few months of life between infants at low and high altitudes and in different populations at high altitude. Figure 26.1 shows the Sa,O_2 during the first 4 months of life in quietly sleeping infants at various altitudes and in different populations. Infants at sea level have a saturation of 96–98% within the first few hours after birth and reach a slightly higher level with less variability over the next few months as their cardiorespiratory control goes through the transition from fetal to young infant settings. At Denver (1610 m) there is a small drop from 24 to 48 h after birth and the Sa,O_2 then remains constant. The same population at the altitude of Leadville (3100 m) shows a profound drop 24–48 h after birth and then a rise over the next 2 months. Han Chinese infants in Lhasa (3658 m) show a similar drop but then a continued decline over 4 months. Tibetan infants also at Lhasa have a rather higher Sa,O_2 at birth than Chinese infants but a similar drop, which then remains steady. Andean infants (not shown) have results intermediate between Tibetan and Han Chinese. The mechanisms behind these observations are complex and include changes and differences in control of breathing, maturation of the lung and control of pulmonary vascular pressures. It seems likely that hypoxia interferes with the normal transition of responses that occurs after birth (Parkins *et al.* 1998) It is the Han Chinese infants, of course, who, with their profound hypoxemia, are particularly prone to symptomatic high altitude pulmonary hypertension (previously called sub-acute mountain sickness) (Sui *et al.* 1988), described in Chapter 22.

Yaron *et al.* (2003) reported the physiological responses to altitude of children aged 3 to 36 months. The comparison was between Denver (1610 m) and an altitude of 3109 m. After 24 h at altitude the children showed tachypnea, relative hypoxia, hypocarbia and a reduction in cerebral tissue oxygenation (by near-infrared spectroscopy). These changes were similar to those seen in adults. However, the reduction in cerebral oxygenation was age dependant with lower values being seen in the younger subjects. AMS symptoms were scored but there was no correlation between AMS scores and any physiological measurement. In another part of the same study, sleep was monitored. They found that, as in adults, sleep was disturbed especially during the first night at altitude (3109 m) (Yaron *et al.* 2004).

26.2.3 Sudden infant death at altitude

In view of the quite severe desaturation in infants at altitude (Fig. 26.1) and the known effect of an acute respiratory infection to lower Sa,O_2 still further, it would seem likely that altitude must be a risk factor for sudden infant death syndrome (SIDS). However, there is very little evidence. One study that did address this question was by Kohlendorfer and colleagues (1998) who carried out a case–control study in Austria of SIDS deaths. They found that higher altitude districts did have higher rates of SIDS but these districts also had higher rates for the practice of placing infants in the prone position for sleep. This effect largely accounted for the difference in

rate of SIDS. The possibility that altitude is a risk factor for SIDS cannot be ruled out at present, especially at altitudes higher than in this study.

26.2.4 Diagnosis of AMS in children

In older children, the diagnosis of AMS can be made on symptoms as in adults. The diagnostic problems are much the same. Those feeling cold, miserable and depressed may exaggerate while those (usually boys in a group) who consider it 'sissy' to admit to symptoms will minimize them. However, in younger children who cannot articulate their feelings the problems are worse. In them AMS symptoms cannot be distinguished from other causes of ill health. In the setting of a recent increase in altitude, the only safe course is to assume a young child's fractiousness is due to AMS unless there are signs clearly pointing to some other cause. Yaron *et al.* (1998) have proposed a 'fussiness score' in such pre-verbal children, analogous to the Lake Louise score for AMS (section 18.8). They studied 23 children aged 3–36 months in Colorado at Denver (1609 m), Fort Collins (1615 m) and Keystone Summit Lodge (3488 m), taking 4 days to reach there. There were 45 accompanying adults and 20% of these had AMS at Keystone. Using their score, 21% of the infants were diagnosed as having AMS. Fussiness is scored on a scale of 0 to 6 for both amount and intensity. This equates to the headache symptom in the Lake Louise system. Other symptoms are then scored 0 to 3 for, 'How well has your child eaten?', 'How playful is your child today?' and 'How has the child napped today?' This system may also be found as an appendix to the ISMM consensus statement. The fussiness, or 'Children's Lake Louise score' was further evaluated by Yaron and colleagues (2002). They found it to be robust, in that there was good inter-observer agreement in the scoring.

26.2.5 Incidence of AMS in children

There have been a few surveys of children at altitude. Wu (1994b) studied adults and children as they traveled the Qinghai–Tibet highway to Lhasa. He surveyed 5355 adults and 464 children at the overnight stop, Tuo-Tuo (4550 m). These people were lowland Han Chinese. The diagnosis was made on symptoms and on the response to oxygen breathing. HAPE was also diagnosed by chest radiograph. The incidences for AMS and HAPE respectively were 38.2% and 1.27% in adults and 34.1% and 1.51% in children. In Colorado, Theis *et al.* (1993) found an incidence of AMS of 28% at an altitude of 2835 m for children aged 9–14 years, but there was no comparable figure for adults. This may seem rather high for this altitude but a control group at sea level had a 20% incidence of these symptoms, so some symptoms may have been due to the travel itself. A more recent paper (Yaron *et al.* 2002) also found similar incidence of AMS in young children as in adults: 19 and 24%, respectively. From these studies (including that of Yaron *et al.* 1998 above) it would seem that children probably have about the same susceptibility to AMS and HAPE as adults. One paper also suggests that, as in adults, respiratory infection predisposes to HAPE in children (Durmowicz *et al.* 1997). There seem to have been no reported cases of HACE in children.

26.2.6 Management of AMS in children

The management of AMS in children is the same as in adults (section 18.7). The crucial first step is to have a high index of suspicion in the setting of a recent gain in altitude. The essential step is to get the child down to a lower altitude. Only in the mildest cases is a 'wait and see' policy justified. If there is any suspicion of AMS further ascent is out of the question. There have been no formal trials of any drugs in children in this setting but it is assumed that the same medication can be used in children as in adults. The dosage suggested for drugs used in AMS is shown in Table 26.1.

The management of HAPE (and HACE) is similar to that in adults (Chapters 19 and 20). There is a report of the successful use of the Gamow bag in a 3.5-year-old child with severe AMS (Taber 1994).

26.2.7 Children, cold and heat

Children are not only smaller than adults but have a larger surface-to-weight ratio, so as a result, cool faster in cold and heat up more quickly in hot conditions (Kennedy and Gentle 1995). Thermal balance

Table 26.1 Dosage for drugs used in children for acute mountain sickness, high altitude pulmonary edema and high altitude cerebral edema

Drug	Dose	Route
Paracetamol	12 mg kg^{-1} every 6 h	Oral
Dexamethasone	0.15 mg kg^{-1} every 4 h	Oral or i.v.
Acetazolamide	5 mg kg^{-1} every 8–12 h; max. 350 mg	Oral
Nifedipine	0.5 mg kg^{-1} every 8 h; max 20 mg for caps, 40 mg for tabs	Oral

Aspirin should be avoided because of the slight risk of Reye's syndrome.
Source: after Pollard and Murdoch (1997).

is less efficient in children, and during exercise they generate more metabolic heat for a unit mass than adults, have lower cardiac output and gain heat more rapidly from the environment. They also acclimatize to heat more slowly in hot conditions. In addition to their larger surface to mass ratio, they have less subcutaneous fat and may have an underdeveloped shivering mechanism. For all these reasons, they are at greater risk than adults of hypothermia in a cold environment and of overheating in hot environments.

In cold or wet conditions a windproof and waterproof garment is essential, and particular attention should be paid to the head from which proportionally more heat is lost than in an adult. It should also be remembered that a child who is being carried is not generating heat in the way the adult carrier is and so needs more clothing.

Overheating can occur when on a glacier or snowfield in sunny conditions because of direct and reflected heat. Eyes must be protected by goggles and the exposed skin by sunblock cream. Adequate fluid must be given, especially in hot conditions, to prevent dehydration (Pollard and Murdoch 1997).

26.2.8 Conclusions

Although children are at no greater risk of AMS than adults at the same altitude, the fact that young children have difficulty in articulating their symptoms means that diagnosis is more difficult and may be delayed. The fact that in most cases an altitude holiday is also a holiday in a part of the world where medical help is far away and gastrointestinal infections and other diseases are common must be borne in mind. Also, it is true that children with these problems can progress from being perfectly healthy to being seriously ill at an alarming rate. Finally, it is questionable if young children really appreciate the mountain environment in the way adults do, so the rewards of such a holiday, as compared with a more conventional bucket and spade or low altitude country holiday, are less. On the other hand family travel is undoubtedly a valuable experience. On balance we would concur with Pollard *et al.* (1998) in a cautious approach in advising families considering high altitude trips. They suggest that, with children under 2 years of age, parties should not sleep at over 2000 m and no higher than 3000 m for children of 2–10 years. The latter may be too conservative since children of say 6–10 years, who can express their symptoms, could well enjoy higher altitudes with probably little more risk than adults.

26.3 ELDERLY PEOPLE

26.3.1 Introduction

The increased numbers of people going to high altitude, mainly for recreation, include a large proportion of elderly people. People are living longer and in general are fitter than in previous decades. Many retired men and women have the money, time and inclination to enjoy sightseeing or treks to the great ranges, to ski and to attend conferences. Doctors are often asked questions about risks involved. In Chapter 24 specific pre-existing conditions are considered which are frequently encountered in elderly patients. Saito *et al.* (2002) found that over 70% of Japanese trekkers were over 50 years old. Many were over 70 and of these 75% had some pre-existing medical problem! However, in this section we consider the apparently fit elderly person at altitude.

The effects of altitude on cardiovascular and pulmonary problems have been studied in elderly people, and a survey of over 1900 visitors to Keystone, Colorado (2783 m), revealed that 48% were aged 40–60 years and 15% were over 60. Approximately 10% of trekkers in Nepal were 50 years of age or

older (Hultgren 1992) and a few mountaineers of this age have climbed Everest using supplementary oxygen (Gillman 1993).

26.3.2 Performance

All bodily functions deteriorate with age and this includes the maximum oxygen uptake both at sea level and at altitude (Pugh *et al.* 1964). However, the effect of age on $V_{O_2,max}$ is very variable (Dill *et al.* 1964). West *et al.* (1983c) reported the results of measurements of $V_{O_2,max}$ on two subjects. There was only a moderate deterioration in performance over a 20-year period (aged 31–51 years). Stathokostas *et al.* (2004) found a 14% decline in $V_{O_2,max}$ over a decade in men with a mean age of 73 years, whilst in a group of women, of a similar age, the decline was only 7%.

With increasing age skeletal muscles gradually decrease in volume, mainly due to a reduced number of motor units (Porter *et al.* 1995). This in turn may be due to drop-out of anterior horn cells as part of the loss of neurons throughout the CNS. Conley and colleagues (2000) measured the reduction in cross-sectional area of the large muscles involved in cycling together with performance, measured as $V_{O_2,max}$ in a group of elderly subjects (mean age 69 years), compared with a group of younger subjects (mean age 39 years). They also measured the oxidative capacity of the quadriceps muscle. They found that the volume of the exercising muscles in the elderly was only 67% of that in the younger group. The oxidative capacity was reduced to 53% of the younger group and the $V_{O_2,max}$ was only 45% of the younger group. They conclude that the oxidative capacity decline with age resulted from a reduction in both muscle volume and capacity per unit volume and was an important determinant of the age-related reduction in $V_{O_2,max}$.

Exercise can make a big difference to the rate of decline in performance. Kasch *et al.* (1995) carried out a follow-up of a group of men for 28 years. Twelve continued to exercise over this period and 12 dropped out of exercising. The rates of decline were 5 and 19%, respectively. Interestingly, the blood pressure in the exercising group remained unchanged at 119/75 whilst in the drop-out group it rose from 128/85 to 149/90. A study by Macaluso *et al.* (2003) showed that in healthy women aged 65 to 74, an 8-week exercise training program increases muscle strength, power and functional ability (there was no further improvement with a further 8 weeks' training).

The ability to go to altitude depends more on an individual's degree of fitness than on age. Fit men of 75 years who normally live at sea level have spent months at 5000 m without difficulty and a peak of 6000 m has been climbed by an 80-year-old mountaineer. However, their ability to carry loads is reduced. No one should be discouraged from going to altitude on grounds of age alone, but rapid ascent and undue exertion will place more strain on those in the older age group than on those who are younger. However, their greater experience will enable them to pace themselves so that given time they can often achieve worthwhile objectives. Levine *et al.* (1997) studied 20 subjects with a mean age of 68 years attending a veterans' reunion at a resort at 2500 m. They found the expected decrease in Pa,O_2, Sa,O_2 and $VO_{2,max}$ and increase in pulmonary artery pressure of 43% due to the effect of hypoxic vasoconstriction and sympathetic activation. The induction of a 1 mm depression of the S–T segment occurred at a lower exercise rate at altitude but this returned to sea level values after 5 days at altitude. They conclude that elderly men acclimatize well at this altitude and regain sea level performance after 5 days.

26.3.3 Age and acclimatization

There are very few data on the effect of age on rate and degree of acclimatization. There is no evidence that age has an effect on minute ventilation or PCO_2. PO_2 declines with age at sea level and also at altitude due to reduced pulmonary efficiency. Burtscher *et al.* (2001) found that ventilatory adaptation to high altitude in the elderly (55–77-year-old men) was complete within the first 2 days at an altitude of 2000 m. The fact that the elderly are no more susceptible to AMS than the young (see below) also suggests that they acclimatize as fast and as well as young people.

26.3.4 Age and AMS

It might be assumed that older people would be more prone to AMS, but there is no evidence that this is the case. Anecdotal evidence suggests that

older mountaineers do better than the young but this may be because they do not climb so fast and therefore are at lower risk of AMS. Surveys such as that by Kayser (1991) find no significant age effect on the incidence of AMS. Although it is true that older people have more pre-existing disease, especially heart and lung disease, it seems that this does not increase the risk of AMS (Roach *et al.* 1995); nor does the fact that with age, the sensitivity of the ventilatory response to hypoxia (HVR) declines (Kronenberg and Drage 1973, Poulin *et al.* 1993, Serebrovskaya *et al.* 2000). Also arterial oxygen saturation is lower in older people due to declining lung function as well as lower HVR yet the incidence of AMS is no higher. There is a hypothesis, at present unproved, that AMS is due to cerebral edema increasing intra-cranial pressure. Subjects with a large brain in relation to their skull will have a rapid rise in pressure with only a small degree of cerebral edema. Those with a smaller brain in relation to their skull capacity will have less rise in pressure for a given degree of edema (Ross 1985). The elderly, who have lost a proportion of their neurons, will have more space within their skulls than the young. This could explain the apparent resistance to AMS in older subjects and provide a rare example of the advantage of growing old.

26.3.5 Conclusions and advice

The evidence that we have indicates that age alone is no bar to a fit person going to altitude. Exercise capacity is reduced in elderly people as it is in young people, and the itinerary should be planned accordingly, but the risk of AMS is no greater. However, 'age never comes alone' and the presence of pre-existing conditions, which might reduce one's enjoyment of a holiday at best and be life threatening at worst, should give pause for thought. Some of these conditions are considered in Chapter 27. However, anyone who can manage a full day walking on hills at low altitude without undue strain is likely to be able to enjoy a standard Himalayan trek. In a situation of having to go rapidly to altitude, for instance having to fly into an airport at high altitude, it is probably more important for elderly people than for young people that they should give themselves 2–3 days to acclimatize before undertaking any strenuous activity (Levine *et al.* 1997).

27

Commuting to high altitude for commercial and other activities

SUMMARY

Increasingly, large numbers of people are commuting to high altitude for commercial, scientific and other activities. Several mines are now situated at altitudes of 4000–6000 m. In some cases, the miners live at sea level and are bussed up to the mine where they spend a working period such as 7 days. They then return to their families at sea level for a further 7 days, and the cycle is repeated indefinitely. This pattern raises interesting questions about acclimatization and also how best to select people for this work. Telescopes are being sited at an altitude of 4200 m in Mauna Kea (Hawaii), and even higher at altitudes of 5000 m or more in Chajnantor in north Chile. In Mauna Kea, some of the workers commute daily from sea level. For the Chajnantor project, many workers will live at an altitude of about 2400 m and commute to the telescope though some will sleep at 5050 m. Military operations have now been conducted at altitudes up to 7000 m in the dispute between India and Pakistan with some soldiers moving rapidly to high altitudes and down again. A new railway to Lhasa, Tibet from Golmad, Qinghai Province, China reaches as high as 5000 m. Some athletes now commute to high altitude to improve their performance. An important innovation is the use of oxygen-enriched rooms at high altitude to relieve the hypoxia and reduce the equivalent altitude. Each 1% increase of oxygen concentration reduces the equivalent altitude by 300 m. Oxygen enrichment has been shown to improve neuropsychological function during the day and enhance sleep at night. The use of oxygen-enriched modules at the Chajnantor site shows great promise. The same technology is also being used at lower altitudes especially to improve sleeping.

27.1 INTRODUCTION

Currently one of the most challenging and interesting topics in high altitude medicine and physiology relates to the increasing number of people who commute to high altitude for commercial or scientific activities. The two main areas are high altitude mining and high altitude astronomy. Mining at high altitude goes back several hundred years, although the modern practice of having miners commute from much lower altitudes, even sea level, is relatively recent. Siting telescopes at high altitudes, for example over 4000 m, is also a more recent activity. Some of the most interesting problems arise in connection with placing telescopes at altitudes of 5000 m or above in north Chile. In addition, military operations at high altitudes, new railways, and training regimes for athletes involve intermittent exposure to high altitude.

This chapter overlaps somewhat with previous chapters. The use of intermittent hypoxia training is referred to in Chapter 11. The value of oxygen enrichment of room air to improve sleep at high altitude was briefly discussed in Chapter 13. The improvement of neuropsychological function at an altitude of 5000 m as a result of oxygen enrichment of room air was referred to in Chapter 16.

27.2 HISTORICAL

Mining activities at high altitude are very old. For example, gold has been mined in west Tibet for centuries. The open cast mines at Thok Jalung (Thok is Tibetan for gold) were investigated in 1867 by Nain Singh, one of the early pundits, the clandestine native explorers of the Survey of India (Waller 1990). Chinese sources suggest that Tibetans worked as high as 6000 m in the Tanggula range of central Tibet mining quartz, and chromate mines are also found in central Tibet (Ward 1990). In several areas of the South American Andes, there is evidence that mining activities were carried out by the Incas before the Spanish conquest. The Spanish conquistadors founded the imperial city of Potosí (4060 m) in Bolivia, the site of an enormous silver mine, in the 1540s. According to one historian quoted by Monge, M. (1948) there were 100 000 natives and 20 000 Spaniards in Potosí at one time. However, little information remains about the actual mining activities.

An informative description of the mining practices in Cerro de Pasco, Peru (4340 m), was given by Barcroft *et al.* (1923) in their account of the International High Altitude Expedition to Cerro de Pasco which took place in 1921–22. Although most of the studies carried out by the physiologists were on themselves, many interesting observations were made on the native miners. One mine was 250 ft (76 m) below the surface, and the staircase which

led down to it was 600 ft (183 m) in length. The porters who carried up the loads of ore from the mine varied greatly in age and stature. One boy who was said to be 10 years of age carried a load of 40 lb (18 kg) (Fig. 27.1). Another porter who was thought to be 19 years old brought up a load of about 100 lb (45 kg). The physiologists noted that the exercise was spasmodic. The climb was very slow and consisted of the ascent of a few steps, followed by a long pause during which the porter regained his breath. They noted that the panting of the porters could be heard far down the staircase, before they came into view. The miners enjoyed sports, for example soccer, when they were not working. Each period of the game was 15 min long.

More recently, the extraordinary physical activity of miners at the Aucanquilcha mine (5950 m) in north Chile has been described (McIntyre 1987). The photograph on page 455 of that article shows

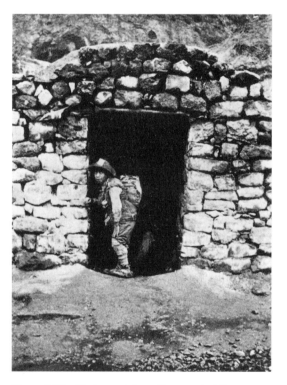

Figure 27.1   Photograph from the report of the 1921–22 International High Altitude Expedition to Cerro de Pasco, Peru, showing a young boy, said to be 10 years old, carrying a load of 18 kg, which he has just brought up from the mine 250 ft (76 m) below the surface. (From Barcroft *et al.* 1923.)

the miners shattering boulders of sulfur ore using sledgehammers. The caretakers of this mine lived indefinitely at this altitude, and they were probably the highest inhabitants in the world (West 1986a). The mine is no longer working.

27.3 MINING

Table 27.1 lists the altitudes of some of the most important commercial activities at high altitude. All of these are mines, except for two telescope sites. It can be seen that many of the mines are above 4000 m in altitude, with the highest being Aucanquilcha at 5950 m, although, as indicated earlier, this mine is no longer operating.

The mines fall into two categories. Many of the old mines, such as those at Cerro de Pasco and Morococha, have complete communities near the mine itself. This means that the families are located there and, in particular, the children are raised at these high altitudes. Many people now question the wisdom of this because there is some evidence that children grow more slowly at high altitude (Frisancho and Baker 1970), although the issue is somewhat controversial (see Chapter 26). Certainly the central nervous system is exquisitely sensitive to hypoxia, as discussed in Chapter 16, and, other things being equal, one would prefer to see children brought up in a more normal ambient P_{O_2}.

Another disadvantage of having whole communities at the site of the high altitude mine is that a large amount of infrastructure has to be provided. This includes schools, medical facilities and meeting halls, all of which increases the expenses of the mine. These considerations have led many modern mining operations to develop a commuting pattern where the families live at or near sea level and the miners commute to the mine itself where they spend a period of 7–10 days.

As an example of a modern mine based on the commuting pattern, the mine at Collahuasi will be briefly described. This is a very large, open-cut copper mine in north Chile at a latitude of 21°S. Mining operations in this area were carried out in pre-Spanish times. It is interesting that Thomas H. Ravenhill (1881–1952), who gave the first accurate clinical descriptions of high altitude pulmonary edema (HAPE) and high altitude cerebral edema (HACE) (Ravenhill 1913), was the medical officer at this mine in 1909–11 (West 1996b). The working areas of the mine are at altitudes of 4400–4600 m, though the mining camp where the miners sleep is at an altitude of 3800 m. There are currently several thousand people working at the mine, which makes it one of the largest copper mines in the world. Copper is a major export of Chile.

The miners' families live in Iquique on the coast in accommodation supplied by the mining company. The miners are transported to the mine by

Table 27.1 Examples of commercial and scientific activities at altitudes of 3500–6000 m

Country/state	Facility	Altitude (m)	Latitude	Product or activity
Chile	Andina	3400–4200	33°S	Copper
	Aucanquilcha[a]	5950	21°S	Sulfur
	Choquelimpie	4500	20°S	Silver
	Collahuasi	4400–4600	21°S	Copper
	El Indio	3800–4000	30°S	Copper, gold, silver
	Quebrada Blanca	4400	21°S	Copper
	Chajnantor	5000	23°S	Telescope site
Peru	Cerro de Pasco	4330	11°S	Copper, gold, lead, zinc
	Morococha	4550	12°S	Copper
Bolivia	Potosí	4060	20°S	Silver, tin
Hawaii	Mauna Kea	4200	20°N	Telescope site
Colorado	Climax	4350	39°N	Molybdenum
	Summitville	4050	37°N	Gold

[a] This mine is not operating at present.

special buses which take a few hours for the trip on a new road built by the mining company. A typical schedule is that the miners spend 7 days at the mine, where they work for up to 12 h per day, and then sleep in the mining camp at an altitude of 3800 m. At the end of 7 days they are bussed down to Iquique, where they spend the next 7 days with their families. The cycle is repeated indefinitely.

Richalet and colleagues (2002) have studied a group of 29 of these miners aged 25 ± 5 years over a period of 2.5 years. The subjects were extensively tested at sea level prior to their exposure to high altitude including a physical examination, ECG, hematology, maximal exercise, ventilatory and cardiac responses to an inhaled oxygen concentration of 11.4% both at rest and exercise, pulmonary vascular response to hypoxia using echocardiography, and 24 h monitoring of ECG and arterial pressure. Measurements at high altitude included a daily acute mountain sickness score, sleep characteristics, and 24 h monitoring of the ECG and arterial pressure. All the measurements were repeated after periods of about 12, 19 and 31 months.

It was found that the hematocrit increased, measured at both sea level and high altitude, after 12 and 19 months (Fig. 27.2), but interestingly it returned to values similar to the initial preexposure values at the end of 31 months of chronic intermittent hypoxia. In every instance there was an increase in hematocrit on acute exposure to high altitude which continued over the 31 months and presumably can be attributed to a reduced plasma volume. Perhaps surprisingly, body weight and body composition did not change significantly over the 31 months. This may be related to the fact that although the miners were exposed to high altitude which often causes a weight loss, they had excellent food at the living facility. Mean systemic arterial pressure both during the day and night were increased at high altitude compared with sea level. The sea level pressures tended to decrease with time. Another interesting finding was that the systolic pulmonary artery pressures, measured by echocardiography, both in normoxia and after challenge with 11.4% oxygen at sea level, did not change significantly over the first 19 months although the pressure following an acute hypoxic challenge was less after 31 months. There was a small increase in end-diastolic diameter of the right ventricle as measured by echocardiography from 18.6 ± 3 mm

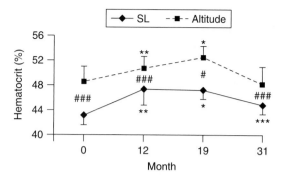

Figure 27.2 Hematocrit of miners before (0) and after 12, 19 and 31 months of exposure to chronic intermittent hypoxia. Seven days were spent at an altitude of 3800–4600 m followed by 7 days at sea level and the cycle was repeated for the whole 31 months. Mean ± SD. Time *vs.* 0: *, **, ***: $p < 0.05$, 0.01, 0.001, respectively. Altitude *vs.* sea level (SL): #, ##, ###: $p < 0.05$, 0.01, 0.001, respectively. (From Richalet *et al.* 2002.)

to 22.4 ± 2.4 mm after 19 months of exposure to chronic intermittent hypoxia.

Unexpectedly, maximal exercise as measured at sea level was found to be decreased by 12.3% at the end of 31 months of chronic intermittent hypoxia. This was accompanied by a decrease in maximal heart rate of 6.8%. When the arterial oxygen saturation during exercise was measured following exposure to the hypoxic mixture, the saturation was found to be lower at the end of 12 months of chronic intermittent hypoxia than in the prehypoxia measurements but it remained stable thereafter. On the other hand the ventilatory response to hypoxia increased after 12 months of exposure and remained elevated. Interestingly, symptoms of acute mountain sickness were similar throughout the period of exposure to chronic intermittent hypoxia, the score always being higher on the first or second day following ascent to altitude. Consistent with this the quality of sleep was impaired during the first two nights at high altitude (being worse on the second night) and remained unaltered during the 31 months of chronic intermittent hypoxia.

This was the first study of this pattern of chronic intermittent hypoxia and showed that some degree of acclimatization occurred during the 31 months but that, not surprisingly, the changes were less than in a group of people permanently exposed to an altitude of 4000 m. However, it was interesting

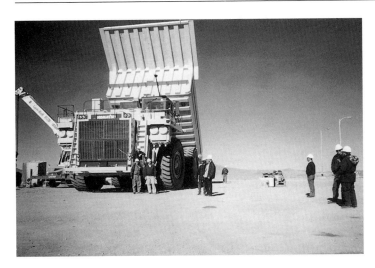

Figure 27.3 Enormous diesel electric truck at the modern Collahuasi mine in north Chile. This can transport 240 tons of copper ore.

that the symptoms of acute mountain sickness and the impairment of sleeping at high altitude persisted during the whole of the 31 months. Incidentally, it had been hoped to extend this study for a total of 5 years but apparently the mining company that supported the work felt that sufficient information had been obtained for their purposes after 31 months.

The 7 by 7-day schedule referred to above is not universally employed in the high altitude mines that use commuting. Periods at high altitude as long as 10–14 days have been tried. It clearly does not make much sense from a physiological point of view to have a period at high altitude of less than 7 days because there is evidence that the ventilatory acclimatization continues for at least this period of time (Lahiri 1972, Dempsey and Forster 1982). Other features of high altitude acclimatization, such as the development of polycythemia, take several weeks to reach a steady state. On the other hand, the physiological value of polycythemia is now less clear than it was earlier thought to be (Winslow and Monge C. 1987).

Another important question is the time course of deacclimatization. Ideally, the workers should not lose all the acclimatization that they have developed at high altitude during their period with their families at sea level. Relatively little information about the rate of deacclimatization is available, although some measurements suggest that the rate of change of the ventilatory response during deacclimatization is slower than during acclimatization (Lahiri 1972). Deacclimatization is discussed further in section 4.4.4.

Finally, although the physiological aspects of scheduling are important, it may be that social factors will be dominant. Experience has shown that miners are reluctant to leave their homes for more than 7–10 days, and it is probable that a schedule of 7 days of high altitude followed by 7 days at sea level, or alternatively 10 by 10 days, will be the most acceptable.

Reference was made above to the miners at Aucanquilcha (5950 m) who were breaking large pieces of sulfur ore using sledgehammers. However, the activities at a modern mine such as Collahuasi are quite different. The ore is dislodged using explosives, and then it is picked up by enormous diesel electric front-end loaders that can scoop up 80 tons of ore at a time. Three scoops are then placed in a gigantic diesel electric truck, which can carry 240 tons (Fig. 27.3). Of course, considerable skill is necessary to operate these very large pieces of equipment, and substantial damage can be done to people or machines if the equipment is not operated correctly.

The highly skilled nature of modern mining is one reason why, in mines like Collahuasi, none of the miners are people indigenous to the high altitudes. Another reason is that there is not a large indigenous high altitude population in Chile. This is in contrast to the situation in many mines in Peru where, for example at Cerro de Pasco and Morococha, there are large indigenous populations who can provide relatively cheap, unskilled labor for the mines.

Another challenging problem of these high altitude mines is the selection of workers. Certainly not everybody is able to work effectively at altitudes of 4400–4500 m. There is considerable interest in possible medical tests that could predict who will be able to work well at altitude or, perhaps more important, who will be unable to tolerate the altitude. One possible test is the ventilatory response to hypoxia, during both rest and exercise (Rathat *et al.* 1992). As pointed out in Chapter 12, there is evidence that tolerance to extreme altitude requires a reasonable level of hypoxic ventilatory response in order to defend the alveolar P_{O_2} at a viable level. However, whether this will be a useful prognostic test for working at altitudes of 4000–5000 m is not clear. Probably the best predictor at the present time is whether a prospective worker has previously worked effectively at high altitude.

Even if workers have been shown to tolerate these high altitudes reasonably well, it is clear that they cannot accomplish the same amount of physical work as at sea level. The decline in maximal oxygen consumption with increasing altitude was discussed in Chapter 11, where it was pointed out that the $\dot{V}_{O_2,max}$ of an acclimatized subject at an altitude of 5000 m is only about 70% of the sea level value. Another way of looking at this is that the work force would have to be increased by about 40% at high altitude to accomplish the same amount of physical work. It is interesting that this inefficiency is not confined to human beings, but is also seen in mechanical equipment. Table 27.2 shows that, at an altitude of 4000 m, the amount of equipment to produce the same amount of work as at sea level has to be increased by 25 to 85% (Jimenez 1995).

27.4 TELESCOPES

27.4.1 Mauna Kea

As indicated previously, there have been mines at altitudes over 4000 m in the South American Andes for many years, even before the Spanish conquest. However, the practice of siting telescopes at high altitude is much more recent, mostly within the last 50 years. There are several advantages in placing telescopes at high altitudes. One is that the instrument is then above much of Earth's atmosphere, which otherwise absorbs some of the optical and radio waves. Another advantage is that in some areas, for example Chajnantor (see below), the

Table 27.2 Increase in mine equipment size at 3000 m and 4000 m to achieve the same output as at sea level

Equipment	Output unit	Increase at altitude (%)	
		3000 m	4000 m
Diesel engines	Brake horsepower	40	55
Compressors	Airtool work	55	75
Vacuum filters	Tons solids h^{-1}	30	45
Vacuum pumps	Intake volume	30	40
Transmission lines	MVA km^{-1}	20	30
Transformers	MVA	15	25
Electrical machines	kW	15	25
Flotation	tons h^{-1}	35	50
Leach vessels	tons h^{-1}	50	85

Source: modified from Jimenez (1995).

atmosphere is extremely dry and absorption of radio waves by water vapor is therefore much less. Finally, remote mountain sites tend to have little light or radio wave pollution, although this advantage can also be achieved in other remote areas at lower altitudes.

Two telescope sites will be considered here. One is the extinct volcano at Mauna Kea in the big island of Hawaii. The summit is at an altitude of 4200 m and at least 10 instruments are located either on the summit or not far below it. A feature of Mauna Kea is that it is close to the city of Hilo, which is at sea level, and it is possible to drive from one site to the other in a couple of hours. There is also an intermediate station with dormitories at 3000 m at Hale Pohaku, and some newcomers can spend a night there before going to the summit. However, the majority of the staff who operate the telescopes commute from sea level every day. The barometric pressure at the summit is about 465 mmHg, so the P_{O_2} of moist inspired gas is only 87 mmHg, as against 150 mmHg at sea level. The hypoxic stress is therefore severe.

Forster (1986) studied the incidence of acute mountain sickness (AMS) and the arterial blood gases of some of the workers on the United Kingdom Infrared Telescope (UKIRT) on the summit of Mauna Kea. These shift workers spent 40 days working at sea level at Hilo, followed by a 5-day shift at high altitude. The first night of the shift was spent in the dormitories at 3000 m, and following that 4 days were spent on the summit of Mauna Kea, with the workers returning to 3000 m for each night. It was found that 80% of the shift workers had symptoms of AMS on their first day at the summit. Apart from breathlessness, headache was the most frequent complaint, and this affected 41% of shift workers at the start of their high altitude shift. Other common symptoms were insomnia, lethargy, poor concentration, poor memory and unsteadiness of gait. The frequency of symptoms decreased over the 5 days of the shift, and at the end 60% of the workers were asymptomatic.

Arterial blood gases were measured in 27 UKIRT shift workers. On day 1 at 4200 m, the mean arterial P_{O_2} was 42 mmHg, rising to 44 mmHg on day 5. The arterial P_{CO_2} was 29 mmHg on the first day, falling to 27 mmHg on the fifth day. Arterial pH was 7.49 on day 1, falling to 7.48 on day 5.

It is interesting that there was no difference in the incidence of AMS between shift workers who worked at the summit after a brief sojourn at sea level (mean 4 days), compared to a protracted rest period (mean 37 days) at sea level. This suggests that in this group, the acclimatization to high altitude achieved during 5 days on Mauna Kea was lost within a few days of return to sea level. High altitude pulmonary edema (HAPE) was infrequently seen at Mauna Kea, with only one case in 41 shift workers during a 2-year study period. Also only one worker on Mauna Kea had an episode of high altitude cerebral edema (HACE).

An interesting problem related to the astronomers near the summit of Mauna Kea is their reluctance to admit that the hypoxia is affecting them, and their resistance to using oxygen enrichment of room air which is discussed in section 29.8. As Fig. 6.2 showed, the alveolar P_{O_2} for acute exposure to the barometric pressure on the summit of Mauna Kea is about 45 mmHg. This increases to as much as about 53 mmHg if the subject is fully acclimatized although this never happens on Mauna Kea because astronomers never stay there long enough. Note that these values for alveolar P_{O_2} agree well with the arterial P_{O_2} values cited above when the arterial P_{O_2} was 42 mmHg on day 1 rising to 44 mmHg on day 5.

This is a severe degree of oxygen deprivation. As was pointed out in section 6.3, Fig. 6.2 also shows

that if a patient with chronic obstructive pulmonary disease has a P_{O_2} below 55 mmHg, he is entitled to continuous oxygen therapy under Medicare. Clearly, the Mauna Kea astronomers are well below that level which unquestionably reduces physical and mental powers. It would be easy to alleviate some of this severe hypoxia using oxygen enrichment of room air, but for some curious reasons some of the astronomers are adamantly against this. This macho attitude is inexplicable.

27.4.2 Chajnantor

The other telescope site that will be discussed here is Chajnantor in north Chile, southeast of San Pedro de Atacama, at a latitude of 23°S and an altitude of about 5000 m. This is a remarkable site because it is fairly flat, covers a large area, and is easily accessible by road from San Pedro (altitude 2440 m). The first part of the road is an international highway leading from Chile to Bolivia and Argentina, and the final 15 km is now also paved. The drive from San Pedro to Chajnantor takes only about 1 h. There must be few places in the world where it is possible to reach an altitude of 5000 m so easily.

Several small radio telescopes have been sited at Chajnantor or nearby. The California Institute of Technology has had a radio telescope for studying the cosmic microwave background radiation for several years. However, part of the interest of Chajnantor is that it is the site of an enormous multinational radio telescope, construction of which is far advanced. When finished it will be the largest radio telescope in the world, with a cost of several hundred million dollars. Since the barometric pressure at the site, altitude 5050 m, is about 420 mmHg, the inspired P_{O_2} is only 78 mmHg, so the degree of hypoxic stress is substantial. The large amount of construction work required to complete the telescope, and the number of workers who will be at the site to run it, means that this is a remarkably challenging problem in high altitude medicine.

27.5 MILITARY OPERATIONS

To paraphrase Winston Churchill, never have so many lowlanders been transported to such high altitudes for such long periods (and it might be added, to so little avail) as in the dispute between India and Pakistan over the Jammu–Kashmir region. The unhappy result is that large numbers of soldiers have been stationed at altitudes up to 7000 m for substantial periods of time. Many of these soldiers come from altitudes near sea level such as the plains of India. A fascinating account of some of the problems was given by Anand (2001). Indeed this conflict was responsible for the appearance of a new medical condition initially called adult subacute mountain sickness (Anand *et al.* 1990) in which young soldiers develop right heart failure with peripheral edema somewhat reminiscent of brisket disease in cattle at high altitude (see Chapter 21). Jha and his colleagues (2002) reported the high incidence of stroke in these young soldiers at these great altitudes. There have been previous military operations at high altitudes, for example in the Soviet Union during World War II, but the altitudes near the Siachen Glacier where the India–Pakistan dispute has taken place are far above these.

27.6 RAILWAYS

Railways have been built at high altitude for many years. For example the central railway of Peru was completed to Aroya in 1893 and this included crossing the Andean crest at Ticlio at an altitude of 4800 m. Slightly earlier the cog railway up to the summit of Pikes Peak in Colorado (4300 m) was finished in 1891. However, a modern railway from Golmud in Qinghai Province, China to Lhasa, Tibet has posed enormous challenges not only for the engineers and construction workers, but indeed for the passengers. The length of the rail link is over 1100 km with more than three-quarters of the distance above 4000 m altitude. In fact the track crosses some of the highest ranges on the Tibetan plateau, the highest altitude being just over 5000 m. Some 30 000 to 50 000 construction workers are reported to have been used to put in the track, and although the medical facilities were impressive, there were many cases of mountain sickness. Indeed it could be argued that Chinese physicians probably have more experience of high altitude problems (including their prevention and management) than any other group in the world.

An interesting problem is how to help the train passengers to tolerate these altitudes. Tibetans are not likely to be seriously affected because they live so high. However, Chinese boarding the train at Beijing near sea level will soon be exposed for many hours to altitudes over 4000 m and up to 5000 m. Possible solutions include having oxygen masks available for each passenger, pressurizing the railway cars as in aircraft, or using oxygen enrichment of room air as described in section 27.8. In any event the Golmud–Lhasa railway is undoubtedly one of the most ambitious engineering challenges at high altitude in the history of the world.

27.7 ATHLETIC TRAINING

As described in Chapter 11 a popular method of training for athletics now is to live high and train low. This can be accomplished by having the athlete physically commute between the two altitudes, or now increasingly, living or just sleeping in a low oxygen environment provided by a nitrogen-enriched house, apartment, or even a tentlike structure around the bed.

27.8 OXYGEN ENRICHMENT OF ROOM AIR TO RELIEVE THE HYPOXIA OF HIGH ALTITUDE

Partly in response to the burgeoning of commercial and scientific activities at high altitude, considerable work has been done on the feasibility and value of raising the oxygen concentration of room air at high altitude in order to relieve the hypoxia. The possibility of doing this was suggested by Cudaback (1984) and, at one stage, plans were made to oxygen-enrich the control room of the Keck telescope at Mauna Kea, although these were never carried out at the time.

The principle of oxygen enrichment is simple. Oxygen, ideally from a concentrator or possibly from a cryogenic source, is added to the ventilation of a room, thus increasing the oxygen concentration from 21% to a higher value. The reason why oxygen enrichment is so powerful is that relatively small degrees of oxygen enrichment result in large reductions of equivalent altitude. The term 'equivalent altitude' refers to the altitude at which the moist inspired P_{O_2}, when a subject is breathing ambient air, is the same as the inspired P_{O_2} in the

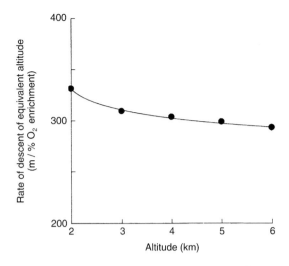

Figure 27.4 Degree of reduction of equivalent altitude (meters of descent per 1% oxygen enrichment) plotted against the altitude at which the enrichment is made. Note that at altitudes up to about 6000 m, each 1% of oxygen enrichment results in an altitude reduction of more than 300 m. (From West 1995.)

oxygen-enriched environment. Figure 27.4 shows that, between altitudes of 3000 and 6000 m, each 1% of oxygen enrichment results in a reduction of equivalent altitude by about 300 m. In other words, if we oxygen enrich a room at the Chajnantor site, altitude 5000 m, by 6% (that is, we increase the oxygen concentration from 21 to 27%), the equivalent altitude is reduced by about 6×300 m, or 1800 m. Therefore we effectively go from an altitude of 5000 m to one of 3200 m, which is much more easily tolerated.

When this idea was originally proposed, some people argued that it would be impossible to maintain an enriched-oxygen atmosphere within the room because of inevitable leaks. However, in practice, oxygen enrichment is relatively simple and reliable. The room does not have to be gas tight. Large potential leaks such as window surrounds are taped, and a double door is provided so that there is an air lock. However, oxygen-enriched air is blown into the room and escapes through small leaks, and in practice it is easy to control the oxygen level within 0.25%.

Oxygen enrichment of rooms has become feasible largely because large quantities of oxygen can now be produced relatively cheaply. The simplest way to do this is to use an oxygen concentrator; thousands of these are now used in homes to provide oxygen for patients with chronic lung disease. The principle is that air is pumped at high pressure through a nonflammable synthetic zeolite which absorbs nitrogen from the air. The result is that the effluent gas has a high oxygen concentration, typically 90–95%. After 20–30 s, the zeolite is unable to absorb more nitrogen and the compressed air is then switched to another cylinder containing the same material. The original cylinder is then purged of nitrogen by blowing air through it at normal pressures. In this way, a continuous supply of 90–95% oxygen is available. A typical unit provides 5 L min^{-1} of over 90% pure oxygen at a power consumption of 350 W. It is also possible to provide the oxygen from liquid oxygen tanks, but this is more expensive and less convenient because the tanks need to be replenished.

An important issue is what level of ventilation to use in the room. Clearly, the higher the ventilation, the larger the amount of oxygen that must be produced to maintain a given degree of oxygen enrichment. This topic has been discussed extensively elsewhere (West 1995). We use the 1975 American Society of Heating, Refrigeration and Air-Conditioning Engineers (ASHRAE) standard of 8.5 m^3 person^{-1} h^{-1}, which corresponds to 142 L min^{-1}. This is calculated to maintain the carbon dioxide concentration in the room below 0.24%, based on a carbon dioxide production rate per person of 0.3 L min^{-1}. This concentration of carbon dioxide was chosen by ASHRAE as a measure of acceptable ventilation levels. Substantially higher concentrations of carbon dioxide can exist without people being aware of them. However, the carbon dioxide concentration is a useful objective marker of adequacy of ventilation, and higher levels tend to be associated with awareness of body odor.

It should be added that in 1989, ASHRAE increased the minimum standard of ventilation by three- to four-fold. This was a somewhat controversial decision, and was partially based on the possibilities that there may be smokers in the room, there are health variations among people, and some types of room furniture cause outgassing, which may be injurious. In designing a facility for use at high altitude, it can be assumed that people will not be allowed to smoke in the room, and it is also possible to choose furniture that does not result in outgassing hazards.

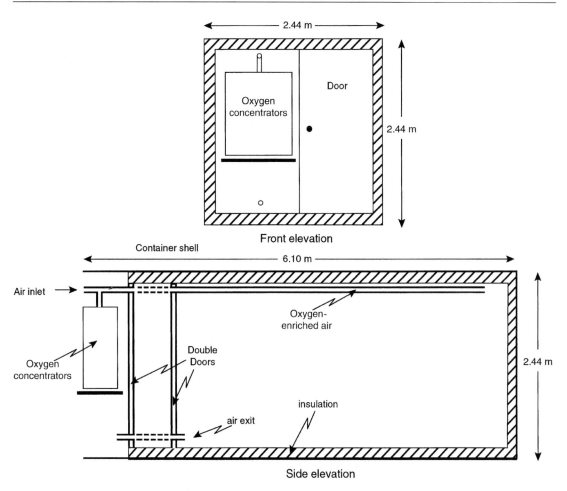

Figure 27.5   A self-contained oxygen-enriched module suitable for field work at high altitude. The module uses a standard shipping container 20 ft (6.10 m) long and 8 ft (2.44 m) wide and high. These oxygen-enriched modules are being used at the California Institute of Technology radio telescope at Chajnantor, altitude 5050 m.

Figure 27.5 shows a sketch of a module that can be used for oxygen enrichment in the field. In this instance, a standard shipping container of dimensions 20 ft (6.1 m) long, 8 ft (2.44 m) wide and 8 ft high is fitted out as a living space with beds, or a laboratory or a machine shop. A larger laboratory can be housed in a standard shipping container of dimensions 40 ft (12.19 m) long by 8 ft wide by 8 ft high. Such containers are currently in use at the Chajnantor site, in connection with the CalTech radio telescope. The oxygen is provided from oxygen concentrators, and the concentrations of both oxygen and carbon dioxide are continually monitored inside the rooms.

The experience of the astronomers with oxygen enrichment has been very satisfactory (West and Readhead 2004). There have been few technical problems in maintaining the target oxygen concentration of 27%, and the carbon dioxide concentration is typically less than 0.25%. The CalTech project was a particularly valuable field test of oxygen enrichment because, for the first 2 weeks, the astronomers were working in ambient air conditions. They found this extremely tiring, despite the fact that they slept every night at San Pedro (altitude 2440 m). When the oxygen enrichment modules were set up, they noticed an immediate improvement in work productivity and efficiency. In fact, they soon instituted a rule that no one was allowed to control the telescope or use power tools unless using oxygen enrichment. When the astronomers were not in the oxygen-enriched modules, they used portable oxygen in order to provide oxygen enrichment. They also reported that it was feasible to sleep at the Chajnantor site in the oxygen-enriched rooms. This had not proved to be possible while breathing ambient air because of the poor quality of sleep.

Several studies have now been carried out on the physiological effects of oxygen enrichment of room air at high altitude. The first studies were performed at the Barcroft facility of the White Mountain Research Station (altitude 3800 m) in California, where the oxygen concentration of the test room was raised from 21 to 24% (Luks *et al.* 1998). This reduced the equivalent altitude to about 2900 m. In a double-blind study, it was shown that oxygen enrichment during the night resulted in fewer apneas and less time spent in periodic breathing with apneas. Subjective assessments of sleep quality showed significant improvement. There was also a lower AMS score during the morning after oxygen-enriched sleep. An unexpected finding was that there was a larger increase in arterial oxygen saturation from evening to morning after oxygen-enriched sleep than after sleeping in ambient air (Fig. 27.6). Of course, both measurements of arterial oxygen saturation were made with the subject breathing ambient air.

In another study, the mechanism of the unexpected increase in arterial oxygen saturation the following morning was investigated (McElroy *et al.* 2000). Because this could have been caused by a change in the control of ventilation, the ventilatory responses to hypoxia and to carbon dioxide were measured in the evening and in the morning after sleeping both in the oxygen-enriched environment and in ambient air. No effect of oxygen enrichment on the control of ventilation was found. An alternative explanation is that the increase in arterial oxygen saturation seen following sleep in the oxygen-enriched environment might have been the result of less subclinical pulmonary edema, compared with sleeping in ambient air. An additional observation that might support this explanation was that the increase in arterial oxygen saturation was transient, so that by midday the difference between the oxygen-enriched and ambient air treatments on oxygen saturation was abolished.

A final study was carried out on the effects of oxygen enrichment on neuropsychological function at a simulated altitude of 5000 m, as referred to briefly in Chapter 16. Again, the Barcroft facility,

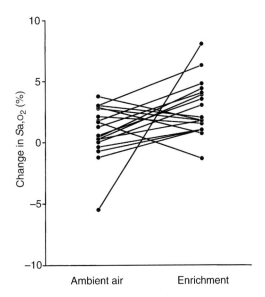

Figure 27.6 Change in arterial oxygen saturation from evening to morning for subjects sleeping in ambient air, compared with the same subjects sleeping in 24% oxygen enrichment, at an altitude of 3800 m. The measurements of oxygen saturation were made by pulse oximetry, with the subjects breathing ambient air. The increase was greater after sleep in oxygen enrichment ($p < 0.05$). (From Luks *et al.* 2000.)

at an altitude of 3800 m, was used, and the concentration of oxygen in the room was manipulated to simulate ambient air at an altitude of 5000 m, and an oxygen concentration of 27% at an altitude of 5000 m. A large battery of neuropsychological tests was performed in a double-blinded manner, and it was found that there were significant improvements in reaction times, hand–eye coordination, and mood (Gerard *et al.* 2000). These findings are directly relevant to the project of oxygen enrichment at the Chajnantor site.

An important consideration when oxygen is added to air is whether the fire hazard is increased, compared with sea level. This has been analyzed carefully (West 1997) and it has been shown that, with the levels of oxygen enrichment considered here, the fire hazard is less than at sea level. The basic reason is that, although the P_{O_2} is increased by oxygen enrichment at high altitude, it is still far below the value at sea level. Although it is true that the reduction of the partial pressure of nitrogen at altitude also increases the fire hazard to a small extent because of the reduced extinguishing effect of this inert gas, it remains true that the fire hazard using the degrees of oxygen enrichment described here is less than at sea level. As an example, the National Fire Protection Association (NFPA 1993) defines an oxygen-enriched atmosphere as having an increased fire hazard, in the sense that it will support an increased burning rate of materials, if the percentage concentration of oxygen is greater than $23.45/(P_f^{0.5})$, where P_f is the total barometric pressure expressed as a fraction of the sea level pressure. For the Chajnantor site, $P_f = 0.55$, so that if the oxygen concentration is greater than 31.6% it would exceed the NFPA threshold. The oxygen concentration of 27% is well below this value.

Up to the present time, most of the interest in oxygen enrichment of room air has been for commercial or scientific activities above 4000 m. However, it is likely that the same technique could be valuable at substantially lower altitudes associated with ski or mountain resorts. Many people who visit these places have difficulties especially with sleeping during the first 2 or 3 days. Oxygen enrichment of room air can greatly improve sleep quality. Indeed, people who build houses at altitudes above 2000 m have shown interest in oxygen enrichment of bedrooms for the same reason. A study of the appropriate oxygen concentrations at these moderate altitudes indicates that considerable alleviation of the hypoxia can be brought about without incurring a fire hazard (West 2002b).

It could be argued that oxygen enrichment of room air represents a new attitude to living and working at high altitude. Until now, most people have accepted hypoxia as something that has to be endured. However, this proactive attitude of raising oxygen concentration of the rooms to reduce the equivalent altitude could represent a major advance.

28

Athletes and altitude

SUMMARY

It is only recently that athletes have used high altitude training to enhance sea level performance, but many remarkable feats of endurance have been recorded in mountains. One of the most remarkable was the first ascent of Everest without supplemental oxygen in 1978 which has been followed by a number of phenomenally fast ascents to extreme altitude without supplemental oxygen.

In athletic competitions at altitude lower times are recorded in sprint events because of lowered air resistance, whilst in endurance events, because of a lower $V_{O_2,max}$, times are slower.

The paradox is that acclimatization to altitude results in central and peripheral adaptation that enhances oxygen delivery and utilization, but hypoxia decreases the intensity of training and may even cause detraining.

As polycythemia increases the $V_{O_2,max}$ and endurance performance, this might indicate that the higher the athlete goes to train the better, but this is not the case as an increased hematocrit carries its own disadvantages, as well as the problem of decreased exercise capacity resulting in decreased training intensity.

There is some evidence that athletes who live at moderate altitude (2500 m) and train at low altitude (1500 m) improve their endurance performance. However, there is considerable individual variation in the results of the 'live high, train low' method, and in one series, sea level $V_{O_2,max}$ did not improve, yet race times improved by about 6%. Recently, there also has been much interest in the use of intermittent exposure to hypoxic environments in both human and animal models to see if benefits for performance can be attained this way.

For maximal sea level performance it is still not clear how long or how high the athlete should live at altitude or how long they should remain at sea level before racing, and these techniques have become the focus of intense debates in the governing bodies who oversee international sport. There is even a controversy on the 'legality' of athletes using exposure to hypoxic environments as an ergogenic aid and thus the use of 'unfair means.'

Unfortunately, few trials have adequate sea level controls to compare with altitude training. Until this is done much information will remain largely anecdotal.

28.1 INTRODUCTION

In 1965, Pugh (1965) suggested that athlete performance at altitude would result in lower times in sprint events due to decreased air resistance that parallels barometric pressure; by contrast in distance events times would be increased because the maximum oxygen uptake falls with altitude.

Comparing the times of athletes in the 1965 Pan-American games held in Mexico (2250 m) with those of the Melbourne Olympics of 1956 at sea level, he showed that there was an increase in time of 2.6% in the 800 m and 14.9% in the 10 000 m events. In the 100 m and 400 m, but not the 200 m, race times at altitude were faster than at sea level.

When the Olympic games were held in Mexico City in 1968, several world records in short and sprint events were broken whilst in the longer endurance events times were slower than at sea level. This was due to the reduced $V_{O_{2},max}$ which at this altitude is 84% of sea level values. However, the times were not as slow as had been predicted. In one of the most important races in those games, in an upset, Kip Keino who was born and raised at approximately 2300 m in Kenya beat the heavily favored Jim Ryan from the United States. This race was the beginning of heated debates about the value of altitude training on athletic performance. There was little note that Keino not only lived at altitude but also had grown up running many miles back and forth to school as a child!

Marathon performance at altitude is affected mainly by a lowered $V_{O_{2},max}$ which decreases by about 1.5–3.5% for every 300 m of ascent above 1500 m (Roi *et al.* 1999).

28.2 THE MOUNTAINEER AS AN ATHLETE

The first mountaineers who could be called athletes were Habler and Messner (Messner 1979). In 1978, they made the first ascent of Everest without supplemental oxygen, and this focused attention on their birth, upbringing and training at intermediate altitude in the European Alps. A number of high altitude natives have repeated this feat on Everest, but then so have mountaineers born and bred at sea level.

Habler and Messner's training, which included long distance running and very rapid alpine ascents up to 4875 m and later rapid ascents in the Himalaya, played a major role in their exceptional fitness and subsequent success.

With training, outstanding feats of endurance have been recorded. In 1899, a Ghurka soldier born and bred at intermediate altitude in Nepal ascended and descended a 800 m peak in Scotland and crossed 4 miles of scree and bog in 55 min. A hundred years

later in 1999, this feat was repeated by a trained athlete (a fell runner) in 53 min 45 s (*The Times* 1999).

Other outstanding endurance feats at low and high altitude are recorded. For instance, a 49-year-old man ran 391 miles in 7 days 1 h and 25 min over Lakeland Hills up to 850 m in the UK. This involved a total ascent of 37 000 m, an average of over 5000 m per day (Brasher 1986). In June 1988, 76 summits in the same region were reached in 24 h involving an ascent and descent of 12 000 m (Brasher 1988). At intermediate altitude all 54 of the peaks over 4300 m in Colorado, USA were climbed in 21 days (Boyer 1978) and the ascent of Mont Blanc (4807 m) from Chamonix, with return to Chamonix (1050 m) was made in 5.5 h (Smyth 1988). At high altitude, one ascent was made from 4900 m to 8047 m with return to 4900 m in 22 h (Wielicki 1985) and from 3000 m to 6000 m in 19 h (Rowell 1982).

In 1986 an ascent and descent of Everest (8848 m) in 2 days by a new route on the North face was completed from the head of the West Rongbuck Glacier (5800 m); supplementary oxygen was not used (Everest 1987). In 1990, Marc Batard ascended from Base Camp to the summit of Everest in 22.5 h also without the use of supplementary oxygen (Gillman 1993). An astounding ascent by Sherpa Pemba Dorji from Base Camp to the summit was reported to be 8 h 10 min (www.mounteverest.net/news)!

28.3 HYPOXIC TRAINING

To achieve optimum physical performance in middle and long distance events at altitude, it is clear that adequate acclimatization to hypoxia, or better still being born and bred at altitude, is essential. Most evidence suggests that after a period of training at altitude, performance improves upon returning to sea level, but the timing, i.e. altitude and duration at altitude for maximum sea-level performance after altitude training is not clear. However, altitude training or exposure to simulated hypoxic environments at low altitude is frequently used by competition athletes to improve their sea level performance. On the one hand, acclimatization to high altitude results in central and peripheral adaptations that improve oxygen delivery and utilization. Hypoxic exercise may increase the stimulus of training thus magnifying the effect of endurance training. On the other hand, the hypoxia of altitude limits the intensity of training and may result in detraining.

Some of the best endurance runners have been born and bred in East Africa, living at an altitude of 1500–2000 m, and this upbringing will contribute to their continued success. However, Weston et al. (1999) compared elite African 10 km runners and their Caucasian counterparts, both of whom lived at sea level. The African runners had a greater resistance to fatigue, and higher oxidative enzyme activity, combined with a lower accumulation of lactate. With the difference between winning and losing an event being often so small, the psychological effects of altitude training should not be discounted.

Numerous anecdotal reports suggest that endurance athletes benefit from altitude training; however, when appropriate controls have been included in studies, the results are less impressive. Additionally, there have been several altitudes used such that it is difficult to know if there is a minimal altitude, above which a benefit is gained. Using controls, Roskamm et al. (1969) found subjects who trained at 2250 m improved their $V_{O_{2,max}}$ by comparison with sea level subjects and those at 3450 m, but Hanson et al. (1967) also with sea level controls and starting with unfit subjects ($V_{O_{2,max}} < 40\,mL\,min^{-1}\,kg^{-1}$) found no advantage in training at an altitude of 4300 m. In well-trained subjects too, the picture is not clear. A well-controlled study by Adams et al. (1975) using a cross-over design in experienced trained athletes ($V_{O_{2,max}}$ 73 mL min^{-1} kg^{-1}) showed no significant differences in performance between altitude (2300 m) and sea level training.

Because so many hypoxic training studies have been completed without normoxic controls, it is difficult to determine whether the physiological changes noted are due to hypoxia alone or a training effect. In one series with controls 10 elite middle to long distance runners trained for 10 weeks at the same exercise rate at sea level and at a stimulated altitude of 4000 m. There was no improvement in $V_{O_{2,max}}$, yet personal best times over 10 km improved by about 6% (Asano et al. 1986). Is it possible that this was due to a psychological effect? Anaerobic performance may also improve after returning to sea level, following a stay at altitude; however, many studies have shown no improvement (Martin and Pyne 1998).

Some investigators have utilized 'doses' of hypoxia during training to effect a training advantage. Ventura et al. (2003) trained athletes for 6 weeks at high intensity with bouts of simulated 3200 m and found no change in performance. Brugniaux et al. (2006) had well-trained athletes sleep at simulated altitudes of 1200, 2500, 3000 and 3500 m for 13–18 days and found that 3000 m was safe and induced a degree of ventilatory acclimatization. Truijens et al. (2003) trained accomplished swimmers in a flume in an intense interval protocol at either low altitude or while inspiring air consistent with 2500 m altitude for 5 weeks and then measured performance at 100 and 400 m swims and found no difference. In another study, cyclists trained for 4 weeks at either sea level or simulated 2750 m three times per week in 10 intervals at 80% of maximum (Morton and Cable 2005). Without an increase in hemoglobin, the subjects increased their endurance but not their maximum work intensity, but there was no difference between the hypoxic or sea level-trained athletes. These studies suggest that short-term exposure to hypoxic air during intense training has no discernible benefit for performance.

28.4 LIVING–TRAINING HYPOXIC PARADIGMS

In the late 1990s a number of elegant studies were undertaken to investigate the various living–training environments in which athletes could realistically be exposed during a period of intense training. In other words, athletes lived high and trained low, lived and trained high, lived low and trained high, and trained and lived low. These studies were designed to take advantage of a number of physiologic responses of acclimatization which might convey an advantage in physical performance.

Levine and Stray-Gundersen (1997) suggested that if athletes were acclimatized to a moderate altitude (2500 m) and trained at lower altitude (1500 m) for 6 weeks they could get the best of both worlds and improve their performance more than an equivalent control group at sea level or altitude. A 5000 m run time trial was the main measure of performance while they also undertook an additional number of physiologic measurements. The trained runners who 'lived high, trained low' showed an increase above sea level performance. Sea level performance was not improved in those who lived and trained at moderate altitude nor in those who lived and trained at sea level only.

There was, however, considerable individual variation in the response to altitude training, and some do not respond to the 'live high, train low regime'. (Chapman *et al.* 1998). The 'responders' had the highest rise in erythropoietin and thus hematocrit, suggesting that the improved endurance was conveyed by the higher oxygen-carrying capacity in that group, but no genetic markers to elucidate this variability could be found (Jedlickova *et al.* 2003). Elite (world championship qualifiers) male and female runners were studied over 4 weeks at 2500 m during continued training; and although there was variability in the results, these already highly trained athletes showed improvement in all variables of performance (Stray-Gundersen *et al.* 2001). Attempts to have similar responses at the same altitude, but for shorter periods of time (5, 10 and 15 days), were unsuccessful in improving exercise performance (Roberts *et al.* 2003).

In attempts to gain advantage with shorter periods of exposure, the concept of 'intermittent hypoxic training' was entertained in a study which was based on discernible physiologic changes noted in animal models. This approach exposed athletes to short periods (70 min) of hypoxia at rest for 4 weeks (Julian *et al.* 2004). There were no changes in any of the hematologic, physiologic or performance variables. Human and animal studies, such as this one, have led to much debate about the 'dose response' of the hypoxic exposure and the subsequent gain or lack thereof in performance (Stray-Gundersen *et al.* 2001, Levine and Stray-Gundersen 2006, Levine 2005). Attempts to find a competitive edge has led to the utilization of hypoxic tents and sleeping chambers where the athlete can gain the benefit of 'living high, training low' in the comfort of sea level living. The entire concept of a performance advantage with various constructs of hypoxic exposure has recently incited an intense debate between athletes, investigators and international regulatory agencies which is far from being resolved.

28.5 PRESUMED MECHANISM OF HYPOXIC EXPOSURE

As is well described in ealier Chapters, exposure to high altitude incites a number of physiologic responses which optimize the transport of oxygen from the air to the mitochondria. With respect to

hypoxia and training, the following studies give us some insight into the mechanism of the modest benefit.

28.5.1 Ventilation

Over 4 weeks Townsend *et al.* (2002, 2004) exposed two groups of subjects to simulated 2650 m altitude and one to sea level for 20 nights, 4×5 nights with 2 nights off, and low altitude and found that hypoxic ventilatory response was increased in both altitude groups (greater in the 20 consecutive night group) with a corresponding decrease in resting P_{CO_2}.

28.5.2 Cardiac response

Two weeks of nocturnal exposure to 1980 m resulted in an improvement in left ventricular function as measured by echocardiography in 10 well-trained athletes as compared to low altitude controls (Liu *et al.* 1998). Athletes undergoing a live high, train low (LHTL) protocol at 2500–3000 m for 13 days demonstrated greater heart rate variability during hypoxic challenge than low altitude controls (Povea *et al.* 2005). Heart rate variability is a marker of autonomic tone associated with aerobic fitness (Povea *et al.* 2005). These two studies suggest that LHTL training can improve cardiac function, but more work needs to be done in this area.

28.5.3 Hematologic response

Up to about 2500 m polycythaemia increases the $V_{O_2,max}$ and endurance performance (Levine and Stray-Gundersen 1992). For this reason the use of erythropoietin by subcutaneous injection or autologous blood transfusion, both of which create a transient increase in red cell mass, has been banned for athletic events. The effect of autologous erythrocyte infusion on exercise performance at high altitude (4300 m) was studied by Pandolf *et al.* (1998). No significant improvement in a 3.2 km run at sea level was found after infusion and at altitude times were only slightly faster.

Hypoxia stimulates the release of erythropoietin and in turn the bone marrow is stimulated to produce more red cells. The process, however, takes weeks rather than days and the initial rise in hemoglobin and hematocrit on going to altitude is almost entirely due to a reduction in plasma volume (Chapter 8). The increase in hematocrit is advantageous as it increases the oxygen-carrying capacity of the blood. However, the resulting reduction in blood volume may be part of the reason for the reduction in cardiac output found at an early stage of altitude exposure. For the sea level athletes training at altitude, this decrease in plasma volume on ascent is rapidly reversed on descent and any advantage in terms of hematocrit is quickly lost. In a person resident at altitude for many months or years, the red cell mass may be increased by as much as 50% of its normal sea level value. On descent to sea level this increased cell mass is retained for some weeks which could be an advantage in endurance events.

It is still not clear what the optimum altitude is at which athletes should be taken to maximize their performance.

Considering the inverse relationship between P_{O_2} and hemoglobin concentration it might be thought that the higher the athlete can go, the better, but work (Gore et al. 1998) suggests that altitude training at 2650 m does not increase $V_{O_2,max}$ or hemoglobin. Further studies show varying results with respect to the erythropoietic response which is secondary to altitude and time there. Ashenden et al. (1999) utilized a 'nitrogen house' to simulate 3000 m in which they exposed six subjects for 23 nights. Parameters of red cell production did not increase with this protocol. These same authors (1999) also found no change in reticulocytosis in elite female cyclists exposed to 2650 m for 12 consecutive nights. Well-trained runners exposed to five nights of 2650 m showed an increase of erythropoietin but not in reticulocytes (Ashenden et al. 1999b). Two weeks of nocturnal exposure to training triathletes showed a temporary increase in erythropoietin but no other hematologic variables (Dehnert et al. 2002). Eighteen nights at 2500 m, however, resulted in significant increases in erythrocytosis and aerobic performance in elite middle-distance runners. These studies suggest that there is a threshold in time and altitude that will result in a significant improvement in red blood cell volume and aerobic performance.

Also, when sea level dwellers spend long periods over 5000 m physical and mental deterioration occurs, associated with loss of appetite, loss of weight and reduction of muscle mass (Ward 1954). In addition a high hematocrit carries with it the danger of transient or permanent vascular episodes and possible death secondary to excessive viscosity.

28.5.4 Tissue adaptations

Mathieu-Costello (2001) and Hoppeler and Vogt (2001) reviewed the cellular adaptations that occur with prolonged exposure to high altitude and describe studies which show an increase in both capillary and mitochondrial density, both adaptations which improve oxygen flux at the cellular level and presumably improve exercise performance. Subjects trained at 3850 m simulated altitude showed molecular adaptations in muscle biopsies which are markers of improved oxidative metabolism (Vogt et al. 2001). The investigators found increased levels of mRNA concentrations of HIF-1α, myoglobin and vascular endothelial growth factor (VEGF), as well as augmented oxidative enzymes.

Increased mitochondrial and capillary length density were correlated with the hypoxic exposure and intensity of training in previously untrained subjects exposed to a LHTL regimen compared to the control study groups which also resulted in an increase in $V_{O_2,max}$.

28.6 CRITICAL P_{O_2} FOR HEMATOLOGICAL ADAPTATION

In one study of elite cross-country skiers, 3 weeks' training at an altitude of 1900 m was sufficient to raise the hematocrit by 5% (Ingier and Myhre 1992). However, the scarcity of similar studies does not allow any definite conclusion to be made.

It has been suggested that the longer the period at altitude the greater the hemopoietic response. However, during the Silver Hut Expedition 1960–61, when 3 months were spent at 5800 m and above, the hemoglobin concentration leveled off after about 6 weeks.

Obviously hypoxia increases the demand for iron and athletes training at altitude may prove to be iron deficient, particularly female athletes. Again few studies have been made but differences in iron status may explain differences in individual hematological response (Ingier and Myhre 1992).

On descent from altitude hemoglobin levels return to normal quite quickly. In Operation Everest III (COMEX) after 30 days in a chamber ascending to the equivalent height of the summit of Everest, the [Hb] was back to normal values after 4 days at sea level pressure (Richalet *et al.* 1999). Also after a long period at altitude individuals feel physically 'slack' and less energetic for the first few days. Therefore most coaches advise return to low altitude at least 2 to 3 days before an important race.

28.7 DETRAINING AND HYPOXIA

It has recently been seen that in elite endurance athletes, $V_{O_2,max}$ can be reduced at altitudes as low as 610 m (Gore *et al.* 1996). This occurred in about 50% of trained subjects with $V_{O_2,max}$ above $65 \, mL \, min^{-1} kg^{-1}$ (Anselme *et al.* 1992), and they appeared to develop a more severe level of arterial hypoxaemia during maximal and submaximal exercise than more sedentary controls under hypoxic and normoxic conditions (Lawler *et al.* 1988, Koistenen *et al.* 1995). This might have been due to a detraining effect (Saltin 1967). However, it has also been suggested that intermittent exposure to altitudes between 2300–3300 m maximizes the balance between acclimatization and intensity of training (Daniels and Oldridge 1970). It is also possible that the intensity of training at sea level could produce as good a result as intermittent visits to altitude.

28.8 IMMUNE RESPONSE AT ALTITUDE

The effect of training at high altitude and even at sea level upon one's inherent immune responses and host defenses is a hotly debated subject, as is the topic of immunity and altitude per se. However, the possibility that training at altitude may cause some defect in the immune system is possible. A defect in B-cell function has been suggested but not proved (Meehan 1987). On Operation Everest II when individuals ascended to the 'summit' of Everest in a decompression chamber, results suggested that T-cell activation was blunted during exposure to severe hypoxia whereas B-cell function and mucosal immunity were not (Meehan *et al.* 1988).

Athletes frequently complain of recurrent minor infections and mountaineers at high altitude find that cuts and infections seem to improve more rapidly on return to lower altitude. Bailey *et al.* (1998) in two studies with a total of 24 elite endurance athletes training at altitudes between 1500 and 2000 m found a 50% increase in the frequency of upper respiratory and gastrointestinal tract infections during the altitude period. They also recorded a reduction in plasma glutamine concentration at rest. Glutamine is important as a substrate for macrophages and lymphocytes and a reduction in its concentration might indicate impairment of immune defence against opportunistic infections. A decrease in secretory immunoglobulin A (sIgA) was noted in subjects undergoing an 18-day LHTL protocol at approximately 3000 m which did not recover after 2 weeks (Tiollier *et al.* 2005). Certain strategies have been suggested for athletes to maintain immunocompetence (Pyne *et al.* 2000). These measures involve simple monitoring of physiologic, psychological, environmental and performance variables to minimize the possibility of over-training.

28.9 IS ALTITUDE TRAINING WORTH IT?

Is it worthwhile for athletes to train at altitude? At present there is no clear answer to this question. The disadvantages are the risk of acute mountain sickness and high altitude pulmonary and cerebral oedema. The reduction of $V_{O_2,max}$ and the earlier onset of fatigue means that altitude training is less intense than at sea level. However, living high and training low has shown improved performance in a 5 km time trial.

On the strength of this and other trials, it would seem that for distance events it would be better to live at 2500 m and train at less than 1500 m. Bailey and Davis (1997) reviewed the available evidence for the efficacy of altitude training for sea level events and concluded,

> Scientific evidence to support the claim that either continuous or intermittent hypoxic training will enhance sea level performance remains at present equivocal.

But many authorities would contest their skepticism and agree that careful modulation of hypoxic exposure and training is beneficial for aerobic exercise performance.

The optimum time of stay at altitude is still not clear, but to increase red cell mass at least 4 weeks at altitude may be necessary, but the associated reduction in training intensity would not be advantageous. To obtain maximum performance after the athlete descends to lower levels, the timing of the event is also not clear: a minimum of 2–3 days with a maximum of 14–21 days has been suggested (Suslov 1994).

29

Clinical lessons from high altitude

SUMMARY

The study of healthy subjects at altitude has given valuable insights into the effects of hypoxia on human physiology and pathology. In this chapter we consider the similarities and differences between humans at high altitude and patients at sea level with various medical conditions. Altitude-acclimatized humans are a very good model for the hypoxia suffered by patients with lung diffusion limitation due to conditions such as fibrosing alveolitis where there is little or no airway obstruction. Chronic obstructive lung diseases (chronic bronchitis, emphysema and chronic asthma) have many similarities to acclimatized humans but differ in that such patients have normal or raised P_{CO_2} whereas acclimatized humans have a low P_{CO_2}. Healthy subjects at altitude have some similarities to patients with cardiac conditions which limit the heart in its response to exercise. The sensation of fatigue in the working muscles is similar and is experienced by both. It is probably due to insufficient oxygen supply in both cases. Anemia gives rise to the same sensation due to oxygen lack though through different mechanisms. The problems of patients with cyanotic heart disease are also reflected in acclimatized humans.

At a more fundamental level, altitude physiology has influenced clinical medicine through concepts such as the importance of partial pressure of gases, especially of oxygen and carbon dioxide and, by extension, of anesthetic gases, and of acid–base balance and oxygen dissociation curves. Much early work in these areas was stimulated by interest in humans and animals at altitude. In hematology the very early work on polycythemia of altitude provided a stimulus to work on erythropoiesis. In cardiology the raised pulmonary artery pressure found at altitude has stimulated work on the control of pressure in the lesser circulation. Individual or population differences in response to hypoxia are often genetically determined. This fact has stimulated research in both the altitude and genetics communities.

29.1 INTRODUCTION

High altitude medicine and physiology constitute a legitimate subject for study in their own right and if, like any branch of science, such study casts light on other fields, including clinical medicine, that is a bonus.

However, it is often argued that a justification for human studies at high altitude is that the knowledge so gained may be applied in clinical medicine. Patients hypoxic because of pulmonary or cardiovascular disease present a complex picture in which hypoxia is only one of their many problems. In the study of humans at high altitude one can study the effects of hypoxia alone in otherwise healthy subjects. The stimulus, hypoxia, can be applied in a measurable controlled way at a time to suit the scientist, so that controlled measurements can be made before and after hypoxia.

The insight so gained can be applied to the more complicated uncontrolled situation of the hypoxic patient. This chapter discusses how good a model human subjects at high altitude are for the hypoxic patient, and the similarities and the differences between these two situations. It also reviews the extent to which high altitude physiology has illuminated clinical medicine.

29.2 CHRONIC OBSTRUCTIVE LUNG DISEASE

Probably the commonest cause of hypoxia in medicine is chronic obstructive pulmonary disease (COPD). Within this category are included patients with chronic obstructive bronchitis and emphysema. Patients with long-standing severe deformity, such as kyphoscoliosis, also develop hypoxia in the later stages of their disease. Table 29.1 lists the similarities and differences between a patient with COPD and a subject at high altitude.

29.2.1 Symptoms

The similarities include the symptoms of dyspnea, especially on exertion, and the limitation of work capacity. Dyspnea is a difficult sensation to describe and probably the term includes more than one sort of sensation. Patients with asthma, for instance, say that the sensation during an attack is quite different from the breathlessness they feel at the end of a run when free of asthma. The dyspnea of an individual at high altitude is probably more like the latter; the sensation is of needing to hyperventilate and being quite free to do so. Patients with COPD, on the other hand, probably suffer a rather different sensation, akin to that of the asthmatic patient in an attack, which is described as a difficulty in 'getting the breath' or of suffocation.

The reduction in work or exercise capacity is very similar in both patients and high altitude subjects. In both, the dyspnea is felt to play a part but

Table 29.1   Comparison of clinical aspects of chronic obstructive pulmonary disease with findings in people at high altitude

Symptom/finding	At high altitude	Chronic obstructive pulmonary disease
Dyspnea on exertion	Yes	Yes
Limited work capacity	Yes	Yes
Peripheral edema	Seen in AMS	Frequent
Polycythemia	Yes	Yes
Red cell mass	Increased	Increased
Arterial P_{O_2}	Reduced	Reduced
Arterial P_{CO_2}	Reduced	Normal or raised
Arterial pH	Raised	Normal or reduced
Bicarbonate level in blood, CSF	Reduced	Raised
Work of breathing L^{-1}	Reduced	Increased
Work of breathing, total	Increased	Increased
CO_2 ventilatory response	Shift to left and steepened	Shift to right and flattened
Cerebral blood flow	Increased/normal	Increased
Pulmonary arterial pressure	Raised	Raised
Weight loss	Yes (variable)	Yes (in some cases)

CSF, cerebrospinal fluid; AMS, acute mountain sickness.

both also complain that work is limited by a sensation of the legs 'giving out' or 'feeling like lead'. This is for large muscle mass dynamic work such as walking, cycling, and climbing stairs. If the strength of a small muscle mass is tested (e.g. hand grip), it is found to be largely unimpaired in both cases. The possibility that the central nervous system may play a role in limiting exhaustive exercise fatigue at altitude has been proposed (Kayser *et al.* 1993b). Could this also apply to patients with COPD?

In the patient with COPD the work of breathing (per liter) is increased because of airway obstruction. The total ventilation may be increased as well, even if there is alveolar hypoventilation, because of the increased dead space; thus the total work of breathing is further increased. At high altitude, the work of breathing per liter is modestly decreased because of the reduction in air density at reduced barometric pressure; however, the total work of breathing is increased due to the marked hyperventilation especially on exercise (Chapter 11).

29.2.2 Blood gases and acid–base balance

Subjects at high altitude and patients with COPD both have reduced PO_2. At high altitude this is due to low inspired PO_2 whereas in COPD patients it is caused by gas transfer problems due to ventilation/perfusion ratio inequalities (Chapter 6.8). In both cases, the hypoxemia is made worse by exertion.

The PCO_2 level, however, is different. In patients with COPD the Pa,CO_2 is either normal or, in more severe cases, raised. The pH is consequently lowered; respiratory acidosis and secondary renal compensation result in elevated blood bicarbonate concentration. The cerebrospinal fluid (CSF) bicarbonate concentration is also elevated and there follows a shift to the right of the ventilatory carbon dioxide response line and the response becomes flattened (i.e. blunted). In contrast, at high altitude the Pa,CO_2 is reduced, pH elevated, blood and CSF bicarbonate concentration reduced, and the carbon dioxide response shifts to the left and becomes more brisk (Chapter 5). These differences in acid–base will affect the oxygen dissociation curve as discussed in Chapter 9. The left shift in climbers at extreme altitude is probably beneficial. In COPD patients the respiratory acidosis due to high PCO_2 is normally compensated by increased bicarbonate but in acute exacerbations may not be and the rightward shift of the dissociation curve will add to the hypoxemia suffered by these patients.

29.2.3 Hematological changes

At high altitude and in COPD patients there is an increase in red cell mass. This invariably results in polycythemia at high altitude where it is accompanied at first by a reduced plasma volume (Chapter 8). In COPD the plasma volume is usually increased, for reasons which are unclear, so that polycythemia is often not seen until red cell mass is considerably increased by a more extreme hypoxia. In both cases the increase is due to more erythropoiesis, stimulated by increased levels of erythropoietin. After the first few days at a given high altitude, levels of erythropoietin fall to within the normal or control range (Chapter 8) and similarly, in over half the patients with polycythemia due to hypoxic lung disease, erythropoietin levels are within the normal range (Wedzicha *et al.* 1985).

Plasma volume, as already mentioned, is increased in COPD. Plasma volume is decreased on first going to altitude but returns towards normal after about 3 months (Chapter 8). In high altitude residents plasma volume is decreased by about 27% compared with sea level residents (Sanchez *et al.* 1970).

29.2.4 Fluid balance and peripheral edema

Patients with COPD are at risk of developing peripheral edema, mainly dependent, and raised venous pressure. They have been shown to have a defect of sodium and water handling; they fail to excrete a water load at the normal rate if they have a high PCO_2 (Farber *et al.* 1975, Stewart *et al.* 1991a). COPD patients have a reduced effective renal plasma flow and urinary sodium excretion. They may have raised plasma renin activity and aldosterone levels. The development of peripheral edema may take place without increase in body weight (Campbell *et al.* 1975), suggesting a transfer of fluid from intracellular to extracellular compartments. This is in contrast to edema formation in cardiac failure when, as expected, it is associated with weight gain. How these findings can be fitted into a coherent account of the mechanism of this condition is still not clear.

The fluid balance in people at high altitude is also far from clear. It seems likely that the development of acute mountain sickness (AMS) is associated with fluid retention, whereas the healthy response on going to high altitude is a diuresis. Peripheral edema frequently occurs in AMS, often affecting the periorbital regions and hands as well as the ankles. The headache is probably caused by cerebral edema. Pulmonary edema and cerebral edema are the serious forms of AMS and clearly there is pathological edema in these conditions (Chapters 18–20). In the acclimatized subject there is no evidence of any problem in fluid handling.

Whether there are analogies between the mechanisms of AMS and cor pulmonale are questions for future research in both fields. For instance, it is the COPD patients with high Pa,CO_2 who are likely to develop cor pulmonale, and in subjects at altitude higher Pa,CO_2 may be associated with AMS although this is thought not to be an important factor.

29.2.5 The circulation

The systemic circulation is not importantly affected by either COPD or altitude. There is often mild elevation of the blood pressure in both cases, but there are important changes in the pulmonary circulation in both patients with COPD and those at high altitude. There is increased pulmonary resistance, resulting in raised pulmonary artery and right ventricular pressures in both COPD and the healthy subject at altitude and similar electrocardiographic (ECG) changes (i.e. right axis deviation) (Chapter 7).

29.2.6 Cerebral blood flow (CBF)

In patients with COPD the CBF is increased due to the cerebral vasodilatory effects of both hypoxia and hypercarbia. On going to altitude the CBF is normally modestly increased at first, then tends to fall towards sea level values (Severinghaus *et al.* 1966b). This is due to the low Pa,CO_2, which tends to reduce CBF opposing the effect of hypoxia. Polycythemia, as it develops in both COPD patients and those at high altitude, will tend to reduce CBF. Very low CBF values have been inferred from the large arteriovenous

cerebral oxygen difference in Andean altitude residents with marked polycythemia (Milledge and Sorensen 1972), whereas patients with COPD are to a degree protected from cerebral hypoxia by their hypercapnia, which causes increased CBF.

29.2.7 Alimentary system

There has been little work on the effect of hypoxia on bowel function in either patients or individuals at high altitude. Milledge (1972) showed that small bowel absorption, as measured by the xylose absorption test, was reduced in patients with either hypoxic lung disease or cyanotic heart disease, when the saturation fell below about 70%. It was suggested that this finding might explain the loss of weight which often characterizes patients with severe emphysema towards the end of the course of their disease.

Subjects at high altitude tend to lose weight and, although much of this weight reduction is due to reduced energy intake, there has been uncontrolled evidence that at altitudes above about 5500 m there is continued weight loss even with adequate energy intake (Pugh 1962a). During the American Medical Research Expedition to Everest (AMREE) in 1981, there was a significant reduction in both fat and xylose absorption in subjects at 6300 m (Blume 1984). Dinmore *et al.* (1994) found that absorption of both D-xylose and 3-O-methyl-D-glucose was reduced in subjects at 6300 m, and Travis *et al.* (1993) also found a reduction in the ratio of these carbohydrates at 5400 m, indicating impairment of absorption (Chapter 14). Westerterp *et al.* (1994) on Mount Sajama (6542 m) found that gross energy digestibility decreased to 85%, indicating some malabsorption, though most of the weight loss was attributable to low food intake. On the other hand in Operation Everest III, Westerterp *et al.* (2000) found a normal energy digestibility of 94% at 7000 m simulated altitude. Contributing to this weight loss is the increased metabolic rate at altitude. It seems that in COPD there is also an increased metabolic rate which is not compensated for by increased dietary intake. The cause of this elevated metabolism is a matter of much debate and several factors have been implicated (Decramer *et al.* 2005).

It now seems likely that malabsorption, due to hypoxia, if it exists, is only a minor factor in the weight loss seen at altitude which is predominantly due to a negative energy balance. Similarly there is loss of appetite in COPD and there has been some work looking for the cause amongst the various humeral factors thought to influence appetite, e.g. ghrelin (Luo *et al.* 2005), tumor necrosis factor-α (Pitsiou *et al.* 2002) or increased muscle apoptosis (Agusti *et al.* 2002).

29.2.8 Mental effects

Patients with hypoxia due to COPD frequently have disturbance of mental function, especially during exacerbations, when their P_{O_2} falls to very low levels. In the milder stages these disturbances may be quite subtle but, as hypoxia becomes severe, patients become irritable, restless and confused. Motor function may become impaired with ataxia. These changes are very similar to those observed in healthy subjects exposed to acute hypoxia in decompression chambers. However, in acclimatized subjects, very low saturations may be seen, especially on exercise, with very little mental disturbance, though at extreme altitude and with AMS these mental problems may be seen (Chapter 16).

29.2.9 Molecular and genetic mechanisms

Amongst the molecular and genetic mechanisms underlying the adaptation to the chronic hypoxia in both COPD patients and healthy subjects at altitude is the rise in levels of hypoxia inducible factor 1 (HIF-1). This in turn induces a whole range of genes including erythropoietin and genes involved in metabolism. Raguso *et al.* (2004) review the common mechanisms between COPD and altitude with respect to the effect on nutrition and metabolism. HIF-1 induces gene expression of fructose-2-6-biphosphatase, for instance, an enzyme switching glucose metabolism towards glycolysis, allowing energy production in anaerobic conditions. They point out the possible importance of HIF-1 polymorphism and interaction with other molecules, especially estrogens in the clinical evolution of the disease. These considerations may also underlie the differing individual susceptibility to the effects of altitude hypoxia in healthy subjects.

29.2.10 Summary

Table 29.1 summarizes the similarities and differences between patients with COPD and those at high altitude. Healthy people at altitude differ in a number of important respects from patients with hypoxia due to COPD. Most of these differences are attributable to the one being hypocapnic and the other hypercapnic. However, the hypoxia is similar and results in similar effects on a number of bodily systems, including erythropoiesis, muscles, the alimentary system, metabolism (weight loss) and mental function. Providing the carbon dioxide effect is borne in mind, persons at high altitude can be considered as a model for the hypoxia of COPD.

29.3 INTERSTITIAL LUNG DISEASE

Within this category are included such conditions as sarcoidosis, fibrosing alveolitis, allergic alveolitis (farmer's lung, etc.), pneumoconiosis (including silicosis) and other causes of diffuse pulmonary fibrosis. Some types of pneumonia, for instance that due to *Pneumocystis pneumoniae*, which are diffuse rather than lobar, present similar pathophysiology. In all these conditions the main problem is an impairment of gas exchange. There usually develops some restriction of lung volumes as well but, unlike COPD, there is little or no airways obstruction. The result is that hypoxia develops without any rise in $Pa,_{CO_2}$. Indeed, the $Pa,_{CO_2}$ is characteristically decreased as it is in subjects at high altitude.

The dominant symptom in these patients is breathlessness on exertion and, later, even at rest. The arterial desaturation becomes worse on exertion just as it does in those at extreme altitudes (Chapter 12). The cause of the hypoxemia in these patients is a defect of gas transfer. This is due to ventilation/perfusion ratio inhomogeneity and an increase in the diffusion path length, that is, a thickening of the alveolar capillary membrane by cellular infiltrate or fibrosis. In most cases the ventilation/perfusion mismatch problem is the more important. These conditions usually develop over a period of months and a subject well acclimatized to high altitude is a very good model for the hypoxia of a patient with interstitial lung disease.

29.4 CYANOTIC HEART DISEASE

Most patients in this group have congenital cardiac defects which result in right to left shunts and therefore in cyanosis. Diagnoses include tetralogy of Fallot, ventricular and atrial septal defects with reversed shunts, patent ductus arteriosus with reversed shunt, and most forms of anomalous venous drainage.

These patients, often hypoxic from birth, sometimes have most extreme cyanosis with severe polycythemia. Pa,CO_2 is usually in the normal range but may be low as is found at high altitude. Those with extreme polycythemia, in whom the hematocrit can be up to 70%, resemble cases of chronic mountain sickness and may suffer the same symptoms of lethargy, poor concentration, being easily fatigued, etc. (Chapter 21). Though these patients do get out of breath on exertion, dyspnea is not a prominent symptom, perhaps because the condition has been present since birth. Again, like chronic mountain sickness and the 'blue bloater' type of COPD patient, it may be due to a blunted respiratory drive. The histopathology of the pulmonary circulation of children with cyanotic heart disease is comparable to that of high altitude residents (Heath and Williams 1995, pp. 121–39). The normal demuscularization of pulmonary arteries after birth is retarded so that the wall thickness, especially of the resistance arterioles, is increased compared with the normal pulmonary arterial tree (Chapter 17).

Children with cyanotic heart disease have retarded growth, as do children at altitude (Chapter 17). If their defect can be corrected by surgery, growth accelerates and they catch up with their peers. If their arterial saturation is below about 70% they will have impaired small bowel absorption which may contribute to their growth retardation. Surgical repair of the defect relieves the cyanosis and the small bowel absorption improves (Milledge 1972). In this respect they resemble those at high altitude (Chapter 14).

29.5 LOW OUTPUT CARDIAC CONDITIONS

Ischemic heart disease and cardiomyopathy can result in low cardiac output. In milder forms of this condition the output at rest is normal but there is failure of the normal response to exercise of an increase in cardiac output. Patients are symptom free at rest but find that their exercise tolerance is markedly diminished; they can only walk slowly and the slightest uphill slope causes them to stop and rest. They are not limited by dyspnea but by fatigue in the leg muscles. In these patients the Pa,O_2 is normal, but blood flow is limited, which reduces oxygen delivery and results in tissue hypoxia. The tissues most affected are those which have a high extraction of oxygen and which increase their oxygen demand on exercise, that is, the working muscles. The mixed venous Pa,O_2 is very low but Pa,CO_2 is normal.

The subject at high altitude is obviously not such a good model for this type of patient, but, especially at extreme altitude, there are physiological similarities. The maximum cardiac rate and output are limited to some degree (Chapter 12), so that, during large muscle mass dynamic exercise, oxygen delivery to the working muscles is limited. There is certainly tissue hypoxia, especially of these muscles, due to a reduction in delivery of oxygen and possibly also to limitation of oxygen diffusion at the tissue level (Chapter 12). As mentioned in section 29.2.1, the sensation of work being limited by 'the legs giving out' rather than dyspnea alone is common both to individuals at high altitude and to these patients.

29.6 CHRONIC ANEMIA

Patients with chronic anemia have a very similar pathophysiology to patients with low cardiac output. The oxygen delivery to the tissues is reduced in their case by the reduced oxygen capacity of the blood. Cardiac output increases, partly due to a decreased viscosity of the blood, and this partially compensates for the loss of oxygen-carrying capacity. Nevertheless, oxygen delivery is reduced, especially to the working muscles, during exercise. The resulting symptoms are similar to those of low cardiac output and have their analogy in those at extreme altitude.

29.7 HEMOGLOBINOPATHIES WITH ALTERED OXYGEN AFFINITY

The hemoglobinopathies are a rare, but interesting, group of conditions in which patients have a genetic defect resulting in minor changes to their hemoglobin. These changes result in their hemoglobin having either a greater or a reduced affinity for oxygen compared with normal hemoglobin. The oxygen dissociation curve is shifted either to the left (increased affinity) or to the right (decreased affinity).

Patients with increased affinity hemoglobin experience a degree of tissue hypoxia because oxygen is not readily unloaded in the tissues. This evidently stimulates erythropoietin production since these patients are typically polycythemic.

Conversely, patients with decreased affinity hemoglobin are anemic, presumably because their tissue PO_2 is higher than normal, as evidenced by the ease with which oxygen is unloaded there. At moderate altitude this may confer some advantage, though this has not been demonstrated, and on exercise the difficulty of oxygen loading in the lungs would probably outweigh any advantage in the tissues. At higher altitude the difficulty in loading oxygen into the blood in the lungs would certainly be a disadvantage.

Indeed, increased oxygen affinity is probably beneficial, since, at high altitude, the advantage in the lungs more than outweighs the disadvantage in the tissues. A study by Hebbel et al. (1978) of two subjects with Hb Andrews-Minneapolis, a high affinity hemoglobin ($P_{50} = 17$ mmHg), found that they had less reduction in exercise capacity on going to altitude than their siblings with normal hemoglobin.

Normal subjects at high altitude, especially at extreme altitudes above 8000 m, have their oxygen dissociation curves shifted to the left by respiratory alkalosis; this is probably advantageous for the above reason (Chapters 9 and 11). Thus, those at high altitude can be a model for some aspects of hemoglobinopathies.

29.8 CONTRIBUTION OF HIGH ALTITUDE PHYSIOLOGY TO CLINICAL MEDICINE

29.8.1 Partial pressure of gases

The importance to clinical medicine of Paul Bert's work published in his landmark La Pression Barométrique (1878) is enormous. This work clearly showed that it is the partial pressure of oxygen, rather than the barometric pressure or oxygen percentage,

that determines the effect of hypoxia in causing mountain sickness and death. Although he did not work at altitude himself he corresponded with and encouraged people who did, and used chambers to reduce the ambient pressure for both human and animal subjects. He can truly be claimed as a father figure for both altitude physiology and aviation medicine. Of course, other physiologists and clinicians after Paul Bert developed the idea of the partial pressure of gases and its importance, including such workers as Haldane, Douglas, FitzGerald, Henderson, Schneider, Bohr, Krogh and Barcroft, all of whose work was stimulated by the problems of altitude physiology.

The concept of the effect of gases on the body being due to their partial pressures (especially of oxygen and carbon dioxide) is fundamental to respiratory medicine and physiology, and to aviation and underwater medicine. In anesthesia the partial pressure of gases extends to all volatile agents.

29.8.2 Hematology

The polycythemia of high altitude was first documented by Viault (1890) and has been extensively studied ever since. As a tool in hematological research, this stimulus to erythropoiesis has been invaluable. Much of the early work on the oxygen dissociation curve, by Haldane, Barcroft and others, owes its stimulus to the question of human survival and acclimatization to high altitude. These 'lessons from high altitude' are amongst the foundation stones of modern hematology, open heart surgery, respiratory medicine, cardiology and anesthetics. More recently, research on 2,3-diphosphoglycerate and its influence on the position of the oxygen dissociation curve has been studied at altitude (Chapter 9) and the results incorporated into the body of hematological knowledge. More recently interest in the mechanism of gene induction by hypoxia of genes such as erythropoietin has resulted in a great volume of research in an ever-increasing number of genes induced by hypoxia. The mechanism is via by the hypoxia inducing factor-α, HIF-1α (Semenza et al. (1998). The other hypoxia-induced genes all have similar core binding sites for HIF-1α which induces the gene by binding to it. Again this has been a two-way stimulus between altitude research and the molecular laboratory.

29.8.3 Respiratory medicine

Work on the effect of altitude acclimatization on the control of breathing (Chapter 5) has helped in the understanding of the changes in control of breathing in patients with COPD with hypercapnia. These patients 'acclimatize' to a high Pa,CO_2 and their carbon dioxide ventilatory response becomes blunted, the opposite of altitude acclimatization. They are then dependent on hypoxia as a drive to ventilation and may have their breathing depressed if given high inspired oxygen mixtures to breathe.

In patients with asthma, as the condition worsens, their Pa,O_2 falls. At first the Pa,CO_2 is reduced because of the hypoxic drive to ventilation; then, with increasing airways resistance, Pa,CO_2 rises to 'normal' and finally rises above normal. Cochrane et al. (1980) have pointed out that the Pa,CO_2 in the middle of these three stages should be below 'normal', depending on the degree of hypoxia. Drawing on altitude data, Wolff (1980) gives a predicted value for Pa,CO_2, dependent on Pa,O_2. The patient should be considered to be in respiratory failure if the Pa,CO_2 is above this value. For instance, a patient with a Pa,O_2 of 60 mmHg has a predicted Pa,CO_2 of 30 mmHg, assuming full acclimatization to this degree of hypoxia.

Study of the increasing arterial desaturation due to diffusion limitations found in climbers on exercise at altitude (Chapter 6) helps in the understanding of the similar problems in patients at sea level with interstitial lung disease and limited diffusing capacity.

29.8.4 Cardiology

The phenomenon of the hypoxic pulmonary pressor response has been studied at sea level and altitude in humans and animals, with results from altitude stimulating work at sea level and vice versa. The insights gained have helped in the understanding of patients with pulmonary hypertension due to hypoxia secondary to heart or lung disease or with primary pulmonary hypertension. The mechanisms involved in pulmonary artery vasoconstriction and remodeling seen in high altitude pulmonary hypertension are likely to be similar, at the cellular level, to those involved in primary pulmonary hypertension.

29.8.5 Genetics

Interest in various aspects of altitude research has stimulated the study of genetics. In the area of human performance at high altitude the work of Montgomery and colleagues (1998) on the ACE gene polymorphism is an example. They showed that subjects who had climbed to over 7000 m without supplemental oxygen had a disproportionate preponderance of the insertion allele. In the same paper, they showed that soldiers with the II genotype had significantly greater improvement in performance after a period of standard physical training than either ID or DD genotypes. This paper stimulated much further work on this 'performance gene'.

The differences in [Hb] between Andean and Tibetan populations has been studied by a number of groups (see section 8.5.2) and particularly in Tibetans there is an important genetic component (Beall et al. 1998). Also the differences in [Hb] between Han Chinese and Tibetans (Wu et al. 2005) must be at least partially genetically determined.

In section 5.5.1 mention was made of the work by Malik et al. (2005) in identifying a possible gene (fos-B) necessary for the increase of the hypoxic ventilatory response (HVR) which is an important part of altitude acclimatization. This family of genes is involved, in the brain, with plasticity of cerebral function, a topic of great current interest in neurophysiology.

29.8.6 Other areas of clinical medicine

High altitude physiology and medicine have lessons for other branches of clinical medicine, for example:

- Small bowel function, which is possibly impaired at altitude as well as in hypoxic patients (Chapter 14)
- Metabolism, in the slower growth of children at altitude, and patients hypoxic due to congenital heart disease

- Reproductive medicine, in the problem of fertility at altitude
- Endocrinology, in the effect of hypoxia on various endocrine systems (Chapter 15), and their counterparts in patients with similar conditions

However, these fields have been less thoroughly explored both by high altitude and by clinical scientists. No doubt high altitude has yet more lessons to teach clinical medicine in the future.

30

Practicalities of field studies

SUMMARY

The practical difficulties of carrying out good research at altitude in the mountains are obvious and are considered in this chapter. However, there are many compensations. The difficulties can be met by careful planning and by choosing projects and techniques that are appropriate for field work.

The advantages and disadvantages of field versus chamber studies, including cost, are discussed. There is a place for both types of study and they are complementary. Most of the techniques of classical cardiorespiratory and exercise physiology have been used at altitude. Blood, urine and saliva samples can be taken, stored and brought back for biochemical and hormonal analysis. Arterial blood samples have been taken at over 8000 m. With the advance of electronics quite sophisticated techniques in sleep studies, audiometry, visual fields, psychometric testing and even Doppler echocardiography and near-infrared spectroscopy have been used in the field. Laptop computers have been used at great altitudes and can be used on-line with the more sophisticated equipment.

In planning either a pure scientific expedition or one in which science is combined with mountaineering, it is important to ensure the support of all members for the scientific program. This is best done by communicating the objectives of the program to everyone in simple terms and giving all members (professional and lay) an active role in the science.

30.1 INTRODUCTION

The problems associated with field research in the great ranges are obvious and include cold, hypoxia, fatigue and lack of amenities of civilization such as piped hot and cold water, reliable electricity supplies, heating, etc. The lack of easy access to specialist advice from service engineers or colleagues can be a severe problem. However, there are compensations. Perhaps the greatest is the elimination of distractions from the work in hand. There is no commuting to work, no committees, no lectures to give or attend, no family commitments and little in the way of social events. Also the camaraderie of the expedition team can be both wonderfully enjoyable and productive. Of course the stresses and strains of living in close proximity with colleagues under sometimes tough conditions can have just the opposite effect. The authors have been fortunate in this respect and this is the more usual experience of medical scientific expeditions. If the site has been well chosen there is the added advantage of living for a while among the grandest and most beautiful scenery on Earth.

30.1.1 Planning, testing and practice

Many of the data referred to in this book have been collected on expeditions to the major mountain regions of the world. Good scientific work under these conditions can be difficult but is perfectly possible, providing adequate time, thought and effort are given to planning and preparation. The preparation time will be at least 3–6 months for a small expedition and 2 years or more for a major scientific expedition.

Increasingly, scientists from Europe and North America are working in collaboration with colleagues in countries with high altitude facilities and populations. This is especially true for the Andean countries, Peru, Bolivia and Chile. For instance the group of J.-P. Richalet from France has worked for many years with the Instituto Boliviano de Biologia de Altura in La Paz, or Schoene's team from USA with the Renal team from Cayetano University, Lima working at Cerro de Pasco, Peru. Similarly teams under the late Jack Reeves and others from Denver have conducted profitable collaborative studies in Tibet with local medical colleagues. There are many other examples and without the active help of local professionals, providing facilities, recruiting subjects, and in many other ways, these studies would not have been possible. As more scientists from these mountainous regions become interested in the problems of high altitude such opportunities for collaboration should increase. In such ventures it is vital that planning be meticulous and that everyone's contribution be adequately acknowledged.

The techniques and apparatus to be used must be tested adequately beforehand. Many studies require control measurements at sea level and these are best carried out using the same equipment as will be used in the field. Not only are results more reliable if the same equipment is used, but problems and deficiencies are identified before leaving for the mountains. Practice with the equipment in the comfort of a standard laboratory is also highly desirable, though not absolutely essential. One of

the authors of this book taught one of the others the technique of gas analysis using the Lloyd–Haldane apparatus during the course of their first Himalayan expedition at 5800 m. Even if study protocols do not demand control measurements before leaving, it is advisable to carry out a complete dummy run of the observations to be made, listing all the equipment needed, down to the last rubber band and needle.

30.1.2 Field versus chamber studies

Although this chapter is concerned with field studies at altitude, much valuable work has been done in decompression chambers. The advantages of chamber studies over field studies are:

- Rate of ascent and descent, and altitude can be controlled to suit the problem under study.
- Other factors such as temperature and humidity can be controlled.
- More invasive procedures can be justified since, in the event of some complication, help is readily available.

The disadvantages are perhaps not so obvious, especially to people who have not been involved with such work. Living for more than a few hours in a decompression chamber is not pleasant. The environment is usually noisy, confined and often smelly – though this is less true of large modern facilities such as the chamber at Natick, MA, operated by the US Army Institute of Environmental Medicine. However, even the largest chamber is cramped compared with being in the mountains and it is difficult and very boring to take much exercise. Acclimatization seems to be slower and less complete in chamber studies than on the mountain. Values for P_{CO_2} are consistently higher for the same altitude in chambers than on the mountain. This may be due to less exercise taken by subjects in chambers or due to other factors or stresses (Rahn and Otis 1949, Houston 1988–9, West 1988b). In studies lasting more than a few hours, boredom, and hence morale, is a problem. A limiting factor for chamber studies is the number of subjects that can be accommodated. This might be less of a drawback for most physiological studies but it would be important in studies of acute mountain sickness

(AMS) where a large number of subjects are needed to ensure that some have symptoms and others are unaffected. Finally, chambers are built with specific tasks in mind; usually their use is geared to short-term experiments on acute hypoxia and so they may not be available to altitude scientists for prolonged experiments.

In comparing the results of studies carried out in the field with those done in low pressure chambers, it is useful to look at the results obtained from the Silver Hut Expedition and the American Medical Research Expedition to Everest (AMREE), and compare these with the two major simulation studies to date, Operation Everest I and II. In many areas, the results of the two types of studies have been very similar. For example, the measurements of maximal oxygen consumption for the inspired P_{O_2} on the summit of Mount Everest were almost identical in AMREE and Operation Everest II. However, the two types of studies have yielded quantitatively different information in some areas, presumably because of the different periods of acclimatization. The main differences are seen in three areas.

ALVEOLAR GAS COMPOSITION

The shorter period of acclimatization in the two low pressure chamber studies to date resulted in very different alveolar P_{O_2} and P_{CO_2} values at extreme altitudes compared with the results from the field studies (see Fig. 12.4). The differences are particularly marked for Operation Everest I and are discussed in section 12.3.3.

BLOOD LACTATE CONCENTRATION

Blood lactate concentrations after maximal exercise were appreciably higher on Operation Everest II than on the AMREE and extensive field measurements made by Cerretelli (1980). These are shown in Fig. 12.5 and discussed in section 12.3.4. Again the differences are presumably due to the shorter period of acclimatization on Operation Everest II. This topic is discussed fully by West (1993b).

EXERCISE VENTILATION AT EXTREME ALTITUDE

As was pointed out in section 11.3, both the Silver Hut Expedition and AMREE found a decrease in ventilation at maximal exercise at extreme altitude (see Fig. 11.3). By contrast, maximal exercise ventilation on Operation Everest II continued to increase with greater altitude. The reason for the differences is not clear; it is presumably related to the different degrees of acclimatization.

30.1.3 Cost

It is often assumed that chamber studies must be cheaper than field studies. This is not necessarily the case, long-term studies can be very expensive. Accounting in both cases is a very inexact science. The cost of a mountaineering expedition is clear, but in many cases the climbers are going to the mountains anyway and the scientific work can be carried out at very little extra cost. Chambers represent a huge capital cost but usually the altitude scientist is not called upon to contribute to this. However, even the running costs of a chamber are not inconsiderable. Apart from the subjects and scientists, chambers have to manned 24 h a day by teams of highly trained technicians whose salaries have to be met. If all expenses are charged realistically to the study, long-term chamber projects are very expensive.

In summary, chambers are very useful in studies of acute and subacute hypoxia lasting a few hours. Their advantage over field studies becomes less as the duration of the study and the number of subjects increase. Thus the two modes of research are complementary.

30.1.4 Personnel management

The psychodynamics of a mountaineering expedition are fascinating and of vital importance in achieving both climbing and scientific goals, but too great an emphasis on psychological factors may well be self-defeating. The essential aspect of leadership of a scientific expedition is to ensure that the whole team is as fully aware of the scientific program as possible and in sympathy with it. Climbers may be suspicious of scientists but can understand quite abstruse scientific argument providing terms and concepts are explained in everyday language. They are naturally interested in topics such as AMS, work performance at altitude and the effect of altitude on various biological systems and can become enthusiastic participants, providing the issues are clearly explained.

Time spent in presenting the scientific program to the whole team is well spent, as was evident from experience on the AMREE, where climbers as well as climbing scientists were enthusiastic about working on the scientific program as well as climbing the mountain. In a large party with a number of scientists it is equally important that the various scientific members understand the relevance of each other's projects and are in sympathy with them.

After presenting the program, the next essential is to delegate responsibility as widely as possible. It is highly desirable that every member of the expedition has a job to do in relation to the scientific program, for two reasons.

WORK LOAD

The programs are usually over-ambitious in terms of what can be achieved in the time available and, by sharing the work out, the load on the main scientists is reduced.

COMMITMENT TO THE SCIENTIFIC PROGRAM

By having a designated job, each member feels he or she is personally committed to the scientific program, with consequent improvement in morale. This is particularly important if nonscientific members are expected to act as subjects. Having a job to do as well as being a subject avoids the feeling, 'they only want me as a guinea-pig'. There are many jobs which can be carried out perfectly well by expedition members who are not scientifically trained, such as measurement of urine volume or body weights, or clerking results as another member reads them off. Even the spinning and pipetting of blood samples can be quickly taught. A further important aspect of delegating work as widely as possible is that it helps to keep the work going should any of the scientific members be unable to function owing to illness or accident.

30.2 LABORATORY WORK IN THE FIELD

30.2.1 Laboratory accommodation

However small the expedition, some form of designated laboratory accommodation is recommended.

For small expeditions this will be a tent; if at all possible it should be of the type high enough to stand up in, and have a folding table and chairs. Cold is a major problem in the mountains. Most types of scientific work cannot be carried out in temperatures below 5–10°C, and certainly not below freezing. Battery operated instruments work poorly below freezing, plastic bags crack easily and venipuncture is difficult because of vasoconstriction. Under severe freezing conditions blood samples will freeze and hemolyse. If there is no space heating available, the time for scientific work will be limited to the warmest hours of the day. However, it must also be said that at high altitude the sun is strong and when it is shining on a tent the temperature rises rapidly inside, even though the outside shade temperature remains well below zero. On the Medical Research Expeditions to Chamlang Base Camp no less than nine frame tents were set up at Base Camp (5000 m) in which up to 12 teams worked successfully. There was also a large dome tent which was used for a mess tent, communications, battery and power control facility.

On a large expedition, good laboratory conditions can be achieved by using a modern 'tent', such as a Weatherport (Hansen Weatherport, Gunniston, CO). This is a tubular aluminum frame with padded plastic cover made in various sizes which proved very satisfactory in the Western Cwm in 1981 (West 1985a). On snow, a good floor is a great asset, we used plywood in the Western Cwm. Heating was provided by a propane stove of the type designed for mobile homes in which a heat exchanger heats the air, which is blown into the tent. In this way there is no possibility of carbon monoxide from the burning propane entering the tent. Carbon monoxide poisoning is a real danger from less sophisticated forms of heating.

The Silver Hut similarly provided almost ideal conditions in 1960–61, though at far greater expense. It was a prefabricated hut made from boxed-up marine plywood members with foam insulation within the box sections. A similar hut but using fiberglass sections was used at Base Camp on the AMREE and was also successful. Work surfaces, seating and lighting should also be provided. In such conditions, the working day can be prolonged into the night if necessary, allowing more work to be carried out than in an unheated laboratory, as well as avoiding the problem of cold as an interfering factor if one is studying the effects of chronic hypoxia.

30.2.2 Electricity supply

Early in the planning of an expedition the decision will have to be made about whether to use mains voltage apparatus or to restrict work to battery operated and non-electrical equipment.

The advantages of mains voltage equipment are obvious, and certain types of equipment are only available as mains operated versions. It is possible to get petrol-powered generators that weigh no more than one porter load, and on a large expedition this a possible chosen option. The disadvantages are not inconsiderable. In order to try to ensure that one generator is working, at least two must be taken; even then it is quite likely that both will break down. Extra spare parts must be taken and at least one expedition member should be a mechanic with knowledge of that particular generator. Altitude affects petrol engines as it does the animal organism and adjustments must be made to the fuel mix, usually by changing the jets in the carburetor. Some generators are available with variable jets, in which case the settings required for various altitudes should be ascertained before the expedition. The power output declines with altitude, as it does in humans, so a more powerful generator must be taken than would be needed for the same equipment at sea level. Petrol and oil must also be carried.

Alternative sources of electrical power have been used. In the Silver Hut Expedition much of the electricity used over the winter was derived from a wind generator and on the AMREE a battery of solar cells gave almost 30 A at 15 V. In both cases this power was fed into 12 V storage batteries and mains voltage was obtained by using converters. These introduced their own degree of inefficiency, as well as further expense and transport penalties. In 1998 on Kangchenjunga we were able to supply almost all our not inconsiderable power needs from solar cells because we were fortunate with the weather. However, this required discipline in the use of power especially in the morning to allow the batteries to charge up in the sun after they had been used at night often for communication by satellite phone. These alternative sources cannot be relied upon and petrol generators are advisable for back-up.

Over the years, electronic equipment has become more efficient in that less power is required. Solar cells have become more efficient, cheaper and lighter. They have also become more robust and can now be flexible so a large panel can be rolled up for transportation. Thus more equipment can be battery operated with cells that can be re-charged from solar panels and the possibility of dispensing with petrol generators is becoming more feasible.

30.3 RESPIRATORY MEASUREMENTS

30.3.1 Classical methods

Classical measurements of ventilation and oxygen consumption using Douglas bags, taps and valves are as easy to carry out in the field as in the laboratory (providing all the bits are remembered, including the nose clip). The gas meter will be of the dry type or a Wright's respirometer (anemometer) can be used if care is taken not to empty the Douglas bag too fast through it (accuracy $\pm 2\%$). The gas analysis is more of a problem for the physiologist used to using a mass spectrometer. If mains voltage is available (section 30.2.2) an infrared carbon dioxide meter and paramagnetic oxygen meter can be used, though calibrating gases will have to be carried. Paramagnetic oxygen analyzers are available as battery operated instruments but carbon dioxide meters are not. Alternatively, one can be really classical and use the Lloyd–Haldane or Scholander apparatus and analyze samples chemically though it takes time to become proficient in their use and the analyses are very time consuming.

Care should be taken with modern Douglas bags. The plastic that is used now for these bags is much less likely to become hard and brittle in the cold than was previously the case but care may be needed if overnight temperatures have been very low. A repair kit should be taken which should include duct (gaffer) tape.

30.3.2 Electronic spirometers and oxygen uptake systems

Ventilation can be recorded using one of a number of electronic spirometers, though the resistance of some commercially available models is not well tolerated at the very high ventilation found in climbers exercising at altitude. Such an electronic spirometer was successfully used by Pizzo near the summit of Everest (West *et al.* 1983c).

The Oxylog was a portable electronic instrument (no longer available) giving a continuous read-out of minute ventilation and oxygen consumption (updated each minute), and the total ventilation and oxygen consumption since it was last reset. The subject wore a mask, into the inspiratory port of which is fitted an electronic spirometer or anemometer. The output (V and Vo_2) could be recorded for hours on a portable tape recorder. It was accurate for sub-maximal work rates (Milledge *et al.* 1983c) but is not suitable for $Vo_{2,max}$ measurements. However, other devices are now on the market, one such is the Viasys Oxycon Mobile which does the same job and, of course, has added features and associated software for downloading to a computer. It can be used up to maximum work and ventilation rates for measurements of $Vo_{2,max}$. It has been tested in a chamber to 5500 m and in temperatures from -10 to $+50°C$ but has not been used at altitude on the mountain yet.

30.3.3 Alveolar gas sampling

Alveolar or end-tidal gas samples have been taken from subjects at altitude on a number of expeditions, in 1981 from the summit of Everest itself.

Glass ampoules were successfully used on a number of expeditions, including the Silver Hut Expedition, when samples were brought back from 7830 m. These were of 50 mL capacity and had a stem with two necks in it. The ampoules were pre-evacuated before leaving. In the field, a Haldane–Priestley sample was delivered down a tube with the ampoule attached to a side arm by a short length of pressure tubing. Surgical forceps were then used to break the glass within the pressure tube and the sample entered the ampoule. With the rubber tube clamped the ampoule was brought back to base where, with a suitable gas flame, the ampoule was sealed at the lower neck and transported back for analysis.

On the AMREE 1981, 20 mL aerosol cans of the type used in asthma inhalers were used. These cans, supplied by the pharmaceutical industry, had the metering device removed and were then pre-evacuated. They were shown to hold their vacuum for at least 6 months. In the field, the simplest apparatus involved merely a T-shaped piece of tubing into the stem of which the can was fitted with its nozzle resting on a shoulder. The subject delivered a Haldane–Priestley alveolar sample across the T to which was added a soft, wide-bore tube; the can was then depressed, which opened its valve, and the sample entered the can. Releasing the can sealed it again and it was then transported back for analysis.

The actual device used on the summit of Everest was rather more complicated (West 1985a); it held six pre-evacuated cans in a rotating cylinder to which two handles were attached. The subject exhaled across the top of the cylinder through two one-way valves and the end-tidal gas was caught between them. On squeezing the handles, one can was opened and a sample taken. On releasing the handles the can was closed; the cylinder rotated to present the next can for a second sample (Maret *et al.* 1984).

Analysis at the home institute was by mass spectrometry using a special inlet device which would accept the aerosol can. The sample volume at sea level pressure would be only 5–7 mL but adequate for analysis.

If rapid carbon dioxide and oxygen analyzers are taken, end-tidal gases can be measured over sufficient time to be sure of a steady state.

30.3.4 Pulse oximetry

The pulse oximeter allows the easy measurement of arterial oxygen saturation with a very lightweight battery powered instrument. There are many models on the market now and most are accurate and reliable. They also read heart rate. Many also have data storage facilities and data can be downloaded into laptop computers. This allows them to be readily used for sleep studies. They are not suitable for ambulatory measurements, though they can be used during exercise on a cycle ergometer. The sensors are made for use either on the finger or earlobe, the former being usually preferred. It is essential for the finger to be warm in order to get a good signal.

30.4 CARDIOLOGICAL MEASUREMENTS

30.4.1 Electrocardiography (ECG)

The ECG is easy to record at altitude, either the classical 12-lead ECG at rest, or ambulatory recording over many hours. Such recordings have been made on Everest climbers (West *et al.* 1983c). The pulse rate can be obtained from such recordings. Computer analysis can be carried out looking for arrhythmia and spectral analysis of R–R intervals, etc. Care is needed in the electrode placement and attachment (as at sea level).

30.4.2 Echocardiography

Until recently the size, weight and complexity of ultrasound machines for conducting echocardiography were such that there was no question of using this technique in the field. However, machines are getting smaller, lighter and more reliable and it can now be considered as a possibility. Such a machine was used by Dubowitz at the Himalayan Rescue Association Clinic at Pheriche (4243 m) to complete a study measuring pulmonary artery pressure by Doppler echocardiography in trekkers on their way to Everest Base Camp (Dubowitz and Peacock 1999). The same machine was taken to Kangchenjunga Base Camp (5100 m) but unfortunately developed a fatal electrical fault soon after the study started but was used successfully on the Chamlang Expedition (Dubowitz *et al.* 2004). There are now machines which weigh as little as 4 kg.

30.4.3 Cardiac catheterization

More invasive cardiac techniques, such as right heart and pulmonary artery catheterization, have been discussed and, though possible under field conditions with mains voltage electricity available, are probably not justified, though this is debatable. Catheterization has been carried out in chamber studies, most extensively in Operation Everest II (Houston *et al.* 1987); in skilled hands it carries very little risk.

30.5 SLEEP STUDIES

Sleep studies have been carried out on a number of expeditions where mains voltage was provided (Chapter 13). ECGs, electroencephalograms (EEGs), electro-oculograms, ear and pulse oximetry and respiratory movements have all been monitored simultaneously and recorded on tape and paper while the subject was asleep. Most of this monitoring can now be carried out with battery operated instruments but it is important that some way of monitoring the signals during the recording is provided, even if the analysis from tape is left until after the expedition. One such system is the Vivometrics Lifeshirt® (Vivometrics; Ventura, CA, USA). It uses the principle of inductive plethysmography first developed by Dr F. Stott (Milledge and Stott 1977) to record chest and abdominal movement and hence tidal volume, respiratory rate and ventilation. ECG and other sensors are available to provide additional physiological monitoring. This system was used on the recent Cho Oyu Expedition (2005) mentioned below. It worked well, except when an attempt was made to use it on the summit day when it failed, possible due to the cold.

30.6 BLOOD SAMPLING AND STORAGE

30.6.1 Venipuncture

There is little problem in performing venipuncture in the field. Two physician climbers took samples from each other on the South Col of Everest the morning after climbing to the summit (Winslow *et al.* 1984). 'Vacutainer' systems using pre-evacuated tubes and double-ended needles are particularly convenient, as the sampling tubes are used for centrifuging. They fill (from the vein) perfectly well at altitude.

30.6.2 Centrifuging blood samples

If mains voltage is available, a small electrical centrifuge can be used and this presents no problem. Hand centrifuges can be used but require quite a lot of muscle power. They need to be spun very vigorously for 15–20 min; even then the cells are not as tightly packed as by even the lowest powered electrical centrifuge. This means that the yield of plasma is less, typically a maximum of 5 mL from 10 mL of blood. When subjects become polycythemic the problem becomes worse.

These hand centrifuges usually take four 10 mL tubes compared with six or eight in the small electrical centrifuges; they are really intended for spinning urine samples and are not designed for such vigorous spinning. Older designs with brass gears and cast metal casings stand up better than do modern models with nylon gears and plastic cases. A firm bench on which to clamp the centrifuge is essential. However, with all these drawbacks, hand centrifuging of blood is possible if mains voltage is unavailable. A dry-battery centrifuge is not a viable possibility.

30.6.3 Arterial blood sampling and analysis

If the usual precautions are taken and if the doctor is experienced in the procedure, there should be no problem in arterial puncture in a base camp setting. Arterial cannulation is more hazardous and its justification in the field is debatable.

There has been recent interest in the possibility of obtaining arterial blood samples at extreme altitude and even on the summit of Mount Everest (Catron *et al.* 2006). In preparation for attempting this on an expedition in 2007 (Xtreme Everest Project), a group from the same team went to Cho Oyu in the autumn of 2005. They ascended the mountain with Sherpas and on the flat summit erected a small tent. In it, one climber breathing oxygen at $4\,L\,min^{-1}$ successfully carried out a femoral artery puncture on another climber, obtaining a good sample of arterial blood. Both operator and subject were doctors. The sample was transported to Camp 1 (6100 m) in ice, within 4 h by a Sherpa. A full report, with practical details, is available. (www.Xtreme-everest.co.uk). The apparatus used by the Cho Oyu team was the i-STAT. The i-STAT Blood Gas Analyzer is a portable hand-held unit designed to analyze blood chemistries and blood gases. The unit uses cartridges and a very small amount of blood to analyze various parameters in the blood depending upon the cartridge being used. The unit runs on two 9 V lithium batteries and weighs about 570 g. It has been shown to give comparable results to that of a conventional laboratory blood gas analyzer (Sediame *et al.* 1999). The storage of the cartridges presented problems because they have to be kept at refrigerator temperatures. The system worked well up to Advanced Base Camp (5700 m) but failed at Camp 1 probably as a result of damage to the cartridge, so Po_2 from the summit

sample was not obtained though arterial pH and Pco_2 were.

30.6.4 Sample storage

Plasma, serum and urine samples can be deep frozen, stored and transported back to the home laboratory by using liquid nitrogen in a suitable container. In previous editions of this book we described how a portable deep-freeze container could be made by using a 28 L liquid nitrogen flask (often called a Dewar flask) and packing it with dry ice (solid carbon dioxide). This gave up to 130 days of use. However, dry ice is no longer readily obtainable (presumably because of the ready availability of freezers) so this method has now been abandoned. There was also the disadvantage that, although the necks of these flasks were quite narrow, they could not be tightly sealed because the nitrogen could not evolve and there would be danger of explosion. Therefore there was always the potential for spillage of liquid nitrogen and harm to porters, though I know of no such accident ever happening.

However, systems have now been developed for the safe transport of deep-frozen samples using liquid nitrogen trapped in an absorbent matrix inside a vacuum container. One such commercial system is called a Cryopak. Much of the capacity of the flask is taken up with the filler material and there is quite a small well for the samples. The makers supply a vial holder or canister, which slides into this well and takes sample vials. This allows vials to be removed, inspected, sampled and replaced but further reduces the capacity of the flask. Alternatively the canister can be dispensed with and vials just thrown into the well. This allows more samples, but at the risk of losing labels, and makes sorting more of a problem. There is a range of flask sizes with capacity ranging from 30 to 324 2-mL vials. The gross weight when charged with nitrogen ranges from 7.3 to 22.7 kg. The static holding time (full of liquid nitrogen) is 30 days but the working time (absorbed nitrogen only, empty well) is only 21 days. The flask, of course, can be topped up with liquid nitrogen. This system is safer than the previous one, since once any excess liquid nitrogen has evolved, there is no risk of spillage. This means that they can be freighted on aircraft as normal, instead of going as 'dangerous goods' and, of course, they are safer as porter loads. This system was used on the 1998 Kangchenjunga Expedition. The more limited time available is a disadvantage and without the benefit of helicopter freight and topping up we would have had difficulty in keeping our samples frozen until return to London.

Samples should be taken into PTFE tubes with good screw caps. Tubes should have a matt surface for labeling, which should be done in pencil; they should then be covered in low temperature adhesive tape. During transportation (if the canister or holder is dispensed with) these tubes are constantly chafed together, and unless the labels are firm they will come off or run and all will be lost. It was found that pencil under low temperature clear adhesive tape was safe.

For shorter periods of up to 1–2 weeks, it may be adequate to use polystyrene boxes of dry ice. Although the newer Cryopak flasks are not treated as 'dangerous goods', airline regulations are frequently changed and anyone planning to use these or other systems should check the current regulations with the airline they are using, including the container requirements in force. Airlines are usually familiar with handling 'medical samples' in this way but expect to deal with recognized shippers. The bureaucracy and expense of such a shipment are not inconsiderable; delays of a few days at each end can be anticipated and must be allowed for in calculating the time available at deep-freeze temperature.

30.7 HEMATOLOGY

Much hematology can be done with quite simple equipment in the field. Battery operated micro centrifuges for packed cell volume are available commercially. Hemoglobin can be measured by the cyanmethemoglobin method and a battery operated spectrometer. Cell count can be carried out by classical microscopy techniques. With mains voltage electricity and PO_2 electrodes, the oxygen dissociation curve and P_{50} can be measured (Winslow *et al.* 1984).

30.8 COMPUTERS

Laptop or notebook computers are now commonplace on expeditions. They are now reasonably reliable and robust and, compared with much scientific equipment, they are quite cheap. Their power requirements are not great. If generators are being taken there is no problem; otherwise their batteries can be recharged from solar panels if necessary. Therefore there need be no hesitation in including computers in expedition equipment. Like all battery operated apparatus they work better at comfortable temperatures but are no more fussy than ECG machines, for instance. Computers have many applications, from writing reports to online control of other equipment. They are good for storing data, on- or off-line with back-up on discs. If more than one computer is to be taken, as is likely, it is worth ensuring that the same programs are installed on all of them so that one can act as a back-up for any other machine.

30.9 OTHER AREAS OF SCIENTIFIC STUDY

The areas of research mentioned are the classical ones for altitude research. As more workers from different fields have become interested in the effects of altitude hypoxia on other systems of the body, more techniques have been used in the mountains. Psychomotor testing equipment has changed from clipboard, stopwatch and pencil to computers. Visual field testing, retinal photography, audiometry and measurement of balance or sway have been made using computer based systems. Overnight cough frequency has been monitored with voice activated battery tape recorders and cough threshold measured with nebulized citric acid solutions. Even near-infrared spectroscopy has been used to measure brain oxygenation at altitude in the field (Imray *et al.* 2000, Chan *et al.* 2005). All these applications of modern electronics, and others, show how the possibilities for research at altitude have expanded. The future of the subject is only limited by the imagination of researchers and should be bright indeed.

References

Acosta, I. de (1590) *Historia Natural y Moral de las Indias*, Lib 3, Cap. 9, Iuan de Leon, Seville. Section of English translation of 1604 (1604), Edward Blount and William Aspley, London. Reprinted in *High Altitude Physiology* (ed. J.B. West), Hutchinson Ross Publishing Company, Stroudsburg, PA, 1981.

Adam, J.M. and Goldsmith, R. (1965) Cold climates, in *Exploration Medicine* (eds. O.G. Edholm and A.L. Bacharach), Wright, Bristol, pp. 245–77.

Adams, W.C., Bernauer, E.M., Dill, D.B., and Bowmar, J.B. Jr (1975) Effects of equivalent sea-level and altitude training on VO$_2$ max and running performance. *J. Appl. Physiol.* **39**, 262–6.

Adams, W.H. and Strang, L.J. (1975) Haemoglobin levels in persons of Tibetan ancestry living at high altitude. *Proc. Soc. Exp. Biol. Med.* **149**, 1036–9.

Adnot, S., Chabrier, P.E., Brun-Buisson, C., Voissat, I. and Braguet, P. (1988) Atrial natriuretic factor attenuates the pulmonary pressor response to hypoxia. *J. Appl. Physiol.* **65**, 1975–83.

Adzaku, F., Mohammed, S., Annobil, S. and Addae, S. (1993) Relevant laboratory findings in patients with sickle cell disease living at high altitude. *J. Wilderness Med.* **4**, 374–83.

Agostoni, P., Cattadori, G., Guazzi, M. *et al.* (2000) Effects of simulated altitude-induced hypoxia on exercise capacity in patients with chronic heart failure. *Am. J. Med.* **109**, 450–5.

Agusti, A.G., Sauleda, J., Miralles, C. *et al.* (2002) Skeletal muscle apoptosis and weight loss in chronic obstructive pulmonary disease. *Am. J. Respir. Crit. Care Med.* **166**, 485–9.

Ahle, N.W., Buroni, J.R., Sharp, M.W. and Hamlet, M.P. (1990) Infrared thermographic measurement of circulatory compromise in trenchfoot-injured Argentine soldiers. *Aviat. Space Environ. Med.* **61**, 247–50.

Aigner, A., Berghold, F. and Muss, N. (1980) Investigations on the cardiovascular system at altitudes up to a height of 7,800 meters. *Z. Kardiol.* **69**, 604–10.

Albrecht, P.H. and Littell, J.K. (1972) Plasma erythropoietin in men and mice during acclimatization to different altitudes. *J. Appl. Physiol.* **32**, 54–8.

Aldashev, A.A., Sarybaev, A.S., Sydykov, A.S. *et al.* (2002) Characterization of high-altitude pulmonary hypertension in the Kyrgyz: association with angiotensin-converting enzyme genotype. *Am. J. Respir. Crit. Care Med.* **166**, 1396–402.

Aldeshev, A.A., Kojonazarov, B.K., Amatov, T.A. *et al.* (2005) Phosphodiesterase type 5 and high altitude pulmonary hypertension. *Thorax* **60**, 683–7.

Alexander, J. (1995) Age, altitude, and arrhythmia. *Texas Heart Inst. J.* **22**, 308–16.

Alexander, J.K. (1999) Cardiac arrhythmia at high altitude: the progressive effect of aging. *Texas Heart Inst. J.* **26**, 258–63.

Alexander, J.K., Hartley, L.H., Modelski, M. and Grover, R.F. (1967) Reduction of stroke volume during exercise in man following ascent to 3100 m altitude. *J. Appl. Physiol.* **23**, 849–58.

Alexander, L. (1945) *The Treatment of Shock from Prolonged Exposure to Cold Especially in Water*, Combined Intelligence Objective Sub-Committee, Item No. **24**, File No. 24–37.

Allegra, L., Cogo, A., Legnani, D., Diano, P.L., Fasano, V. and Negretto, G.G. (1995) High altitude exposure reduces bronchial responsiveness to hypo-osmolar aerosols in lowland asthmatics. *Eur. Respir. J.* **8**, 1842–6.

Alpert, M.A. (2001) Obesity cardiomyopathy: pathophysiology and evolution of the clinical syndrome. *Am. J. Med. Sci.* **321**, 225–36.

Altman, P.L. and Dittmer, D.S. (1966) Erythrocyte values at altitude; Part 1 Man., in *Environmental Biology* (eds. P.L. Altman and D.S. Dittmer), Fed. Am. Soc. Exper. Biol., Bethesda, pp. 351–5.

American Physiological Society (1995) Standards for the diagnosis and care of patients with chronic obstructive pulmonary disease. *Am. J. Respir. Crit. Care Med.* **152**: S77–120.

Anand, I.S. (2001) Letter from the field: letter from Siachen Glacier. *High Alt. Med. Biol.* **2**, 553–7.

Anand, I.S., Harris, E., Ferrari, R., Pearce, P. and Harris, P. (1986) Pulmonary haemodynamics of the yak, cattle and cross breeds at high altitude. *Thorax* **41**, 696–700.

Anand, I.S., Malhotra, R.M., Chandrashekhar, Y. *et al.* (1990) Adult subacute mountain sickness – a syndrome of congestive heart failure in man at very high altitude. *Lancet* **335**, 561–5.

Anand, I.S., Chandrashekhar, Y., Rao, S.K. *et al.* (1993) Body fluid compartments, renal blood flow, and hormones at 6000 m in normal subjects. *J. Appl. Physiol.* **74**, 1234–9.

Anand, I.S., Prasad, B.A., Chugh, S.S. *et al.* (1998) Effect of inhaled nitric oxide and oxygen in high-altitude pulmonary edema. *Circulation* **98**, 2441–5.

Andersen, P. and Henriksson, J. (1977) Capillary supply of the quadriceps femoris muscle of man: adaptive response to exercise. *J. Physiol. (Lond.)* **270**, 677–90.

Anderson, J.V., Struthers, A.D., Payne, N.N., Slater, J.D. and Bloom, S.R. (1986) Atrial natriuretic peptide inhibits the aldosterone response to angiotensin II in man. *Clin. Sci.* **70**, 507–12.

Anderson, S., Herbring, B.G. and Widman, B. (1970) Accidental profound hypothermia (case report). *Br. J. Anaesth.* **42**, 653–5.

Andrew, H.G. (1963) Work in extreme cold. *Trans. Assoc. Indust. Med. Off.* **13**, 16–19.

Andrew, M., O'Brodovitch, H. and Sutton, J. (1987) Operation Everest II; coagulation system during prolonged decompression to 282 torr. *J. Appl. Physiol.* **63**, 1262–7.

Anholm, J.D., Poweles, AC., Downey, R.D. *et al.* (1992) Operation Everest II: arterial oxygen saturation and sleep at extreme simulated altitude. *Am. Rev. Respir. Dis.* **145**, 817–26.

Anholm, J.D., Milne, E.N., Stark, P., Bourne, J.C. and Friedman, P. (1999) Radiographic evidence of interstitial pulmonary edema after exercise at altitude. *J. Appl. Physiol.* **86**, 503–9.

Anonymous (1990) Kiss of life for a cold corpse (Editorial). *Lancet* **335**, 1435.

Anooshiravani, M., Dumont, L., Mardirosoff, C., Soto-Debeuf, G. and Delavelle, J. (1999) Brain magnetic resonance imaging (MRI) and neurological changes after a single high altitude climb. *Med. Sci. Sports Exerc.* **31**, 969–72.

Another Ascent of the World's Highest Peak – Qomolangma (1975) Foreign Languages Press, Peking.

Anselme, F., Caillaud, C., Courret, I. and Prefaut, C. (1992) Exercise induced hypoxaemia and histamine excretion in extreme athletes. *Int. J. Sports Med.* **13**, 80–1.

Antezana, A.-M., Richalet, J.-P., Noriega, I., Galarza, M. and Antezana, G. (1995) Hormonal changes in normal and polycythemic high-altitude natives. *J. Appl. Physiol.* **79**, 795–800.

Antezana, A.M., Antezana, G., Aparicio, O., Noriega, I., Velarde, F.L. and Richalet, J.-P. (1998) Pulmonary hypertension in high altitude chronic hypoxia: response to nifedipine. *Eur. Respir. J.* **12**, 1181–5.

Antezana, G., Leguia, G., Guzman, A.M., Coudert, J. and Spielvogel, H. (1982) Hemodynamic study of high altitude pulmonary edema (12200 ft), in *High Altitude Physiology and Medicine* (eds. W. Brendel and R.A. Zink), Springer-Verlag, New York, pp. 232–41.

Anthony, A., Ackerman, E. and Strother, G.K. (1959) Effects of altitude acclimatization on rat myoglobin. Changes in myoglobin content of skeletal and cardiac muscle. *Am. J. Physiol.* **196**, 512–16.

Aoki, V.S. and Robinson, S.M. (1971) Body hydration and the incidence and severity of acute mountain sickness. *J. Appl. Physiol.* **31**, 363–7.

Appell, H.-J. (1978) Capillary density and patterns in skeletal muscle. III. Changes of the capillary pattern after hypoxia. *Pflügers Arch.* **377**, R53 (abstract).

Appleton F.M. (1967) Possible influence of altitude on blood pressure (abstract). *Circ.* **36(Suppl. 2)**, 55.

Araki, T. (1891) Ueber die Bildung von Milchsäure und Glycose im Organismus bei Sauerstoffmangel. *Z. Physiol. Chem.* **15**, 335–70.

Araneda, O.F., Garcia, C., Lagos, N. *et al.* (2005) Lung oxidative stress as related to exercise and altitude. Lipid peroxidation evidence in exhaled breath condensate: a possible predictor of acute mountain sickness. *Eur. J. Appl. Physiol.* **95**, 383–90. E-pub 30 September 2005.

Archer, S.L., Tolins, J.P., Raij, L. and Weir, E.K. (1989) Hypoxic pulmonary vasoconstriction is enhanced by inhibition of the synthesis of an endothelium derived relaxing factor. *Biochem. Biophys. Res. Commun.* **164**, 1198–205.

Arias-Stella, J. (1969) Human carotid body at high altitudes (abstract). *Am. J. Pathol.* **55**, 82.

Arias-Stella, J. (1971) Chronic mountain sickness: pathology and definition, in *High Altitude Physiology: Cardiac and Respiratory Aspects,* Ciba Foundation

Symposium (eds. R. Porter and J. Knight), Churchill Livingstone, Edinburgh, pp. 31–40.

Arias-Stella, J. and Recavarren, S. (1962) Right ventricular hypertrophy in native children living at high altitude. *Am. J. Pathol.* **41**, 55–64.

Arias-Stella, J. and Saldaña, M. (1962) The muscular arteries in people native to high altitude. *Med. Thorac.* **19**, 55–64.

Arias-Stella, J. and Kruger, H. (1963) Pathology of high altitude pulmonary edema. *Arch. Pathol.* **76**, 147–57.

Arias-Stella, J. and Saldaña, M. (1963) The terminal portion of the pulmonary arterial tree in people native to high altitudes. *Circulation* **28**, 915–25.

Arias-Stella, J. and Topilsky, M. (1971) Anatomy of the coronary circulation at high altitude, in *High Altitude Physiology: Cardiac and Respiratory Aspects* (eds. R. Porter and J. Knight), Churchill Livingstone, London, pp. 149–57.

Arias-Stella, J., Kruger, H. and Recavarren, S. (1973) Pathology of chronic mountain sickness. *Thorax* **28**, 701–8.

Armstrong, L.S. and Maresh, C.M. (1991) The induction and decay of heat acclimatisation in trained athletes. *Sports Med.* **12**, 302–12.

Asaji, T., Sakurai, E., Tanizaki, Y. *et al.* (1984) Report on medical aspects of Mount Lhotse and Everest expedition in 1983: with special reference to a case of cerebral venous thrombosis in the altitude. *Jpn. J. Mount. Med.* **4**, 91–8.

Asano, K., Sub, S., Matsuzaka, A. *et al.* (1986) The influence of simulated high altitude training on work capacity and performance in middle and long distance runners. *Bull. Inst. Health Sports Med.* **9**, 1195–202.

Asano, M., Kaneoka, K., Nomura, T. *et al.* (1998) Increase in serum vascular endothelial growth factor levels during altitude training. *Acta. Physiol. Scand.* **162**, 455–9.

Asemu, G., Papousek, F., Ostadal, B. and Kolar, F. (1999) Adaptation to high altitude hypoxia protects the rat heart against ischemia-induced arrhythmias. Involvement of mitochondrial K(ATP) channel. *J. Mol. Cell. Cardiol.* **31**, 1821–31.

Asemu, G., Neckar, J., Szarszoi, O. *et al.* (2003) Decrease in peak rate with acute hypoxia in relation to sea level. *Physiol. Res.* **49**, 597–606.

Ashack, R., Farber, M.O., Weinberger, M.H., Robertson, G.L., Fineberg, N.S. and Manfredi, F. (1985) Renal and hormonal responses to acute hypoxia in normal individuals. *J. Lab. Clin. Med.* **106**, 12–16.

Ashenden, M.J., Gore, C.J., Martin D,T., Dobson, G.P. and Hahn, A.G. (1999a) Effects of a 12-day 'live high, train low' camp on reticulocyte production and haemoglobin mass in elite female road cyclists. *Eur. J. Appl. Physiol. Occup. Physiol.* **80**, 472–8.

Ashenden, M.J., Gore, C.J., Dobson, G.P. and Hahn, A.G. (1999b) 'Live high, train low' does not change the total haemoglobin mass of male endurance athletes sleeping at a simulated altitude of 3000 m for 23 nights. *Eur. J Appl. Physiol. Occup. Physiol.* **80**, 479–84.

Asmussen, E. and Consolazio, F.C. (1941) The circulation in rest and work on Mount Evans (4,300 m). *Am. J. Physiol.* **132**, 555–63.

Aste-Salazar, H. and Hurtado, A. (1944) The affinity of hemoglobin for oxygen at sea level and at high altitudes. *Am. J. Physiol.* **142**, 733–43.

Astrup, P. and Severinghaus, J.W. (1986) *The History of Blood Gases, Acids and Bases*, Munksgaard, Copenhagen.

Atrial natriuretic peptide [editorial]. (1986) *Lancet* **2**, 371–2.

Au, J., Brown, J.E., Lee, M.R. and Boon, N.A. (1990) Effect of cardiac tamponade on atrial natriuretic peptide concentrations: influence of stretch and pressure. *Clin. Sci.* **79**, 377–80.

Aughey, R.J., Gore, C.J., Hahn, A.G. *et al.* (2005) Chronic intermittent hypoxia and incremental cycling exercise independently depress muscle in vitro maximal Na^+-K^+-ATPase activity in well-trained athletes. *J. Appl. Physiol.* **98**, 186–92. E-pub 19 March 2004.

Ayton, J.M. (1993) Polar hands: spontaneous skin fissures closed with cyanoacrylate (Histoacryl Blue) tissue adhesive in Antarctica. *Arctic Med. Res.* **52**, 127–30.

Babcock, M.A., Pegelow, D.F., McClaran, S.R., Suman, O.E. and Dempsey, J.A. (1995) Contribution of diaphragmatic power output to exercise-induced diaphragm fatigue. *J. Appl. Physiol.* **78**, 1710–19.

Backer, H.D., Shopes, E. and Collins, S.L. (1993) Hyponatemia in recreational hikers in Grand Canyon national Park. *Wild. Environ. Med.* **4**, 391–406.

Baddeley, A.D., Cuccaro, W.J., Egstrom, G.H. and Willis, M.A. (1975) Cognitive efficiency of divers working in cold water. *Hum. Factors* **17**, 446–54.

Baertschi, A.J., Hausmaninger, C., Walsh, R.S. *et al.* (1986) Hypoxia-induced release of atrial natriuretic factor (ANF) from isolated rat and rabbit heart. *Biochem. Biophys. Res. Commun.* **140**, 427–33.

Bailey, D.M. and Davies, B. (1997) Physiological implications of altitude training for endurance performance at sea level: a review. *Br. J. Sports Med.* **31**, 183–90.

Bailey, D.M., Davies, B., Romer, L. *et al.* (1998) Implications of moderate altitude training for sea-level endurance in elite distance runners. *Eur. J. Appl. Physiol.* **78**, 360–8.

Bailey, D.M., Davies, B., Milledge, J.S. *et al.* (2000) Elevated plasma cholecystokinin at high altitude: metabolic implications for the anorexia of acute mountain sickness. *High Alt. Med. Biol.* **1**, 9–23.

Bailey, D.M., Davies, B., Young, I.S., Hullin, D.A. and Seddon, P.S. (2001) A potential role for free radical-mediated skeletal muscle soreness in the pathophysiology of acute mountain sickness. *Aviat. Space Environ. Med.* **72**, 513–21.

Bailey, D.M., Davies, B., Castell, L.M. *et al.* (2003) Symptoms of infection and acute mountain sickness; associated metabolic sequelae and problems in differential diagnosis. *High Alt. Med. Biol.* **4**, 319–31.

Bailey, D.M., Ainslie, P.N., Jackson, S.K., Richardson, R.S. and Ghatei, M. (2004) Evidence against redox regulation of energy homoeostasis in humans at high altitude. *Clin. Sci.* **107**, 589–600.

Bailey, D.M., Roukens, R., Knauth, M. *et al.* (2005) Free radical-mediated damage to barrier function is not associated with altered brain morphology in high-altitude headache. *J. Cereb. Blood Flow Metab.* **26**, 99–111.

Bailey, F.M. (1957) *No Passport to Tibet.* Hart Davis, London, p. 261.

Baker, P.T. (1966) Microenvironment cold in a high altitude Peruvian population, in *Human Adaptability and Its Methodology* (eds. H. Yoshimura and J.S. Weiner), Japanese Society for the Promotion of Sciences, Tokyo, pp. 67–77.

Baker, P.T. (1978) *The Biology of High Altitude Peoples.* Cambridge University Press, Cambridge.

Baker, P.T. and Dutt, J.S. (1972) Demographic variables as measures of biological adaptation: a case study of high altitude population, in *The Structure of Human Populations* (eds. G.A. Harrison and A.J. Boyce), Clarendon Press, Oxford, pp. 352–78.

Bakewell, S.E., Hart, N.D., Wilson, C.M. *et al.* (1999) A randomised, double blind placebo controlled trial of the effect of inhaled nedocromil sodium or slameterol xinafoate on the citric acid cough threshold in subjects travelling to high altitude (abstract), in *Hypoxia: Into the Next Millennium*

(eds. R.C. Roach, P.D. Wagner and P.H. Hackett), Plenum/Kluwer Academic Publishing, New York, p. 362.

Banchero, N. (1982) Long term adaptation of skeletal muscle capillarity. *Physiologist* **25**, 385–9.

Bandopadhyay, P. and Selvamurthy, W. (2003) Suggested predictive indices for high altitude pulmonary oedema. *J. Assoc. Phys. India* **48**, 290–329.

Bangham, C.R.M. and Hackett, P.H. (1978) Effects of high altitude on endocrine function in the Sherpas of Nepal. *J. Endocrinol.* **79**, 147–8.

Banner, A.S. (1988) Relationship between cough due to hypotonic aerosol and the ventilatory response to CO_2 in normal subjects. *Am. Rev. Respir. Dis.* **137**, 647–50.

Barash I.A., Beatty C., Powell F.L., Prisk G.K. and West J.B. (2001) Nocturnal oxygen enrichment of room air at 3800 meter altitude improves sleep architecture. *High Alt. Med. Biol.* liebertonline.com

Barber, S.G. (1978) Drugs and doctoring for trans-Saharan travellers. *BMJ* **2**, 404–6.

Barclay, J.K. (1986) A delivery-independent blood flow effect on skeletal muscle fatigue. *J. Appl. Physiol.* **61**, 1084–90.

Barcroft, J. (1911) The effect of altitude on the dissociation curve of blood. *J. Physiol. (Lond.)* **42**, 44–63.

Barcroft, J. (1925) *The Respiratory Function of the Blood. Part I. Lessons from High Altitudes*, Cambridge University Press, Cambridge.

Barcroft, J. and King, W.O.R. (1909) The effect of temperature on the dissociation curve of blood. *J. Physiol. (Lond.)*, **39**, 374–84.

Barcroft, J. and Orbeli, L. (1910) The influence of lactic acid upon the dissociation curve of blood. *J. Physiol. (Lond.)*. **41**, 355–67.

Barcroft, J., Camis, M., Mathison, C.G., Roberts, F.F. and Ryffel, J.H. (1914) Report of the Monte Rosa Expedition of 1911. *Philos. Trans. R. Soc. Lond. Ser. B* **206**, 49–102.

Barcroft, J., Cooke, A., Hartridge, H., Parsons, T.R. and Parsons, W. (1920) The flow of oxygen through the pulmonary epithelium. *J. Physiol. (Lond.)* **53**, 450–72.

Barcroft, J., Binger, C.A., Bock, A.V. *et al.* (1923) Observations upon the effect of high altitude on the physiological processes of the human body, carried out in the Peruvian Andes, chiefly at Cerro de Pasco. *Philos. Trans. R. Soc. Lond. Ser. B* **211**, 351–480.

Barer, G.R., Howard, P. and Shaw, J.W. (1970) Stimulus–response curves for the pulmonary vascular bed to hypoxia and hypercapnia. *J. Physiol. (Lond.)* **211**, 139–55.

Barnard, P., Andronikou, S., Pokorski, M. *et al.* (1987) Time-dependent effect of hypoxia on carotid body chemosensory function. *J. Appl. Physiol.* **63**, 684–91.

Barry, P.B., Mason, N.M. and Collier, D.J. (1995) Sex differences in blood gases during acclimatization, in *Hypoxia and the Brain* (eds. J.R. Sutton, C. S Houston and G. Coates), Queen City Printers, Burlington, VA, p. 314.

Barry, P.W., Mason, N.P., Riordan, M. and O'Callaghan, C. (1997a) Cough frequency and cough receptor sensitivity are increased in man at high altitude. *Clin. Sci.* **93**, 181–6.

Barry, P.W., Mason, N.P. and O'Callaghan, C. (1997b) Nasal mucociliary transport is impaired at altitude. *Eur. Respir. J.* **10**, 35–7.

Barry, P.W., Mason, N.P., Nicol, A. *et al.* (1997c) Cough receptor sensitivity and dynamic ventilatory response to carbon dioxide in man acclimatized to high altitude (Abstract), in *Women at Altitude* (eds. C.S. Houston and G. Coates), Queens City Press, Burlington, VA, p. 303.

Bartlett, D. Jr and Remmers, J.E. (1971) Effects of high altitude exposure on the lungs of young rats. *Respir. Physiol.* **13**, 116–25.

Bärtsch, P., Schmidt, E.K. and Straub, P.W. (1982) Fibrinopeptide A after strenuous physical exercise at high altitude. *J. Appl. Physiol.* **53**, 40–3.

Bärtsch, P., Waber, U., Haeberli, A., Gnädinger, M.P. and Weidmann, P. (1987) Enhanced fibrin formation in high-altitude pulmonary edema. *J. Appl. Physiol.* **63**, 752–7.

Bärtsch, P., Shaw, S., Franciolli, M. *et al.* (1988) Atrial natriuretic peptide in acute mountain sickness. *J. Appl. Physiol.* **65**, 1929–37.

Bärtsch, P., Lämmle, B., Huber, I. *et al.* (1989) Contact phase of blood coagulation is not activated in edema of high altitude. *J. Appl. Physiol.* **67**, 1336–40.

Bärtsch, P., Baumgartner, R.W., Waber, U., Maggiorini, M. and Oelz, O. (1990) Comparison of carbon dioxide enriched, oxygen enriched, and normal air in treatment of acute mountain sickness. *Lancet* 336, 772–5.

Bärtsch, P., Pfluger, N., Audetat, M.S. *et al.* (1991a) Effects of slow ascent to 4559 m on fluid homeostasis. *Aviat. Space Environ. Med.* **62**, 105–10.

Bärtsch, P., Maggiorini, M., Ritter, M., Noti, C., Vock, P. and Oelz, O. (1991b) Prevention of high-altitude pulmonary edema by nifedipine. *N. Engl. J. Med.* **325**, 1284–9.

Bärtsch, P., Merki, B., Hofsetter, D., Maggiorini, M., Kayser, B. and Oelz, O. (1993) Treatment of acute mountain sickness by simulated descent: a randomised controlled trial. *BMJ* **306**, 1098–101.

Bärtsch, P., Swenson, E.R., Paul, A., Julg, B. and Hohenhause, E. (2002) Hypoxic ventilatory response, ventilation, gas exchange, and fluid balance in acute mountain sickness. *High Alt. Med. Biol.* **3**, 361–76.

Bascom, D.A., Clement, I.D., Cunningham, D.A., Painter, R. and Robins, P.A. (1990) Changes in peripheral chemoreceptor sensitivity during sustained isocapnic hypoxia. *Respir. Physiol.* **82**, 161–76.

Basnyat, B. (1997) Seizure and hemiparesis at high altitudes outside the setting of acute mountain sickness. *J. Wilderness Environ. Med.* **8**, 221–2.

Basnyat, B. (2001) Isolated facial and hypoglossal nerve palsies at high altitude. *High Alt. Med. Biol.* **2**, 301–3.

Basnyat, B., Leomaster, J. and Litch, J.A. (1999) Everest or bust: a cross sectional, epidemiological survey of acute mountain sickness at 4234 m in the Himalaya. *Aviat. Space Environ. Med.* **70**, 867–73.

Basnyat, B., Sleggs, J. and Spinger, M. (2000a) Seizures and delirium in a trekker: the consequences of excessive water drinking? *Wild. Environ. Med.* **11**, 69–70.

Basnyat, B., Subedi, D., Sleggs, J. *et al.* (2000b) Disoriented and ataxic pilgrims: an epidemiological study of acute mountain sickness and high-altitude cerebral edema at a sacred lake at 4300 m in the Nepal Himalayas. *Wild. Environ. Med.* **11**, 89–93.

Basnyat, B., Gertsch, J.H., Johnson, E.W., Castro-Marin, F., Inoue, Y. and Yeh, C. (2003) Efficacy of low-dose acetazolamide (125 mg BID) for the prophylaxis of acute mountain sickness: a prospective, double-blind, randomized, placebo-controlled trial. *High Alt. Med. Biol.* **4**, 45–52.

Basnyat, B., Wu, T.Y. and Certsch, J.H. (2004) Neurological conditions at altitude that fall outside the definition of altitude illness. *High Alt. Med. Biol.* **5**, 171–9.

Basnyat, B., Gertsch, J.H., Holck, P.S. *et al.* (2006) Acetazolamide 125 mg BD is not significantly different from 375 mg BD in the prevention of acute mountain sickness: the prophylactic acetazolamide dosage comparison for efficacy (PACE) trial. *High Alt. Med. Biol.* **7**, 17–27.

Bauer, A., Demetz, F., Bruegger, D. *et al.* (2006) Effect of high altitude and exercise on microvascular parameters in acclimatized subjects. *Clin. Sci. (Lond).* **110**, 207–15.

Baumgartner, R.W., Bärtsch, P., Maggiorini, M., Waber, U. and Oelz, O. (1994) Enhanced cerebral blood flow in acute mountain sickness. *Aviat. Space Environ. Med.* **65**, 726–9.

Baumgartner, R.W., Spyridopoulos, I., Bartsch, P., Maggiorini, M. and Oelz, O. (1999) Acute mountain sickness is not related to cerebral blood flow: a decompression chamber study. *J. Appl. Physiol.* **86**, 1578–82.

Bayliss, R.I.S. (1987) Endocrine manifestations of non-endocrine disease, in *Oxford Textbook of Medicine,* 2nd edn (eds. D.J. Weatherall, J.G.G. Leadingham and D.A. Warrell), Oxford University Press, Oxford, pp. 101–19.

Bazett, H.C. and McGlone, B. (1927) Temperature gradients in the tissues of man. *Am. J. Physiol.* **82**, 415–51.

Beall, C.M., Goldstein, M.C. and the Tibetan Academy of Sciences (1987) Hemoglobin concentration of pastoral nomads permanently resident at 4850–5450 meters in Tibet. *Am. J. Phys. Anthropol.* **73**, 433–8.

Beall, C.M., Blangero, J., Williams-Blangero, S. and Goldstein, M.C. (1994) Major gene for percent of oxygen saturation of arterial hemoglobin in Tibetan highlanders. *Am. J. Phys. Anthropol.* **95**, 271–6.

Beall, C.M., Strohl, K.P., Blangero, J. *et al.* (1997a) Ventilation and hypoxic ventilatory response of Tibetan and Aymara high altitude natives. *Am. J. Anthropol.* **104**, 427–47.

Beall, C.M., Strohl, K.P., Blangero, J. *et al.* (1997b) Quantitative genetic analysis of arterial oxygen saturation in Tibetan highlanders. *Hum. Biol.* **69**, 597–604.

Beall C.M., Brittenham, G.M., Strohl, K.P. *et al.* (1998) Hemoglobin concentration of high-altitude Tibetans and Bolivian Aymara. *Am. J. Anthropol.* **106**, 385–400.

Beall, C.M., Almasy, L.A., Blangero, J. *et al.* (1999) Percent of oxygen saturation of arterial hemoglobin among Bolivian Aymara at 3,990–4,000 m. *Am. J. Phys. Anthropol.* **108**, 41–51.

Beall, C.M., Decker, M.J., Brittenham, G.M., Kushner, I., Gebremedhin, A. and Strohl, K.P. (2002) An Ethiopian pattern of human adaptation to high-altitude hypoxia. *Proc. Natl. Acad. Sci. USA.* **99**, 17215–8. E-pub 5 December 2002.

Beall, C.M., Song, K., Elston, R.C. and Goldstein, M.C. (2004). Higher offspring survival among Tibetan women with high oxygen saturation genotypes residing at 4,000 m. *PNAS* **101**, 14300–4.

Beaumont, M., Goldenberg, F., Lejeune, D., Marotte, H., Horf, A. and Lofaso, F. (1996) Effect of zolpidem on sleep and ventilatory patterns at simulated altitude of 4,000 meters. *Am. J. Respir. Crit. Care Med.* **153**, 1864–9.

Beidleman, B.A., Muza, S.R., Rock, P.B. *et al.* (1997) Exercise responses after altitude acclimatization are retained during reintroduction to altitude. *Med. Sci. Sports Exerc.* **29**, 1588–95.

Beidleman, B.A., Rock, P.B., Muza, S.R. *et al.* (1999) Exercise VE and physical performance at altitude are not affected by menstrual cycle phase. *J. Appl. Physiol.* **86**, 1519–26.

Bell, C. (1928) *The People of Tibet,* Oxford University Press, Oxford, p. 197.

Bencowitz, H.Z., Wagner, P.D. and West, J.B. (1982) Effect of change in P_{50} on exercise tolerance at high altitude: a theoretical study. *J. Appl. Physiol.* **53**, 1487–95.

Bender, P.B., DeBehnke, D.J., Swart, G.L. and Hall, K.N. (1995) Serum potassium concentration as a predictor of resuscitation outcome in hypothermic cardiac arrest. *Wilderness Environ. Med.* **6**, 273–82.

Benesch, R. and Benesch, R.E. (1967) The effect of organic phosphates from the human erythrocyte on the allosteric properties of hemoglobin. *Biochem. Biophys. Res. Commun.* **26**, 162–7.

Benoit, H., Busso, T., Castells, J., Geyssant, A. and Denis, C. (2000) Decrease in peak rate with acute hypoxia in relation to sea level Vo_{2max}. *Eur. J. Appl. Physiol.* **90**, 514–9.

Benson, H., Lehmann, J.W., Malhotra, M.S. *et al.* (1982) Body temperature changes during the practice of g-tum-mo yoga. *Nature* **295**, 234–6.

Berg, B.W., Dillard, T.A., Rajagopal, K.R. and Mehm, W.J. (1992) Oxygen supplementation during air travel in patients with chronic obstructive lung disease. *Chest* **101**, 638–41.

Berg, J.T., Fu, Z., Breen, E.C., Tran, H.-C., Mathieu-Costello, O. and West, J.B. (1997) High lung inflation increases mRNA levels of ECM components and growth factors in lung parenchyma. *J. Appl. Physiol.* **83**, 120–8.

Berg, J.T., Breen, E.C., Fu, Z., Mathieu-Costello, O. and West, J.B. (1998) Alveolar hypoxia causes increased gene expression of extracellular matrix proteins and platelet-derived growth factor B in lung parenchyma. *Am. J. Respir. Crit. Care Med.* **158**, 1920–8.

Berger, J., Aguayo, V.M., Tellez, W., Lujan, C., Traissac, P. and San Miguel, J.L. (1997) Weekly iron supplementation is as effective as 5 day per week iron supplementation in Bolivian school children living at high altitude. *Eur. J. Clin. Nutr.* **51**, 381–6.

Berger, M.M., Hesse, C., Dehnert, C. *et al.* (2005) Hypoxia impairs systemic endothelial function in individuals prone to high-altitude pulmonary edema. *Am. J. Respir. Crit. Care. Med.* **172**, 763–7.

Bergeron, M., Gidday, J.M., Yu, A.Y. *et al.* (2000) Role of hypoxia-inducible factor-1 in hypoxia-induced ischemic tolerance in neonatal rat brain. *Ann. Neurol.* **48**, 285–96.

Berlin, N.I., Reynafarje, C. and Lawrence, J.H. (1954) Red cell life span in the polycythemia of high altitude. *J. Appl. Physiol.* **7**, 271–2.

Bernardi, L., Road, R.C., Keyl, C. *et al.* (2003) Ventilation, autonomic function, sleep and erythropoietin. Chronic mountain sickness of Andean natives. *Ad. Exper. Med. Biol.* **543**, 161–75.

Bernaudin, M., Nedelec, A.S., Divoux, D. *et al.* (2002) Normobaric hypoxia induces tolerance to focal permanent cerebral ischemia in association with an increased expression of hypoxia-inducible factor-1 and its target genes, erythropoietin and VEGF, in the adult mouse brain. *J. Cereb. Blood Flow Metab.* **22**, 393–403.

Berner, G., Froelicher, V.F. and West, J.B. (1988) Trekking in Nepal: safety after coronary artery bypass. *JAMA* **259**, 3184.

Bernhard, W.N., Schalick, I.M., Delaney, P.A. *et al.* (1998) Acetazolamide plus dexamethasone is better than acetazolamide alone to ameliorate symptoms of acute mountain sickness. *Aviat. Space Environ. Med.* **69**, 883–6.

Berre, J., Vachiery, J.L., Moraine, J.J. and Naeije, R. (1999) Cerebral blood flow velocity responses to hypoxia in subjects who are susceptible to high-altitude pulmonary oedema. *Eur. J. Appl. Physiol.* **80**, 260–3.

Berssenbrugge, A., Dempsey, J., Iber, C., Skatral, J. and Wilson, P. (1983) Mechanisms of hypoxia-induced periodic breathing during sleep in humans. *J. Physiol. (Lond.)* **343**, 507–26.

Bert, P. (1878) *La Pression Barométrique.* Masson, Paris. English translation by M.A. Hitchcock and F.A. Hitchcock, College Book Co., Columbus, OH, 1943.

Bestle, M.H., Olsen, N.V., Poulsen, T.D. *et al.* (2002) Prolonged hypobaric hypoxemia attenuates vasopressin secretion and renal response to osmostimulation in men. *J. Appl. Physiol.* **92**, 1911–22.

Bhaumik, G., Purkayastha, S.S., Selvamurthy, W. and Banerjee, P.K. (2003) Oxygen saturation response to exercise Vo_2 at 2100 m and 4350 m in women mountaineering trainees. *Indian J. Physiol. Pharmacol.* **47**, 43–51.

Bigard, A.X., Douce, P., Merino, D. *et al.* (1996a) Changes in dietary protein fail to prevent decrease in muscle growth induced by severe hypoxia in rats. *J. Appl. Physiol.* **80**, 208–15.

Bigard, A.X., Lavier, P., Ullman, L. *et al.* (1996b) Branched-chain amino acid supplementation during repeated prolonged skiing exercises at altitude. *Int. J. Sport Nutr.* **6**, 295–306.

Bircher, H.P., Eichenberger, U., Maggiorini, M., Oelz, O. and Bärtsch, P. (1993) Relationship of mountain sickness to physical fitness and exercise intensity during ascent. *J. Wilderness Med.* **5**, 302–11.

Birgegard, G. and Sandhagen, B. (2001) Erythropoietin treatment can increase 2,3-diphosphoglycerate levels in red blood cells. *Scand. J. Clin. Lab. Invest.* **61**, 337–40.

Birks, J.W., Klassen, L.W. and Curney, C.W. (1975) Hypoxia induced thrombocytopenia in mice. *J. Lab. Clin. Med.* **86**, 230–8.

Birmingham Medical Research Expeditionary Society Mountain Sickness Study Group (1981) Acetazolamide in control of acute mountain sickness. *Lancet* **1**, 180–3.

Biscoe, T.J. and Duchen, M.R. (1990) Cellular basis of transduction in carotid body chemoreceptors. *Am. J. Physiol.* **258**, L270–8.

Bisgard, G.E., Busch, M.A. and Forster, H.V. (1986) Ventilatory acclimatization to hypoxia is not dependent on cerebral hypocapnic alkalosis. *J. Appl. Physiol.* **60**, 1011–14.

Bishop, R.A., Litch, J.A. and Stanton, J.M. (2000) Ketamine anesthesia at high altitude. *High Alt. Med. Biol.* **1**, 111–14.

Bjurstrom, R.L. and Schoene, R.B. (1986) Ventilatory control in elite synchronized swimmers. *Am. Rev. Respir. Dis.* **133** (Suppl.), A134.

Black, C.P. and Tenney, S.M. (1980) Oxygen transport during progressive hypoxia in high-altitude and sea-level waterfowl. *Respir. Physiol.* **39**, 217–39.

Blauw, G.J., Westerterp, R.G., Srivastava, N. *et al.* (1995) Hypoxia induced arterial endothelin does not influence peripheral vascular tone. *J. Cardiol. Pharm.* **3**, S242–3.

Bledsoe, S.W. and Hornbein, T.F. (1981) Central chemosensors and the regulation of their chemical environment, in *Regulation of Breathing, Part I* (ed. T.F. Hornbein), Marcel Dekker, New York, pp. 347–428.

Bligh, J. and Chauca, D. (1978) The effects of intracerebroventricular injections of carbachol and noradrenaline in cold induced pulmonary artery hypertension in sheep. *J. Physiol.* **284**, 53P.

Bligh, J. and Chauca, D. (1982) Effects of hypoxia, cold exposure and fever on pulmonary artery pressure and their significance for Arctic residents, in *Circum Polar Health 1981* (eds. B. Harvald and J.B. Hart Hansen), Report **32**, Nordic Council for Arctic Medical Research, Copenhagen, pp. 606–7.

Blows from the winter wind (editorial) (1980) *BMJ* **1**, 137–8.

Blume, F.D. (1984) Metabolic and endocrine changes at altitude, in *High Altitude and Man* (eds. J.B. West and S. Lahiri), American Physiological Society, Bethesda, MD, pp. 37–45.

Blume, F.D. and Pace, N. (1967) Effect of translocation to 3800 m altitude on glycolysis in mice. *J. Appl. Physiol.* **23**, 75–9.

Blume, F.D. and Pace, N. (1971) The utilisation of ^{14}C-labelled palmitic acid, alanine and aspartic acid at high altitude. *Environ. Physiol.* **1**, 30–6.

Blume, F.D., Boyer, S.J., Braverman, L.E. and Cohen, A. (1984) Impaired osmoregulation at high altitude. *JAMA* **252**, 524–6.

Bocqueraz, O., Koulmann, N., Guigas, B., Jimenez, C. and Melin, B. (2004) Fluid-regulatory hormone responses during cycling exercise in acute hypobaric hypoxia. *Med. Sci. Sports Exerc.* **36**, 1730–6.

Bodary, P.F., Pate, R.R., Wu, Q.F. and McMillan, G.S. (1999) Effects of acute exercise on plasma erythropoietin levels in trained runners. *Med. Sci. Sports Exerc.* **31**, 543–6.

Boero, J.A., Ascher, J., Arregui, A., Rovainen, C. and Woolsey, T.A. (1999) Increased brain capillaries in chronic hypoxia. *J. Appl. Physiol.* **86**, 1211–9.

Bogaard, H.J., Hopkins, S.R., Yamaya, Y. *et al.* (2002) Role of the autonomic nervous system in the reduced maximal cardiac output at altitude. *J. Appl. Physiol.* **93**, 271–9.

Bohn, D.J. (1987) Treatment of hypothermia in hospital, in *Hypothermia and Cold* (eds. J.R. Sutton, C.S. Houston and G. Coates), Prager, New York, pp. 286–305.

Bohr, C. (1885) *Experimentale Untersuchungen über die Sauerstoffaufnahme des Blutfarbstoffes*, O.C. Olsen, Copenhagen.

Bohr, C. (1891) Über die Lungenatmung. *Skand. Arch. Physiol.* **2**, 236–68. English translation in *Translations in Respiratory Physiology* (ed. J.B. West), Hutchinson Ross, Stroudsburg, PA, 1981.

Bohr, C. (1909) Über die spezifische Tätigkeit der Lungen bei der respiratorischen Gasaufnahme und ihr Verhalten zu der durch die Alveolarwand stattfindenden Gasdiffusion. *Skand. Arch. Physiol.* **22**, 221–80. English translation in *Translations in Respiratory Physiology* (ed. J.B. West), Hutchinson Ross, Stroudsburg, PA, 1981.

Bohr, C., Hasselbalch, C.B.K. and Krogh, A. (1904) Ueber einen in biologischer Beziehung wichtigen Einfluss, den die Kohlensäurespannuny des Blutes auf dessen Sauerstoffbinding übt. *Skand. Arch. Physiol.* **16**, 402–12.

Bonelli, J., Waldhausl, W., Magometschnigg, D. *et al.* (1977) Effect of exercise and of prolonged administration of propranolol on haemodynamic variables, plasma renin concentration, plasma aldosterone and c-AMP. *Eur. J. Clin. Invest.* **7**, 337–43.

Boner, A.L., Comis, A., Schiassi, M., Venge, P. and Piacentini, G.L. (1995) Bronchial reactivity in asthmatic children at high and low altitude. Effect of budesonide. *Am. J. Respir. Crit. Care Med.* **151**, 1194–200.

Bonvalot, G. (1891) *Across Thibet,* Cassell, London.

Borgström, L., Johannsson, H. and Siesjö, B.K. (1975) The relationship between arterial P_{O2} and cerebral blood flow in hypoxic hypoxia. *Acta Physiol. Scand.* **93**, 423–32.

Bouchama, A. and De Vol, E.B. (2001) Acid–base alterations in heatstroke. *Intensive Care Med.* **27**, 680–5.

Bouchama, A. and Knochel, J.P. (2002) Medical progress: heat stroke. *New Engl. J. Med.* **346**, 1978–88.

Bouissou, P., Peronnet, F., Brisson, C. *et al.* (1986) Metabolic and endocrine responses to graded exercise under acute hypoxia. *Eur. J. Appl. Physiol.* **55**, 290–4.

Bouissou, P., Guezennec, C.Y., Galen, F.X. *et al.* (1988) Dissociated response of aldosterone from plasma renin activity during prolonged exercise under hypoxia. *Horm. Metab. Res.* **20**, 517–21.

Bouissou, P., Richalet, J.-P., Galen, F.X., Lartigue, M., Larmignet, P., Devaux, F. *et al.* (1989) Effect of β-adrenoreceptor blockade on renin–aldosterone and σ-ANF during exercise at altitude. *J. Appl. Physiol.* **67**, 141–6.

Boulos, P., Kouroukis, C. and Blake, G. (2000) Superior sagittal sinus thrombosis occurring at high altitude associated with protein C deficiency. *Acta Haematol.* **102**, 104–6.

Boussuges, A., Molenat, F., Burnet, H. *et al.* (2000) Operation Everest III (Comex '97): modifications of cardiac function secondary to altitude-induced hypoxia – An echocardiographic and Doppler study. *Am. J. Resp. Crit. Care Med.* **161**, 264–70.

Boutellier, U., Howald, H., di Prampero, P.E., Giezendanner, D. and Cerretelli, P. (1983) Human muscle adaptations to chronic hypoxia. *Prog. Clin. Biol. Res.* **136**, 273–85.

Boycott, A.E. and Haldane, J.S. (1908) The effects of low atmospheric pressures on respiration. *J. Physiol. (Lond.)* **37**, 355–77.

Boyer, S.J. (1978) Endurance test on Colorado's 14,000 ft peaks. *Summit Magazine* **24**, 30–5.

Boyer, S.J. and Blume, F.D. (1984) Weight loss and changes in body composition at high altitude. *J. Appl. Physiol.* **57**, 1580–5.

Boyle, R. (1660) *New Experiments Physico-Mechanicall, Touching the Spring of the Air, and its Effects*. H. Hall for Tho. Robinson, Oxford.

Boyle, R. (1662) *New Experiments Physico-Mechanical, Touching the Air: Whereunto is Added a Defence of the Authors Explication of the Experiments, Against the Objections of Franciscus Linus, and, Thomas Hobbes*. H. Hall for T. Robinson, Oxford. Relevant pages reprinted in *High Altitude Physiology* (ed. J.B. West), Hutchinson Ross, Stroudsburg, PA, 1981.

Bozzini, C.E., Barcelo, A.C., Conti, M.C., Martinez, M.P. and Alippi, R.M. (2005) Enhanced erythropoietin production during hypobaric hypoxia in mice under treatments to keep the erythrocyte mass from rising: implication for the adaptive role for poycythemia. *High Alt. Med. Biol.* **6**, 238–46.

Bradwell, A.R. and Delamere, J.P. (1982) The effect of acetazolamide on the proteinuria of altitude. *Aviat. Space Environ. Med.* **53**, 40–3.

Bradwell, A.R., Dykes, P.W., Coote, J.H. *et al.* (1986) Effect of acetazolamide on exercise performance and muscle mass at high altitude. *Lancet* **1**, 1001–5.

Bradwell, A.R., Winterbourn, M., Wright, A.D. *et al.* (1988) Acetazolamide treatment in acute mountain sickness. *Clin. Sci.* 74 (Suppl. 18), 62P.

Brasher, C. (1986) Wizard of the peaks. *Observer* (London) 29 June.

Brasher, C. (1988) Ascent of superman. *Observer* (London) 26 June.

Brauer, H., Gens, A., Ledderhos, C. *et al.* (1996) Cardiorespiratory and renal responses to arterial chemoreceptor stimulation by hypoxia or almitrine in men. *Clin. & Exper. Pharm. & Physiol.* **23**, 1021–7.

Braun, B. (1997) Substrate Utilization During Rest and Exercise at High Altitude, in *Women at Altitude* (eds.

C.S. Houston and G. Coates), Queen City Printers, Inc., Burlington, VT, pp. 20–34.

Braun, B., Butterfield, G.E., Dominick, S.B. *et al.* (1998) Women at altitude: changes in carbohydrate metabolism at 4,300 m elevation and across the menstrual cycle. *J. Appl. Physiol.* **85**, 1966–73.

Braun, B., Mawson, J.T., Muza, S.R. *et al.* (2000) Women at altitude: carbohydrate utilization during exercise at 4300 m. *J. Appl. Physiol.* **88**, 246–56.

Braun, B., Rock, P.B., Zamudio, S. *et al.* (2001) Women at altitude: Short-term exposure to hypoxia and/or alpha1-adrenergic blockade reduces insulin sensitivity. *J. Appl. Physiol.* **91**, 623–31.

Braun, P. (1985) Pathophysiology and treatment of hypothermia, in *High Altitude Deterioration* (eds. J. Rivolier, P. Cerretelli, J. Foray and P. Segantini), Karger, Basel, pp. 140–8.

Breen, E.C., Johnson, E.C., Wagner, H., Tseng. H.M., Sung, L.A. and Wagner, P.D. (1996) Angiogenic growth factor mRNA responses in muscle to a single bout of exercise. *J. Appl. Physiol.* **81**, 355–61.

Brendel, W. (1956) Anpassung von Atmung, Hämoglobin, Körpertemperatur und Kreislauf bei langfristigem Aufenthalt in grossen Höhen (Himalaya). *Pflügers Arch.* **263**, 227–52.

Brennan, P.J., Greenberg, G., Miall, W.E. and Thompson, S.G. (1982) Seasonal variation in arterial blood pressure. *BMJ* **2**, 919–23.

Brenner, I.K.M., Castellani, J.W., Gabaree, C. *et al.* (1999) Immune changes in humans during cold exposure: effects of prior heating and exercise. *J. Appl. Physiol.* **87**, 699–710.

Brent, P. (1974) *Captain Scott and the Antarctic Tragedy,* Weidenfeld and Nicolson, London.

Brodal, P., Ingjer, F. and Hermansen, L. (1977) Capillary supply of skeletal muscle fibers in untrained and endurance-trained men. *Am. J. Physiol.* **232**, H705–12.

Brooks, G.A., Butterfield, G.E., Wolfe, R.R. *et al.* (1991) Increased dependence on blood glucose after acclimatization to 4300 m. *J. Appl. Physiol.* **70**, 919–27.

Brooks, G.A., Wolfel, E.E., Butterfield, G.E. *et al.* (1998) Poor relationship between arterial [lactate] and leg net release during exercise at 4,300 m altitude. *Am. J. Physiol.* **275**, R1192–201.

Broom, J.R., Stoneham, M.D., Beeley, J.M., Milledge, J.S. and Hughes, A.S. (1994) High altitude headache: treatment with ibuprofen. *Aviat. Space Environ. Med.* **65**, 19–20.

Brown, J.M. and Page, J. (1952) The effect of chronic exposure to cold or temperature and blood flow of the hands. *J. Appl. Physiol.* **5**, 221–7.

Bruce, C.G. (1923) *The Assault on Mt. Everest.* E. Arnold & Co. London.

Brunt, D. (1952) *Physical and Dynamical Meteorology,* 2nd edn, Cambridge University Press, Cambridge, p. 379.

Brutsaert, T.D., Parra, E.J., Shriver, M.D. *et al.* (2003) Spanish genetic admixture is associated with larger V(O2) max decrement from sea level to 4338 m in Peruvian Quechua. *J. Appl. Physiol.* **95**, 519–28. E-pub 11 April 2003.

Budd, G.M. (1984) Daily fluid balance. International Biomedical Expedition to the Antarctic. *6th International Symposium on Circum Polar Health,* Anchorage, May 1984, pp. 59–60.

Buettner, K.J.K. (1969) The effect of natural sunlight on human skin, in *The Biologic Effects of Ultraviolet Radiation, with Special Emphasis on the Skin* (ed. F. Urbach), Pergamon Press, Oxford, pp. 237–49.

Buguet, A.G.C., Livingstone, S.D. and Reed, L.D. (1979) Skin temperature changes in paradoxical sleep in man in the cold. *Aviat. Space Environ. Med.* **50**, 567–70.

Buick, F., Gledhill, N., Froese, A. *et al.* (1980) Effects of induced erythrocythemia on aerobic work capacity. *J. Appl. Physiol.* **48**, 636–42.

Bulow, K. (1963) Respiration and wakefulness in man. *Acta Physiol. Scand.* **59** (Suppl. 209), 1–110.

Burch, G.E. (1945) Rate of water loss from the respiratory tract of normal subjects in a subtropical climate. *Arch. Int. Med.* **76**, 315–27.

Burgess, K.R., Johnson, P.L. and Edwards, N. (2004) Central and obstructive sleep apnoea during ascent to high altitude. *Respirology* **9**, 222–9.

Burr, R.E. (1993) Trench foot. *J. Wilderness Med.* **4**, 348–52.

Burri, P.H. and Weibel, E.R. (1971) Morphometric estimation of pulmonary diffusion capacity. II. Effect of P_{O2} on the growing lung; adaption of the growing rat lung to hypoxia and hyperoxia. *Respir. Physiol.* **11**, 247–64.

Burton, A.C. and Edholm, O.G. (1955) *Man in a Cold Environment,* Arnold, London.

Burtscher, M., Bachman, O., Hatzl, T. *et al.* (2001) Cardiopulmonary and metabolic responses to healthy elderly humans during a 1 week hiking program at high altitude. *Eur. J. Appl. Physiol.* **84**, 379–86.

Burtscher, M., Flatz, M. and Faulhaber, M. (2004) Prediction of susceptibility to acute mountain sickness by SaO2 values during short-term exposure to hypoxia. *High Alt. Med. Biol.* **5**, 335–40.

Burtscher, M.B., Likar, R., Nachbauer, W. and Philadelphy, M. (1998) Aspirin for prophylaxis against headache at high altitudes: randomised, double blind, placebo controlled trial. *BMJ* **316**, 1057–8.

Burtscher, M.B., Philadelphy, M., Likar, R. and Nachbauer, W. (1999) Aspirin versus diamox plus aspirin for headache during physical activity at high altitude (abstract), in *Hypoxia: Into the Next Millennium* (eds. R.C. Roach, P.D. Wagner and P.H. Hackett), Plenum/Kluwer, New York, p. 133.

Busch, T., Bartsch, P., Pappert, D. *et al.* (2001) Hypoxia decreases exhaled nitric oxide in mountaineers susceptible to high-altitude pulmonary edema. *Am. J. Respir. Crit. Care. Med.* **345**, 107–14.

Buschke, H. (1973) Selective reminding for analysis of memory and learning. *J. Verb. Learn. Verb. Behav.* **13**, 543–50.

Buskirk, E.R. (1977) Temperature regulation with exercise. *Exerc. Sport Sci. Rev.* **5**, 45–88.

Buskirk, E.R. (1978) Work capacity of high-altitude natives, in *The Biology of High Altitude Peoples* (ed. P.T. Baker), Cambridge University Press, Cambridge, pp. 173–87.

Butson, A.R.C. (1949) Acclimatization to cold in Antarctica (Letter). *Nature* **163**, 132–3.

Butson, A.R.C. (1975) Effects and prevention of frostbite in wound healing. *Can. J. Surg.* **18**, 145–8.

Butterfield, G. (1997) Energy requirements of Women at Altitude, in *Women at Altitude* (eds. C.S. Houston and G. Coates), Queen City Printers, Inc., Burlington, VT, pp. 8–19.

Butterfield, G.E., Gates, J., Fleming, S. *et al.* (1992) Increased energy intake minimizes weight loss in men at high altitude. *J. Appl. Physiol.* **72**, 1741–8.

Byrne-Quinn, E., Weil, J.V., Sodal, I.E. *et al.* (1971) Ventilatory control in the athlete. *J. Appl. Physiol.* **30**, 91–8.

Cabanac, M. and LeBlanc, J. (1983) Physiological conflict in humans: fatigue vs. cold discomfort. *Am. J. Physiol.* **244**, R621–8.

Cabrera de Leon, A., Gonzalez, D.A., Mendez, L.I. *et al.* (2004) Leptin and altitude in the cardiovascular diseases. *Obes. Res.* **12**, 1492–8.

Cahoon, R.L. (1972) Simple decision making at high altitude. *Ergonomics* **15**, 157–63.

Cain, S.M. and Dunn, J.E. (1965) Increase of arterial oxygen tension at altitude by carbonic anhydrase inhibition. *J. Appl. Physiol.* **20**, 882–4.

Calbet, J.A. (2003) Chronic hypoxia increases blood pressure and noradrenalin spillover in healthy subjects. *J. Physiol. (Lond.)* **551**, 379–86.

Calbet, J., Radegran, G., Boushel, R., Sondergaard, H., Saltin, B. and Wagner, P.D. (2002) Effect of blood haemoglobin concentration on VO_2max and cardiovascular function in lowlanders acclimatized to 5260 m. *J. App. Physiol.* **545**, 715–28.

Calbet, J.A., Radegran, G., Boushel, R., Sondergaard, H., Saltin, B. and Wagner, P.D. (2004) Plasma volume expansion does not increase maximal cardiac ouput or VO_2 max in lowlanders acclimatized to altitude. *Am. J. Physiol Heart Circ. Physiol.* **287**, H1214–24.

Campbell, R.H.A., Brand, H.L., Cox, J.R. and Howard, P. (1975) Body weight and body water in chronic cor pulmonale. *Clin. Sci. Mol. Med.* **49**, 323–35.

Caplan, C.E. (1999) The big chill: diseases exacerbated by exposure to cold. *Can. Med. Assoc. J.* **160**, 88.

Cargill, R.I., Kiely, D.G., Clark, R.A. and Lipworth, B.J. (1995) Hypoxaemia and release of endothelin-1. *Thorax* **50**, 1308–10.

Carlsten, C., Swenson, E.R. and Ruoss, S. (2004) A dose–response study of acetazolamide for acute mountain sickness prophylaxis in vacationing tourists at 12,000 feet (3630 m). *High Alt. Med. Biol.* **5**, 33–9.

Carpenter, T.C., Reeves, J.T. and Durmowicz, A.G. (1998) Viral respiratory infection increases susceptibility of young rats to hypoxia-induced pulmonary edema. *J. Appl. Physiol.* **84**, 1048–54.

Carrillo, C. (1996) Pregnancy at high altitude (abstract). *Acta Andina* **5**(2), 67.

Cassin, S.R., Gilbert, R.D., Bunnell, C.E. and Johnson, E.M. (1971) Capillary development during exposure to chronic hypoxia. *Am. J. Physiol.* **220**, 448–51.

Castellani, J.W., Young, A.J., Sawka, M.W. *et al.* (1998) Amnesia during cold water immersion. A case report. *Wilderness Environ. Med.* **9**, 153–5.

Castellani, J.W., Young, A.J., Kain, J.E. and Sawka, M.W. (1999a) Thermo regulatory responses to cold water at different times of day. *J. Appl. Physiol.* **87**, 243–6.

Castellani, J.W., Young, A.J., Kain, J.E. *et al.* (1999b) Thermoregulation during cold exposure: effects of prior exercise. *J. Appl. Physiol.* **87**, 247–52.

Castellini, M.A. and Somero, G.N. (1981) Buffering capacity of vertebrate muscle – correlations with potentials for anaerobic function. *J. Comp. Physiol.* **143**, 191–8.

Castilla, E.E., Lopez-Camelo, J.S. and Campana, H. (1999) Altitude as a risk factor for congenital anomalies. *Am. J. Med. Genet.* **86**, 9–14.

Catron, T.F., Powell, F.L. and West, J.B. (2006) A Strategy for determining arterial blood gasses on the summit of Mt Everest. *BMC Phsyiol.* **6**, 3.

Cattermole, T.J. (1999) The epidemiology of cold injury in Antarctica. *Aviat. Space Environ. Med.* **70**, 135–40.

Cauchy, E., Chetaille, E., Marchand, V. and Marsigny, B. (2001) Retrospective study of 70 cases of severe frostbite lesion: a proposed new classification scheme. *Wild. Environ. Med.* **12**, 248–55.

Cavaletti, G. and Tredici, G. (1993) Long-lasting neuropsychological changes after a single high altitude climb. *Acta Neurol. Scand.* **87**, 103–5.

Cavaletti, G., Moroni, R., Garavaglia, P. and Tredici, G. (1987) Brain damage after high-altitude climbs without oxygen. *Lancet* **1**, 101.

Cerretelli, P. (1976a) Limiting factors to oxygen transport on Mount Everest. *J. Appl. Physiol.* **40**, 658–67.

Cerretelli, P. (1976b) Metabolismo ossidativo ed anaerobico nel soggetto acclimatato all'altitudine. Rilievi sperimentali nel corso della spedizione italiana all'Everest. *Minerva Med.* **67**, 2331–46.

Cerretelli, P. (1980) Gas exchange at high altitude, in *Pulmonary Gas Exchange,* Vol. II (ed. J.B. West), Academic Press, New York, pp. 97–147.

Cerretelli, P. (1987) Extreme hypoxia in air breathers: some problems, in *Comparative Physiology of Environmental Adaptations,* Vol. 2: *Adapatations to Extreme Environments* (ed. P. Dejours), Karger, Basel.

Cerretelli, P. (1992) Energy sources for muscular exercise. *Int. J. Sports Med.* **13**(Suppl 1), S106–10.

Cerretelli, P. and Hoppeler, H. (1996) Morphologic and metabolic response to chronic hypoxia: the muscle system, in *Handbook of Physiology*, Section 4: *Environmental Physiology,* Vol. II (eds. M.J. Fregly and C.M. Blatteis), American Physiological Society, New York, pp. 1155–81.

Cerretelli, P. and Whipp, B.J. (1980) *Exercise Bioenergetics and Gas Exchange.* Elsevier/North-Holland Biomedical Press, Amsterdam.

Cerretelli, P., Marconi, C., Dériaz, O. and Giezendanner, D. (1984) After effects of chronic hypoxia on cardiac output and muscle blood flow at rest and exercise. *Eur. J. Appl. Physiol.* **53**, 92–6.

Chan, C., Hoar, H., Pattinson, K. *et al.* (2005) Effect of sildenafil and acclimatization on cerebral oxygenation at altitude *Clin. Sci.* **109**, 319–24.

Chance, B. (1957) Cellular oxygen requirements. *Fed. Proc.* **16**, 671–80.

Chance, B., Cohen, P., Jobsis, F. and Schoener, B. (1962) Intracellular oxidation-reduction states *in vivo*. *Science* **137**, 499–508.

Chandrashekhar, Y., Anand, I.S., Rao, K.S. and Malhotra, R.M. (1992) Continuous ambulatory electrocardiographic changes after rapid ascent to extreme altitudes. *Indian Heart J.* **44**, 403–5.

Chang, C., Chen, N., Coward, M.P. *et al.* (1986) Preliminary conclusions of the Royal Society and Academic Sinica 1985 Geotraverse of Tibet. *Nature* **323**, 501–7.

Chanutin, A. and Curnish, R.R. (1967) Effect of organic and inorganic phosphates on the oxygen equilibrium of human erythrocytes. *Arch. Biochem. Biophys.* **121**, 96–102.

Chapman, F.S. (1938) *Lhasa. The Holy City*, Chatto and Windus, London, p. 241.

Chapman, J.A., Grant, I.S., Taylor, G. *et al.* (1972) Endemic goitre in the Gilgit Agency, West Pakistan. *Philos. Trans. R. Soc. Lond. Ser. B* **263**, 459–91.

Chapman, K.R. and Cherniack, N.S. (1986) Aging effects on the interaction of hypercapnia and hypoxia as ventilatory stimuli. *Am. Rev. Respir. Dis.* **133** (Suppl. A), 137.

Chapman, R.F., Stray-Gundersen, J. and Levine, B.D. (1998) Individual variation in response to altitude training. *J. Appl. Physiol.* **85**, 1448–56.

Chatterji, J.C., Ohri, V.C., Das, B.K. *et al.* (1982) Platelet count, platelet aggregation and fibrinogen levels following acute induction to high altitude (3200 and 3771 metres). *Thromb. Res.* **26**, 177–82.

Chavez, J.C., Agani, F., Pichiule, P. and LaManna, J.C. (2000) Expression of hypoxia-inducible factor-1alpha in the brain of rats during chronic hypoxia. *J. Appl. Physiol.* **89**, 1937–42.

Chen, Q.H., Ge, R.L., Wang, X.Z. *et al.* (1997) Exercise performance of Tibetan and Han adolescents at altitudes of 3,417 and 4,300 m. *J. Appl. Physiol.* **83**, 661–7.

Chen, Y.C., Wong, L.Z., Mung, Z.H. and Fung, G.Y. (1982) An analysis of 300 cases of high altitude heart disease in adults [in Chinese]. *Zhonghua Xin Xue Guan Bing Za Zhi* **10**, 256–8.

Chernow, B., Lake, C.R., Zaritsky, A. *et al.* (1983) Sympathetic nervous system 'switch off' with severe hypothermia. *Crit. Care Med.* **11**, 677–80.

Chesner, I.M., Small, N.A. and Dykes, P.W. (1987) Intestinal absorption at high altitude. *Postgrad. Med. J.* **63**, 173–5.

Cheyne, J. (1818) A case of apoplexy in which the fleshy part of the heart was converted into fat. *Dublin Hosp. Rep.* **2**, 216–23.

Chiodi, H. (1957) Respiratory adaptations to chronic high altitude hypoxia. *J. Appl. Physiol.* **10**, 81–7.

Chouker, A., Demetz, F., Martignoni, A. *et al.* (2005) Strenuous physical exercise inhibits granulocyte activation induced by high altitude. *J. Appl. Physiol.* **98**, 640–7.

Chrenko, F.A. and Pugh, L.G.C.E. (1961) The contribution of solar radiation to the thermal environment of man in Antarctica. *Proc. R. Soc. Lond. Ser. B* **155**, 243–65.

Christensen, C.C., Ryg, M., Refvem, O.K. and Skjonsberg, O.H. (2000) Development of severe hypoxaemia in chronic obstructive pulmonary disease patients at 2,438 m (8,000 feet). *Eur. Respir. J.* **15**, 635–9.

Christensen, E.H. (1937) Sauerstoffaufnahme und Respiratorische Funktionen in Grossen Höhen. *Skand. Arch. Physiol.* **76**, 88–100.

Christensen, E.H. and Forbes, W.H. (1937) Der Kreislauf in grossen Höhen. *Skand. Arch. Physiol.* **76**, 75–87.

Cibella, F., Cuttitta, G., Romano, S., Grassi, B., Bonsignore, G. and Milic-Emili, J. (1999) Respiratory energetics during exercise at high altitude. *J. Appl. Physiol.* **86**, 1785–92.

Clark, C.F., Heaton, R.K. and Wiens, A.N. (1983) Neuropsychological functioning after prolonged high altitude exposure in mountaineering. *Aviat. Space Environ. Med.* **54**, 202–7.

Clark, I.M., Awburn, M.M., Cowden, W.B. and Rockett, K.A. (1999) Can excessive iNOS induction explain much of the illness of acute mountain sickness, in *Hypoxia: Into the Next Millennium* (eds. R.C. Roach, P.D. Wagner and P.H. Hackett), Plenum/Kluwer, New York, p. 373.

Clark, R.T., Criscuolo, D. and Coulson, D.K. (1952) Effects of 20,000 feet simulated altitude on myoglobin content of animals with and without exercise. *Fed. Proc.* **11**, 25.

Clarke, C. and Duff, J. (1976) Mountain sickness, retinal haemorrhages, and acclimatization on Mount Everest in 1975. *BMJ* **2**, 495–7.

Clarke, C.R.A. (1983) Cerebral infarction at extreme altitude, in *Hypoxia, Exercise and Altitude* (eds. J.R. Sutton, C.S. Houston and N.L. Jones), Liss, New York, pp. 453–4.

Claybaugh, J.R., Wade, C.E., Sato, A.K. *et al.* (1982) Antidiuretic hormone responses to eucapnic and hypocapnic hypoxia in humans. *J. Appl. Physiol. Respir. Environ. Exerc. Physiol.* **53**, 815–23.

Claydon, V.E., Norcliffe, L.J., Moore, J.P. *et al.* (2005) Cardiovascular responses to orthostatic stress in healthy altitude dwellers and altitude residents with chronic mountain sickness. *Exper. Physiol.* **90**, 103–10.

Clegg, E.J. (1978) Fertility and early growth, in *The Biology of High Altitude Peoples* (ed. P.T. Baker), Cambridge University Press, Cambridge, pp. 65–115.

Clini, E., Bianchi, L., Foglio, K., Vitacca, M. and Ambrosino, N. (2002) Exhaled nitric oxide and exercise tolerance in severe COPD patients. *Respir. Med.* **96**, 312–6.

Cochrane, G.M., Prior, J.G. and Wolff, C.B. (1980) Chronic stable asthma and the normal arterial pressure of carbon dioxide in hypoxia. *BMJ* **301**, 705–7.

Cogo, A., Basnyat, B., Legnani, D. and Allegra, L. (1997) Bronchial asthma and airway hyperresponsiveness at high altitude. *Respiration* **64**, 444–9.

Cogo, A., Fischer, R. and Schoene, R. (2004) Respiratory diseases and high altitude. *High Alt. Med. Biol.* **5**, 435–44.

Cold hypersensitivity (editorial) (1975) *BMJ* **1**, 643–4.

Colice, C.L. and Ramirez, C. (1986) Aldosterone response to angiotensin II during hypoxemia. *J. Appl. Physiol.* **61**, 150–4.

Collier, D.J., Nickol, A., Milledge, J.S. *et al.* (1995) Dynamic chemosensitivity to carbon dioxide increases with acclimatisation to chronic hypoxia in man. *J. Physiol. (Lond.)* **487**, 109P.

Collier, D., Wolff, C.B., Nathan, J. *et al.* (1997a) Benzolamide, acidosis and acute mountain sickness, in *Hypoxia: Women at Altitude* (eds. C.S. Houston and G. Coates), Queen City Printers, Burlington, VA. p. 307

Collier, D.J., Collier, C.J., Dubowitz, G., and Rosenberg, M. (1997b) Gender and weight loss at altitude (abstract), in *Hypoxia: Women at Altitude* (eds. C.S. Houston and G. Coates), Queen City Printers, Burlington, VA, p. 308.

Colquohoun, W.P. (1984) Effects of personality on body temperature and mental efficiency following transmeridian flight. *Aviat. Space Environ. Med.* **55**, 493–6.

Comroe, J.H. (1938) The location and function of the chemoreceptors of the aorta. *Am. J. Physiol.* **127**, 176–91.

Conley, K.E., Esselman, P.C., Jubrias, S.A. *et al.* (2000) Ageing, muscle properties and maximal O_2 uptake rate in humans. *J. Physiol.* **526**, 211–7.

Connaughton, J.J., Douglas, N.J., Morgan, A.D. *et al.* (1985) Almitrine improves oxygenation when both awake and asleep in patients with hypoxia and carbon dioxide retention caused by chronic bronchitis and emphysema. *Am. Rev. Respir. Dis.* **132**, 206–10.

Consolazio, C.F., Matoush, L.O., Johnson, H.L. and Daws, T.A. (1968) Protein and water balances of young adults during prolonged exposure to high altitude (4300 m). *Am. J. Clin. Nutr.* **21**, 134–61.

Consolazio, C.F., Matoush, L.O., Johnson, H.L. *et al.* (1969) Effects of high carbohydrate diets on performance and clinical symptomatology after rapid ascent to high altitude. *Fed. Proc.* **28**, 937–43.

Consolazio, C.F., Johnson, H.L., Krzywicki, H.J. and Daws, T.A. (1972) Metabolic aspects of acute altitude exposure (4300 m) in adequately nourished humans. *Am. J. Clin. Nutr.* **25**, 23–9.

Cook, J.D., Boy, E., Flowers, C. and Daroca Mdel, C. (2005) The influence of high-altitude living on body iron. *Blood* **106**, 1441–6. E-pub 3 May 2005.

Coppin, E.G., Livingstone, S.P. and Kuehn, L.A. (1978) Effects on hand grip strength due to arm immersion in a 10°C water bath. *Aviat. Space Environ. Med.* **49**, 1319–26.

Cornolo, J., Brugniaux, J.V., Macarlupu, J.L., Privat, C., Leon-Velarde, F. and Richalet, J.P. (2005) Autonomic adaptations in andean trained participants to a 4220-m altitude marathon. *Med. Sci. Sports Exerc.* **37**, 2148–53.

Cosby, R.L., Sophocles, A.M., Durr, J.A. *et al.* (1988) Elevated plasma atrial natriuretic factor and vasopressin in high-altitude pulmonary edema. *Ann. Intern. Med.* **109**, 796–9.

Costello, M.L., Mathieu-Costello, O. and West, J.B. (1992) Stress failure of alveolar epithelial cells studied by scanning electron microscopy. *Am. Rev. Respir. Dis.* **145**, 1446–55.

Costil, D.L., Coyle, E., Dalsky, G. *et al.* (1977) Effect of elevated plasma FFA and insulin on muscle glycogen usage during exercise. *J. Appl. Physiol.* **43**, 695–9.

Cotes, J.E. (1954) Ventilatory capacity at altitude and its relation to mask design. *Proc. R. Soc. (Lond). Ser. B* **143**, 32–9.

Coward, W.A. (1991) Measurement of energy expenditure: the doubly labelled water method in clinical practice. *Proc. Nutr. Soc.* **50**, 227–37.

Crawford, J.P. (1979) Endogenous anxiety and circadian rhythms. *BMJ* **1**, 662.

Crawford, R.D. and Severinghaus, J.W. (1978) CSF pH and ventilatory acclimatization to altitude. *J. Appl. Physiol.* **44**, 274–83.

Cremona, G., Asnaghi, R., Baderna, P. *et al.* (2002) Pulmonary extravascular fluid accumulation in recreational climbers: a prospective study. *Lancet* **359**, 303–9.

Crognier, E., Villena, M. and Vargas, E. (2002) Reproduction in high altitude Aymara: physiological stress and fertility planning? *J. Biosoc. Sci.* **34**, 463–73.

Cruden, N.L.M., Newby, D.E., Ross, J.A., Johnston, N.R. and Webb, D.J. (1998) Effect of high altitude, cold and exercise on plasma endothelin-1 and markers of endothelial function in man. (Abstract) *Clin. Sci.* **94**, p. 20.

Cruden, N.L.M., Newby, D.E., Ross, J.A. *et al.* (1999) Effect of cold exposure, exercise and high altitude on plasma endothelin-1 and endothelial cell markers in man. *Scott. Med. J.* **44**, 143–6.

Cruz, J.C., Diaz, C., Marticorena, E. and Hilario, V. (1979) Phlebotomy improves pulmonary gas exchange in chronic mountain polycythemia. *Respiration* **38**, 305–13.

Cruz, J.C., Reeves, J.T., Grover, R.F. *et al.* (1980) Ventilatory acclimatization to high altitude is prevented by CO_2 breathing. *Respiration* **39**, 121–30.

Cudaback, D.M. (1984) Four-km altitude effects on performance and health. *Publ. Astronom. Soc. Pacif.* **96**, 463–77.

Cumbo, T.A., Basnyat, B., Graham, J., Lescano, A.G. and Gambert, S. (2002) Acute mountain sickness, dehydration, and bicarbonate clearance: preliminary field data from the Nepal Himalaya. *Aviat. Space Environ. Med.* **73**, 898–901.

Cummings, P. and Lysgaard, M. (1981) Cardiac arrhythmia at high altitude. *West. J. Med.* **135**, 66–8.

Cunningham, D.J.C., Cormack, R.S., O'Riordan, J.L.H., Jukes, M.G. and Lloyd, B.B. (1957) Arrangement for studying the respiratory effect in man of various factors. *Q. J. Exp. Physiol.* **42**, 294–303.

Cunningham, D.J.C., Patrick, J.M. and Lloyd, B.B. (1964) The respiratory response of man to hypoxia, in *Oxygen in the Animal Organism* (eds. F. Dickens and E. Niel), Pergamon, Oxford, pp. 277–93.

Cunningham, W.L., Becker, E.J. and Kreuzer, F. (1965) Catecholamine in plasma and urine at high altitude. *J. Appl. Physiol.* **20**, 607–10.

Curran, L.S., Zhuang, J., Droma, T. *et al.* (1995) Hypoxic ventilatory response in Tibetan residents of 4400 m compared with 3658 m. *Respir. Physiol.* **100**, 223–30.

Curran, L.S., Zhuang, J., Sun, S.F. and Moore, L.G. (1997) Ventilation and hypoxic ventilatory responsiveness in Chinese-Tibetan residents at 3,658 m. *J. Appl. Physiol.* **83**, 2098–104.

Curran, L.S., Zhuang, J., Droma, T. and Moore, L.G. (1998) Superior exercise performance in lifelong Tibetan residents of 4,400 m compared with Tibetan residents of 3,658 m. *Am. J. Phys. Anthropol.* **105**, 21–31.

Currie, T.T., Carter, P.H., Champion, W.L. *et al.* (1976) Spironolactone and acute mountain sickness. *Med. J. Aust.* **2**, 168–70.

Cymerman, A., Lieberman, P., Hochstadt, J., Rock, P.B., Butterfield, G.E. and Moore, L.G. (2002) Speech motor control and acute mountain sickness. *Aviat. Space Environ. Med.* **73**, 766–72.

Dagg, K.D., Thomson, L.J, Clayton, R.A. *et al.* (1997) Effect of acute alterations in inspired oxygen tension on methacholine induced bronchoconstriction. *Thorax* **52**, 453–7. (thorax.bmjjournals.com)

Daleau, P., Morgardo, D.C., Iriartem C.A. and Desbiens, R. (2006) New epilepsy seizure at high altitude without signs of acute mountain sickness or high altitude cerebral edema. *High Alt. Med. Biol.* **7**, 81–3. (ncbi.nlm.nih.gov)

Dang, S., Yan, H., Yamamoto, S., Wang, X. and Zeng, L. (2004) Poor nutritional status of younger Tibetan children living at high altitudes. *Eur. J. Clin. Nutr.* **58**, 938–46.

Daniels, J. and Oldridge, N. (1970) The effects of alternate exposure to altitude and sea level on world class middle distance runners. *Med. Sci. Sports Exerc.* **2**, 107–112.

Danzl, D.F., Pozos, R.S. and Hamlet, M.P. (1995) Accidental hypothermia, in *Wilderness Medicine* (ed. P.S. Auerbach), Mosby, St Louis, Mo, pp. 51–103.

Das, B.K., Tewari, S.C., Parashar, S.K. *et al.* (1983) Electrocardiographic changes at high altitude. *Indian Heart J.* **35**, 30–3.

Das, S.C. (1902) *Journey to Lhasa and Central Tibet,* John Murray, London, pp. 257–60.

Datta, A.K. and Nickol, A. (1995) Dynamic chemoreceptiveness studied in man during moderate exercise breath by breath, in *Modeling and Control of Ventilation* (eds. S.J.G. Semple, L. Adams, and B.J. Whipp), Plenum Press, New York, pp. 235–8.

Davies, R.O., Edwards, M.W. Jr and Lahiri, S. (1982) Halothane depresses the response of carotid body chemoreceptors to hypoxia and hypercapnia in the cat. *Anesthesiology* **57**, 153–9.

Dawson, A. (1972) Regional lung function during early acclimatization to 3,100 m altitude. *J. Appl. Physiol.* **33**, 218–23.

De Angelis, C., Ferri, C., Urbani, L. and Ferrace, S. (1996) Effect of acute exposure to hypoxia on electrolyes and water metabolism regulatory hormones. *Aviat. Space Environ. Med.* **67**, 746–50.

Deasy, H.H.P. (1901) *In Tibet and Chinese Turkestan,* T. Fisher Unwin, London, pp. 2–73.

Decramer, M., De Benedetto, F., Del Ponte, A. and Marinari, S. (2005) Systemic effects of COPD. *Respir. Med.* **99**(Suppl B), S3–10.

Deem, S., Hedges, R.G., Kerr, M.E. and Swenson, E.R. (2000) Acetazolamide reduces hypoxic pulmonary vasoconstriction in isolated perfused rabbit lungs. *Respir. Physiol.* **123**, 109–19.

De Filippi, F. (1912) *Karakoram and Western Himalaya, 1900,* Constable, London.

De Glinsezinski, J., Crampes, F., Harant, I., *et al.* (1999) Decrease in subcutaneous adipose tissue lipolysis after exposure to hypoxia during a simulated ascent of Mt Everest. *Eur. J. Physiol.* **439**, 134–40.

DeGraff, A.C., Jr, Grover, R.F., Johnson, R.L., Jr, Hammond, J.W., Jr and Miller, J.M. (1970) Diffusing capacity of the lung in Caucasians native to 3,100 m. *J. Appl. Physiol.* **29**, 71–6.

Dehnert, C., Weymann, J., Montgomery, H.E. *et al.* (2002a) No association between high-altitude tolerance and the ACE I/D gene polymorphism. *Med. Sci. Sports. Exerc.* **34**, 1928–33.

Dehnert, C., Hutler, M., Liu, Y. *et al.* (2002b) Erythropoiesis and performance after two weeks of living high and training low in well trained triathletes. *Int. J. Sports Med.* **23**, 561–6.

De Jong, G.F. (ed.) (1968) *Demography of High Altitude Populations,* WHO/PAHO/IBP Meeting of Investigators on Population Biology of Altitude, Pan American Health Organization, Washington DC.

Dejours, P., Girard, F., Labrousse, Y. and Teillac, A. (1959) Etude de al régulation de la ventilation de repos chez l'homme en haute altitude. *Rev. Franc. Etudes Clin. et Biol.* **4**, 115–27.

del Pilar Valle, M., Garcia-Godos, F., Marticirena J.M. *et al.* (2006) Improvement of myocardial perfusion in coronary patients after intermittent hypoxia. *J. Nucl. Cardiol.* **13**, 69–74.

de Meer, K., Heymans, H.S. and Zijlstra, W.G. (1995) Physical adaptation of children to life at high altitude. *Eur. J. Ped.* **154**, 263–72.

De Pay, A.W. (1982) Medical treatment of hypothermic victims, in *Unterkuhlung im Seenotfall,* 2nd Symposium Deutsche Gesellschaft zur Rettung

Schiffbruchiger (eds. P. Koch and M. Kohfahl), Cuxhaven, Germany pp. 146–53.

de Saussure, H.-B. (1786–7) *Voyages Dans Les Alpes,* 4 volumes, Barde, Manget, Geneva.

Dempsey, J.A. (1983) Ventilatory regulation in hypoxic sleep: introduction, in *Hypoxia, Exercise, and Altitude* (eds. J.R. Sutton, C.S. Houston and N.L. Jones), Liss, New York, pp. 61–3.

Dempsey, J.A. and Forster, H.V. (1982) Mediation of ventilatory adaptations. *Physiol. Rev.* **62**, 262–346.

Dempsey, J.A., Reddan, W.G., Birnbaum, M.L. *et al.* (1971) Effects of acute through life-long hypoxic exposure on exercise pulmonary gas exchange. *Respir. Physiol.* **13**, 62–89.

Dempsey, J.A., Forster, H.V., Chosy, L.W., Hanson, P.G. and Reddan, W.G. (1978) Regulation of CSF [HCO_3^-] during long-term hypoxic hypocapnia in man. *J. Appl. Physiol.* **44**, 175–82.

Dempsey, J.A., Forster, H.V., Bisgard, G.E. *et al.* (1979) Role of cerebrospinal fluid [H^+] in ventilatory deacclimatization from chronic hypoxia. *J. Clin. Invest.* **64**, 199–204.

Denison, D.M., Ledwith, F. and Poulton, E.C. (1966) Complex reaction times at simulated cabin altitudes of 5,000 feet and 8,000 feet. *Aerosp. Med.* **37**, 1010–13.

Denjean, A., Roux, C., Herve, P. *et al.* (1988) Mild isocapnic hypoxia enhances the bronchial response to methacholine in asthmatic subjects. *Am. Rev. Respir. Dis.* **138**, 789–93.

Desideri, L. (1712–27) Journey across the great desert of Nguari Giongar, and assistance rendered by a Tartar princess and her followers, in *An Account of Tibet* (ed. F. de Filippi), Routledge, London, 1932, p. 87.

Desplanches, D., Hoppeler, H., Linossier, M.T. *et al.* (1993) Effects of training in normoxia and normobaric hypoxia on human muscle structure. *Pflügers Arch.* **425**, 263–7.

Dickinson, J., Heath, D., Gosney, J. and Williams, D. (1983) Altitude related deaths in seven trekkers in the Himalayas. *Thorax* **38**, 646–56.

Dickinson, J.G. (1979) Severe acute mountain sickness. *Postgrad. Med. J.* **55**, 454–8.

Dickinson, J.G. (1982) Terminology and classification of acute mountain sickness. *BMJ* **285**, 720–1.

Diffey, B.L. (1991) Solar ultraviolet radiation effects on biological systems. *Phys. Med. Biol.* **36**, 299–328.

Dill, D.B., Edwards, H.T., Fölling, A., Oberg, S.A., Pappenheimer, A.M. Jr and Talbott, J.H. (1931)

Adaptations of the organism to changes in oxygen pressure. *J. Physiol. (Lond.)* **71**, 47–63.

Dill, D.B., Talbott, J.H. and Consolazio, W.V. (1937) Blood as a physiochemical system. XII. Man at high altitudes. *J. Biol. Chem.* **118**, 649–66.

Dill, D.B., Robinson, S., Balke, B. and Newton, J.L. (1964) Work tolerance: age and altitude. *J. Appl. Physiol.* **19**, 483–8.

Dillard, T.A. and Ewald Jr., F.W. (2004) The use of pulmonary function testing in piloting, air travel, mountain climbing, and diving. *Clin. Chest Med.* **22**, 795–816.

Dillard, T.A., Berg, B.W., Rajagopal, K.R. *et al.* (1989) Hypoxemia during air travel in patients with chronic obstructive pulmonary disease. *Ann. Intern. Med.* **111**, 362–7.

Dillard, T.A., Beninati, W.A. and Berg, B.W. (1991) Air travel in patients with chronic obstructive pulmonary disease. *Arch. Intern. Med.* **151**, 1793–5.

Dillard, T.A., Rosenberg, A.P. and Berg, B.W. (1993) Hypoxemia during altitude exposure. A meta-analysis of chronic obstructive pulmonary disease. *Chest* **103**, 422–5.

Dillard, T.A., Rajagopal, K.R., Slivka, W.A. *et al.* (1998) Lung function during moderate hypobaric hypoxia in normal subjects and patients with chronic obstructive pulmonary disease. *Aviat. Space Environ. Med.* **69**, 979–85.

Dillard, T.A., Khosla, S., Ewald, F.W. Jr, Kaleem, M.A. (2005) Pulmonary function testing and extreme environments. *Clin. Chest Med.* (S. Ruoss and R.B. Schoene, eds.) **26**, 485–507.

Dinmore, A.J., Edwards, J.S.A., Menzies, I.S. and Travis, S.P.L. (1994) Intestinal carbohydrate absorption and permeability at high altitude (5730 m). *J. Appl. Physiol.* **76**, 1903–7.

Dombret, M.C., Rouby, J.J., Smeijan, J.M. *et al.* (1987) Pulmonary oedema during pulmonary embolism. *Br. J. Dis. Chest,* **81**, 407–10.

Donaldson, G.C., Tchernjavski, V.E., Ermakov, S.P. *et al.* (1998a) Winter mortality and cold stress in Yekaterinburg, Russia: interview survey. *BMJ* **316**, 514–18.

Donaldson, G.C., Ermakov, S.P., Komarov, Y. *et al.* (1998b) Cold related mortalities and protection against cold in Yakutsk, eastern Siberia: observation and interview study. *BMJ* **317**, 978–82.

Donayre, J., Guerra-Garcia, R., Moncloa, F. and Sobrevilla, L.A. (2003) Endocrine studies at high altitude. *J. Reprod. Fertil.* **16**, 55–8.

Donnelly, D.F. and Carroll, J.L. (2005) Mitochondrial function and carotid body transduction (Review). *High Alt. Med. Biol.* **6**, 121–32.

Dor, Y., Porat, R. and Keshet, E. (2001) Vascular endothelial growth factor and vascular adjustments to perturbations in oxygen homeostasis. *Am. J. Physiol. Cell Physiol.* **280**, C1367–74.

Douglas, C.G. and Haldane, J.S. (1909) The causes of periodic or Cheyne–Stokes breathing. *J. Physiol. (Lond.)* **38**, 401–19.

Douglas, C.G., Haldane, J.S., Henderson, Y. and Schneider, E.C. (1913) Physiological observations made on Pike's Peak, Colorado, with special reference to adaptation to low barometric pressures. *Phil. Trans. R. Soc. (Lond). Ser. B* **203**, 185–381.

Drinking and drowning (editorial) (1979) *BMJ* **1**, 70–1.

Droma, Y., Hayano, T., Takabayashi, Y. *et al.* (1996a) Endothelin-1 and interleukin-8 in high altitude pulmonary oedema. *Eur. Respir. J.* **9**, 1947–9.

Droma, Y., Ge, R.L., Tanaka, M. *et al.* (1996b) Acute hypoxic pulmonary vascular response does not accompany plasma endothelin-1 elevation in subjects susceptible to high altitude pulmonary edema. *Int. Med.* **35**, 257–60.

Droma, Y., Hanaoka, M., Ota, M. *et al.* (2002) Positive association of the endothelial nitric oxide synthase gene polymorphisms with high-altitude pulmonary edema. *Circulation* **106**, 826–30.

Dubas, F. (1980) Aspects de medicaux de l'accident par avalanche. Hypotherme et gelure. *Z. Unfallmed. Berfskr.* **73**, 164–7.

Dubas, F., Henzwlin, R. and Michelet, J. (1991a) Avalanche prevention and rescue, in *A Colour Atlas of Mountain Medicine* (eds. J. Vallotten and F. Dubas), Wolfe, London, pp. 104–12.

Dubas, F., Henzwlin, R. and Michelet, J. (1991b) Rescue in crevasses, in *A Colour Atlas of Mountain Medicine* (eds. J. Vallotten and F. Dubas), Wolfe, London, pp. 112–16.

Dubowitz, G. (1998) Effect of temazepam on oxygen saturation and sleep quality at high altitude: randomised placebo controlled crossover trial. *BMJ* **21**, 587–9.

Dubowitz, G. and Peacock, A.J. (1999) Pulmonary artery pressure variation measured by Doppler echocardiography in healthy subjects at 4250 m (abstract), in *Hypoxia: Into the Next Millennium* (eds. R.C. Roach, P.D. Wagner and P.H. Hackett), Plenum/Kluwer, New York, p. 378.

Dubowitz, G., Bickler, P. and Schiller, N. (2004) Patent foramen ovale at high altitude (abstract). *High Alt. Med. Biol.* **5**, 482.

Dudley, G.A., Tullson, P.C. and Terjung, R.L. (1987) Influence of mitochondrial content on the sensitivity of respiratory control. *J. Biol. Chem.* **262**, 9109–14.

Duff, J. (1999a) Observations while treating altitude illness (Letter). *Wilderness Environ. Med.* **10**, 274.

Duff, J. (1999b) The Tibetan tuck: a dry land cold condition survival position equivalent to that used in cold water. *Wilderness Environ. Med.* **10**, 206–7.

Duke, H.N. (1954) Site of action of anoxia on the pulmonary blood vessels of the cat. *J. Physiol. (Lond.)* **125**, 373–82.

Duplain, H., Vollenweider, L., Delabeys, A. *et al.* (1999a) Augmented sympathetic activation during short-term hypoxia and high-altitude exposure in subjects susceptible to high-altitude pulmonary edema. *Circulation* **99**, 1713–8.

Duplain, H., Lepori, M., Sartori, C. *et al.* (1999b) Inflammation does not contribute to high altitude pulmonary edema. *Am. J. Respir. Crit. Care* **159**, A345 (abstract).

Duplain, H., Sartori, C., Lepori, M. *et al.* (2000) Exhaled nitric oxide in high-altitude pulmonary edema: role in the regulation of pulmonary vascular tone and evidence for a role against inflammation. *Am. J. Respir. Crit. Care Med.* **162**, 221–4.

Durand, J. and Martineaud, J.P. (1971) Resistance and capacitance vessels of the skin in permanent and temporary residents at high altitude, in *High Altitude Physiology: Cardiac and Respiratory Aspects,* Ciba Foundation (eds. R. Porter and J. Knight), Churchill Livingstone, London, pp. 159–70.

Durand, J. and Raynaud, J. (1987) Limb blood and heat exchange at altitude, in *Hypoxia and Cold* (eds. J.R. Sutton, C.S. Houston and G. Coates), Praeger, New York, pp. 100–13.

Durand, F., Kippelen, P., Ceugniet, F. *et al.* (2005) Undiagnosed exercise-induced bronchoconstriction in ski-mountaineers. *Int. J. Sports Med.* **26**, 233–7.

Durig, A. (1911) Ergebnisse der Monte Rosa Expedition vom Jahre 1906 von Prof. Dr. A. Durig. Über den Gaswechsel beim Gehen. *Denkschr. d. Mathem. - Naturw. Kl.* **86**, 293–347.

Durmowicz, A.G., Noordeweir, E., Nicholas, R. and Reeves, J.T. (1997) Inflammatory processes may predispose children to high altitude pulmonary edema. *J. Pediatr.* **130**, 838–40.

Duteil, L., Queille-Roussel, C., Lorenz, B., Thieroff-Ekerdt, R. and Ortonne, JP. (2002) A randomized, controlled study of the safety and efficacy of topical corticosteroid treatments of sunburn in healthy volunteers. *Clin. Exp. Dermatol.* **27**, 314–8.

Dwinell, M.R. and Powell, F.L. (1999) Chronic hypoxia enhances the phrenic nerve response to arterial chemoreceptor stimulation in anaesthetized rats. *J. Appl. Physiol.* **87**, 817–23.

Eady, R.A.J., Bentley-Phillips, C.B., Keahey, T.M. and Greaves, M.W. (1978) Cold urticaria vasculitis. *Br. J. Dermatol.* **99** (Suppl. 16), 9–10.

Eaton, J.W., Skelton, T.D. and Berger, E. (1974) Survival at extreme altitude: protective effect of increased hemoglobin-oxygen affinity. *Science* **183**, 743–4.

Eckardt, K., Boutellier, U., Kurtz, A. *et al.* (1989) Rate of erythropoietin formation in humans in response to acute hypobaric hypoxia. *J. Appl. Physiol.* **66**, 1785–8.

Edwards, H.T. (1936) Lactic acid in rest and work at high altitude. *Am. J. Physiol.* **116**, 367–75.

Eger, E.I., Kellogg, R.H., Mines, A.H. *et al.* (1968) Influence of CO_2 on ventilatory acclimatization to altitude. *J. Appl. Physiol.* **24**, 607–14.

Egli-Sinclair. (1893) Sur le mal de montagne. *Annals de Observatoire Météorologique, Physique et Glaciaire du Mont Blanc* **1**, 109–30.

Eichenberger, U., Weiss, E., Riemann, D., Oelz, O. and Bartsch, P. (1996) Nocturnal periodic breathing and the development of acute high altitude illness. *Am. J. Respir. Crit. Care Med.* **154**, 1748–54.

Ekblom, B., Goldbarg, A.N. and Gullbring, B. (1972) Response to exercise after blood loss and reinfusion. *J. Appl. Physiol.* **33**, 175–80.

Ekelund, L.G. (1967) Circulatory and respiratory adaptation during prolonged exercise. *Acta Physiol. Scand.* **292**(Suppl.), 1–38.

Eldridge, M.W., Podolsky, A., Richardson, R.S. *et al.* (1996) Pulmonary haemodynamic response to exercise in subjects with prior high-altitude pulmonary edema. *J. Appl. Physiol.* **81**, 911–21.

Eldridge, W.E., Braun, R.K., Yoneda, K.Y. *et al.* (1998) Lung injury after heavy exercise at altitude. *Chest* **114**, 66S–67S.

Elliott, A.R., Fu, Z., Tsukimoto, K. *et al.* (1992) Short-term reversibility of ultrastructural changes in pulmonary capillaries caused by stress failure. *J. Appl. Physiol.* **73**, 1150–8.

Elliott, M.E. and Goodfriend, T.L. (1986) Inhibition of aldosterone synthesis by atrial natriuretic factor. *Fed. Proc.* **45**, 2376–81.

Ellsworth, A.J., Meyer, E.F. and Larson, E.B. (1991) Acetazolamide or dexamethasone use versus placebo to prevent acute mountain sickness on Mount Rainier. *West. J. Med.* **154**, 289–93.

Elterman, L. (1964) *Atmospheric Attenuation Model, 1964, in the Ultraviolet, Visible, and Infrared Regions for Altitudes to 50 km*, Environmental Research Papers No. **46**, L.G. Hanscom Field, MA, Air Force Cambridge Research Laboratories, Office of Aerospace Research, AFCRL-64-740.

Enander, A. (1984) Performance and sensory aspects of work in cold environments – a review. *Ergonomics* **27**, 365–78.

English, J.S.C. (1987) High altitude and the skin, in *Abstracts of the UIAA Mountain Medicine Conference*, Mountain Medicine Data Centre, St Bartholomew's Hospital, London, p. 20.

Engwall, M.J.A. and Bisgard, G.E. (1990) Ventilatory response to chemoreceptor stimulation after hypoxic acclimatization in awake goats. *J. Appl. Physiol.* **69**, 1236–43.

Ennemoser, O., Ambach, W. and Flora, G. (1988) Physical assessment of heat insulation of rescue foils. *Int. J. Sports Med.* **9**, 179–82.

Erba, P., Anastasi, S., Senn, O., Maggiorirni, M. and Bloch, K.E. (2004) Acute mountain sickness is related to nocturnal hypoxemia but not to hypoventilation. *Eur. Respir. J.* **24**, 303–8.

Erdman, J., Sun, K.T., Masar, P. and Niederhauser, H. (1998) Effects of exposure to altitude on men with coronary artery disease and impaired left ventricular function. *Am. J. Cardiol.* 81, 266–70.

Erslev, A. (1987) Erythropoietin coming of age. *N. Engl. J. Med.* **316**, 101–3.

Evans, R.C. (1956) *Kanchenjunga. The Untrodden Peak,* Hodder and Stoughton, London.

Eversman, T., Gottsman, M., Uhlich, E. *et al.* (1978) Increased secretion of growth hormone, prolactin, antidiuretic hormone and cortisol induced by the stress of motion sickness. *Aviat. Space Environ. Med.* **49**, 53–7.

Fagan, K.A. and Weil, J.V. (2001) Potential genetic contribution to control of the pulmonary circulation and ventilation at high altitude. *High Alt. Med. Biol.* **2**, 165–71.

Fâ-Hien (399–414) *A Record of Buddhistic Kingdoms, Being an Account by the Chinese Monk Fâ-Hien of his Travels in India and Ceylon (AD 399–414) in Search of the Buddhist Books of Discipline.* Translated and annotated with a Korean recension of the Chinese text by J. Legge, Dover Publications, New York (1965), pp. 40–1 (p. 12 of the Korean text).

Falk, B., Bar-Or, J., Smolander, J. and Frost, G. (1994) Response to rest and exercise in the cold: the effect of age and aerobic fitness. *J. Appl. Physiol.* **76**, 72–8.

Faraci, F.M. (1986) Circulation during hypoxia in birds. *Comp Biochem Physiol A* **85**, 613–20.

Faraci, F.M. and Fedde, M.R. (1986) Regional circulatory responses to hypocapnia and hypercapnia in bar-headed geese – *Am. J. Physiol.* **250**, (3 Pt 2), R499–504.

Farber, M.O., Bright, T.P., Strawbridge, R.A. *et al.* (1975) Impaired water handling in chronic obstructive lung disease. *J. Lab. Clin. Med.* **85**, 41–9.

Fatemian, M., Nieuwenhuijs, D.J., Teppema, L.J. *et al.* (2003) The respiratory response to carbon dioxide in humans with unilateral and bilateral resections of the carotid bodies. *J. Physiol.* **549**, 965–73.

Feldman, K.W. and Herndon, S.P. (1977) Positive expiratory pressure for the treatment of high altitude edema. *Lancet* **1**, 1036–7.

Fencl, V., Miller, T.B. and Pappenheimer, J.R. (1966) Studies on the respiratory response to disturbances of acid–base balance, with deductions concerning ionic composition of cerebral interstitial fluid. *Am. J. Physiol.* **210**, 449–72.

Fencl, V., Gabel, R.A. and Wolfe, D. (1979) Composition of cerebral fluids in goats adapted to high altitude. *J. Appl. Physiol.* **47**, 408–13.

Ferrara, N. and Davis-Smyth, T. (1997) The biology of vascular endothelial growth factor. *Endocr. Rev.* **18**, 4–25.

Ferrazzini, G., Maggiorini, M., Kriemler, S., Bärtsch, P. and Oelz, O. (1987) Successful treatment of acute mountain sickness with dexamethasone. *BMJ* **294**, 1380–2.

Ferri, C., Bellini, C., De Angelis, C. *et al.* (1995) Circulating endothelin-1 concentrations in patients with chronic hypoxia. *J. Clin. Path.* **48**, 519–24.

Ferrus, L., Guenard, H., Vardon, G. and Varene, P. (1980) Respiratory water loss. *Respir. Physiol.* **39**, 367–81.

Ferrus, L., Commenges, D., Gire, J. and Varene, P. (1984) Respiratory water loss as a function of ventilatory or environmental factors. *Respir. Physiol.* **56**, 11–20.

Fineman, J.R., Heymann, M.A. and Soifer, S.J. (1991) N^{ω}-nitro-L-arginine attenuates endothelium-dependent pulmonary vasodilation in lambs. *Am. J. Physiol.* **260**, H1299–306.

Finisterer, J. (1999) High altitude illness induced by tooth root infection. *Postgrad. Med. J.* **75**, 227–9.

Fiorenzano, G., Papalia, M.A., Parrivicini, M. *et al.* (1997) Prolonged ECG abnormalities in a subject with high altitude pulmonary edema (HAPE). *J. Sports Med. Phys. Fitness* **37**, 292–6.

Firth, P.G. and Bolay, H. (2004) Transient high altitude neurological dysfunction: an origin in the temporoparietal cortex. *High. Alt. Med. Biol.* **5**, 71–5.

Fischer, A.P., Stumpe, F. and Vallotton, J. (1991) Hypothermia in an avalanche: a case report, in *A Colour Atlas of Mountain Medicine* (eds. J. Vallotton and F. Du Bas), Wolfe, London, pp. 96–7.

Fischer, R., Vollmar, C., Thiere, M. *et al.* (2004) No evidence of cerebral oedema in severe acute mountain sickness. *Cephalalgia* **24**, 66–71.

Fischer, R. *et al.* (2005) Lung function in adults with cystic fibrosis at altitude: impact on air travel. *Eur. Respir. J.* **25**, 718–24.

Fischer S., Clauss M., Wiesnet M. *et al.* (1999) Hypoxia induces permeability in brain microvessel endothelial cells via VEGF and NO. *Am. J. Physiol. Cell. Physiol.* **276**, C812–20.

Fisher, J.W. and Langston, J.W. (1967) The influence of hypoxia and cobalt on erythropoietin production in the isolated perfused dog kidney. *Blood* **29**, 114–25.

Fisher, R., Lang, S.M., Bergner, A. and Huber, R.M. (2005) Monitoring of expiratory flow rates and lung volumes during a high altitude expedition. *Eur. J. Med. Res.* **10**, 469–74.

Fishman, A.P. (1985) Pulmonary circulation, in *Handbook of Physiology,* Section 3: *The Respiratory System,* Vol. 1: *Circulation and Nonrespiratory Functions* (eds. A.P. Fishman and A.B. Fisher), American Physiological Society, Bethesda, MD, pp. 93–165.

Fishman, R.A. (1975) Brain edema. *N. Engl. J. Med.* **293**, 706–11.

Fitch, R.F. (1964) Mountain sickness: a cerebral form. *Ann. Intern. Med.* **60**, 871–6.

FitzGerald, M.P. (1913) The changes in the breathing and the blood at various altitudes. *Philos. Trans. R. Soc. Lond. Ser. B* **203**, 351–71.

FitzGerald, M.P. (1914) Further observations on the changes in the breathing and the blood at various high altitudes. *Proc. Roy. Soc. Lond. Ser. B.* **88**, 248–58.

Fitzgerald, F.T. and Jessop, C. (1982) Accidental hypothermia. A report of 22 cases and review of the literature. *Adv. Intern. Med.* **27**, 127–50.

Flora, G. (1985) Secondary treatment of frostbite, in *High Altitude Deterioration* (eds. J. Rivolier, P. Cerretelli, J. Foray and P. Segantini), Karger, Basel, pp. 159–69.

Folsom A.R. *et al.* (2002) Protein C, antithrombin, and venous thromboembolism incidence: a prospective population-based study. *Arterscler. Thromb. Vasc. Biol.* **22**, 1018–22.

Foray, J. and Cahen, C. (1981) Les hypothermies de montagne. *Chirurgie* **107**, 255–310.

Foray, J. and Salon, F. (1985) Casualties with cold injuries: primary treatment, in *High Altitude Deterioration* (eds. J. Rivolier, P. Cerretelli, J. Foray and P. Segantini), Karger, Basel, pp. 149–58.

Forbes, C.B. and Drenick, E.J. (1979) Loss of body nitrogen of fasting. *Am. J. Clin. Nutr.* **32**, 1370–4.

Forsling, M.L. and Milledge, J.S. (1977) Effect of hypoxia on vasopressin release in man. *J. Physiol.* **267**, 22–23P.

Forsling, M.L. and Milledge, J.S. (1980) The effect of simulated altitude (4000 m) on plasma cortisol and vasopressin concentration in man. *Proc. Int. Union Physiol. Sci.* **14**, 414.

Forster, H.V., Dempsey, J.A. and Chosy, L.W. (1974) Incomplete compensation of CSF [H$^+$] in man during acclimatization to high altitude (4300 m). *J. Appl. Physiol.* **38**, 1067–72.

Forster, H.V., Bisgard, G.E. and Klein, J.P. (1981) Effect of peripheral chemoreceptor denervation on acclimatization of goats during hypoxia. *J. Appl. Physiol.* **40**, 392–8.

Forster, P. (1984) Reproducibility of individual response to exposure to high altitude. *BMJ* **289**, 1269.

Forster, P. (1986) Telescopes in high places, in *Aspects of Hypoxia* (ed. D. Heath), Liverpool University Press, Liverpool, pp. 217–33.

Forsyth, T.D. (1875) *Report of a Mission to Yarkund in 1873.* Foreign Department Press, Calcutta, pp. 66–9.

Forwand, S.A., Landowne, M., Follansbee, J.N. and Hansen, J.E. (1968) Effect of acetazolamide on acute mountain sickness. *N. Engl. J. Med.* **279**, 839–45.

Fox, V.F. (1967) Human performance in the cold. *Hum. Factors* **9**, 203–90.

Francis, T.J.R. and Golden, F. St C. (1985) Non-freezing cold injury: the pathogenesis. *J. R. Nav. Med. Serv.* **71**, 3–8.

Franz, D.R., Berberich, J.J., Blake, S. and Mills, W.J. (1978) Evaluation of fasciotomy and vasodilators for the treatment of frostbite in the dog. *Cryobiology* **15**, 659–69.

Fraser, J.B. (1820) *Journal of a Tour Through Part of the Snowy Range of the Himala Mountains, and to the Sources of the Rivers Jumna and Ganges,* Rodwell and Martin, London, p. 349.

Frayser, R., Houston, C.S., Bryan, A.C., Rennie, I.D. and Gray, G. (1970) Retinal hemorrhage at high altitude. *N. Engl. J. Med.* **282**, 1183–4.

Frayser, R., Rennie, I.D., Gray, G.W. and Houston, C.S. (1975) Hormonal and electrolyte response to exposure to 17,500 ft. *J. Appl. Physiol.* **38**, 636–42.

Fred, H.L., Schmidt, A.M., Bates, T. and Hecht, H.H. (1962) Acute pulmonary edema of altitude. Clinical and physiologic observations. *Circulation* **25**, 929–37.

Freeman. K., Shalit. M. and Stroh. G. (2004) Use of the Gamow bag by EMT-basic park rangers for treatment of high-altitude pulmonary edema and high-altitude cerebral edema. *Wild. Environ. Med.* **15**, 198–201.

Freitas, J., Costa, O., Carvalho, M.J. and Falcao de Freitas, A. (1996) High altitude-related neurocardiogenic syncope. *Am. J. Cardiol.* **77**, 1021.

Freund, B.J., O'Brien, C. and Young, A.J. (1994) Alcohol ingestion and temperature regulation during cold exposure. *J. Wilderness Med.* **5**, 88–98.

Friedman, N.B. (1945) The pathology of trench foot. *Am. J. Pathol.* **21**, 387–433.

Frisancho, A.R. (1978) Human growth and development among high-altitude populations, in *The Biology of High Altitude Peoples* (ed. P.T. Baker), Cambridge University Press, Cambridge, pp. 117–71.

Frisancho, A.R. (1988) Origins of differences in hemoglobin concentration between Himalayan and Andean populations. *Respir. Physiol.* **72**, 13–18.

Frisancho, A.R. and Baker, P.T. (1970) Altitude and growth: a study of the patterns of physical growth of a high altitude Peruvian Quechua population. *Am. J. Phys. Anthropol.* **32**, 279–92.

Froese, G. and Burton, A.C. (1957) Heat loss from the human head. *J. Appl. Physiol.* **10**, 235–41.

Frostell, C.G., Blomqvist, H., Hedenstierna, G., Lundberg, J. and Zapol, W.M. (1993) Inhaled nitric oxide selectively reverses human hypoxic pulmonary vasoconstriction without causing systemic vasodilation. *Anesthesiology* **78**, 427–35.

Fu, Z., Costello, M.L., Tsukimoto, K. *et al.* (1992) High lung volume increases stress failure in pulmonary capillaries. *J. Appl. Physiol.* **73**, 123–33.

Fudge, B.W., Westerterp, K.R., Kiplamai, F.K. *et al.* (2006) Evidence of negative energy balance using doubly labelled water in elite Kenyan endurance runners prior to competition. *Br. J. Nutr.* **95**, 59–66.

Fuhrer-Haimendorf, C. von (1964) *The Sherpas of Nepal: Bhuddist Highlanders*, John Murray, London.

Fujimaki, T., Matsutani, M. Asai, A., Kohno, T. and Koike, M. (1986) Cerebral venous thrombosis due to

high altitude polycythemia. Case report. *J. Neurosurg.* **64**, 148–50.

Fujimoto, K., Matsuzawa, Y., Hirai, K. *et al.* (1989) Irregular nocturnal breathing patterns at high altitude in subjects susceptible to high-altitude pulmonary edema (HAPE): a preliminary study. *Aviat. Space Environ. Med.* **60**, 786–91.

Fukushima, M., Yasaki, K., Shibamoto, T. *et al.* (1983) Findings of brain computed tomography in patients with high altitude pulmonary edema, in *Hypoxia, Exercise and Altitude* (eds. J.R. Sutton, C.S. Houston and N.L. Jones), Liss, New York, pp. 456–7.

Fulco, C.S., Rock, P.B. and Cymerman, A. (1998) Maximal and submaximal exercise performance at altitude (Review). *Aviat. Space Environ. Med.* **69**, 793–801.

Gabry, A.L., Ledoux, X., Mozziconacci, M. and Martin, C. (2003) High-altitude pulmonary edema at moderate altitude (<2,400 m; 7,870 feet): a series of 52 patients. *Chest* **123**, 49–53.

Gaillard, S., Dellasanta, P., Loutan, L. and Kayser, B. (2004) Awareness, prevalence, medication use, and risk factors of acute mountain sickness in tourists trekking around the Annapurnas in Nepal: a 12-year follow-up. *High Alt. Med. Biol.* **5**, 410–9.

Gale, G.E., Torre-Bueno, J.R., Moon, R.E. *et al.* (1985) Ventilation–perfusion inequality in normal humans during exercise at sea level and simulated altitude. *J. Appl. Physiol.* **58**, 978–88.

Galeotti, G. (1904) Les variations de l'alcalinité du sang sur le sommet du Mont Rosa. *Arch. Ital. Biol.* **41**, 80–92.

Galileo, G. (1638) *Dialogues Concerning Two New Sciences.* English translation of relevant pages in *High Altitude Physiology* (ed. J.B. West), Hutchinson Ross, Stroudsburg, PA, 1981.

Galton, V.A. (1978) Environmental effects, in *The Thyroid*, 4th edn (eds. S.C. Werner and S.H. Ingbar), Harper Row, New York, pp. 247–52.

Gamboa, A., León-Velarde, F., Rivera-Ch, M., Vargas, M., Palacios, J.A. and Monge-C, C. (2001) Ventilatory and cardiovascular responses to hypoxia and exercise in Andean natives living at sea level. *High Alt. Med. Biol.* **2**, 341–7.

Gamboa, A., León-Velarde, F., Rivera-ch, M. *et al.* (2003) Acute and sustained ventilatory responses to hypoxia in high-altitude natives living at sea level. *J. Appl. Physiol.* **94**, 1253–62. E-pub 27 November 2002.

Ganfornina, M.D. and Lopez-Barneo, J. (1991) Single K channels in membrane patches of arterial chemoreceptor cells are modulated by O_2 tension. *Proc. Natl. Acad. Sci. USA* **88**, 2927–30.

Garcia, N., Hopkins, S.R. and Powell, F.L. (1999) Effects of intermittent vs. continuous hypoxia on the isocapnic ventilatory hypoxic response in man. *Am. J. Crit. Care Respir. Med.* **159**, A44.

Garcia, N., Hopkins, S.R. and Powell, F.L. (2000) Effects of intermittent hypoxia on the isocapnic ventilatory hypoxic response and erythropoiesis in humans. *Respir. Physiol.* **123**, 39–49.

Garcia, N., Hopkins, S.R., Elliott, A.R. *et al.* (2001) Ventilatory response to 2-h sustained hypoxia in humans. *Respir. Physiol.* **124**, 11–22.

Garrido, E., Castello, A., Ventura, J.L., Capdevila, A. and Rodriguez, F.A. (1993) Cortical atrophy and other brain magnetic resonance imaging (MRI) changes after extremely high-altitude climbs without oxygen. *Int. J. Sports Med.* **14**, 232–4.

Garrido, E., Rodas, G., Javierre, C., Segura, R., Estruch, A. and Ventura, J.L. (1997) Cardiorespiratory response to exercise in elite Sherpa climbers transferred to sea level. *Med. Sci. Sports Exerc.* **29**, 937–42.

Garrow, J.S. (1987) Are liquid diets (VLCD) safe or necessary? in *Recent Advances in Obesity Research, V* (eds. E.M. Berry, S.H. Blondheim, H.E. Eliahou and E. Shafrir), Food and Nutrition Press, Westport, CT, pp. 312–16.

Gautier, H., Peslin, R., Grassino, A. *et al.* (1982) Mechanical properties of the lungs during acclimatization to altitude. *J. Appl. Physiol.* **52**, 1407–15.

Gautier, H., Bonora, M., Schultz, S.A. and Remmers, J.E. (1987) Hypoxia induced changes in shivering and body temperature. *J. Appl. Physiol.* **62**, 2577–81.

Gazenco, O.G. (1987) *Physiology of Man at High Altitude* [in Russian], Nauka, Moscow.

Ge, R.L. and Helun, G.W. (2001) Current concept of chronic mountain sickness: pulmonary hypertension-related high-altitude heart disease. *Wilder. Environ. Med.* **12**, 190–4.

Ge, R.L., Chen, Q.H., Wang, L.H. *et al.* (1994) Higher exercise performance and lower VO2max in Tibetan than Han residents at 4,700 m altitude. *J. Appl. Physiol.* **77**, 684–91.

Ge, R.L., Matsuzawa, Y., Takeoka, M. *et al.* (1997) Low pulmonary diffusing capacity in subjects with acute mountain sickness. *Chest* **111**, 58–64.

Ge, R.L., Kubo, K., Kobayashi, T., Sekiguchi, M. and Honda, T. (1998) Blunted hypoxic pulmonary vasoconstrictive response to the rodent *Ochotona*

curzoniae (pika) at high altitude. *Am. J. Physiol. Heart Circ. Physiol.* **274**, H1792–9.

Ge, R-L., Shai, H-R., Takaoka, M. *et al.* (2001) Atrial natriuretic peptide and red cell 2,3-diphosphoglyceride in patients with chronic mountain sickness. *Wild. Envion. Med.* **12**, 2–7.

Gehr, P., Bachofen, M. and Weibel, E.R. (1978) The normal human lung: ultrastructure and morphometric estimation of diffusion capacity. *Respir. Physiol.* **32**, 121–40.

Geiser, J., Vogt, M., Billeter, R., Zuleger, C., Belforti. and Hoppeler, H. (2001) Training high–living low: changes of aerobic performance and muscle structure with training at simulated altitude. *Int. J. Sports Med.* **22**, 579–85.

Gerard, A.B., McElroy, M.D., Taylor M.J. *et al.* (2000) Six percent oxygen enrichment of room air at simulated 5000 m altitude improves neuropsychological function. *High Alt. Med. Biol.* **1**, 51–61.

Gerlach, H., Clauss, M., Ogawa, S. and Stern, D.M. (1992) Modulation of endothelial coagulant properties and barrier function by factors in the vascular microenvironment, in *Endothelial Cell Dysfunctions* (ed. N. Simoniescu and M. Simoniescu), Plenum, New York, pp. 525–45.

Gertsch, J.H., Seto, T.B., Mor, J. and Onopa, J. (2002) Ginkgo biloba for the prevention of severe acute mountain sickness (AMS) starting one day before rapid ascent. *High Alt. Med. Biol.* **3**, 29–37.

Gertsch, J.H., Basnyat, B., Johnson, E.W., Onopa, J. and Holck, P.S. (2004) Randomised, double blind, placebo controlled comparison of ginkgo biloba and acetazolamide for prevention of acute mountain sickness among Himalayan trekkers: the prevention of high altitude illness trial (PHAIT). *BMJ* **328**, 797. E-pub 11 March 2004.

Ghofrani, H.A., Reichenberger, F., Kohstall, M.G. *et al.* (2004) Sildenafil increased exercise capacity during hypoxia at low altitudes and at Mount Everest base camp: a randomized, double-blind, placebo-controlled crossover trial. *Ann. Intern. Med.* **141**, 169–77.

Giesbrecht, G.E., Goheen, M.S.L., Johnston, C.E. *et al.* (1997) Inhibition of shivering increases core temperature after drop and attenuates rewarming in hypothermic humans. *J. Appl. Physiol.* **83**, 1630–4.

Gilbert, D.L. (1983) The first documented report of mountain sickness: the China or Headache Mountain story. *Respir. Physiol.* **52**, 315–26.

Gilbert, D.L. (1991) The Pariacaca or Tullujoto story: political realism? *Respir. Physiol.* **86**, 147–57.

Gill, M.B. and Pugh, L.G.C.E. (1964) Basal metabolism and respiration in men living at 5,800 m (19000 ft). *J. Appl. Physiol.* **19**, 949–54.

Gill, M.B., Milledge, J.S., Pugh, L.G.C.E. and West, J.B. (1962) Alveolar gas composition at 21,000 to 25,700 ft (6400–7830 m). *J. Physiol. (Lond.)* **163**, 373–7.

Gill, M.B., Poulton, E.C., Carpenter, A., Woodhead, M.M. and Gregory, M.H.P. (1964) Falling efficiency at sorting cards during acclimatization at 19,000 ft. *Nature* **203**, 436.

Gillman, P. (1993) *Everest*, Little Brown, Boston.

Glazier, J.B. and Murray, J.F. (1971) Sites of pulmonary vasomotor reactivity in the dog during alveolar hypoxia and serotonin and histamine infusion. *J. Clin. Invest.* **50**, 2550–8.

Glazier, J.B., Hughes, J.M.B., Maloney, J.E. and West, J.B. (1969) Measurements of capillary dimensions and blood volume in rapidly frozen lungs. *J. Appl. Physiol.* **26**, 65–76.

Goldberg, S.V., Schoene, R.B., Haynor, D. *et al.* (1992) Brain tissue pH and ventilatory acclimatization to high altitude. *J. Appl. Physiol.* **72**, 58–63.

Golden, F. St C. (1973) Recognition and treatment of immersion hypothermia. *Proc. R. Soc. Med.* **66**, 1058–61.

Golden, F. St C. (1983) Rewarming, in *The Nature and Treatment of Hypothermia* (eds. R.S. Pozos and L.E. Wittmers), Croom Helm, London/University of Minnesota Press, Minneapolis, pp. 194–208.

Golden, F. St C. and Hervey, G.R. (1981) The 'after drop' and death after rescue from immersion in cold water, in *Hypothermia Ashore and Afloat* (ed. J.N. Adams), Aberdeen University Press, Aberdeen, pp. 37–56.

Goldenberg, F., Richalet, J.P., Onnen, I., and Antezana, A.M. (1992) Sleep apneas and high altitude newcomers. *Int. J. Sports Med.* **13**, S34–6.

Goldsmith, R. and Minard, D. (1976) Cold, cold work, in *Occupational Health and Safety*, Vol. 1, International Labour Office, Geneva, pp. 319–20.

Goldstein, M.C. and Beall, C.M. (1989) *Nomads of Western Tibet*, Serindia, London.

Gollnick, P.D. and Saltin, B. (1982) Significance of skeletal muscle oxidative enzyme enhancement with endurance training. *Clin. Physiol.* **2**, 1–12.

Goñez, C., Villena, A. and Gonzales, G.F. (1993) Serum levels of adrenal androgens up to adrenarche in Peruvian children living at sea level and at high altitude. *J. Endocrinol.* **136**, 517–23.

Gong Jr., H., Tashkin, D.P., Lee, E.Y. and Simmons, M.S. (1984) Hypoxia–altitude simulation test. Evaluation of patients with chronic airway obstruction. *Am. Rev. Respir. Dis.* **130**, 980–6.

Gonzales, G.F. and Salirrosas, A. (2005) Arterial oxygen saturation in healthy newborns delivered at term in Cerro de Pasco (4340 m) and Lima (150 m). *Reprod. Biol. Endocrinol.* **3**, 46.

Gonzales, G.F., Villena, A., Escuderl, F and Coyotupa, J. (1996) Reproduction in the Andes (Abstract). *Acta Andina* **5**(2), 68–9.

Gonzalez, N.C. and Wood, J.G. (2001) Leukocyte–endothelial interactions in environmental hypoxia (Review). *Adv. Exp. Med. Biol.* **502**, 39–60.

Gonzalez, N.C., Albrecht, T., Sullivan, L.P. and Clancy, R.L. (1990) Compensation of respiratory alkalosis induced after acclimation to simulated altitude. *J. Appl. Physiol.* **69**, 1380–6.

Goodenough, R.D., Royle, G.T., Nadel, E.R. *et al.* (1982) Leucine and urea metabolism in acute human cold exposure. *J. Appl. Physiol.* **53**, 367–72.

Goodman, L. (1964) Oscillatory behavior of ventilation in resting man. *IEEE Trans. Biomed. Elec.* **11**, 82–93.

Gore, C., Craig, N., Hahn, A. *et al.* (1998) Altitude training at 2690 m does not increase total haemoglobin mass or sea level VO$_2$ max in world champion track cyclists. *J. Sci. Med. Sport.* **1**, 156–70.

Gore, C.J., Hahn, A.G., Watson, D.B. *et al.* (1996) VO$_2$ max and arterial oxygen saturation at sea level and 610 m. *Med. Sci. Sports Exerc.* **27**, Abstract 42.

Gorlin, R. (1966) Physiology of the coronary circulation, in *The Heart* (eds. J.W. Hurst and R.B. Logan), McGraw-Hill, New York, pp. 653–8.

Gosney, J. (1986) Histopathology of the endocrine organs in hypoxia, in *Aspects of Hypoxia* (ed. D. Heath), Liverpool University Press, Liverpool, pp. 131–45.

Gosney, J., Heath, D., Williams, D. and Rios-Dalenz, J. (1991) Morphological changes in the pituitary–adrenocortical axis in natives of La Paz. *Int. J. Biometeorol.* **35**, 1–5.

Graham, L.E. and Basnyat, B. (2001) Cerebral edema in the Himalayas: too high, too fast! *Wild. Environ. Med.* **12**, 62.

Graham, W.G.B. and Houston, C.S. (1978) Short-term adaptation to moderate altitude. Patients with chronic obstructive pulmonary disease. *JAMA* **240**, 1491–4.

Grahn, D. and Kratchman, J. (1963) Variations in neonatal death rate and birth weight in the United States and possible relations to environmental radiation, geology and altitude. *Am. J. Hum. Genet.* **15**, 329–52.

Gray, D. (1987) Survival after burial in an avalanche. *BMJ* **294**, 611–12.

Gray, G.W. (1983) High altitude pulmonary edema. *Semin. Respir. Med.* **5**, 141–50.

Green, H.J., Sutton, J.R., Cymerman, A., Young, P.M. and Houston, C.S. (1989) Operation Everest II: adaptations in human skeletal muscle. *J. Appl. Physiol.* **66**, 2454–61.

Green, R.L., Huntsman, R.G. and Serjeant, G.R. (1971) The sickle-cell and altitude. *Br. Med. J.* **4**, 593–5.

Green, S.P.T. (1992) The 1991 Everest marathon and the Namche Bazaar dental clinic. *J. R. Nav. Med. Serv.* **78**, 165–71.

Greene, R. (1934) Observations on the composition of alveolar air on Mt. Everest. *J. Physiol. (Lond.)* **32**, 481–5.

Greene, R. (1943) The immediate vascular changes in true frostbite. *J. Pathol. Bacteriol.* **55**, 259–68.

Gregory, I.C. (1974) The oxygen and carbon monoxide capacities of foetal and adult blood. *J. Physiol.* **236**, 625–34.

Grenard, F. (1904) *Tibet,* Hutchinson, London.

Grissom, C.K., Roach, R.C., Sarnquist, F.H. and Hackett, P.H. (1992) Acetazolamide in the treatment of acute mountain sickness: clinical effect on gas exchange. *Ann. Intern. Med.* **116**, 461–5.

Grissom, C.K., Albertinae, K.H. and Elstsda, M.R. (2000) Alveolar haemorrhage in a case of high altitude pulmonary oedema. *Thorax* **55**, 167–9.

Grissom, C.K., Richer, L.D. and Elstad, M.R. (2005) The effects of a 5-lipoxygenase inhibitor on acute mountain sickness and urinary leukotriene E4 after ascent to high altitude. *Chest* **127**, 565–70.

Groechenig, E. (1994) Treatment of frostbite with iloprost. *Lancet* **394**, 1152–3.

Grollman, A. (1930) Physiological variations of the cardiac output of man. VII. The effect of high altitude on the cardiac output and its related functions: an account of experiments conducted on the summit of Pikes Peak, Colorado. *Am. J. Physiol.* **93**, 19–40.

Gronbeck, C. (1984) Chronic mountain sickness at an elevation of 2000 metres. *Chest* **85**, 577–8.

Grootendorst, D.C., Dahlen, S.E., Van Den Bos, J.W. *et al.* (2001) Benefits of high altitude allergen avoidance in atopic adolescents with moderate to severe asthma, over and above treatment with high dose inhaled steroids. *Clin. Exp. Allergy* **31**, 400–8.

Grover, R.F. (1980) Speculations on the pathogenesis of high-altitude pulmonary edema. *Adv. Cardiol.* **27**, 1–5.

Grover, R.F., Lufschanowski, R. and Alexander, J.K. (1970) Decreased coronary blood flow in man following ascent to high altitude. *Adv. Cardiol.* **5**, 72–9.

Groves, B.M., Reeves, J.T., Sutton, J.R. *et al.* (1987) Operation Everest II: elevated high-altitude pulmonary resistance unresponsive to oxygen. *J. Appl. Physiol.* **63**, 521–30.

Groves, B.M., Droma, T., Sutton, J.R. *et al.* (1993) Minimal hypoxic pulmonary hypertension in normal Tibetans at 3,658 m. *J. Appl. Physiol.* **74**, 312–18.

Grunig, E., Mereles, D., Hildebrandt, W. *et al.* (2000) Stress Doppler echocardiography for identification of susceptibility to high altitude pulmonary edema. *J. Am. Coll. Cardiol.* **35**, 980–7.

Guerra-Garcia, R. (1971) Testosterone metabolism in men exposed to high altitude. *Acta Endocrinol. Panama* **2**, 55–9.

Guezennec, C.Y. and Pesquies, P.C. (1985) Biochemical basis for physical exercise fatigue, in *High Altitude Deterioration* (eds. J. Rivolier, P. Cerretelli, J. Foray and P. Segantini), Karger, Basel, pp. 79–89.

Guilleminault, C., Connolly, S., Winkle, R., Melvin, K. and Tilkian, A. (1984) Cyclical variation of the heart rate in sleep apnoea syndrome. Mechanisms, and usefulness of 24 h electrocardiography as a screening technique. *Lancet* **1**, 126–31.

Guleria, J.S., Pande, J.N. and Khanna, P.K. (1969) Pulmonary function in convalescents of high altitude pulmonary edema. *Dis. Chest* **55**, 434–7.

Guleria, J.S., Pande, J.N., Sethi, P.K. and Roy, S.B. (1971) Pulmonary diffusing capacity at high altitude. *J. Appl. Physiol.* **31**, 536–43.

Gunga, H-C., Kirsch, K., Rocker, L., and Schobersberger, W. (1994) Time course of erythropoietin, triiodothyronine, thyroxin, and thyroid-stimulating hormone at 2315 m. *J. Appl. Physiol.* **76**, 1068–72.

Gupta, M.L., Rao, K.S., Andand, I.S., Banerjee, A.K. and Boparai, M.S. (1992) Lack of smooth muscle in the small pulmonary arteries of the native Ladakhi. *Am. Rev. Respir. Dis.* **145**, 1201–4.

Gustafsson, T., Puntschart, A., Kaijser, L., Jansson, E. and Sundberg, C.J. (1999) Exercise-induced expression of angiogenesis-related transcription and growth factors in human skeletal muscle. *Am. J. Physiol. Heart Circ. Physiol.* **276**, 679–85.

Guttman, R. and Gross, M.M. (1956) Relationship between electrical and mechanical changes in muscle caused by cooling. *J. Coll. Comp. Physiol.* **48**, 421–30.

Guyton, A.C., Jones, C.E. and Coleman, T.C. (1973) *Cardiac Output and its Regulation,* 2nd edn, Saunders, Philadelphia, p. 396.

Haab, P., Perret, C. and Piiper, J. (1965) La capacité de diffusion pulmonaire pour l'oxygène chez l'homme normal jeune. *Helv. Physiol. Acta* **23**, C23–5.

Haas, J.D. (1976) Prenatal and infant growth and development, in *Man in the Andes* (eds. P.T. Baker and M.A. Little), Dowden, Hutchinson & Ross, Stroudsburg, PA, pp. 161–78.

Habeler, P. (1979) *Everest: Impossible Victory,* Arlington, London.

Haberman, S., Capildeo, R. and Rose, F. (1981) The seasonal variation in mortality from cerebro-vascular disease. *J. Neurol. Sci.* **52**, 25–36.

Hackett, P.H. (1999) The cerebral etiology of high-altitude cerebral edema and acute mountain sickness. *Wilderness Environ. Med.* **10**, 97–109.

Hackett, P.H. (2000) Subarachnoid cyst and ascent to high altitude – a problem? *High Alt. Med. Biol.* **1**, 337–9.

Hackett, P.H. (2001) High altitude and common medical conditions, In *High Altitude: an Exploration of Human Adaptation* (eds. T.F. Hornbein and R.B. Schoene), Marcel Decker, New York, pp. 839–85.

Hackett, P.H. and Rennie, D. (1976) The incidence, importance and prophylaxis of acute mountain sickness. *Lancet* **2**, 1149–54.

Hackett, P.H. and Rennie, D. (1979) Râles, peripheral edema, retinal hemorrhage and acute mountain sickness. *Am. J. Med.* **67**, 214–18.

Hackett, P.H. and Rennie, D. (1982) Cotton wool spots: a new addition to high altitude retinopathy, in *High Altitude Physiology and Medicine* (eds. W. Brendel and R.A. Zink), Springer-Verlag, New York, pp. 215–16.

Hackett, P.H. and Roach, R.C. (2001) Current concepts: high-altitude illness. *N. Engl. J. Med.* **345**, 107–14.

Hackett, P.H., Rennie, D. and Levine, H.D. (1976) The incidence, importance and prophylaxis of acute mountain sickness. *Lancet* **2**, 1149–54.

Hackett, P.H., Forsling, M.L., Milledge, J. and Rennie, D. (1978) Release of vasopressin in man at altitude. *Horm. Metab. Res.* **10**, 571.

Hackett, P.H., Creagh, C.E., Grover, R.F. *et al.* (1980a) High altitude pulmonary edema in persons without the right pulmonary artery. *N. Engl. J. Med.* **302**, 1070–3.

Hackett, P.H., Reeves, J.T., Reeves, C.D. *et al.* (1980b) Control of breathing in Sherpas at low and high altitude. *J. Appl. Physiol.* **49**, 374–9.

Hackett, P.H., Rennie, D., Grover, R.F. and Reeves, J.T. (1981) Acute mountain sickness and the edemas of high altitude: a common pathogenesis? *Respir. Physiol.* **46**, 383–90.

Hackett, P.H., Rennie, D., Hofmeister, S.E., Grover, R.F., Grover, E.B. and Reeves, J.T. (1982) Fluid retention and relative hypoventilation in acute mountain sickness. *Respiration* **43**, 321–9.

Hackett, P.H., Schoene, R.B., Winslow, R.M., Peters, R.M. and West, J.B. (1985) Acetazolamide and exercise in sojourners to 6,300 m – a preliminary study. *Med, Sci. Sports Exerc.* **17**, 593–7.

Hackett, P.H., Bertman, J. and Rodriguez, G. (1986) Pulmonary edema fluid protein in high-altitude pulmonary edema. *JAMA* **256**, 36.

Hackett, P.H., Roach, R.C., Harrison, C.L., Schoene, R.B. and Miles, W.J., Jr (1987a) Respiratory stimulants and sleep periodic breathing at high altitude. Almitrine versus acetazolamide. *Am. Rev. Respir. Dis.* **135**, 896–8.

Hackett, P.H., Hollingshead, K.F., Roach, R.B. *et al.* (1987b) Arterial saturation during ascent predicts subsequent acute mountain sickness (abstract), in *Hypoxia and Cold* (eds. J.R. Sutton, C.S. Houston and G. Coates), Praeger, New York, p. 544.

Hackett, P.H., Hollingshead, K.F., Roach, R.B. *et al.* (1987c) Cortical blindness in high altitude climbers and trekkers – a report of six cases (abstract), in *Hypoxia, and Cold* (eds. J.R. Sutton, C.S. Houston and G. Coates), Praeger, New York, p. 536.

Hackett, P.H., Swenson, E.R., Roach, R.C. *et al.* (1988a) 250 mg acetazolamide intravenously does not increase cerebral blood flow at high altitude (abstract), in *Hypoxia the Tolerable Limits* (eds. J.R. Sutton, C.S. Houston and G. Cotes), Benchmark Press, Indianapolis, p. 383.

Hackett, P.H., Roach, R.C., Schoene, R.B. *et al.* (1988b) Abnormal control of ventilation in high-altitude pulmonary edema. *J. Appl. Physiol.* **64**, 1268–72.

Hackett, P.H., Roach, R.C., Hartig, G.S. *et al.* (1992) The effect of vasodilators on pulmonary hemodynamics in high altitude pulmonary edema: a comparison. *Int. J. Sports Med.* **13**, S68–S71.

Hackett, P.H., Yarnell, P.R., Hill, R. *et al.* (1998) High-altitude cerebral edema evaluated with magnetic resonance imaging. *JAMA* **280**, 1920–5.

Haddad, G.G. and Jiang, C. (1993) O_2 deprivation in the central nervous system: on mechanisms of neuronal response, differential sensitivity and injury. *Progr. Neurobiol.* **40**, 277–318.

Hahn, A.G., Gore, C.J., Martin, D.T. *et al.* (2001) An evaluation of the concept of living at moderate altitude and training at sea level. *Comp. Biochem. Physiol. A Mol. Integr. Physiol.* **128**, 777–89.

Haight, J.S.J. and Keatinge, W.R. (1973) Failure of thermoregulation in the cold during hypoglycaemia induced by exercise and ethanol. *J. Physiol. (Lond).* **229**, 87–97.

Haldane, J.S. and Priestley, J.G. (1935) Oxygen secretion in the lungs, in *Respiration,* 2nd edn, Yale University Press, New Haven, CT, pp. 250–96.

Haldane, J.S. and Priestley, J.G. (1935) *Respiration*, 2nd edn, Yale University Press, New Haven, CT.

Haldane, J. and Smith, J. Lorrain (1897) The absorption of oxygen by the lungs. *J. Physiol. (Lond.)* **22**, 231–58.

Haldane, J.S., Kellas, A.M., and Kennaway, E.L. (1919) Experiments on acclimatisation to reduced atmospheric pressure. *J. Physiol. (Lond.)* **53**, 181–206.

Halhuber, M.J., Humpeler, E., Inama, A.K. and Jungmann, H. (1985) Does altitude cause exhaustion of the heart and circulatory system? Indications and contra-indications for cardiac patients in altitudes, in *High Altitude Deterioration* (eds. R.J. Rivolier, P. Cerretelli, J. Foray and P. Segantini), Karger, Basel, pp. 192–202.

Hall, F.G. (1936) The effect of altitude on the affinity of hemoglobin for oxygen. *J. Biol. Chem.* **115**, 485–90.

Hall, F.G., Dill, D.B. and Guzman-Barron, E.S. (1936) Comparative physiology in high altitudes. *J. Cell. Comp. Physiol.* **8**, 301–13.

Halperin, B.D., Sun, S., Zhuang, J., Droma, T. and Moore, L.G. (1998) ECG observations in Tibetan and Han residents of Lhasa. *J. Electrocardiol.* **31**, 237–43.

Hamilton, R.S. and Paton, B.C. (1996) The diagnosis and treatment of hypothermia by mountain rescue teams: a survey. *Wilderness Environ. Med.* **7**, 28–37.

Hamilton, S.J.C. (1980) Hypothermia and unawareness of mental impairment. *BMJ* **1**, 565.

Hamlet, M.P. (1983) Fluid shifts in hypothermia, in *The Nature and Treatment of Hypothermia* (eds. R.S. Pozos and L.E. Wittmers), Croom Helm, London/ University of Minnesota Press, Minneapolis, pp. 94–9.

Hamlet, M.P., Veghte, J., Bowers, W.D. and Boyce, J. (1977) Thermographic evaluation of experimentally produced frostbite of rabbit feet. *Cryobiology* **14**, 197–204.

Hammel, H.T. (1964) Terrestrial animals in the cold. Recent studies in primitive man, in *Handbook of Physiology: Adaptation to the Environment,* American Physiological Society, Washington DC, pp. 413–34.

Hammond, M.D., Gale, G.E., Kapitan, K.S., Ries, A. and Wagner, P.D. (1986) Pulmonary gas exchange in humans during normobaric hypoxic exercise. *J. Appl. Physiol.* **61**, 1749–57.

Han, J.L., Chen, D.X. and Chen, G.I. (1985) The investigation of nail fold microcirculation in 1–13 year old healthy children at different altitudes, in *Abstracts of the Second High Altitude Medicine Symposium,* Department of High Altitude Science, Xining, Quinghai, China, p. 44.

Hanaoka, M., Tanaka, M., Ge, R.L. *et al.* (2000) Hypoxia-induced pulmonary blood redistribution in subjects with a history of high-altitude pulmonary edema. *Circulation* **101**, 1418–22.

Handley, A.J., Golden, F. St C., Keatinge, W.R. *et al.* (1993) *Report of the Working Party on Out of Hospital Management of Hypothermia*, Medical Commission on Accident Prevention, UK.

Hann, J. von (1901) *Lehrbuch der Meteorologie*, Tauchnitz, Leipzig. English translation by R.D.C. Ward, MacMillan, New York, 1903, p. 222.

Hannon, J. (1966) High altitude acclimatization in women, in *The Effects of Altitude on Physical Performance* (ed. R. Goddard), Athletic Institute, Chicago, pp. 37–44.

Hannon, J. (1978) Comparative adaptability of young men and women, in *Environmental Stress: Individual Human Adaptation* (eds. L. Folinsby, J. Wagner, J. Borgia *et al.*) Academic Press, New York, pp. 335–60.

Hannon, J.P., Klain, G.J., Sudman, D.M. and Sullivan, F.J. (1976) Nutritional aspects of high-altitude exposure in women. *Am. J. Clin. Nutr.* **29**, 604–13.

Hanoka, M., Kubo, K., Yamazaki, Y. *et al.* (1998) Association of high altitude pulmonary edema with the major histocompatibility complex. *Circulation* **97**, 1124–8.

Hansen, J.E. and Evans, W.O. (1970) A hypothesis regarding the pathophysiology of acute mountain sickness. *Arch. Environ. Health* **21**, 666–9.

Hansen, J. and Sander, M. (2003) Sympathetic neural overactivity in healthy humans after prolonged exposure to hypobaric hypoxia. *J. Physiol (Lond.)* **546**, 921–9.

Hanson, J.E., Vogel, J.A., Stelter, G.P. and Consolazio, F. (1967) Oxygen uptake in man during exhaustive work at sea level and high altitude. *J. Appl. Physiol.* **23**, 511–22.

Harber, M.J., Williams, J.D. and Morton, J.J. (1981) Antidiuretic hormone excretion at high altitude. *Aviat. Space Environ. Med.* **52**, 38–40.

Harbinson, M.J. (1999) William Harvey, hypothermia and battle injuries. *BMJ* **319**, 1561.

Harms, C.A., Babcock, M.A., McClaran, S.R. *et al.* (1997) Respiratory muscle work compromises leg blood flow during maximal exercise. *J. Appl. Physiol.* **82**, 1573–83.

Harms, C.A., Wetter, T.J., St. Croix, C.M., Pegelow, D.F., and Dempsey, J.A. (2000) Effects of respiratory muscle work on exercise performance. *J. Appl. Physiol.* **89**, 131–8.

Harnett, R.M., Pruitt, J.R. and Sias, F.R. (1983) A review of the literature concerning resuscitation from hypothermia, Part II. Selected rewarming protocols. *Aviat. Space Environ. Med.* **54**, 487–95.

Harper, A.M. and Glass, H.I. (1965) Effect of alterations in the arterial carbon dioxide tension on the blood flow through the cerebral cortex at normal and low arterial blood pressures. *J. Neurol. Neurosurg. Psychiatry* **28**, 449–52.

Harris, P. (1986) Evolution, hypoxia and high altitude, in *Aspects of Hypoxia* (ed. D. Heath), Liverpool University Press, Liverpool, pp. 207–16.

Harris, P., Castillo, Y., Gibson, K. *et al.* (1970) Succinic and lactic dehydrogenase activity in myocardial homogenates from animals at high and low altitude. *J. Mol. Cell. Cardiol.* **1**, 189–93.

Harrison, G.A., Kuchemann, C.F., Moore, M.A.S. *et al.* (1969) The effects of altitudinal variation in Ethiopian populations. *Philos. Trans. R. Soc. Lond. Ser. B* **256**, 147–82.

Harrison, M.H. (1985) Effects of thermal stress and exercise on blood volume in humans. *Physiol. Rev.* **65**, 149–208.

Hartung, G.H., Myhre, L.G., Nunnerly, S.A. and Tucker, D.M. (1984) Plasma substrate response in men and women during marathon running. *Aviat. Space Environ. Med.* **55**, 128–31.

Harvey, T.C., Raichle, M.E., Winterborn, M.H. *et al.* (1988) Effect of carbon dioxide in acute mountain sickness: a rediscovery. *Lancet* **2**, 639–41.

Hashmi, M.A., Bokjari, S.A.H., Rashid, M. *et al.* (1998) Frostbite: epidemiology at high altitude in the Karakoram mountains. *Ann. R. Coll. Surg.* **80**, 91–5.

Hatcher, J.D. (1965) Acute anoxic anoxia, in *The Physiology of Human Survival* (eds. O.G. Edholm and A.L. Bacharach), Academic Press, London, pp. 81–120.

Hathorn, M.K.S. (1971) The influence of hypoxia on iron absorption in the rat. *Gastroenterology,* **60**, 76–81.

Hayward, J.S. (1997) Inhibition of shivering increases core temperature after-drop and attenuates rewarming in hypothermic humans. *J. Appl. Physiol.* **83**, 1030–4.

Hayward, J.S., Eckerson, J.D. and Kemna, D. (1984) Thermal and cardiovascular changes during three methods of resuscitation from mild hypothermia. *Resuscitation* **11**, 21–33.

Hayward, M.G. and Keatinge, W.R. (1979) Progressive symptomless hypothermia in water. Possible cause of diving accidents. *BMJ* **1**, 1222.

Heath, D. (1986) Carotid body hyperplasia, in *Aspects of Hypoxia* (ed. D. Heath), Liverpool University Press, Liverpool, pp. 61–74.

Heath, D. and Williams, D.R. (1995) *High-Altitude Medicine and Pathology,* 4th edn, Oxford University Press, Oxford.

Heath, D., Edwards, C., Winson, M. and Smith, P. (1973) Effects on the right ventricle, pulmonary vasculature, and carotid bodies of the rat of exposure to, and recovery from, simulated high altitude. *Thorax* **28**, 24–8.

Heaton, J.M. (1972) The distribution of brown adipose tissue in the human. *J. Anat.* **112**, 35–9.

Hebbel, R.P., Eaton, J.W., Kronenberg, R.S. *et al.* (1978) Human llamas: adaptation to altitude in subjects with high hemoglobin oxygen affinity. *J. Clin. Invest.* **62**, 593–600.

Hecht, H.H., Lang, R.L., Carnes, W.H. *et al.* (1959) Brisket disease. I. General aspects of pulmonary hypertensive heart disease in cattle. *Trans. Assoc. Am. Physiol.* **72**, 157–72.

Hecht, H.H., Kuida, H., Lange, R.L., Horne, J.L. and Brown, A.M. (1962) Brisket disease. III. Clinical features and hemodynamic observations in altitude-dependent right heart failure of cattle. *Am. J. Med.* **32**, 171–83.

Heggers, J.P., Phillips, L.G., McAuley, R.L. and Robson, M.C. (1990) Frostbite: experimental and clinical evaluation of treatment. *J. Wilderness Med.* **1**, 27–32.

Hellems, H.K., Ord, J.W., Talmers, F.N. and Christensen, R.C. (1957) Effects of hypoxia on coronary blood flow and myocardial metabolism in normal human subjects (abstract). *Circ.* **16**, 893.

Henderson, A.F., Heaton, R.W., Dunlop, L.S. and Costello, J.F. (1983) Effects of nifedipine on antigen-induced bronchoconstriction. *Am. Rev. Respir. Dis.* **127**, 549–53.

Henderson, Y. (1919) The physiology of the aviator. *Science* **49**, 431–41.

Henderson, Y. (1939) The last thousand feet on Everest. *Nature* **143**, 921–23.

Hepple, R.T., Agey, P.J., Szewczak, J.M. *et al.* (1998) Increased capillarity in leg muscle of finches living at altitude. *J. Appl. Physiol.* **85**, 1871–6.

Hepple, R.T., Hogan, M.C., Stary, C. *et al.* (2000) Structural basis of muscle O_2 diffusing capacity: evidence from muscle function *in situ*. *J. Appl. Physiol.* **88**, 560–6.

Herman, J.K., O'Halloran, K.D. and Bisgard, G.E. (2001) Effect of 8-OH DPAT and detanserin on the ventilatory acclimatization to hypoxia in awake goats. *Respir. Physiol.* **124**, 95–104.

Hernandez, M.J. (1983) Cerebral circulation during hypothermia, in *The Nature and Treatment of Hypothermia* (eds. R.S. Pozos and L.E. Wittmers), Croom Helm, London/University of Minnesota, Minneapolis, pp. 61–8.

Herschkowitz, M. (1977) Penile frostbite: an unforeseen hazard of jogging (letter). *N. Engl. J. Med.* **296**, 178.

Hertzman, A.B. (1957) Individual differences in regional sweating patterns. *J. Appl. Physiol.* **10**, 242–8.

Hervey, G.R. (1973) Physiological changes encountered in hypothermia. *Proc. R. Soc. Med.* **66**, 1053–7.

Hervey, G.R. and Tobin, G. (1983) Luxuskonsumption. Diet-induced thermogenesis and brown fat: a critical review. *Clin. Sci.* **64**, 7–22.

Hetzel, B.S. (1989) *The Story of Iodine Deficiency,* Oxford Medical Publications, Oxford.

Heyman, A., Patterson, J.L. and Duke, T.W. (1952) Cerebral circulation and metabolism in sickle cell and other chronic anemias, with observations on the effects of oxygen inhalation. *J. Clin. Invest.* **31**, 824–8.

Heymans, J.-F. and Heymans, C. (1925) Sur le mécanisme de l'apnée réflexe ou pneumogastrique. *Comptes Rendus Soc. Biol.* **92**, 1335–8.

Heymans, J.-F. and Heymans, C. (1927) Sur les modifications directes et sur la regulation reflexe de l'activité du centre respiratoire de la tête isolée du chien. *Arch. Intern. Pharmacodyn.* **33**, 273–370.

Hildebrandt, W., Ottenbacher, A., Schuster, M., Swenson, E.R. and Bärtsch, P. (2000) Diuretic effect of hypoxia, hypocapnia, and hyperpnea in humans: relation to hormones and O_2 chemosensitivity. *J. Appl. Physiol.* **88**, 599–610.

Hildebrandt, W., Alexander, S., Bärtsch, P. and Draöge, W. (2002) Effect of *N*-acetyl-cysteine on the hypoxic ventilatory response and erythropoietin production: linkage between plasma thiol redox state and O_2 chemosensitivity. *Blood* **99**, 1552–6.

Hill, A.V. (1928) The diffusion of oxygen and lactic acid through tissues. *Proc. R. Soc. Lond. Ser. B* **104**, 39–96.

Hill, L. (1934) Foreword, in *Oxygen and Carbon Dioxide Therapy* (eds A. Campbell and E.P. Poulton), Oxford University Press, London.

Hinchliff, T.W. (1876) *Over the Sea and Far Away,* Longmans Green, London.

Hirata, K., Matsuyama, S. and Saito, A. (1989) Obesity as a risk factor for acute mountain sickness. *Lancet* **2**, 1040–1.

Hirvonen, J. (1982) Accidental hypothermia, in *Report 30*, Nordic Council for Arctic Medical Research, Copenhagen, pp. 15–19.

Hochachka, P.W., Clark, C.M., Stanley, C., Uqurbil, K. and Menon, R.S. (1996) ^{31}P Magnetic resonance spectroscopy of the Sherpa heart: a phosphocreatine/adenosine defence against hypobaric hypoxia. *Proc. Natl. Acad. Sci. USA* **93**, 1215–20.

Hoff, C.J. and Abelson, A.E. (1976) Fertility, in *Man in The Andes, A Multidisciplinary Study of High-Altitude Quechua* (eds. P.T. Baker and M.A. Little), Dowden, Hutchinson & Ross, Stroudsburg, PA, pp. 128–46.

Hoffman, R.C. and Wittmers, L.E. (1990) Cold vasodilatation, pain and acclimatization in Arctic explorers. *J. Wilderness Med.* **1**, 225–34.

Hogan, R.P., Kotchen, T.A., Boyd, A.E. and Hartley, L.H. (1973) Effect of altitude on the renin–aldosterone system and metabolism of water and electrolytes. *J. Appl. Physiol.* **35**, 385–90.

Hogan, M.C., Roca, J., Wagner, P.D. and West, J.B. (1988a) Limitation of maximal O_2 uptake and performance by acute hypoxia in dog muscle *in situ. J. Appl. Physiol.* **65**, 815–21.

Hogan, M.C., Roca, J., West, J.B., and Wagner, P.D. (1988b) Dissociation of maximal O_2 uptake from O_2 delivery in canine gastrocnemius *in situ. J. Appl. Physiol.* **66**, 1219–26.

Hogan, M.C., Bebout, D.E. and Wagner, P.D. (1991) Effect of increased Hb-O_2 affinity on Vo_{2max} at constant O_2 delivery in dog muscle in situ. *J. Appl. Physiol.* **70**, 2656–62.

Hohenhaus, E., Niroomand, F.G., Goerre, S., *et al.* (1994) Nifedipine does not prevent acute mountain sickness. *Am. J. Respir. Crit. Care* **150**, 857–60.

Hohenhaus, E., Paul, A., McCullough, R.E. *et al.* (1995) Ventilatory and pulmonary vascular response to hypoxia and susceptibility to high altitude pulmonary oedema. *Eur. Respir. J.* **8**, 1825–33.

Höhne, C., Pickerodt, P.A., Francis, R.C.E., Boemke, W. and Swenson, E.R. (2006) Pulmonary vasodilation by acetazolamide during acute hypoxia is not related to carbonic anhydrase inhibition. *Am. J. Physiol. Lung Cell Mol. Physiol.* doi:10.1152/ajplung.00205.2006.

Höhne, C., Krebs, M.O., Seiferheld, M., Boemke, W., Kaczmarczyk, G. and Swenson, E.R. (2004) Acetazolamide prevents hypoxic pulmonary vasoconstriction in conscious dogs. *J. Appl. Physiol.* **97**, 515–21.

Hoit, B.D., Dalton, N.D., Erzurum, S.C., Laskowski, D., Strohl, K.P. and Beall, C.M. (2005) Nitric oxide and cardiopulmonary hemodynamics in Tibetan highlanders. *J. Appl. Physiol.* **99**, 1796–801. E-pub 14 July 2005.

Holden, J.E., Stone, C.K., Clark, M. *et al.* (1995) Enhanced cardiac metabolism of plasma glucose in high-altitude natives: adaptation against chronic hypoxia. *J. Appl. Physiol.* **79**, 222–8.

Holditch, T. (1907) *Tibet the Mysterious,* Alston Rivers, London, pp. 242–3.

Holloszy, J.O. and Coyle, E.F. (1984) Adaptations of skeletal muscle to endurance exercise and their metabolic consequences. *J. Appl. Physiol.* **56**, 831–8.

Holm, P. (1997) Endothelin in the pulmonary circulation with special reference to hypoxic pulmonary vasoconstriction. *Scand. Cardiovasc. J.* Suppl. **46**, 1–40.

Homik, L.A., Bshouty, Z., Light, R.B. and Younes, M. (1988) Effect of alveolar hypoxia on pulmonary fluid filtration in *in-situ* dog lungs. *J. Appl. Physiol.* **65**, 46–52.

Hong, S.I. and Nadel, E.R. (1979) Thermogenic control during exercise in a cold environment. *J. Appl. Physiol.* **47**, 1084–9.

Hong, S.K. (1973) Pattern of cold adaptation in women divers of Korea. *Fed. Proc.* **32**, 1414–22.

Honig, A. (1983) Role of arterial chemoreceptors in the reflex control of renal function and body fluid volumes in acute arterial hypoxia, in *Physiology of the Peripheral Arterial Chemoreceptors* (eds. H. Acher and R.C. O'Regan), Elsevier, Amsterdam, pp. 395–429.

Honig, A. (1989) Peripheral arterial chemoreceptors and reflex control of sodium and water homeostasis. *Am. J. Physiol.* **257**, R1282–302.

Honig, C.R. and Tenney, S.M. (1957) Determinants of the circulatory response to hypoxia and hypercapnia. *Am. Heart J.* **53**, 687–98.

Honig, C.R., Gayeski, T.E.J. and Groebe, K. (1991) Myoglobin and oxygen gradients, in *The Lung: Scientific Foundations* (eds. R.G. Crystal and J.B. West), Raven Press, New York, pp. 1489–96.

Honigman, B., Thesis, M.K., Koziol-McLain, J. *et al.* (1993) Acute mountain sickness in a general tourist population at moderate altitude. *Ann. Intern. Med.* **118**, 587–92.

Honigman, B., Noordewier, E., Kleinman, D. and Yaron, M. (2001) High altitude retinal hemorrhages in a Colorado skier. *High Alt. Med. Biol.* **2**, 539–44.

Hoon, R.S., Sharma, S.C., Balasubramanian, V. and Chadha, K.S. (1977) Urinary catecholamine excretion on induction to high altitude (3658 m) by air and road. *J. Appl. Physiol.* **42**, 728–30.

Hopkins, S.R., Garg, J., Bolar, D.S., Balouch, J. and Levin, D.L. (2005) Pulmonary blood flow heterogeneity during hypoxia and high-altitude pulmonary edema. *Am. J. Resp. Crit. Care Med.* **171**, 83–7.

Hoppeler, H. (1999) Vascular growth in hypoxic skeletal muscle. *Adv. Exp. Med. Biol.* **474**, 277–86.

Hoppeler, H. and Michael Vogt, M. (2001) Muscle tissue adaptations to hypoxia. *J. Exp. Biol.* **204**, 3133–9 .

Hoppeler, H., Kayar, S.R., Claassen, H., Uhlmann, E. and Karas, R.H. (1987) Adaptive variation in the mammalian respiratory system in relation to energetic demand: III. Skeletal muscles: setting the demand for oxygen. *Respir. Physiol.* **69**, 27–46.

Hoppeler, H., Howald, H. and Cerretelli, P. (1990) Human muscle structure after exposure to extreme altitude. *Experientia* **46**, 1185–7.

Hoppeler, H., Vogt, M., Weibel, R. and Flück, M. (2003) Response of skeletal muscle mitochondria to hypoxia. *Exp. Physiol.* **88**, 109–19.

Horio, T., Kohno, M., Yokokawa, K. *et al.* (1991) Effect of hypoxia on plasma immunoreactive endothelin-1 concentration in anaesthetized rats. *Metabolism* **40**, 999–1001.

Hornbein, T.F., Townes, B.D., Schoene, R.B. *et al.* (1989) The cost to the central nervous system of climbing to extremely high altitude. *N. Engl. J. Med.* **321**, 1714–19.

Horton, B.T. and Brown, G.E. (1929) Systemic histamine like reactions in allergy due to cold. *Am. J. Med. Sci.* **198**, 191–202.

Horvath, S.M. (1981) Exercise in a cold environment. *Exercise Sports Sci. Rev.* **9**, 191–263.

Hossmann, K.A. (1999) The hypoxic brain. Insights from ischemia research. *Adv. Exp. Med. Biol.* **474**, 155–69.

Hotta, J., Hanaoka, M., Droma, Y. *et al.* (2004) Polymorphisms of renin–angiotensin system genes with high-altitude pulmonary edema in Japanese subjects. *Chest* **126**, 825–30.

Houk, V.N. (1959) Transient pulmonary insufficiency caused by cold. *US Armed Forces Med. J.* **10**, 1354–7.

Houston, C.S. (1987) Transient visual disturbance at high altitude (abstract), in *Hypoxia and Cold* (eds. J.R. Sutton, C.S. Houston and G. Coates), Praeger, New York, p. 536.

Houston, C.S. (1988–9) Operation Everest II – 1985. *Alpine J.* **93**, 196–200.

Houston, C.S. and Bates, R. (1979) *K2, The Savage Mountain.* McGraw-Hill, New York, pp. 180–99.

Houston, C.S. and Dickinson, J. (1975) Cerebral form of high-altitude illness. *Lancet* **2**, 758–61.

Houston, C.S. and Riley, R.L. (1947) Respiratory and circulatory change during acclimatization to high altitude. *Am. J. Physiol.* **149**, 565–88.

Houston, C.S., Sutton, J.R., Cymerman, A. and Reeves, J.T. (1987) Operation Everest II: man at extreme altitude. *J. Appl. Physiol.* **63**, 877–82.

Houston, C.S., Cymerman, A. and Sutton, J.R. (1991) *Operation Everest II: Final Days*, US Army Research Institute of Environmental Medicine, Natick, MA, p. 96.

Howald, H. and Hoppeler, H. (2003) Performing at extreme altitude: muscle cellular and subcellular adaptations. *Eur. J. Appl. Physiol.* **90**, 360–4.

Howald, H., Pette, D., Simoneau, J.A., Uber, A., Hoppler, H. and Cerretelli, P. (1990) Effect of chronic hypoxia on muscle enzyme activities. *Int. J. Sports Med.* **11** (Suppl. 1), S10–14.

Howard, L.S.G.E. and Robbins, P.A. (1995) Alterations in respiratory control during 8 h of isocapnic and poikilocapnic hypoxia in humans. *J. Appl. Physiol.* **78**, 1089–107.

Howard-Bury, C.K. (1922) *Mt. Everest: The Reconnaissance, 1921,* Arnold, London.

Howarth, M. (1999) High altitude cerebral oedema – a rescue. *ISMM Newsletter* **9**(4), 15–17.

Hsu, A.R., Barnholt, K.E., Grundmann, N.K., Lin, J.H., McCallum, S.W. and Friedlander, A.L. (2006) Sildenafil improves cardiac output and exercise performance during acute hypoxia, but not normoxia. *J. Appl. Physiol.* **100**, 2031–40. E-pub 2 February 2006.

Hu, S.T., Huang, W.Y., Chu, S.C. and Pa, C.F. (1982) Chemoreflexive ventilatory response at sea level in subjects with past history of good acclimatization and severe acute mountain sickness, in *High Altitude Physiology and Medicine* (eds. W. Brendel and R.A. Zink), Springer-Verlag, New York, pp. 28–32.

Huang, S.Y., Ning, X.H., Zhou, Z.N. *et al.* (1984) Ventilatory function in adaptation to high altitude: studies in Tibet, in *High Altitude and Man* (eds. J.B. West and S. Lahiri), American Physiological Society, Bethesda, MD, pp. 173–7.

Huang, S.Y., Moore, L.G., McCullough, R.E. *et al.* (1987) Internal carotid and vertebral arterial flow velocity in men at high altitude. *J. Appl. Physiol.* **63**, 395–400.

Huang, S.Y., Tawney, K.W., Bender, P.R. *et al.* (1991) Internal carotid flow velocity with exercise before and after acclimatization to 4300 m. *J. Appl. Physiol.* **71**, 1469–76.

Huang, S.Y., Sun, S., Droma, T. *et al.* (1992) Internal carotid arterial flow velocity during exercise in Tibetan and Han residents of Lhasa (3,658 m). *J. Appl. Physiol.* **73**, 2638–42.

Hubbard, R.W., Gaffin, S.L. and Squire, D.L. (1995) Heat related illness, in *Wilderness Medicine* (ed. P.S. Auerbach), Mosby, St Louis, pp. 167–212.

Huddleston, B., Ataman, E. and Fè de'Ostiane L (2003) Towards a GIS-based analysis of mountain environments and populations. Working paper #10, UN, FAO, Rome. Available on www. fao.org.

Hudson, J.G., Bowen, A.L., Navia, P. *et al.* (1999) The effect of high altitude on platelet counts, thrombopoietin and erythropoietin levels in young Bolivian airmen visiting the Andes. *Int. J. Biometrol.* **43**, 85–90.

Hüfner, C.G. (1890) Uber das Gesetz der Dissociation des Oxyhämoglobins und über einige daran sich knüpfende wichtige Fragen aus der Biologie. *Arch. Pathol. Anat. Physiol.* 1–27.

Huicho, L. and Niermeyer, S. (2006) Cardiopulmonary pathology among children resident at high altitude in Tintaya, Peru: a cross-sectional study. *High Alt. Med. Biol.* **7**, 168–79.

Hultgren, H., Spickard, W. and Lopez, C. (1962) Further studies of high altitude pulmonary edema. *Br. Heart J.* **24**, 95–102.

Hultgren, H.N. (1969) High altitude pulmonary edema, in *Biomedicine Problems of High Terrestrial Altitude* (ed. A.H. Hegnauer), Springer-Verlag, New York, pp. 131–41.

Hultgren, H.N. (1970). Reduction of systemic arterial blood pressure at high altitude. *Adv. Cardiol.* (Basel) **5**, 49–55.

Hultgren, H.N. (1978) High altitude pulmonary edema, in *Lung Water and Solute Exchange* (ed. N.C. Staub), Dekker, New York, pp. 437–69.

Hultgren, H.N. (1992) Effect of altitude on cardio-vascular diseases. *J. Wilderness Med.* **3**, 301–8.

Hultgren, H.N. (1997) *High Altitude Medicine,* Hultgren Publications, Stanford, CA, p. 12.

Hultgren, H.N. and Marticorena, E.A. (1978) High altitude pulmonary edema. Epidemiologic observations in Peru. *Chest* **74**, 372–6.

Hultgren, H.N., Lopez, C.E., Lundberg, E. and Miller, H. (1964) Physiologic studies of pulmonary edema at high altitude. *Circulation* **29**, 393–408.

Hultgren, H.N., Robison, M.C. and Wuerflein, R.D. (1966) Over perfusion pulmonary edema. *Circulation* **34** (Suppl. 3), 132–3.

Hultgren, H.N., Grover, R.F. and Hartley, L.H. (1971) Abnormal circulatory responses to high altitude in subjects with a previous history of high-altitude pulmonary edema. *Circulation* **44**, 759–70.

Hultgren, H.N., Wilson, R. and Kosek, J.C. (1997) Lung pathology in high-altitude pulmonary edema. *Wild. Environ. Med.* **8**, 218–20.

Hunt, J. (1953) *The Ascent of Everest*, Hodder and Stoughton, London.

Hunter, J. (1781) *Original Cases*, Library of Royal College of Surgeons of England, London.

Hunter, J., Kerr, E.H. and Whillans, M.G. (1952) The relation between joint stiffness upon exposure to cold and the characteristics of synovial fluid. *J. Can. Med. Sci.* **39**, 367–77.

Huonker, M., Schmidt-Trucksass, A., Sorichter, S. *et al.* (1997) Highland mountain hiking and coronary artery disease: exercise tolerance and effects on left ventricular function. *Med. Sci. Sports Exerc.* **29**, 1554–60.

Hupperets, M.D., Hopkins, S.R., Pronk, M.G. *et al.* (2004) Increased hypoxic ventilatory responses during 8 weeks at 3800 m altitude. *Respir. Physiol. Neurobiol.* **142**, 145–52.

Hurtado, A. (1942) Chronic mountain sickness. *JAMA* **120**, 1278–82.

Hurtado, A. (1964) Animals in high altitudes: resident man, in *Handbook of Physiology, Section IV, Adaptation to the Environment* (ed. D.B. Dill), American Physiological Society, Washington DC, pp. 843–60.

Hurtado, A. (1971) The influence of high altitude on physiology, in *High Altitude Physiology* (eds. R. Porter and J. Knight), Ciba Foundation Symposium, Churchill Livingstone, Edinburgh, pp. 3–13.

Hurtado, A., Rotta, A., Merino, C. and Pons, J. (1937) Studies of myohemoglobin at high altitude. *Am. J. Med. Sci.* **194**, 708–13.

Hurtado, A., Merino, C. and Delgado, E. (1945) Influence of anoxemia on the hemopoietic activity. *Arch. Intern. Med.* **75**, 284–323.

Hutchinson, S.J. and Litch, J.A. (1997) Acute myocardial infarction at high altitude. *JAMA* **278**, 1661–2.

Hyde, R.W., Forster, R.E., Power, G.G. *et al.* (1966) Measurement of O_2 diffusing capacity of the lungs with a stable O_2 isotope. *J. Clin. Invest.* **45**, 1178–93.

Hyers, T.M., Scoggin, C.H., Will, D.H. *et al.* (1979) Accentuated hypoxemia at high altitude in subjects susceptible to high-altitude pulmonary edema. *J. Appl. Physiol. Respir. Environ. Exercise Physiol.* **46**, 41–6.

Ibbertson, H.K., Tair, J.M., Pearl, M. *et al.* (1972) Himalayan cretinism. *Adv. Exp. Med. Biol.* **30**, 51–69.

ICAO (1964) *Manual of the ICAO Standard Atmosphere*, 2nd edn, International Civil Aviation Organization, Montreal, Canada.

Ignarro, L.J., Buga, GM., Wood, K.S. *et al.* (1987) Endothelium-derived relaxing factor produced and released from artery and vein is nitric oxide. *Proc. Natl. Acad. Sci. USA* **84**, 9265–9.

Ikawa, G., Dos Santos, P.A.L., Yamaguchi, K.T. *et al.* (1986) Frostbite and bone scanning: the use of [99]m-labelled phosphates in demarcating the line of viability in frostbite victims. *Orthopaedics* **9**, 1257–61.

Iliff, L.D. (1971) Extra-alveolar vessels and edema development in excised dog lungs. *Circ. Res.* **28**, 524–32.

Imray, C.H., Chesner, I., Winterbourn, M. *et al.* (1992) Fat absorption at altitude: a reappraisal (abstract). *Int. J. Sports Med.* **13**, 87.

Imray, C.H., Brearey, S., Clarke, T. *et al.* (2000) Cerebral oxygenation at high altitude and the response to carbon dioxide, hyperventilation and oxygen. *Clin. Sci.* **98**, 159–64.

Imray, C.H., Walsh, S., Clarke, T. *et al.* Birmingham Medical Research Expeditionary Society. (2003) Effects of breathing air containing 3% carbon dioxide, 35% oxygen or a mixture of 3% carbon dioxide/35% oxygen on cerebral and peripheral oxygenation at 150 m and 3459 m. *Clin. Sci. (Lond).* **104**, 203–10.

Imray, C.H., Myers, S.D., Pattinson, K.T. *et al.* (2005) Effect of exercise on cerebral perfusion in humans at high altitude. *J. Appl. Physiol.* **99**, 699–706. E-pub 26 May 2005.

Ind, P.W., Maxwell, D.L., Causon, R.C. *et al.* (1984) Hypoxia and catecholamine secretion in normal man. *Clin. Sci.* **67**, 58–59P.

Ingjer, F. and Brodal, P. (1978) Capillary supply of skeletal muscle fibers in untrained and endurance-trained women. *Eur. J. Appl. Physiol.* **38**, 291–9.

Ingjer, F. and Myhre, K. (1992) Physiological effects of altitude training on elite male cross-country skiers. *J. Sports Sci.* **10**, 37–47.

Irwin, M.S., Thorniley, M.S. and Green, C.J. (1994) An investigation into the aetiology of non-freezing cold injury using infrared spectroscopy. *Biochem. Soc. Trans.* **22**, 418S.

Irwin, M.S., Sanders, R., Gren, C.J. and Terenghi, G. (1997) Neuropathy in non-freezing injuries (trench foot). *J. R. Soc. Med.* **90**, 433–8.

Ishizaki, T., Koizumi, T., Ruan, Z. *et al.* (2005) Nitric oxide inhibitor altitude-dependently elevates pulmonary arterial pressure in high-altitude adapted yaks. *Respir. Physiol. Neurobiol.* **146**, 225–30.

ISMM Newsletter (1998) The combined oral contraceptive (COC) at altitude – is it safe? (10 discussants) *ISMM Newsletter* **8**(2), 11–13.

Itskovitz, J., LaCamma, E.F. and Rudolph, A.M. (1987) Effects of cord compression on fetal blood flow distribution and O_2 delivery. *Am. J. Physiol. (Heart Circ. Physiol.)* **21**, H100–9.

Jackson, F. and Davies, H. (1960) The electrocardiogram of the mountaineer at high altitude. *Br. Heart J.* **22**, 671–85.

Jackson, F.S. (1968) The heart at high altitude. *Br. Heart J.* **30**, 291–4.

Jackson, F.S., Turner, R.W.D. and Ward, M.P. (1966) *Report on IBP Expedition to North Bhutan,* Royal Society, London.

Jackson, J.A. (1975) Avoidance of cold injury. Outline of basic principles, in *Mountain Medicine and Physiology* (eds. C. Clarke, M.P. Ward and E.S. Williams), Alpine Club, London, pp. 28–30.

Jain, S.C., Bardhan, J., Swamy, Y.V. *et al.* (1980) Body fluid compartments in humans during acute high-altitude exposure. *Aviat. Space Environ. Med.* **51**, 234–6.

Jain, S.C., Singh, M.V., Sharma, V.M. *et al.* (1986) Amelioration of acute mountain sickness: comparative study of acetazolamide and spironolactone. *Int. J. Biometeorol.* **30**, 293–300.

Jansen, G.F., Krins, A. and Basnyat, B. (1999) Cerebral vasomotor reactivity at high altitude in humans. *J. Appl. Physiol.* **86**, 681–6.

Jansen, G.F., Krins, A., Basnyat, B., Bosch, A. and Odoom, J.A. (2000) Cerebral autoregulation in subjects adapted and not adapted to high altitude. *Stroke* **31**, 2314–8.

Jansson, E., Sylven, C. and Nordevang, E. (1982) Myoglobin in the quadriceps femoris muscle of competitive cyclists and untrained men. *Acta Physiol. Scand.* **114**, 627–9.

Jedlickova, K., Stockton, D.W., Chen, H. *et al.* (2003) Search for genetic determinants of individual variability of the erythropoietin response to high altitude. *Blood Cells Mol. Dis.* **31**, 175–82.

Jefferson, J.A., Escudero, E., Hertardo, M.E., *et al.* (2002a) Hyperuricemia, hypertension and proteinuria associated with high-altitude polycythemia. *Am. J. Kidney Dis.* **39**, 1135–42.

Jefferson, J.A., Escudero, E., Hurtado, M.-E. *et al.* (2002b) Excessive erythrocytosis, chronic mountain sickness, and serum cobalt levels. *Lancet* **359**, 407–8.

Jensen, G.M. and Moore, L.G. (1997) The effect of high altitude and other risk factors on birthweight: independent or interactive effect. *Am. J. Public Health* **87**, 1003–7.

Jensen, J.B., Wright, A.D., Lassen, N.A. *et al.* (1990) Cerebral blood flow in acute mountain sickness. *J. Appl. Physiol.* **69**, 430–3.

Jenzer, G. and Bärtsch, P. (1993) Migraine with aura at high altitude: case report. *J. Wild. Med.* **4**, 412–5.

Jequier, E., Gygax, P-H., Pittet, P. and Vannotti, A. (1974) Increased thermal body insulation: relationship to the development of obesity. *J. Appl. Physiol.* **36**, 674–8.

Jessen, K. and Hagelstein, J.O. (1978) Peritoneal dialysis in the treatment of profound accidental hypothermia. *Aviat. Space Environ. Med.* **49**, 424–9.

Jha, S.K., Anand, A.C., Sharma, V., Kumar, N. and Adya, C.M. (2002) Stroke at high altitude: Indian experience. *High Alt. Med. Biol.* **3**, 21–7.

Jiménez, D. (1995) High altitude intermittent chronic exposure: Andean miners, in *Hypoxia and the Brain* (eds. J.R. Sutton, C.S. Houston and G. Coates), Queen City Printers, Burlington, VT, pp. 284–91.

Joern, A.T., Shurley, J.T., Brooks, R.E., Guenter, C.A., and Pierce, C.M. (1970) Short-term changes in sleep patterns on arrival at the South Polar Plateau. *Arch. Int. Med.* **125**, 649–54.

Johnson, B.D., Babcock, M.A., Suman, O.E. and Dempsey, J.A. (1993) Exercise-induced diaphragmatic fatigue in healthy humans. *J. Physiol.* **460**, 385–405.

Johnson, R.L. Jr., Cassidy, S.S., Grover, R.E. *et al.* (1985) Functional capacities of lungs and thorax in beagles after prolonged residence at 3,100 m. *J. Appl. Physiol.* **59**, 1773–82.

Johnson, T.S., Rock, P.B., Fulco, C.S. *et al.* (1984) Prevention of acute mountain sickness by dexamethasone. *N. Engl. J. Med.* **310**, 683–6.

Jones, N.M. and Bergeron, M. (2001) Hypoxic preconditioning induces changes in HIF-1 target genes in neonatal rat brain. *J. Cereb. Blood Flow. Metab.* **21**, 1105–14.

Joseph, V., Soliz, J., Pequignot, J. *et al.* (2000) Gender differentiation of the chemoreflex during growth at high altitude: functional and neurochemical studies. *Am. J. Physiol. Regul. Integr. Comp. Physiol.* **278**, R806–16.

Josephson, M.E. and Wellens, H.J. (eds.) (1984) *Tachycardia: Mechanisms, Diagnosis, Treatment,* Lea and Febiger, Philadelphia, PA.

Jourdanet, D. (1875) *Influence de la Pression de l'Air sur la Vie de l'Homme,* Masson, Paris.

Jowers, C., Shih, R., James, J., Deloughery, T.G. and Holden, W.E. (2004) Effects of *Ginkgo biloba* on exhaled nasal nitric oxide during normobaric hypoxia in humans. *High Alt. Med. Biol.* **5**, 445–9.

Julian, C.G., Gore, C.J., Wilber, R.L. *et al.* (2004) Intermittent normobaric hypoxia does not alter performance or erythropoietic markers in highly trained distance runners. *J. Appl. Physiol.* **96**, 1800–7.

Juniper, E.F. and Hargreave, F.E. (1986) Airway responsiveness assessed by aerosol inhalation tests: variability in results due to unexpected differences between calibrated nebulizers. *J. Allergy Clin. Immunol.* **78**, 387–91.

Kacimi, R., Richalet, J.-P., Corsin, A. *et al.* (1992) Hypoxia-induced downregulation of β-adrenergic receptors in rat heart. *J. Appl. Physiol.* **73**, 1377–82.

Kamat, S.R. and Banerji, B.C. (1972) Study of cardiopulmonary function on exposure to high altitude. I. Acute acclimatization to an altitude of 3,500 to 4,000 meters in relation to altitude sickness and cardiopulmonary function. *Am. Rev. Respir. Dis.* **106**, 404–13.

Kamin, W., Fleck, B., Rose, D.M., Thews, O. and Thielen, W. (2006) Predicting hypoxia in cystic fibrosis patients during exposure to high altitudes. *J. Cyst. Fibros.* [E-pub 17 May 2006 ahead of print].

Kaminsky, D.A., Irvin, C.G., Gurka, D.A. *et al.* (1995) Peripheral airways responsiveness to cool, dry air in normal and asthmatic individuals. *Am. J. Respir. Crit. Care Med.* **152**, 1784–90.

Kapanci, Y., Assimacopoulos, A., Irle, C. *et al.* (1974) 'Contractile interstitial cells' in pulmonary alveolar septa: a possible regulator of ventilation–perfusion ratio? Ultrastructural, immunofluorescence, and in vitro studies. *J. Cell Biol.* **60**, 375–92.

Kaplan, L.A. (1992) Suntan, sunburn and sun protection. *J. Wilderness Med.* **3**, 173–96.

Kapoor, S.C. (1984) Changes in electrocardiogram among temporary residents at high altitude. *Defence Sci. J.* **34**, 389–95.

Kapoor, A.K., Kshatriya, G.K. and Kapoor, S. (2003) Fertility and mortality differentials among the population groups of the Himalayas. *Hum Biol.* **75**, 729–47.

Kappes, B.W. and Mills, W.J. (1984) Thermal biofeedback training with frostbite patients (abstract). *Sixth International Symposium on Circumpolar Health,* 13–18 May, Anchorage, Alaska, p. 100.

Karagiannidis, C., Hense, G., Rueckert, B. *et al.* (2006) High-altitude climate therapy reduces local airway inflammation and modulates lymphocyte activation. *Scand. J. Immunol.* **63**, 304–10.

Karliner, J., Sarnquist, F.H., Graber, D.J., Peters, R.M. Jr and West, J.B. (1985) The electrocardiogram at extreme altitude: experience on Mt. Everest. *Am. Heart J.* **109**, 505–13.

Kasch, F.W., Boyer, J.L., Van Camp, S., Nettl, F. and Wallace, J.P. (1995) Cardiovascular changes with age and exercise. A 28-year longitudinal study. *Scan. J. Med. Sci. Sports.* **5**, 147–51.

Katayama, K., Sato, Y., Morotome, Y., *et al.* (2001) Intermittent hypoxia increases ventilation and SaO_2 during hypoxic exercise and hypoxic chemosensitivity. *J. Appl. Physiol.* **90**, 1431–40.

Kato, M. and Staub, N.C. (1966) Response of small pulmonary arteries to unilobar hypoxia and hypercapnia. *Circ. Res.* **19**, 426–40.

Kawashima, A., Kubo, K., Kobayashi, T. and Sekiguchi, M. (1989) Hemodynamic response to acute hypoxia, hypobaria and exercise in subjects susceptible to high-altitude pulmonary edema. *J. Appl. Physiol.* **67**, 1982–9.

Kawashima, A., Kubo, K., Matsuwara, Y. *et al.* (1992) Hypoxia-induced ANP secretion in subjects susceptible to high-altitude pulmonary edema. *Respir. Physiol.* **89**, 309–17.

Kay, J.M. and Edwards, F.R. (1973) Ultrastructure of the alveolar-capillary wall in mitral stenosis. *J. Pathol.* **111**, 239–45.

Kay, J.M., Waymire, J.C. and Grover, R.F. (1974) Lung mast cell hyperplasia and pulmonary histamine-forming capacity in hypoxic rats. *Am. J. Physiol.* **226**, 178–84.

Kayser, B. (1991) Acute mountain sickness in western tourists around the Thorong pass (5400 m) in Nepal. *J. Wilderness Med.* **2**, 110–17.

Kayser, B., Hoppeler, H., Desplances, H. and Cerretelli, P. (1991) Muscle ultrastructure and biochemistry of lowland Tibetans. *J. Appl. Physiol.* **70**, 1938–42.

Kayser, B., Acheson, K., Decombaz, J., Fern E. and Carretelli, P. (1992) Protein absorption and energy digestibility at high altitude. *J. Appl. Physiol.* **73**, 2425–31.

Kayser, B., Binzoni, T., Hoppeler, H. *et al.* (1993a) A case of severe frostbite on Mt Blanc: a multi-technique approach. *J. Wilderness Med.* **4**, 167–74.

Kayser, B., Narici, M.V. and Cibella, F. (1993b) Fatigue and performance at high altitude, in *Hypoxia and Molecular Medicine* (eds. J.R. Sutton, C.S. Houston and G. Coates), Queen City Printers, Burlington, VA, pp. 222–34.

Kayser, B., Hoppeler, H., Claassen, C. *et al.* (1996) Muscle structure and performance capacity of Himalayan Sherpas. *J. Appl. Physiol.* **81**, 419–25.

Kearney, M.S. (1973) Ultrastructural changes in the heart at high altitude. *Pathol. Microbiol.* **39**, 258–65.

Keatinge, W.R. and Cannon, P. (1960) Freezing point of human skin. *Lancet* **1**, 11–14.

Keatinge, W.R., Hayward, M.G. and McIver, N.K.I. (1980) Hypothermia during saturation diving in the North Sea. *BMJ* **1**, 291.

Keatinge, W.R., Coleshaw, S.R.K., Cotter, F. *et al.* (1984) Increases in platelet and red cell counts, blood viscosity and arterial pressure during mild surface cooling: factors in mortality from coronary and cerebral thrombosis in winter. *BMJ* **2**, 1405–8.

Keatinge, W.R., Coleshaw, S.R.K., Millard, C.E. and Axelsson, J. (1986) Exceptional case of survival in cold water. *BMJ* **292**, 171–2.

Keighley, J.H. and Steele, G. (1981) The functional and design requirements of clothing. *Alpine J.* **86**, 138–45.

Kellas, A.M. (2001) A consideration of the possibility of ascending Mount Everest. *High Alt. Med. Biol.* **2**, 431–61.

Keller, H.-R., Maggiorini, M., Bärtsch, P. and Oelz, O. (1995) Simulated descent v dexamethasone in treatment of acute mountain sickness: a randomized trial. *BMJ* **310**, 1232–5.

Kellogg, R.H. (1963) The role of CO_2 in altitude acclimatization, in *The Regulation of Human Respiration* (eds. D.J.C. Cunningham and B.B. Lloyd), Blackwell Scientific Publications, Oxford, pp. 379–94.

Kellogg, R.H. (1980) Acid–base balance in high altitude: historical perspective, in *Environmental Physiology: Aging, Heat and Altitude* (eds. S.M. Horvath and M.K. Yousef), Elsevier, New York, pp. 295–308.

Kelman, C.R. (1966a) Digital computer subroutine for the conversion of oxygen tension into saturation. *J. Appl. Physiol.* **21**, 1375–6.

Kelman, C.R. (1966b) Calculation of certain indices of cardio-pulmonary function using a digital computer. *Respir. Physiol.* **1**, 335–43.

Kelman, C.R. (1967) Digital computer procedure for the conversion of P_{CO_2} into blood CO_2 content. *Respir. Physiol.* **3**, 335–43.

Kennedy, B.C. and Gentle, D.A. (1995) Children in the wilderness, in *Wilderness Medicine* (ed. P.S. Auerbach), Mosby, St Louis, pp. 466–89.

Kerem, D. and Elsner, R. (1973) Cerebral tolerance to asphyxial hypoxia in the harbor seal. *Respir. Physiol.* **19**, 188–200.

Kerendi, F., Halkos, M.E., Kin, H. *et al.* (2005) Upregulation of hypoxia inducible factor is associated with attenuation of neuronal injury in neonatal piglets undergoing deep hypothermic circulatory arrest. *J. Thorac. Cardiovasc. Surg.* **130**, 1079.

Kessler, R., Chaoua, A., Schinkewitch, P. *et al.* (2001) The obesity–hypoventilation syndrome revisited. *Chest* **120**, 369–75.

Kety, S.S. (1950) Circulation and metabolism of the human brain in health and disease. *Am. J. Med.* **8**, 205–17.

Keyes, L.E., Armaza, J.F., Niermeyer, S., Vargas, E., Young, D.A. and Moore, L.G. (2003) Intrauterine growth restriction, preeclampsia, and intrauterine mortality at high altitude in Bolivia. *Pediatr. Res.* **54**, 20–5. E-pub 16 April 2003.

Keynes, R.J., Smith, G.W., Slater, J.D.H. *et al.* (1982) Renin and aldosterone at high altitude in man. *J. Endocrinol.* **92**, 131–40.

Keys, A. (1936) The physiology of life at high altitude: the International High Altitude Expedition to Chile 1935. *Sci. Mon.* **43**, 289–312.

Keys, A., Hall, F.G. and Guzman Barron, E.S. (1936) The position of the oxygen dissociation curve of human blood at high altitude. *Am. J. Physiol.* **115**, 292–307.

Keys, A., Stapp, J.P. and Violante, A. (1943) Responses in size, output and efficiency of the human heart to acute alteration in the composition of inspired air. *Am. J. Physiol.* **138**, 763–71.

Khoo, M.C., Anholm, J.D., Ko, S.W. *et al.* (1996) Dynamics of periodic breathing and arousal during sleep at extreme altitude. *Respir. Physiol.* **103**, 33–43.

Khoo, M.C.K., Kronauer, R.E., Strohl, K.P. and Slutsky, A.S. (1982) Factors inducing periodic breathing in humans: a general model. *J. Appl. Physiol.* **53**, 644–59.

Khoury, G.H. and Hawes, C.R. (1963) Primary pulmonary hypertension in children living at high altitude. *J. Pediatrics* **62**, 177–85.

King, A.B. and Robinson, S.M. (1972) Ventilation response to hypoxia and acute mountain sickness. *Aerospace Med.* **43**, 419–21.

Klausen, K. (1966) Cardiac output in man in rest and work during and after acclimatization to 3800 m. *J. Appl. Physiol.* **21**, 609–16.

Kleger, G.-R., Bärtsch, P., Vock, P. *et al.* (1996) Evidence against an increase in capillary permeability in subjects exposed to high altitude. *J. Appl. Physiol.* **81**, 1917–23.

Kline, D.D., Peng, Y.J., Manalo, J., Semenza, G.L. and Prabhakar, H.R. (2002) Defective carotid body function and impaired ventilatory response to chronic hypoxia in mice partially deficient for hypoxia-inducible factor 1α. *Proc. Natl. Acad. Sci. USA* **99**, 821–6.

Klokker, M., Kharazmi, A., Galbo, H. *et al.* (1993) Influence of *in vivo* hypobaric hypoxia on function of lymphocytes, natural killer cells, and cytokines. *J. Appl. Physiol.* **74**, 1100–6.

Knaupp, W., Khilnani, S., Sherwood, J. *et al.* (1992) Erythropoietin response to acute normobaric hypoxia in humans. *J. Appl. Physiol.* **73**, 837–40.

Knill, R.L. and Celb, A.W. (1978) Ventilatory responses to hypoxia and hypercapnia during halothane sedation and anaesthesia in man. *Anesthesiology* **49**, 244–51.

Knochel, J.P. (1989) Heat stroke and related heat stress disorders. *Dis. Mon.* **35**, 301–77.

Kobrick, J.L. (1972) Effects of hypoxia on voluntary response time to peripheral stimuli during central target monitoring. *Ergonomics* **15**, 147–56.

Kobrick, J.L. (1975) Effects of hypoxia on peripheral visual response to dim stimuli. *Percept. Mot. Skills* **41**, 467–74.

Kohlendorfer, U., Kiechl, S. and Sperl. W (1998) Living at high altitude and risk of sudden infant death syndrome. *Arch. Dis. Child.* **79**, 506–9.

Koistinen, P., Takala, T., Martikkala, V. and Leppalouto, J. (1995) Aerobic fitness influences the response of maximal oxygen uptake and lactate threshold in acute hypobaric hypoxia. *Int. J. Sports Med.* **26**, 78–81.

Koistinen, P.Q., Rusko, H., Irjala, K. *et al.* (2000) EPO, red cells, and serum transferring receptor in continuous and intermittent hypoxia. *Med. Sci. Sports Exerc.* **32**, 800–4.

Koizumi, T., Kawashima, A., Kubo, K., Kobayashi, T. and Sekiguchi, M. (1994) Radiographic and hemodynamic changes during recovery from high-altitude pulmonary edema. *Intern Med.* **33**, 525–8.

Koizumi, T., Ruan, Z., Sakai, A. *et al.* (2004) Contribution of nitric oxide to adaptation of Tibetan sheep to high altitude. *Respir. Physiol. Neurobiol.* **140**, 189–96.

Kontos, H.A. and Lower, R.R. (1963) Role of beta-adrenergic receptors in the circulatory response to high altitude hypoxia. *Am. J. Physiol.* **217**, 756–63.

Kontos, H.A., Levasseur, J.E., Richardson, D.W. *et al.* (1967) Comparative circulatory responses to systemic hypoxia in man and in unanesthetized dog. *J. Appl. Physiol.* **23**, 381–6.

Kosunen, K.J. and Pakarinen, A.J. (1976) Plasma renin, angiotensin II, and plasma and urinary aldosterone in running exercise. *J. Appl. Physiol.* **41**, 26–9.

Kotchen, T.A., Mougey, E.H., Hogan, R.P. *et al.* (1973) Thyroid responses to simulated altitude. *J. Appl. Physiol.* **34**, 145–8.

Koyama, S., Kobayashi, T., Kubo, K. *et al.* (1984) Catecholamine metabolism in patients with high altitude pulmonary edema (HAPE). *Jpn. J. Mount. Med.* **4**, 119.

Krakauer, J. (1997) *Into Thin Air*, Macmillan, London, pp. 189–284.

Krarup, N. and Larsen, J.A. (1972) The effect of slight hypothermia on liver function as measured by the elimination rate of ethanol, the hepatic uptake and excretion of indocyanine green and bile formation. *Acta Physiol. Scand.* **84**, 396–407.

Krasney, J.A. (1994) A neurogenic basis for acute altitude illness (Review). *Med. Sci. Sports Exerc.* **26**, 195–208.

Kreuzer, F. and van Lookeren Campagne, P. (1965) Resting pulmonary diffusing capacity for CO and O_2 at high altitude. *J. Appl. Physiol.* **20**, 519–24.

Kristensen, C., Drenk, N.E. and Jordening, H. (1986) Simple system for central rewarming of hypothermic patients. *Lancet* **2**, 1467–8.

Krogh, A. (1910) On the mechanism of the gas-exchange in the lungs. *Skand. Arch. Physiol.* **23**, 248–78.

Krogh, A. (1919) Number and distribution of capillaries in muscles with calculations of the oxygen pressure head necessary to supplying the tissue. *J. Physiol. (Lond.)* **52**, 409–15.

Krogh, A. (1929) *The Anatomy and Physiology of Capillaries*, Yale University Press, New Haven, CT.

Krogh, A. and Krogh, M. (1910) On the tensions of gases in the arterial blood. *Skand. Archiv. Physiol.* **23**, 179–92.

Krogh, M. (1915) The diffusion of gases through the lungs of man. J. *Physiol. (Lond.)* **49**, 271–96.

Kronenberg, R.S. and Drage, C.W. (1973) Attenuation of the ventilatory and heart rate responses to hypoxia and hypercapnia with ageing in normal men. *J. Clin. Invest.* **52**, 1812–19.

Kronenberg, R.S., Safar, P., Lee, J. *et al.* (1971) Pulmonary artery pressure and alveolar gas exchange in man during acclimatization to 12,470 ft. *J. Clin. Invest.* **50**, 827–37.

Kryger, M., McCullough, R., Doekel, R., Collins, D., Weil, J.V. and Grover, R.F. (1978a) Excessive polycythemia of high altitude: role of ventilatory drive and lung disease. *Am. Rev. Respir.* Dis. **118**, 659–66.

Kryger, M., McCullough, R.E., Collins, D., Scoggin, C.H., Weil, J.V. and Grover, R.F. (1978b) Treatment of excessive polycythemia of high altitude with respiratory stimulant drugs. *Am. Rev. Respir. Dis.* **117**, 455–64.

Kubo, K., Hanaoka, M., Hayano, T. *et al.* (1998) Inflammatory cytokines in BAL fluid and pulmonary hemodynamics in high-altitude pulmonary edema. *Respir. Physiol.* **111**, 301–10.

Kuepper, T. Hoefer, M., Gieseler, U. and Netzer, N. (1999) Prevention of acute mountain sickness with theophylline (abstract), in *Hypoxia: Into the Next Millennium* (eds. R.C. Roach, P.D. Wagner and P.H. Hackett), Plenum/Kluwer, New York, p. 400.

Kumar, A.S., Mishra, S., Dorjey, M., Morup, T. and Ali, R. (2005) Cardiac surgery at high altitude. *Nat. Med. J. India* **18**, 137–8.

Kumar, R., Pasha, Q., Khan, A.P. and Gupta, V. (2004) Renin angiotensin aldosterone system and ACE I/D gene polymorphism in high-altitude pulmonary edema. *Aviat. Space Environ. Med.* **75**, 981–3.

Kumar, V.N. (1982) Intractable foot pain following frostbite. *Arch. Phys. Med. Rehabil.* **63**, 284–5.

Kuwahira, I., Moue, Y., Urano, T. *et al.* (2001) Redistribution of pulmonary blood flow during hypoxic exercise. *Int. J. Sports. Med.* **22**, 393–9.

Lafleur, J., Giron, M., Demarco, M., Kennedy, R., BeLue, R. and Shields, C. (2003) Cognitive effects of dexamethasone at high altitude. *Wild. Environ. Med.* **14**, 20–3.

Lahiri, S. (1972) Dynamic aspects of regulation of ventilation in man during acclimatization to high altitude. *Respir. Physiol.* **16**, 245–58.

Lahiri, S. (1977) Physiological responses and adaptations to high altitude, in *International Review of Physiology Environmental Physiology II vol. 14* (ed. D. Robertshaw), University Park Press, Baltimore, MD, pp. 217–51.

Lahiri, S. and Barnard, P. (1983) Role of arterial chemoreflexes in breathing during sleep at high altitude, in *Hypoxia, Exercise and Altitude* (eds. J.S. Sutton, C.S. Houston and N.L. Jones), Liss, New York, pp. 75–85.

Lahiri, S. and Cherniack, N.S. (2001) Cellular and molecular mechanisms of O_2 sensing with special reference to the carotid body, in *High Altitude* (eds. T.F. Hornbein and R.B. Schoene), Lung Biology in Health and Disease, vol 161, Marcel Dekker, New York, pp. 101–30.

Lahiri, S. and Delaney, R.G. (1975) Stimulus interaction in the response of carotid body chemoreceptor single afferent fibres. *Respir. Physiol.* **24**, 267–86.

Lahiri, S. and Milledge, J.S. (1967) Acid–base in Sherpa altitude residents and lowlanders at 4880 m. *Respir. Physiol.* **2**, 323–34.

Lahiri, S., Milledge, J.S., Chattopadhyay, H.P. *et al.* (1967) Respiration and heart rate of Sherpa highlanders during exercise. *J. Appl. Physiol.* **23**, 545–54.

Lahiri, S., Kao, F.F., Velasquez, T. *et al.* (1969) Irreversible blunted sensitivity to hypoxia in high altitude natives. *Respir. Physiol.* **6**, 360–7.

Lahiri, S., Delaney, R.G., Brody, J.S. *et al.* (1976) Relative role of environmental and genetic factors in respiratory adaptation to high altitude. *Nature* **261**, 133–5.

Lahiri, S., Edelman, N.H., Cherniack, N.S. and Fishman, A.P. (1981) Role of carotid chemoreflex in respiratory acclimatization to hypoxemia in goat and sheep. *Respir. Physiol.* **46**, 367–82.

Lahiri, S., Maret, K. and Sherpa, M.G. (1983) Dependence of high altitude sleep apnea on ventilatory sensitivity to hypoxia. *Respir. Physiol.* **52**, 281–301.

Lahiri, S., Maret, K.H., Sherpa, M.G. and Peters, R.M. Jr (1984) Sleep and periodic breathing at high altitude: Sherpa natives versus sojourners, in *High Altitude and Man* (eds. J.B. West and S. Lahiri), American Physiological Society, Bethesda, MD, pp. 73–90.

Lahiri, S., Rozanov, C. and Cherniack, N.S. (2000) Altered structure and function of the carotid body at high altitude and associated chemoreflexes (Review). *High Alt. Med. Biol.* **1**, 63–74.

Lahti, A. (1982) Cutaneous reactions to cold, in *Report* **30**, Nordic Council for Arctic Medical Research, Copenhagen, pp. 32–5.

Lakshminarayan, S. and Pierson, D.J. (1975) Recurrent high altitude pulmonary edema with blunted chemosensitivity. *Am. Rev. Respir. Dis.* **111**, 869–72.

La Manna, J.C., Chavez, J.C. and Pichiule, P. (2004) Structural and functional adaptation to hypoxia in the rat brain. *J. Exp. Biol.* **207**, 3163–9.

Lanfranchi, P.A., Colombo, R., Cremona, G. *et al.* (2005) Autonomic cardiovascular regulation in subjects with acute mountain sickness. *Am. J. Physiol. Heart Circ. Physiol.* **289**, H2364–72. E-pub 29 July 2005.

Lang, S.D.R. and Lang, A. (1971) The Kunde Hospital and a demographic survey of the Upper Khumbu, Nepal. *N.Z. Med. J.* **74**, 1–8.

Laragh, J.H. (1985) Atrial natriuretic hormone, the renin–aldosterone axis, and blood pressure–electrolyte homeostasis. *N. Engl. J. Med.* **313**, 1330–40.

Larsen, E.B., Roach, R.C., Schoene, R.B. and Hornbein, T.F. (1982) Acute mountain sickness and acetazolamide. Clinical efficacy and effect on ventilation. *JAMA* **248**, 328–32.

Larsen, G.L., Webster, R.O., Worthen, G.S. *et al.* (1985) Additive effect of intravascular complement activation and brief episodes of hypoxia in producing increased permeability in the rabbit lung. *J. Clin. Invest.* **75**, 902–10.

Larsen, J.J., Hansen, J.M., Olsen, N.V.,Galbo, H. and Dela, F. (1997) The effect of altitude hypoxia on glucose homeostasis in men. *J. Physiol.* **504**, 241–9.

Laufmann, H. (1951) Profound accidental hypothermia. *JAMA* **147**, 1201–12.

Lawler, J., Powers, S.K., Thompson, D. *et al.* (1988) Linear relationship between VO$_2$ max and VO$_2$ maximum decrement during exposure to acute hypoxia. *J. Appl. Physiol.* **64**, 1486–92.

Lawrence, D.L. and Shenker, Y. (1991) Effect of hypoxic exercise on atrial natriuretic factor and aldosterone regulation. *Am. J. Hypertens.* **4**, 341–7.

Lawrence, D.L., Skatrud, J.B. and Shenker, Y. (1990) Effect of hypoxia on atrial natriuretic factor and aldosterone regulation in humans. *Am. J. Physiol.* **258**, E243–8.

Lawrie, R.A. (1953) Effect of enforced exercise on myoglobin concentration in muscle. *Nature* **171**, 1069–70.

Lechner, A.J., Grimes, M.J., Aquin, L. and Banchero, N. (1982) Adapative lung growth during chronic cold plus hypoxia is age-dependent. *J. Exp. Zool.* **219**, 285–91.

Ledderhos, C., Pongratz, H., Exner, J. *et al.* (2002) Reduced tolerance of simulated altitude (4200 m) in young men with borderline hypertension. *Aviat. Space Environ. Med.* **73**, 1063–6.

Ledingham, I. McA. (1983) Clinical management of elderly hypothermic patients, in *The Nature and Treatment of Hypothermia* (eds. R.S. Pozos and L.E. Wittmers), Croom Helm, London/University of Minnesota Press, Minneapolis, pp. 165–81.

Ledingham, I. McA. and Mone, J.G. (1980) Treatment of accidental hypothermia: a prospective clinical study. *BMJ* **1**, 1102–5.

Lee, W.C., Chen, J.J., Ho, H.Y. *et al.* (2003) Short-term altitude mountain living improves glycemic control *High Alt. Med. Biol.* **4**, 81–91.

Lehman, T., Mairbaurl, H., Pleisch, B., Maggiorini, M., Bartsch, P. and Reinhert, WH. (2006) Platelet count and function at high altitude and in high-altitude pulmonary edema. *J. Appl. Physiol.* **100**, 690–4.

Lehmann, J.F. (1971) Diathermy, in *Handbook of Physical Medicine and Rehabilitation,* 2nd edn, Saunders, Philadelphia, pp. 1397–442.

Lehmuskallio, E. (1999) Cold protecting ointment and frostbite: a questionnaire study of 830 conscripts in Finland. *Acta Dermato-veneredlogica* **79**, 67–70.

Lehmuskallio, E. and Anttonen, H. (1999) Thermal physical effects of ointments in cold: an experimental study with a skin model. *Acta Dermato-veneredlogica* **79**, 33–6.

Lehmuskallio, E., Linholm, H., Koskenvvo, K. *et al.* (1995) Frostbite of the face and ears: an epidemiological study of risk factors in Finnish conscripts. *BMJ* **311**, 1661–3.

Leiberman, P., Protopapas, A. and Kanki, B.G. (1995) Speech production and cognitive defects on Mt. Everest. *Aviat. Space Environ. Med.* **66**, 857–64.

Leigh-Smith, S. (2004) Blood boosting: a review. *Br. J. Sports Med.* **38**, 99–101.

Lenfant, C. (1967) Time-dependent variations of pulmonary gas exchange in normal men at rest. *J. Appl. Physiol.* **22**, 675–84.

Lenfant, C. and Sullivan, K. (1971) Adaptation to high altitude. *N. Engl. J. Med.* **284**, 1298–309.

Lenfant, C., Torrance, J., English, E. *et al.* (1968) Effect of altitude on oxygen binding by hemoglobin and on organic phosphate levels. *J. Clin. Invest.* **47**, 2652–6.

Lenfant, C., Ways, P., Aucutt, C. and Cruz, J. (1969) Effect of chronic hypoxic hypoxia on the O$_2$–Hb dissociation curve and respiratory gas transport in man. *Respir. Physiol.* **7**, 7–29.

Lenfant, C., Torrance, J.D. and Reynafarje, C. (1971) Shift of the O$_2$–Hb dissociation curve at altitude: mechanism and effect. *J. Appl. Physiol.* **30**, 625–31.

Leonard, W.R., DeWalt, K.M., Stansbury, J.P. and McCaston, M.K. (1995) Growth differences between children of highland and coastal Equador. *Am. J. Phys. Anthropol.* **98**, 47–57.

León-Velarde, F. (1998) First International Group on Chronic Mountain Sickness (CMS) in Matsumoto, in *Progress in Mountain Medicine and High Altitude* (eds. H. Ohno, T. Kobayashi, S. Masuyama and M. Nakashima), Press Committee of the 3rd Congress on Mountain Medicine and High Altitude Physiology, Matsumoto, p. 166.

Léon-Velarde, F. and Arregui, A. (1993) Hipoxia: Investigacionas Basicas y Clinicias. *Homenajie a Carlos Monge Cassinelli*, Instituto Frances de Estudios

Andinos Universidad Peruana Cayetano Heredia, Lima, Peru.

León-Velarde, F. and Richalet, J.P. (2006) Respiratory control in residents at high altitude: physiology and pathophysiology. *High Alt. Med. Biol.* **7**, 125–37.

León-Velarde, F., Monge, C.C., Vidal, A. *et al.* (1991) Serum immunoreactive erythropoietin in high altitude natives with and without excessive erythrocytosis. *Exp. Hematol.* **19**, 257–60.

León-Velarde, F., Arregui, A., Monge C.C. and Ruiz, H. (1993) Ageing at high altitude and the risk of chronic mountain sickness. *J. Wilderness Med.* **4**, 183–8.

León-Velarde, F., Arregui, A., Vargas, M. *et al.* (1994) Chronic mountain sickness and chronic lower respiratory tract disorders. *Chest* **106**, 151–5.

León-Velarde, F., Ramos, M.A., Hermandez, J.A. *et al.* (1997) The role of menopause in the development of chronic mountain sickness. *Am. J. Physiol.* **272**, R90–4.

León-Velarde, F., Gamboa, A., Chuquiza, J.A., Esteba, W.A., Rivera-Chira, M. and Monge, C.C. (2000) Hematological parameters in high altitude residents living at 4,355, 4,660, and 5,500 meters above sea level. *High Alt. Med. Biol.* **1**, 97–104.

León-Velarde, F., Maggiorini, M., Reeves, J.T. *et al.* (2005) Consensus statement on chronic and sub-acute high altitude disease. *High Alt. Med. Biol.* **6**, 147–57.

Lepori, M., Hummler, E., Feihl, F. *et al.* (1999) Amiloride sensitive sodium transport dysfunction augments susceptibility to hypoxia induced lung edema (abstract), in *Hypoxia: Into the Next Millennium* (eds. R.C. Roach, P.D. Wagner and P.H. Hackett), Plenum/Kluwer, New York, p. 403.

Leuthold, E., Hartmann, G., Buhlman, R. *et al.* (1975) Medical and physiological investigations on mountaineers. A field study during a winter climb in the Bernese Oberland, in *Mountain Medicine and Physiology* (eds. C. Clarke, M. Ward and E. Williams), Alpine Club, London, pp. 32–7.

Levin, E.R. (1995) Endothelins. *N. Engl. J. Med.* **333**, 356–61.

Levine, B.D. (2005) Point: Positive effects of intermittent hypoxia (live high:train low) on exercise performance are mediated primarily by augmented red cell volume. *J. Appl. Physiol.* **99**, 2053–5.

Levine, B.D. and Stray-Gundersen, J. (1992) a practical approach to altitude training: where to live and train for optimal performance enhancement. *Int. J. Sports Med.* **13**, 5209–12.

Levine, B.D. and Stray-Gundersen, J. (1997) 'Living high–training low': effect of moderate altitude acclimatization with low altitude training on performance. *J. Appl. Physiol.* **83**(1), 102–12.

Levine, B.D. and Stray-Gundersen, J. (2006) Dose-response of altitude training: how much altitude is enough? *Adv. Exp. Med. Biol.* **588**, 233–47.

Levine, B.D., Yoshimura, K., Kobayashi, T. *et al.* (1989) Dexamethasone in the treatment of acute mountain sickness. *N. Engl. J. Med.* **321**, 1707–13.

Levine, B.D., Zuckerman, J.H. and deFilipps, C.R. (1997) Effect of high altitude exposure in the elderly: the Tenth Mountain Division Study. *Circulation* **96**, 1224–32.

Lewin, S., Brittman, L.R. and Holzman, R.S. (1981) Infections in hypothermic patients. *Arch. Intern. Med.* **141**, 920–5.

Lewis, R.B. and Moen, P.W. (1952) Further studies on the pathogenesis of cold induced muscle necrosis. *Surg. Gynecol. Obstet.* **95**, 543–51.

Lewis, R.F. and Rennick, P.M. (1979) *Manual for the Repeatable Cognitive–Perceptual–Motor Battery,* Axon, Grosse Pointe Park, MI.

Lexow, K. (1991) Severe accidental hypothermia: survival after 6 hrs 30 min of cardio-pulmonary resuscitation. *Arctic Med. Res.* **50**, Suppl. 6, 112–14.

Li, Y.Z. (1985) The birth weight, distribution of new born (in percentile) in high altitude (abstract), 2nd High Altitude Symposium, Qinghai, China (unpublished proceedings).

Lichty, J.A., Ting, R.Y., Bruns, P.D. and Dyar, E. (1957) Studies of babies born at high altitude. *Am. Med. Assoc. J. Dis. Child.* **93**, 666–7.

Lilja, G.P. (1983) Emergency treatment of hypothermia, in *The Nature and Treatment of Hypothermia* (eds. R.S. Pozos and L.E. Wittmers), Croom Helm, London/ University of Minnesota Press, Minneapolis, pp. 143–51.

Lim, T.P.K. (1960) Central and peripheral control mechanisms of shivering and its effect on respiration. *J. Appl. Physiol.* **15**, 567–74.

Lindgarde, F., Ercilla, M.B., Correa, L.R. and Ahren, B. (2004) Body adiposity, insulin, and leptin in subgroups of Peruvian Amerindians. *High Alt. Med. Biol.* **5**, 27–31.

Litch, J.A. and Bishop, R.A. (1999) Transient global amnesia at high altitude. *N. Engl. J. Med.* **340**, 1444.

Litch, J.A. and Bishop, R.A. (2000) High altitude global amnesia. *Wilderness Exp. Med.* **11**, 25–8.

Little, M.A. and Hanna, J.M. (1978) The responses of high altitude populations to cold and other stresses, in *The Biology of High Altitude Peoples* (ed. P.T.

Baker), Cambridge University Press, Cambridge, pp. 251–98.

Liu, L., Cheng, H., Chin, W. *et al.* (1989) Atrial natriuretic peptide lowers pulmonary arterial pressure in patients with high altitude disease. *Am. J. Med. Sci.* **298**, 397–401.

Liu, L.S. (1986) Highlights from the national meeting on hypertension: held by the Chinese Medical Association. *Chin. J. Cardiol.* **14**, 2–3.

Liu, Y., Steinacker, J.M., Dehnert, C. *et al.* (1998) Effect of 'living high-training low' on the cardiac functions at sea level. *Int. J. Sports Med.* **19**, 380–4.

Lloyd, B.B., Jukes, M.G.M. and Cunningham, D.J.C. (1958) The relation of alveolar oxygen pressure and the respiratory response to carbon dioxide in man. *Q. J. Exp. Physiol.* **42**, 214–27.

Lloyd, E.L. (1972) Diagnostic problems and hypothermia. *BMJ* **3**, 417.

Lloyd, E.L. (1973) Accidental hypothermia treated by central re-warming through the airway. *Br. J. Anaesth.* **45**, 41–8.

Lloyd, E.L. (1979) Temperature sensations in veins. *Anaesthesia* **34**, 919.

Lloyd, E.L. (1986) *Hypothermia and Cold Stress,* Croom Helm, London.

Lloyd, E.L. (1996) Accidental hypothermia. *Resuscitation* **32**, 111–24.

Lloyd, E.L. and Mitchell, B. (1974) Factors affecting the onset of ventricular fibrillation in hypothermia: a hypothesis. *Lancet* **2**, 1294–6.

Lloyd, T.C. (1965) Pulmonary vasoconstriction during histotoxic hypoxia. *J. Appl. Physiol.* **20**, 488–90.

Lobenhoffer, H.P., Zink, R.A. and Brendel, W. (1982) High altitude pulmonary edema: analysis of 166 cases, in *High Altitude Physiology and Medicine* (eds. W. Brendel and R.A. Zink), Springer-Verlag, New York, pp. 219–31.

Lockhart, A., Zelter, M., Mensch-Dechene, M. *et al.* (1976) Pressure–flow–volume relationships in pulmonary circulation of normal highlanders. *J. Appl. Physiol.* **41**, 449–56.

Loeppky, J.A., Scotto, P., Charlton, G.C. *et al.* (2001) Ventilation is greater in women than men, but the increase during acute altitude hypoxia is the same. *Respir. Physiol.* **125**, 225–37.

Loeppky, J.A., Icenogle, M.V., Maes, D., Riboni, K., Scotto, P. and Roach, R.C. (2003) Body temperature, autonomic responses and acute mountain sickness. *High Alt. Med. Biol.* **4**, 267–73.

Loeppky, J.A., Icenogle, M.V., Maes, D., Riboni, K., Hinghofer-Szalkay, H. and Roach, R.C. (2005a) Early fluid retention and severe acute mountain sickness. *J. Appl. Physiol.* **98**, 591–7. E-pub 22 October 2004.

Loeppky, J.A., Roach, R.C., Maes, D. *et al.* (2005b) Role of hypobaria in fluid balance response to hypoxia. *High Alt. Med. Biol.* **6**, 60–71.

Loewy, A. and Gerhartz, H. (1914) Uber de Termperatur de Expirationsluft und der Lungemluft. *Pflüger's Arch. Ges. Physiol.* **155**, 231–44.

Lomax, P., Thinney, R. and Mondino, B.J. (1991) The effects of solar radiation, in *A Colour Atlas of Mountain Medicine,* (eds. J. Vallotton and F. Dubas), Wolfe, London, pp. 67–71.

Longmuir, I.S. and Betts, W. (1987) Tissue acclimation to altitude. *Fed. Proc.* **46**, 794.

Louie, D. and Pare, P.D. (2004) Physiological changes at altitude in nonasthmatic and asthmatic subjects. *Can. Respir. J.* **11**, 197–9.

Lovering, A.T., Fraigne, J.J., Dunin-Barkowski, W.L., Vidruk, E.H. and Orem, J.M. (2003) Hypocapnia decreases the amount of rapid eye movement sleep in cats. *Sleep* **26**, 961–7.

Lugaresi, E., Coccagna, G., Cirignotta, R. *et al.* (1978) Breathing during sleep in man in normal and pathological conditions, in *The Regulation of Respiration during Sleep and Anesthesia* (eds. R.S. Fitzgerald, H. Cautier and S. Lahiri), Plenum, New York, pp. 35–45.

Luks, A.M., van Melick, H., Batarse, R. *et al.* (1998) Room oxygen enrichment improves sleep and subsequent day-time performance at high altitude. *Respir. Physiol.* **113**, 247–58.

Lundberg, E. (1952) Edema agudo del pulmon en el soroche. Conferencia sustentada en la ascociacion medica de Yauli, Oroya. (Quoted in Hultgren, H.N., Spickard, W.B., Hellriegel, K. and Houston, C.S. (1961) High altitude pulmonary edema. *Medicine,* **40**, 289–313).

Lundby, C. and van Hall, G. (2001) Peak heart rate at extreme altitudes. *High Alt. Med. Biol.* **2**, 41–5.

Lundby, C and van Hall, G. (2002) Substrate utilization in sea level residents during exercise in acute hypoxia and after 4 weeks acclimatization to 4100 m. *Acta. Physiol. Scand.* **176**, 195–201.

Lundby, C. and Damsgaard, R. (2006) Exercise performance in hypoxia after novel erythropoiesis stimulating protein treatment. *Scand. J. Med. Sci. Sports* **16**, 35–40.

Lundby, C., Saltin, B. and van Hall, G. (2000) The 'lactate paradox', evidence for a transient change in the course of acclimatization to severe hypoxia in lowlanders. *Acta Physiologica* **170**, 265–9.

Lundby, C., Araoz, M. and van Hall, G. (2001a) Peak heart rate decreases with increasing severity of acute hypoxia. *High Alt. Med. Biol.* **2**, 369–76.

Lundby, C., Moller, P., Kanstrup, I.-L. and Olsen, N.V. (2001b) Heart rate response to hypoxic exercise: role of dopamine D_2-receptors and effect of oxygen supplementation. *Clinical Sci.* **101**, 377–83.

Lundby, C., Calber, J.A., van Hall, G., Saltin, B. and Sander, M. (2004a) Pulmonary gas exchange at maximal exercise in Danish lowlanders during 8 weeks of acclimatization to 4,100 m and in high-altitude Aymara natives. *Am. J. Physiol.* **287**, R1202–8.

Lundby, C., Pilegaard, H., Andersen, J.L., van Hall, G., Sander, M. and Calbet, J.A.L. (2004b) Acclimatization to 4100 m does not change capillary density or mRNA expression of potential angiogenesis regulatory factors in human skeletal muscle. *J. Exp. Biol.* **207**, 3865–71.

Lundby, C., Sander, M., van Hall, G., Saltin, B. and Calbet, J.A. (2006) Determinants of maximal exercise and muscle oxygen extraction in acclimatizing lowlanders and in high altitude natives. *J. Physiol.* **573**, 535–43.

Luo, F.M., Liu, X.J., Li, S.Q. *et al.* (2005) Circulating Ghrelin in patients with chronic obstructive pulmonary disease. *Nutrition* **21**, 793–8.

Lupi-Herrera, E., Seoane, M., Sandoval, J. and Casanova, J.M. (1980) Behavior of the pulmonary circulation in the grossly obese patient. Pathogenesis of pulmonary arterial hypertension at an altitude of 2240 meters. *Chest* **78**, 553–8.

Lyons, T.P., Muza, S.R., Rock, P.B. and Cymerman, A. (1995) The effect of altitude pre-acclimatization on acute mountain sickness during reexposure. *Aviat. Space Environ. Med.* **66**, 957–62.

MacDonald, D. (1929) *The Land of the Lama,* Seeley Service, London.

MacDougall, J.D., Green, H., Sutton, J.R. *et al.* (1991) Operation Everest II: structural adaptations in skeletal muscle in response to extreme altitude. *Acta Physiol. Scand.* **142**, 421–7.

Maceluso, A., Young, A., Gibb, K.S., Rowe, D.A. and De Vito, G. (2003) Cycling as a novel approach to resistance training increases muscle strength, power and selected functional abilities in healthy older women. *J. Appl. Physiol.* **95**, 2544–53.

MacInnes, C. (1971) Steroids in mountain rescue. *Lancet* **1**, 599.

MacInnes, C. (1979) Treatment of accidental hypothermia. *BMJ* **1**, 130–1.

MacIntyre, B. (1994) Ice-cream comforts girl who survived big freeze. *The Times* (London), 4 March, p. 15.

MacKinnon, P.C.B., Monk-Jones, M.E. and Fotherby, K. (1963) A study of various indices of adrenocortical activity during 23 days at high altitude. *J. Endocrinol.* **26**, 555–6.

MacNeish, R.S. (1971) Early man in the Andes. *Sci. Am.* **224**, 36–46.

MacPhee, G.C. (1936) *Ben Nevis,* Scottish Mountaineering Club, Edinburgh, pp. 6–9.

Mader, T.H. and Tabin, G. (2003) Going to high altitude with preexisting ocular conditions. *High Alt. Med. Biol.* **4**, 419–30.

Mader, T.H. and White, L.J. (1995) Refractive changes at extreme altitude after radial keratotomy. *Am. J. Ophthalmol.* **119**, 733–7.

Mader, T.H., Blanton, C.L., Gilbert, R.N. *et al.* (1996) Refractive changes during 72-hour exposure to high altitude after refractive surgery. *Ophthalmology* **103**, 1188–95.

Magalhaes, J., Ascensao, A., Viscor, G. *et al.* (2004a) Oxidative stress in humans during and after 4 hours of hypoxia at a simulated altitude of 5500 m. *Aviat. Space Environ. Med.* **75**, 16–22.

Magalhaes, J., Ascensao, A., Soares, J.M. *et al.* (2004b) Acute and severe hypobaric hypoxia-induced muscle oxidative stress in mice: the role of glutathione against oxidative damage. *Eur. J. Appl. Physiol.* **91**, 185–91.

Maggiorini, M. (2006) High altitude-induced pulmonary oedema. *Cardiovasc. Res.* **72**, 41–50.

Maggiorini, M., Buhler, B., Walter, M. and Oelz, O. (1990) Prevalence of acute mountain sickness in the Swiss Alps. *BMJ* **301**, 853–5.

Maggiorini, M., Bärtsch, P. and Oelz, O. (1997) Association between body temperature and acute mountain sickness: cross sectional study. *BMJ* **315**, 403–4.

Maggiorini, M., Muller, A., Hofstetter, D. *et al.* (1998) Assessment of acute mountain sickness by different score protocols in the Swiss Alps. *Aviat. Space Environ. Med.* **69**, 1186–92.

Maggiorini, M., Melot, C., Pierre, S. *et al.* (2001) High-altitude pulmonary edema is initially caused by an increase in capillary pressure. *Circulation* **103**, 2078–83.

Maggiorini, M., Brunner-La Rocca, H.-P. and Peth, S. *et al.* (2006) Both tadalafil and dexamethasone may reduce the incidence of high-altitude pulmonary edema: a randomized trial. *Ann. Intern. Med.* **145**, 497–506.

Maher, J.T., Jones, L.G. and Hartley, L.H. (1974) Effects of high-altitude exposure on submaximal endurance capacity of men. *J. Appl. Physiol.* **37**, 895–8.

Maher, J.T., Jones, L.G., Hartley, L.H., Williams, G.H. and Rose, L.I. (1975a) Aldosterone dynamics during graded exercise at sea level and high altitude. *J. Appl. Physiol.* **39**, 18–22.

Maher, J.T., Manchanda, S.C., Cymerman, A. *et al.* (1975b) Cardiovascular responsiveness to β-adrenergic stimulation and blockade in chronic hypoxia. *Am. J. Physiol.* **228**, 477–81.

Maher, J.T., Cymerman, A., Reeves, J.T. *et al.* (1975c) Acute mountain sickness: increased severity in eucapnic hypoxia. *Aviat. Space Environ. Med.* **46**, 826–9.

Maher, J.T., Levine, P.H. and Cymerman, A. (1976) Human coagulation abnormalities during acute exposure to hypobaric hypoxia. *J. Appl. Physiol.* **41**, 702–7.

Maher, J.T., Denniston, J.C., Wolfe, D.L. and Cymerman, A. (1978) Mechanism of the attenuated cardiac response to β-adrenergic stimulation in chronic hypoxia. *J. Appl. Physiol. Respir. Environ. Exerc. Physiol.* **44**, 647–51.

Mahony, B.S. and Githens, J.H. (1979) Sickling crises and altitude. Occurrence in the Colorado patient population. *Clin Pediatr (Phila)* **18**, 431–8.

Mairbaurl, H. (2006) Role of alveolar epithelial sodium transport in high altitude pulmonary edema (HAPE) (Review). *Respir. Physiol. Neurobiol.* **151**, 178–91. E-pub 5 December 2005.

Mairbaurl, H., Schwobel, F., Hoschele, S. *et al.* (2003) Altered ion transporter expression in bronchial epithelium in mountaineers with high-altitude pulmonary edema. *J. Appl. Physiol.* **95**, 1843–50.

Malconian, M.K., Rock, P.B., Hultgren, H.N. *et al.* (1990) The electrocardiogram at rest and exercise during a simulated ascent of Mt. Everest (Operation Everest II). *Am. J. Cardiol.* **65**, 1475–80.

Malconian, M.K., Rock, P.B., Reeves, J.T. and Houston, C.S. (1993) Operation Everest II: gas tensions in expired air and arterial blood at extreme altitude. *Aviat. Space Environ. Med.* **64**, 37–42.

Malik, M.T., Peng, Y.J., Kline, D.D., Adhikary, G. and Prabhakar, H.R. (2005) Impaired ventilatory acclimatization to hypoxia in mice lacking the immediate early gene fos B. *Respir. Physiol. Neurobiol.* **145**, 23–31.

Malik, R.A., Masson, E.A., Sharma, A.K. *et al.* (1990) Hypoxic neuropathy: relevance to human diabetic neuropathy. *Diabetologia* **33**, 311–8.

Maloiy, G.M.O., Heglund, G.M., Prager, N.C. *et al.* (1986) Energetic cost of carrying loads: have African women discovered an economic way? *Nature* **319**, 668–9.

Manier, C., Guenard, H., Castaing, Y. *et al.* (1988) Pulmonary gas exchange in Andean natives with excessive polycythemia – effect of hemodilution. *J. Appl. Physiol.* **65**, 2107–17.

Mansell, A., Powles, A. and Sutton, J. (1980) Changes in pulmonary PV characteristics of human subjects at an altitude of 5366 m. *J. Appl. Physiol.* **49**, 79–83.

Marciniuk, D., McKim, D., Sanii, R. and Younes, M. (1994) Role of central respiratory muscle fatigue in endurance exercise in normal subjects. *J. Appl. Physiol.* **76**, 236–41.

Marconi, C., Marzorati, M., Grassi, B. *et al.* (2004) Second generation Tibetan lowlanders acclimatize to high altitude more quickly than Caucasians. *J. Physiol.* **556**, 661–71. E-pub 6 February 2004.

Marconi, C., Marzorati, M., Sciuto, D., Ferri, A. and Cerretelli, P. (2005) Economy of locomotion in high-altitude Tibetan migrants exposed to normoxia. *J. Physiol.* **569**, 667–75. E-pub 22 September 2005.

Marconi, C., Marzorati, M. and Cerretelli, P. (2006) Work capacity of permanent residents of high altitude. *High Alt. Med. Biol.* **7**, 105–15.

Marcus, P. (1979) The treatment of acute accidental hypothermia. Proceedings of a Symposium held at the RAF Institute of Aviation Medicine. *Aviat. Space Environ. Med.* **50**, 834–43.

Maresh, C.M., Kreamer, W.J., Judelson, A., *et al.* (2004) Effects of high altitude and water deprivation on arginine vasopressin release in man. *Am. J. Physiol Endocrinol. Metab.* **286**, E20–4.

Maret, K.H., Billups, J.O., Peters, R.M. and West, J.B. (1984) Automatic mechanical alveolar gas sampler for multiple sample collection in the field. *J. Appl. Physiol.* **56**, 1435–8.

Margaria, R. (1957) The contribution of hemoglobin to acid-base equilibrium of the blood in health and disease. *Clin. Chem.* **3**, 306–18.

Margaria, R. (ed.) (1967) *Exercise at Altitude,* Excerpta Medica Foundation, Amsterdam.

Marine, D. and Kimball, O.P. (1920) Prevention of simple goiter in man. *Arch. Intern. Med.* **25**, 661–72.

Marinelli, M., Roi, G.S., Giacometti, M., Bonini, P. and Banfi, G. (1994) Cortisol, testosterone and free testosterone in athletes performing a marathon at 4,000 m altitude. *Horm. Res.* **41**, 225–9.

Marsh, A.R. (1983) A short but distant war: the Falklands Campaign. *J. R. Soc. Med.* **76**, 972–82.

Marshall, H.C. and Goldman, R.F. (1976) Electrical response of nerve to freezing injury, in *Circumpolar Health* (eds. R.J. Shephard and S. Itoh), University Press, Toronto, p. 77.

Marsigny, B. (1998) Mountain frostbite. *ISSM Newsletter* **8**, 8–10.

Marti, H.J.H., Bernaudin, M. and Bellail, M. *et al.* (2000) Hypoxia-induced vascular endothelial growth factor expression precedes neovascularization after cerebral ischemia. *Am. J. Pathol.* **156**, 965–76.

Marticorena, E., Severino, J., Peñaloza, A.D. and Neuriegel, K. (1959) Influencia de las grandes alturas en la determinacion de la persistencia del canal arterial. Observaciones realizadas en 3500 escolares de altura a 4300 m. Sombre el niuel dez mar. Primeros resultados operatorios. *Rev. Asoc. Med. Prov. Yauli* Nos 1–2, La Oroya.

Marticorena, E., Tapia, F.A., Dyer, J. *et al.* (1964) Pulmonary edema by ascending to high altitudes. *Dis. Chest* **45**, 273–83.

Marticorena, E., Ruiz, L., Severino, J., Galvez, J. and Penaloza, D. (1969) Systemic blood pressure in white men born at sea level: changes after long residence in high altitudes. *Am. J. Cardiol.* **23**, 364–8.

Martin, B.J., Wiel, J.V., Sparks, K.E. *et al.* (1978) Exercise ventilation corresponds positively with ventilatory chemoresponsiveness. *J. Appl. Physiol.* **44**, 447–84.

Martin, D. and Pyne, D. (1998) Altitude training at 2690 m does not increase total haemoglobin mass or sea level VO_2max in world champion track cyclists. *J. Sci. Med. Sport* **1**, 156–70.

Mason, N.P., Barry, P.W., Despiau, G. *et al.* (1999) Cough frequency and cough receptor sensitivity to citric acid challenge during a simulated ascent to extreme altitude. *Eur. Respir. J.* **13**, 508–13.

Mason, N.P., Petersen, M., Melot, C. *et al.* (2003) Serial changes in nasal potential difference and lung electrical impedance tomography at high altitude. *J. Appl. Physiol.* **94**, 2043–50. E-pub 6 December 2002.

Masuda, A., Kobayashi, T., Honda, Y. *et al.* (1992) Effect of high altitude on respiratory chemosensitivity. *Jpn. J. Mount. Med.* **12**, 177–81.

Masuyama, S., Kohchiyama, S., Shinozako, T. *et al.* (1989) Periodic breathing at high altitude and ventilatory responses to O_2 and CO_2. *Jpn. J. Physiol.* **39**, 523–35.

Mathews, C.E. (1898) *Annals of Mont Blanc,* T. Fisher Unwin, London, p. 82.

Mathieu-Costello, O. (1987) Capillary tortuosity and degree of contraction or extension of skeletal muscle. *Microvasc. Res.* **33**, 98–117.

Mathieu-Costello, O. (1989) Muscle capillary tortuosity in high altitude mice depends on sarcomere length. *Respir. Physiol.* **76**, 289–302.

Mathieu-Costello, O. (2001) Muscle adaptation to altitude: tissue capillarity and capacity for aerobic metabolism (Review). *High Alt. Med. Biol.* **2**, 413–25.

Mathieu-Costello, O., Agey, P.J., Wu, L. *et al.* (1998) Increased fiber capillarization in flight muscle of finch at altitude. *Respir. Physiol.* **111**, 189–99.

Matsuyama, S., Kimura, H., Sugita, T. *et al.* (1986) Control of ventilation in extreme altitude climbers. *J. Appl. Physiol.* **61**, 400–6.

Matsuyama, S., Kohchiyama, S., Shinozaki, T. *et al.* (1989) Periodic breathing at high altitude and ventilatory responses to O_2 and CO_2. *Jpn. J. Physiol.* **39**, 523–35.

Matsuzawa, Y., Fujimoto, K., Kobayashi, T. *et al.* (1989) Blunted hypoxic ventilatory drive in subjects susceptible to high-altitude pulmonary edema. *J. Appl. Physiol.* **66**, 1152–7.

Matthews, B. (1954) Discussion on physiology of man at high altitudes; limiting factors at high altitude. *Proc. R. Soc. Lond. Ser. B* **143**, 1–4.

Matthews, B.H.C. (1932–3) Loss of heat at high altitudes. *J. Physiol.* **77**, 28–9P.

Maugham, R.J. (1984) Temperature regulation during marathon competition. *Br. J. Sports Med.* **22**, 257–60.

Mawson, J.T., Braun, B., Rock, P.B., Moore, L.G., Mazzeo, R. and Butterfield, G.E. (2000) Women at altitude: energy requirement at 4,300 m. *J. Appl. Physiol.* **88**, 272–81.

Mayhew, T. (1986) Morphometric diffusing capacity for oxygen of the human term placenta at high altitude, in *Aspects of Hypoxia* (ed. D. Heath), Liverpool University Press, Liverpool, pp. 181–90.

Mayhew, T.M. (1991) Scaling placental oxygen diffusion to birthweight: studies on placentae from low- and high-altitude pregnancies. *J. Anat.* **175**, 187–94.

Mayhew, T.M. (2003) Changes in fetal capillaries during preplacental hypoxia: growth, shape remodelling and villous capillarization in placentae from high-altitude pregnancies. *Placenta* **24**, 191–8.

Mazzeo, R.S. (2005) Altitude, exercise and immune function (Review). *Exerc. Immunol. Rev.* **11**, 6–16.

Mazzeo, R.S. and Reeves, J.T. (2003) Adrenergic contribution during acclimatization to high altitude: perspectives from Pikes Peak. *Exerc Sport Sci. Rev.* **31**, 13–8.

Mazzeo, R.S., Bender, P.R., Brooks, G.A. *et al.* (1991) Arterial catecholamine responses during exercise with acute and chronic high-altitude exposure. *Am. J. Physiol.* **261**, E419–24.

Mazzeo, R.S., Child, A., Butterfield, G.E. *et al.* (1998) Catecholamine response during 12 days of high-altitude exposure (4,300 m) in women. *J. Appl. Physiol.* **84**, 1151–7.

Mazzeo, R.S., Dubay, A., Kirsch, J. *et al.* (2003) Influence of α-adrenergic blockade on the catecholamine response to exercise at 4,300 meters. *Metabolism* **52**, 1471–7.

McAuliffe, F., Kameta, N., Ratterty, G.F. *et al.* (2003) Pulmonary diffusing capacity in pregnancy at sea level and at high altitude. *Respir. Physiol. Neurobiol.* **134**, 85–92.

McCarrison, R. (1908) Observations on endemic cretinism in the Chitral and Gilgit valleys. *Lancet* **2**, 1275–80.

McCarrison, R. (1913) *The Pathology of Endemic Goitre (Milroy Lectures 1913),* Bale Sons and Danielson, London.

McCauley, R.C., Smith, D.J., Robson, M.C. and Heggers, J.P. (1995) Frostbite and other cold related injuries, in *Wilderness Medicine* (ed. P.S. Auerbach), Mosby, St Louis, Mo, pp. 129–40.

McClung, J.P. (1969) *Effects of High Altitude on Human Birth,* Harvard University Press, Cambridge, MA.

McCormack, P.D., Thomas, J., Malik, M. and Staschen, C. (1998) Cold stress, reverse T3 and lymphocyte function. *Alaska Med.* **40**, 55–62.

McDonough, P., Merrill Dane, D., Hsia, C.C.W., Yilmaz, C. and Johnson Jr., R.L. (2006) Long-term enhancement of pulmonary gas exchange after high-altitude residence during maturation. *J. Appl. Physiol.* **100**, 474–81.

McElroy, M.K., Gerard, A., Powell, F.L. *et al.* (2000) Nocturnal O_2 enrichment of room air at high altitude increases daytime O_2 saturation without changing control of ventilation. *High Alt. Med. Biol.* **1**, 197–206.

McFarland, R.A. (1937a) Psycho-physiological studies at high altitude in the Andes. I. The effects of rapid ascents by aeroplane and train. *Comp. Psychol.* **23**, 191–225.

McFarland, R.A. (1937b) Psycho-physiological studies at high altitude. II. Sensory and motor responses during acclimatization. *Comp. Psychol.* **23**, 227–58.

McFarland, R.A. (1938a) Psycho-physiological studies at high altitude in the Andes. III. Mental and psycho-somatic responses during gradual adaptation. *Comp. Psychol.* **24**, 147–88.

McFarland, R.A. (1938b) Psycho-physiological studies at high altitude. IV. Sensory and circulatory responses of the Andean residents at 17500 feet. *Comp. Psychol.* **24**, 189–220.

McIntyre, L. (1987) The high Andes. *Natl. Geogr.* **171**, 422–59.

McKendry, R.J.R. (1981) Frostbite arthritis. *Can. Med. Assoc. J.* **125**, 1128–30.

Mecham, R.P., Whitehouse, L.A., Wrenn, D.S. *et al.* (1987) Smooth muscle-mediated connective tissue remodeling in pulmonary hypertension. *Science* **237**, 423–6.

Meehan, R., Duncan, U., Neal, L. *et al.* (1988) Operation Everest II: alterations in the immune system at high altitudes. *J. Clin. Immunol.* **8**, 397–406.

Meehan, R.T. (1987) Immune suppression at high altitude. *Ann. Emerg. Med.* **16**, 974–9.

Meerson, F.Z., Ustinova, E.E. and Orlova, E.H. (1987) Prevention and elimination of heart arrhythmias by adaptation to intermittent high altitude hypoxia. *Clin. Cardiol.* **10**, 783–9.

Megirian, D.A., Ryan, A.T. and Sherrey, J.H. (1980) An electrophysiological analysis of sleep and respiration of rats breathing different gas mixtures: diaphragmatic muscle function. *Electroencephalogr. Clin. Neurophysiol.* **50**, 303–13.

Mejia, O.M., Prchal, J.T., León-Velarde, F., Hurtado, A. and Stockton, D.W. (2005) Genetic association analysis of chronic mountain sickness in an Andean high-altitude population. *Haematologica* **90**, 13–9.

Melin, A., Fauchier, L., Dubuis, E., Obert, P. and Bonnet, P. (2003) Heart rate variability in rats acclimatized to high altitude. *High Alt. Med. Biol.* **4**, 375–87.

Menon, N.D. (1965) High altitude pulmonary edema: a clinical study. *N. Engl. J. Med.* **273**, 66–73.

Menzies, I.S. (1984) Transmucosal passage of inert molecules in health and disease, in *Intestinal Absorption and Secretion,* Falk Symposium 36 (eds. E. Skadhauge and K. Heintze), MTP Press, Lancaster, pp. 527–43.

Mercker, H. and Schneider, M. (1949) Uber capillarveranderungen des gehirns bei hohenanpassung. *Pflügers Arch.* **251**, 49–55.

Merino, C.F. (1950) Studies on blood formation and destruction in the polycythaemia of high altitude. *Blood* **5**, 1–31.

Messner, R. (1979) The mountain, in *Everest: Expedition to the Ultimate*. Kaye & Ward, London, pp. 47–217.

Messner, R. (1981) At my limit. *Natl. Geogr.* **160**, 553–66.

Meyrick, B. and Reid, L. (1978) The effect of continued hypoxia on rat pulmonary arterial circulation. An ultrastructural study. *Lab. Invest.* **38**, 188–200.

Meyrick, B. and Reid, L. (1980) Hypoxia-induced structural changes in the media and adventitia of the rat hilar pulmonary artery and their regression. *Am. J. Pathol.* **100**, 151–78.

Michel, C.C. and Milledge, J.S. (1963) Respiratory regulation in man during acclimatization to high altitude. *J. Physiol.* **168**, 631–43.

Milledge, J.S. (1963) Electrocardiographic changes at high altitude. *Br. Heart J.* **25**, 291–8.

Milledge, J.S. (1968) The control of breathing at high altitude, MD thesis, University of Birmingham.

Milledge, J.S. (1972) Arterial oxygen desaturation and intestinal absorption of xylose. *BMJ* **2**, 557–8.

Milledge, J.S. (1992) Respiratory water loss at altitude. *ISMM Newsletter.* **2**, 5–7. (Available www.issmed.org).

Milledge, J.S. and Catley, D.M. (1982) Renin, aldosterone and converting enzyme during exercise and acute hypoxia in humans. *J. Appl. Physiol.* **52**, 320–3.

Milledge, J.S. and Catley, D.M. (1987) Angiotensin converting enzyme activity and hypoxia. *Clin. Sci.* **72**, 149.

Milledge, J.S. and Lahiri, S. (1967) Respiratory control in lowlanders and Sherpa highlanders at altitude. *Respir. Physiol.* **2**, 310–22.

Milledge, J.S. and Sorensen, S.C. (1972) Cerebral arteriovenous oxygen difference in man native to high altitude. *J. Appl. Physiol.* **32**, 687–9.

Milledge, J.S. and Stott, F.D. (1977) Inductive plethysmography – a new respiratory transducer. *J. Physiol. (Lond)* **267**, 4p–5p.

Milledge, J.S., Iliff, L.D. and Severinghaus, J.W. (1968) The site of vascular leakage in hypoxic pulmonary edema, in *Proceedings of the International Union of Physiological Sciences, Abstracts*, vol. 44, *International Congress*, p. 883.

Milledge, J.S., Halliday, D., Pope, C. *et al.* (1977) The effects of hypoxia on muscle glycogen resynthesis in man. *Q. J. Exp. Physiol.* **62**, 237–45.

Milledge, J.S., Bryson E.I., Catley, D.M. *et al.* (1982) Sodium balance, fluid homeostasis and the renin–aldosterone system during the prolonged exercise of hill walking. *Clin. Sci.* **62**, 595–604.

Milledge, J.S., Catley, D.M., Ward, M.P. *et al.* (1983a) Renin–aldosterone and angiotensin-converting enzyme during prolonged altitude exposure. *J. Appl. Physiol.* **55**, 699–702.

Milledge, J.S., Catley, D.M., Blume, F.D. and West, J.B. (1983b) Renin, angiotensin-converting enzyme, and aldosterone in humans on Mount Everest. *J. Appl. Physiol.* **55**, 1109–12.

Milledge, J.S., Ward, M.P., Williams, E.S. and Clarke, C.R. (1983c) Cardiorespiratory response to exercise in men repeatedly exposed to extreme altitude. *J. Appl. Physiol.* **55**, 1379–85.

Milledge, J.S., Catley, D.M., Williams, E.S. *et al.* (1983d) Effect of prolonged exercise at altitude on the renin–aldosterone system. *J. Appl. Physiol.* **55**, 413–18.

Milledge, J.S. and Cotes, P.M. (1985) Serum erythropoietin in humans at high altitude and its relation to plasma renin. *J. Appl. Physiol.* **59**, 360–4.

Milledge, J.S., Thomas, P.S., Beeley, J.M. and English, J.S.C. (1988) Hypoxic ventilatory response and acute mountain sickness. *Eur. Respir. J.* **1**, 948–51.

Milledge, J.S., Beeley, J.M., McArthur, S. and Morice, A.H. (1989) Atrial natriuretic peptide, altitude and acute mountain sickness. *Clin. Sci.* **77**, 509–14.

Milledge, J.S., Beeley, J.M., Broom, J. *et al.* (1991a) Acute mountain sickness susceptibility, fitness and hypoxic ventilatory response. *Eur. Respir. J.* **4**, 1000–3.

Milledge, J.S., McArthur, S., Morice, A. *et al.* (1991b) Atrial natriuretic peptide and exercise-induced fluid retention in man. *J. Wilderness Med.* **2**, 94–101.

Miller, D. (1999) Menstrual cycle abnormalities and the oral contraceptive pill at high altitude (abstract), in *Hypoxia: Into the Next Millennium* (eds. R.C. Roach, P.D. Wagner and P.H. Hackett), Plenum/Kluwer, New York, p. 412.

Mills, W.J. (1973a) Frostbite and hypothermia. Current concepts. *Alaska Med.* **15**, 26–59.

Mills, W.J. (1973b) Frostbite. A discussion of the problem and a review of an Alaskan experience. *Alaska Med.* **15**, 27–47.

Mills, W.J. (1983a) General hypothermia. *Alaska Med.* **25**, 29–32.

Mills, W.J. (1983b) Frostbite. *Alaska Med.* **25**, 33–8.

Mills, W.J. and Rau, D. (1983) University of Alaska, Anchorage. Section of high latitude study, and the Mount McKinley Project. *Alaska Med.* **25**, 21–8.

Mines, A.H. (1981) *Respiratory Physiology*, Raven Press, New York.

Minetti, A.E., Formenti, F. and Ardigo, L.A. (2006) Himalayan porter's specialization: metabolic power, economy and skill. *Proc. Roy. Soc. Series B* **273**, 2791–7.

Mirrakhimov, M.M. (1978) Biological and physiological characteristics of high altitude natives of Tien Shan and the Pamirs, in *The Biology of High Altitude Peoples* (ed. P.T. Baker), Cambridge University Press, Cambridge, p. 313.

Mirrakhimov, M.M. and Meimanaliev, T.S. (1981) Heart rhythm disturbances in the inhabitants of mountainous regions. *Cor. Vasa.* **23**, 359–65.

Mirrakhimov, M., Brimkulov, N., Cieslick, J. *et al.* (1993) Effect of acetazolamide on overnight oxygenation and acute mountain sickness in patients with asthma. *Eur. Respir. J.* **6**, 536–40.

Mitchell, R.A. (1963) The role of the medullary chemoreceptors in acclimatization to high altitude, in *Proceedings: International Symposium Cardiovascular Respiration*, Karger, Basel, pp. 124–44.

Miyamoto, O. and Auer, R.N. (2000) Hypoxia, hyperoxia, ischemia, and brain necrosis. *Neurology* **54**, 362–71.

Møller, K., Strauss, G.I., Thomsen, G., *et al.* (2002) Cerebral blood flow, oxidative metabolism and cerebrovascular carbon dioxide reactivity in patients with acute bacterial meningitis. *Acta Anaes. Scand.* **46**, 567.

Molnar, G.W., Hughes, A.L., Wilson, O. and Goldman, R.F. (1973) Effect of wetting skin on finger cooling and freezing. *J. Appl. Physiol.* **35**, 205–7.

Moncada, S.R., Palmer, M.J. and Higgs, E.A. (1991) Nitric oxide physiology, pathophysiology, and pharmacology. *Pharmacol. Rev.* **43**, 109–42.

Moncloa, F., Donayre, J., Sobrevilla, L.A. and Guerra-Garcia, R. (1965) Endocrine studies at high altitude: I. Adrenal cortical function in sea level natives exposed to high altitudes (4300 m) for two weeks. *J. Clin. Endocrinol. Metab.* **25**, 1640–2.

Monge, C.C. and Whittembury, J. (1976) Chronic mountain sickness. *Johns Hopkins Med. J.* **139**, 87–9.

Monge, C.C., Bonavia, D., Leon-Velard, F. and Arregui, A. (1990) High altitude populations in Nepal and the Andes, in *Hypoxia: the Adaptations* (eds. J.R. Sutton, G. Coates and J.E. Remmers), Decker, Toronto, pp. 53–8.

Monge, M.C. (1925) Sobre el primer caso del policitemia encontrado en el Peru. *Bull. Acad. Méd. Lima*.

Monge, M.C. (1928) *La Enfermedad de los Andes*, Imp. Americana, Lima.

Monge, M.C. (1948) *Acclimatization in the Andes: Historical Confirmations of 'Climatic Aggression' in the Development of Andean Man*, Johns Hopkins University Press, Baltimore, MD.

Montgomery, H., Clarkson, P., Barnard, M. *et al.* (1999) Angiotensin-converting-enzyme gene insertion/deletion polymorphism and response to physical training. *Lancet* **253**, 1884–5.

Montgomery, H.E., Marshal, R., Hemingway, S. *et al.* (1998) Human gene for physical performance. *Nature* **393**, 221.

Mooi, W., Smith, P. and Heath, D. (1978) The ultrastructural effects of acute decompression on the lung of rats: the influence of frusemide. *J. Pathol.* **126**, 189–96.

Moorcroft, W. and Trebeck, G. (1841) Travels in the Himalayan provinces of Hindustan and the Punjab; in Ladakh and Kashmir; in Peshawar, Kabul, Kuduz and Bokhara, in *William Moorcroft, George Trebeck from 1819 to 1825* (ed. H.H. Wilson), vols. 1 and 2, John Murray, London.

Moore, K., Vizzard, N., Coleman, C., McMahon, J., Hayes, R. and Thompson, C.J. (2001) Extreme altitude mountaineering and Type 1 diabetes; the Diabetes Federation of Ireland Kilimanjaro Expedition. *Diabet. Med.* **18**, 749–55.

Moore, L.G. (1997) Women at altitude in hypoxia, in *Women at Altitude* (eds. C.S. Houston and G. Coates), Queen City Printers, Inc., Burlington, VT, pp. 1–7.

Moore, L.G. (2000) Comparative human ventilatory adaptation to high altitude (Review). *Respir. Physiol.* **121**, 257–76.

Moore, L.G. (2001) Human genetic adaptation to high altitude (Review). *High Alt. Med. Biol.* **2**, 257–79.

Moore, L.G., Harrison, G.L., McCullough, R.E. *et al.* (1986) Low acute hypoxic ventilatory response and hypoxic depression in acute mountain sickness. *J. Appl. Physiol.* **60**, 1407–12.

Moore, L.G., Cymerman, A., Huang, S.Y. *et al.* (1987) Propranolol blocks the metabolic rate increase but not ventilatory acclimatization to 4300 m. *Respir. Physiol.* **70**, 195–204.

Moore, L.G., Niermeyer, S. and Zamudio, S. (1998a) Human adaptation to high altitude: regional and life cycle perspectives. *Am. J. Physical. Anthropol. Ybk.* **41**, 25–64.

Moore, L.G., Asmus, I. and Curran, L. (1998b) Chronic mountain sickness: gender and geographical variation, in *Progress in Mountain Medicine and High Altitude* (eds. H. Ohno, T. Kobayashi, S. Masuyama and M. Nakashima), Press Committee of the 3rd Congress on Mountain Medicine and High Altitude Physiology, Matsumoto, p. 114–19.

Moore, L.G., Young, D., McCullough, R.E., Droma, T. and Zamudio, S. (2001a) Tibetan protection from intrauterine growth restriction (IUGR) and reproductive loss at high altitude. *Am. J. Hum. Biol.* **13**, 635–44.

Moore, L.G., Zamudio, S., Zhuang, J., Sun, S. and Droma, T. (2001b) Oxygen transport in tibetan women during pregnancy at 3,658 m. *Am. J. Phys. Anthropol.* **114**, 42–53.

Moore, L.G., Zamudio, S., Zhuang, J., Droma, T. and Shohet, R.V. (2002) Analysis of the myoglobin gene in Tibetans living at high altitude. *High. Alt. Med. Biol.* **3**, 39–47.

Moore, L.G., Shriver, M., Bemis, L. *et al.* (2004) Maternal adaptation to high-altitude pregnancy: an experiment of nature–a review (Review). *Placenta* **25**(Suppl A), S60–71.

Mordes, J.P., Blume, F.D., Boyer, S., Zheng, M. and Braverman, L.E. (1983) High-altitude pituitary–thyroid dysfunction on Mount Everest. *N. Engl. J. Med.* **308**, 1135–8.

Moret, P.R. (1971) Coronary blood flow and myocardial metabolism in man at high altitude, in *High Altitude Physiology: Cardiac and Respiratory Aspects* (eds. R. Porter and J. Knight), Churchill Livingstone, Edinburgh, pp. 131–44.

Morgan, J., Wright, A., Hoar, H., Hale, D. and Imray, C. (1999) Near-infrared spectroscopy to assess cerebral oxygenation at high altitude (abstract), in *Hypoxia: Into the Next Millennium* (eds. R.C. Roach, P.D. Wagner and P.H. Hackett), Plenum/Kluwer, New York, p. 413.

Morganti, A., Giussani, M., Sala, C. *et al.* (1995) Effects of exposure to high altitude on plasma endothelin-1 levels in normal subjects. *J. Hyperten.* **13**, 859–65.

Morice, A., Pepke-Zaba, J., Loysen, E. *et al.* (1988) Low dose infusion of atrial natriuretic peptide causes salt and water excretion in normal man. *Clin. Sci.* **74**, 359–63.

Moro, P.L., Checkley, W., Gilmon, R.H. *et al.* (1999) Gallstone disease in high altitude Peruvian rural populations. *Am. J. Gastroenterol.* **94**, 153–8.

Morocz, I.A., Zientara, G.P. and Gudbjartsson, H. (2001) Volumetric quantification of brain swelling after hypobaric hypoxia exposure. *Exp. Neurol.* **168**, 96–104.

Morpurgo, G., Arese, P., Bosia, A. *et al.* (1976) Sherpas living permanently at high altitude: a new pattern of adaptation. *Proc. Natl. Acad. Sci. USA* **73**, 747–51.

Morrell, N.W., Sarybaev, A.S., Alikhan, A. *et al.* (1999) ACE genotype and risk of high altitude pulmonary hypertension in Kyrghyz highlanders. *Lancet* **353**, 814.

Mortola, J.P., Rezzonico, R., Fisher, J.T. *et al.* (1990) Compliance of the respiratory system in infants born at high altitude. *Am. Rev. Respir. Dis.* **142**, 43–8.

Morton, J.P. and Cable, N.T. (2005) Effects of intermittent hypoxic training on aerobic and anaerobic performance. *Ergonomics* **48**, 1535–46.

Mosso, A. (1897) *Fisiologia dell'uomo sulle Alpi: studii fatti sul Monte Rosa*, Treves, Milan.

Mosso, A. (1898) *Life of Man on the High Alps.* T. Fisher Unwin, London.

Motley, H.L., Cournand, A., Werko, L. *et al.* (1947) Influence of short periods of induced acute anoxia upon pulmonary artery pressure in man. *Am. J. Physiol.* **150**, 315–20.

Moudgil, R., Michelakis, E.D. and Archer, S.L. (2005) Hypoxic pulmonary vasoconstriction (Review). *J. Appl. Physiol.* **98**, 390–403.

Muelleman, R.L., Grandstaff, P.M. and Robinson, W.A. (1997) The use of pegorgotein in the treatment of frostbite. *Wilderness Environ. Med.* **8**, 17–19.

Mulligan, E., Lahiri, S. and Storey, B.T. (1981) Carotid body O_2 chemoreception and mitochondrial oxidative phosphorylation. *J. Appl. Physiol.* **51**, 438–46.

Murata, T., Hori, M., Sakamoto, K., Karaki, H. and Ozaki, H. (2004) Dexamethasone blocks hypoxia-induced endothelial dysfunction in organ-cultured pulmonary arteries. *Am. J. Respir. Crit. Care. Med.* **170**, 647–55.

Murdoch, D. (1995a) Altitude illness among tourists flying to 3740 meters elevation in the Nepal Himalayas. *J. Travel Med.* **2**, 255–6.

Murdoch, D.R. (1994) Lateral rectus palsy at high altitude. *J. Wild. Med.* **5**, 179–81.

Murdoch, D.R. (1995b) Focal neurological defects and migraine at high altitude. *J. Neurol. Neurosurg. Psychiatry* **58**, 637.

Murdoch, D.R. (1996) Focal neurological deficits associated with high altitude. *Wild. Environ. Med.* **7**, 79–82.

Murdoch, D.R. (1999) How fast is too fast? Attempts to define a recommended ascent rate to prevent acute mountain sickness. *ISMM Newsletter* **9**, 3–6.

Mustafa, S., Thulesius, O. and Ismael, H.N. (2003) Hyperthermia-induced vasoconstriction of the carotid artery, a possible causative factor of heatstroke. *J. Appl. Physiol.* **96**, 1875–8.

Muza, S.R., Kaminsky, D., Fulco, C.S., Banderet, L.E. and Cymerman, A. (2004) Cysteinyl leukotriene blockade does not prevent acute mountain sickness. *Aviat. Space Environ. Med.* **75**, 413–9.

Myerson, S., Hemingway, H., Budget, R., Martin, J., Humphries, S. and Hugh Montgomery, H. (1999) Human angiotensin I-converting enzyme gene and endurance performance. *J. Appl. Physiol.* **87**, 1313–16.

Myres, J.E., Malan, M., Shumway, J.B., Rowe, M.J., Amon, E. and Woodward, S.R. (2000) Haplogroup-associated differences in neonatal death and incidence of low birth weight at elevation: a preliminary assessment. *Am. J. Obstet. Gynecol.* **182**, 1599–605.

Nahum, G.G. and Stanislaw, H. (2004) Hemoglobin, altitude and birth weight: does maternal anemia during pregnancy influence fetal growth? *J. Reprod. Med.* **49**, 297–305.

Nair, C.S., Malhotra, M.S. and Gopinarth, P.M. (1971) Effect of altitude and cold acclimatization on the basal metabolism in man. *Aerosp. Med.* **42**, 1056–9.

Nakashima, M. (1983) High altitude medical research in Japan. *Jpn. J. Mount. Med.* **3**, 19–27.

National Fire Protection Association (1993) *Standard for Hypobaric Facilities*, Quincy, MA, NFPA Code 99B.

National Oceanic and Atmospheric Administration (1976) *US Standard Atmosphere*, 1976, NOAA, Washington, DC.

Nattie E.E. (2002) Central chemosensitivity, sleep and wakefulness. *Respir. Physiol.* **129**, 257–68.

Nayak, N.C., Roy, S. and Narayanan, T.K. (1964) Pathologic features of altitude sickness. *Am. J. Pathol.* **45**, 381–7.

Neckar, J., Szarszoi, O., Koten, L. *et al.* (2002) Effects of mitochondrial K (ATP) modulators on cardioprotection induced by chronic high altitude hypoxia in rats. *Cardiovasc. Res.* **55**, 567–75.

Netzer, N.C. and Strohl, K.P. (1999) Sleep and breathing in recreational climbers at an altitude of 4200 and 6400 meters: observational study of sleep and patterning of respiration during sleep in a group of recreational climbers. *Sleep and Breathing* **3**, 75–82.

Newhouse, M.T. *et al.* (1964) Effect of alterations in end-tidal CO_2 tension on flow resistance. *J. Appl. Physiol.* **19**, 745–9.

NHS (1974) *Accidental Hypothermia*. NHS Memorandum No. 1974 (Gen.) 7, Scottish Home and Health Department.

Niazi, S.A. and Lewis, F.J. (1958) Profound hypothermia in man: report of a case. *Ann. Surg.* **147**, 254–6.

Nicholas, M., Thullier-Lestienne, F., Bouquet, C. *et al.* (2000) A study of mood changes and personality during a 31-day period of chronic hypoxia in a hypobaric chamber (Everest-Comex '97). *Psychol. Reports* **86**, 119–26.

Nicholas, R., O'Meara P.D. and Calonge, N. (1992) Is syncope related to moderate altitude exposure? *JAMA* **268**, 904–6.

Nielsen, A.M., Bisgard, G.E. and Vidruk, E.H. (1998) Carotid chemoreceptor activity during acute and sustained hyoxia in goats. *J. Appl. Physiol.* **65**, 1796–1802.

Niermeyer, S. (2003) Cardiopulmonary transition in the high altitude infant. *High Alt. Med. Biol.* **4**, 225–39.

Niermeyer, S., Yang, P., Shanmina, D. *et al.* (1995) Arterial oxygen saturation in Tibetan and Han infants born in Lhasa, Tibet. *N. Engl. J. Med.* **333**, 1248–52.

Noda, M., Suzuki, S., Tsubochi, H. *et al.* (2003) Single dexamethasone injection increases alveolar fluid clearance in adult rats. *Crit. Care Med.* **4**, 1183–9.

Norese, M.F., Lezon, C.E., Alippi, R.M. *et al.* (2002) Failure of polycythemia-induced increase in arterial oxygen content to suppress the anorexic effect of simulated high altitude in the adult rat. *High Alt. Med. Biol.* **3**, 49–57.

Normand, H., Barragan, M., Benoit, O., Balliart, O. and Raynaud, J. (1990) Periodic breathing and O_2 saturation in relation to sleep stages in normal subjects. *Am. J. Respir. Crit. Care Med.* **149**, 229–35.

Norton, E.F. (1925) Norton and Somervell's attempt, in *The Fight for Everest* (ed. E.F. Norton), Arnold, London, pp. 90–119.

Nugent, S.K. and Rogers, M.C. (1980) Resuscitation and intensive care monitoring following immersion hypothermia. *J. Trauma*, **20**, 814–15.

Nukada, H., Pollock, M. and Allpress, S. (1981) Experimental cold injury to nerve. *Brain* **104**, 779–813.

Nummela, A. and Rusko, H. (2000) Acclimatization to altitude and normoxic training improve 400-m running performance at sea level. *J. Sports Sci.* **18**, 411–9.

Nunn, J.F. (1961) Portable anaesthetic apparatus for use in the Antarctic. *BMJ* **1**, 1139–43.

Nusshag, W. (1954) *Hygiene der Haustiere*, Hirzel, Leipzig, p. 86.

Nygaard, E. and Nielsen, E. (1978) Skeletal muscle fibre capillarization with extreme endurance training in man, in *Swimming Medicine IV* (eds. B. Eriksson and B. Furberg), University Park Press, Baltimore, MD.

Oades, P.L., Buchdahl, R.M. and Bush, A. (1994) Prediction of hypoxaemia at high altitude in children with cystic fibrosis. *BMJ* **308**, 15–18.

O'Brien, C., Young, A.J. and Sawka, M.N. (1998) Hypothermia and thermoregulation in cold air. *J. Appl. Physiol.* **83**, 185–9.

O'Donnell, W.J., Rosenberg, M., Niven, R.W. *et al.* (1992) Acetazolamide and furosemide attenuate asthma induced by hyperventilation of cold, dry air. *Am. Rev. Respir. Dis.* **146**, 1518–23.

Oelz, O., Howald, H., di Prampero, P.E. *et al.* (1986) Physiological profile of world-class high-altitude climbers. *J. Appl. Physiol.* **60**, 1734–42.

Oelz, O., Maggiorini, M., Ritter, M. *et al.* (1989) Nifedipine for high altitude pulmonary oedema. *Lancet* **2**, 1241–4.

Ogilvie, J. (1977) Exhaustion and exposure. *Climber and Rambler,* Sept., 34–9; Oct., 52–5.

Ohkuda, K., Nakahara, K., Weidner, W.J. *et al.* (1978) Lung fluid exchange after uneven pulmonary artery obstruction in sheep. *Circ. Res.* **43**, 152–61.

Okumura, A., Fuse, H., Kawauchi, Y., Mizuno, I. and Akashi, T. (2003) Changes in male reproductive function after high altitude mountaineering. *High Alt. Med. Biol.* **4**, 349–53.

Olfert, I.M., Breen, E.C., Mathieu-Costello, O. and Wagner, P.D. (2001) Chronic hypoxia attenuates resting and exercise-induced VEGF, flt-1, and flk-1 mRNA levels in skeletal muscle. *J. Appl. Physiol.* **90**, 1532–8.

Olsen, N.V., Hansen, J.-M., Kanstrup, I., Richalet, J.-P. and Leyssac, P.P. (1993) Renal hemodynamics, tubular function, and the response to low-dose dopamine during acute hypoxia in humans. *J. Appl. Physiol.* **74**, 2166–73.

Omura, A., Roy, R. and Jennings, T. (2000) Inhaled nitric oxide improves survival in the rat model of high-altitude pulmonary edema. *Wilderness Environ. Med.* **11**, 251–6.

Onywera, V.O., Kiplamai, F.K., Boit, M.K. and Pitsiladis, Y.P. (2004) Food and macronutrient intake of elite kenyan distance runners. *Int. J. Sport Nutr. Exerc. Metab.* **14**, 709–19.

Oort, A.H. and Rasmusson, E.M. (1971) *Atmospheric Circulation Statistics*, US Department of Commerce, NOAA, Rockville, MD, pp. 84–5.

Opitz, E. (1951) Increased vascularization of the tissue due to acclimatization to high altitude and its significance of oxygen transport. *Exp. Med. Surg.* **9**, 389–403.

Orr, K.D. and Fainer, D.C. (1951) *Cold Injuries in Korea During Winter 1950–51*, Army Medical Research Laboratory, Fort Knox, KY.

Osborne, J.J. (1953) Experimental hypothermia: respiratory and blood pH changes in relation to cardiac function. *Am. J. Physiol.* **175**, 389–98.

Ou, L.C. and Tenney, S.M. (1970) Properties of mitochondria from hearts of cattle acclimatized to high altitude. *Respir. Physiol.* **8**, 151–9.

Pace, N., Griswold, R.L. and Grunbaum, B.W. (1964) Increase in urinary norepinephrine excretion during 14 days sojourn at 3800 m elevation (abstract). *Fed. Proc.* **23**, 521.

Pandolf, K.B., Young, A.J., Sawka, M.N. *et al.* (1998) Does erythrocyte infusion improve 3.2 km run performance at high altitude? *Eur. J. Appl. Physiol.* **79**, 1–6.

Pappenheimer, J. (1988) Physiological regulation of transepithelial impedance in the intestinal mucosa of rats and hamsters. *J. Membr. Biol.* **100**, 137–48.

Pappenheimer, J.R. (1977) Sleep and respiration of rats during hypoxia. *J. Physiol. (Lond.)* **266**, 191–207.

Pappenheimer, J.R. (1984) Hypoxic insomnia: effects of carbon monoxide and acclimatization. *J. Appl. Physiol.* **57**, 1696–1703.

Pappenheimer, J.R. and Maes, J.P. (1942) A quantitative measure of the vasomotor tone in the hind limb muscles of the dog. *Am. J. Physiol.* **137**, 187–99.

Pappenheimer, J.R., Fencl, V., Heisey, S.R. and Held, D. (1964) Role of cerebral fluids in control of respiration as studied in unanesthetized goats. *Am. J. Physiol.* **208**, 436–40.

Parker, J.C., Breen, E.C. and West, J.B. (1997) High vascular and airway pressures increase interstitial protein mRNA expression in isolated rat lungs. *J. Appl. Physiol.* **83**, 1697–705.

Parkins, K.J., Poets, C.F., O'Brien, L.M., Stebbins, V.A. and Southall, D.R. (1998) Effect of exposure to 15% oxygen on breathing patterns and oxygen saturation in infants: interventional study. *BMJ* **316**, 887–91.

Pascal, B. (1648) *Story of the Great Experiment on the Equilibrium of Fluids.* English translation of relevant pages in *High Altitude Physiology* (ed. J.B. West), Hutchinson Ross, Stroudsburg, PA, 1981.

Paschen, W. (1996) Disturbances of calcium homeostasis within the endoplasmic reticulum may contribute to the development of ischemic cell damage. *Med. Hypotheses* **47**, 283–8.

Passino, C., Bernardi, L., Spadacini, G. *et al.* (1996) Autonomic regulation of heart rate and peripheral circulation: comparison of high altitude and sea level residents. *Clin. Sci.* **91**, 81–3.

Patel, S., Woods, D.R., Macleod, N.J. *et al.* (2003) Angiotensin-converting enzyme genotype and the ventilatory response to exertional hypoxia. *Eur. Resp. J.* **22**, 755–60.

Paton, B.C. (1983) Accidental hypothermia. *Pharmacol. Ther.* **22**, 331–77.

Paton, B.C. (1987) Pathophysiology of frostbite, in *Hypoxia and Cold* (eds. J.R. Sutton, C.S. Houston and G. Coates), Praeger, New York, pp. 329–39.

Paton, B.C. (1991) Hypothermia, in *A Colour Atlas of Mountain Medicine* (eds. J. Vallotton and F. Dubas), Wolfe, London, pp. 92–6.

Pattengale, P.K. and Holloszy, J.O. (1967) Augmentation of skeletal muscle myoglobin by a program of treadmill running. *Am. J. Physiol.* **213**, 783–5.

Patton, J.F. and Doolittle, W.H. (1972) Core rewarming by peritoneal dialysis following induced hypothermia in the dog. *J. Appl. Physiol.* **33**, 800–4.

Paul, M.A. and Fraser, W.D. (1994) Performance during mild acute hypoxia. *Aviat. Space. Environ. Med.* **65**, 891–9.

Pavan, P., Sarto, P., Merlo, L. *et al.* (2004) Metabolic and cardiovascular parameters in type 1 diabetics at extreme altitude. *Med. Sci. Sports Exerc.* **36**, 1283–9.

Peacock, A.J. and Jones, P.L. (1997) Gas exchange at extreme altitude: results from the British 40th Anniversary Everest Expedition. *Eur. Respir. J.* **10**, 1439–44.

Pearn, J.H. (1982) Cold injury complicating trauma in sub-zero environments. *Med. J. Aust.* **1**, 505–7.

Pederson, L. and Benumof, J. (1993) Incidence and management of hypothermia in a rural African hospital. *Anaesthesia* **48**, 67–9.

Pedlar, C., Whyte, G., Emegbo, S., Stanley, N., Hindmarch, I. and Godfrey, R. (2005) Acute sleep responses in a normobaric hypoxic tent. *Med. Sci. Sports Exerc.* **37**, 1075–9.

Pei, S.X., Chen, X.J., Si Ren, B.Z. *et al.* (1989) Chronic mountain sickness in Tibet. *Q. J. Med.* **71**, 555–74.

Peñaloza, D. (1971) Discussion, in *High Altitude Physiology: Cardiac and Respiratory Aspects* (eds. R. Porter and J. Knight), Churchill Livingstone, Edinburgh, p. 169.

Peñaloza, D. and Echevarria, M. (1957) Electrocardiographic observations on ten subjects at sea level and during one year of residence at high altitudes. *Am. Heart J.* **54**, 811–22.

Peñaloza, D. and Sime, F. (1969) Circulatory dynamics during high altitude pulmonary edema. *Am. J. Cardiol.* **23**, 369–78.

Peñaloza, D. and Sime, F. (1971) Chronic cor pulmonale due to loss of altitude acclimatization (chronic mountain sickness). *Am. J. Med.* **50**, 728–43.

Peñaloza, D., Sime, F., Banchero, N. and Gamboa, R. (1962) Pulmonary hypertension in healthy man born and living at high altitudes. *Med. Thorac.* **19**, 449–60.

Peñaloza, D., Sime, F., Banchero, N. *et al.* (1963) Pulmonary hypertension in healthy men born and living at high altitudes. *Am. J. Cardiol.* **11**, 150–7.

Peñaloza, D., Arias-Stella, J., Sime, F., Recavarren, S. and Marticorena, E. (1964) The heart and pulmonary circulation in children at high altitudes: physiological, anatomical, and clinical observations. *Pediatrics* **34**, 568–82.

Peñaloza, D., Sime, F. and Ruiz, L. (1971) Cor pulmonale in chronic mountain sickness: present concept of Monge's disease, in *High Altitude Physiology: Cardiac and Respiratory Aspects,* Ciba Foundation Symposium (eds. R. Porter and J. Knight), Churchill Livingstone, Edinburgh, pp. 41–60.

Perez-Pinzon, M.A., Chan, C.Y., Rosenthal, M. and Sick, T.J. (1992) Membrane and synaptic activity during anoxia in the isolated turtle cerebellum. *Am. J. Physiol.* **263**, R1057–63.

Peroni, D.G., Boner, A.L., Vallone, G. *et al.* (1994) Effective allergen avoidance at high altitude reduces allergen-induced bronchial hyperresponsiveness *Am. J. Respir. Crit. Care Med.* **149**, 1441–6.

Perrill, C.V. (1993) High-altitude sycope: history repeats itself. *JAMA* **269**, 587.

Pesce, C., Leal, C., Pinto, H. *et al.* (2005) Determinants of acute mountain sickness and success on Mount Aconcagua (6962 m). *High Alt. Med. Biol.* **6**, 158–66.

Petetin, D. (1991) Eye protection at high altitude, in *A Colour Atlas of Mountain Medicine* (eds. J. Vallotton and F. Dubas), Wolfe, London, pp. 71–2.

Petit, J.M., Milic-Emili, J. and Troquet, J. (1963) Travail dynamique pulmonaire et altitude. *Rev. Med. Aerosp.* **2**, 276–9.

Peyronnard, J.M., Pednault, M. and Aquayo, A.J. (1977) Neuropathies due to cold. Quantitative studies of structural changes in human and animal nerves, in *Proceedings of the 11th World Congress of Neurology,* Amsterdam, pp. 308–29.

Pham, I., Uchida, T., Planes, C. *et al.* (2002) Hypoxia upregulates VEGF expression in alveolar epithelial cells in vitro and in vivo. *Am. J. Physiol., Lung Cell. Mol. Physiol.* **283**, L1133–42.

Phillipson, E.A., Sullivan, C.E., Read, D.J.C. *et al.* (1978) Ventilatory and waking responses to hypoxia in sleeping dogs. *J. Appl. Physiol. Respir. Environ. Exerc. Physiol.* **44**, 512–20.

Pichiule, P. and LaManna, J.C. (2002) Angiopoietin-2 and rat brain capillary remodeling during adaptation and deadaptation to prolonged mild hypoxia. *J. Appl. Physiol.* **93**, 1131–9.

Pickering, B.G., Bristow, G.K. and Craig, D.B. (1977) Core rewarming by peritoneal irrigation in accidental hypothermia. *Anesth. Analg.* **56**, 574–7.

Picon-Reategui, E. (1961) Basal metabolic rate and body composition at high altitudes. *J. Appl. Physiol.* **16**, 431–4.

Pierre, B. and Aulard, C. (1985) *Escalades et Randonnés du Hoggar et dans les Tassilis,* Arthaud, Paris, p. 153.

Piiper, J. and Scheid, P. (1980) Blood–gas equilibration in lungs, in *Pulmonary Gas Exchange,* vol. 1, *Ventilation, Blood Flow, and Diffusion* (ed. J.B. West), Academic Press, New York, pp. 131–71.

Piiper, J. and Scheid, P. (1986) Cross-sectional P_{O_2} distributions in Krogh cylinder and solid cylinder models. *Respir. Physiol.* **64**, 241–51.

Pines, A. (1978) High altitude acclimatization and proteinuria in East Africa. *Br. J. Dis. Chest* **72**, 196–8.

Pines, A., Slater, J.D.H. and Jowett, T.P. (1977) The kidney and aldosterone in acclimatization at altitude. *Br. J. Dis. Chest,* **71**, 203–7.

Pison, U., López, F.A., Heidelmeyer, C.F. *et al.* (1993) Inhaled nitric oxide reverses hypoxic pulmonary vasoconstriction without impairing gas exchange. *J. Appl. Physiol.* **74**, 1287–92.

Pitsiou, G., Kyriazis, G., Hatzizisi, O. *et al.* (2002) Tumor necrosis factor-alpha serum levels, weight loss and tissue oxygenation in chronic obstructive pulmonary disease. *Respir. Med.* **96**, 594–698.

Pitt, P. (1970) *Surgeon in Nepal,* Murray, London, p. 135.

Planes, C., Escoubet, B., Blot-Chabaud, M. *et al.* (1997) Hypoxia downregulates expression and activity of epithelial sodium channels in rat alveolar epithelial cells. *Am. J. Respir. Cell. Mol. Biol.* **17**, 508–18.

Plata, R., Cornejo, A., Arratia, C., *et al.* (2002) Angiotensin-converting-enzyme inhibition therapy in altitude polycythemia: a prospective randomized trial. *Lancet* **359**, 663–6.

Plutarch (46–120) Alexander and Caesar. *Loeb Classics,* vol. 7. (1971) Heinemann, London, p. 389.

Podolsky, A., Eldridge, M.W., Richardson, R.S. *et al.* (1996) Exercise-induced VA/Q inequality in subjects with prior high-altitude pulmonary edema. *J. Appl. Physiol.* **81**, 922–32.

Poiani, G.J., Tozzi, C.A., Yohn, S.E. *et al.* (1990) Collagen and elastin metabolism in hypertensive pulmonary arteries of rats. *Circ. Res.* **66**, 968–78.

Pollard, A.J. and Murdoch, D.R. (1997) Children at altitude, in *The High Altitude Medicine Handbook,* 2nd edn, Radcliffe Medical Press, Oxford, pp. 39–49.

Pollard, A.J., Barry, P.W., Mason, N.P. *et al.* (1997) Hypoxia, hypocapnia and spirometry at altitude. *Clin. Sci.* **92**, 593–8.

Pollard, A.J., Murdoch, D.R. and Bärtsch, P. (1998) Children at altitude. *BMJ* **316**, 874–5.

Pollard, A.J., Niermeyer, S., Barry, P. *et al.* (2001) Children at altitude: an international consensus statement by an *ad hoc* committee of the International Society for Mountain Medicine. *High Alt. Med. Biol.* **2**, 389–403.

Poole, D.C. and Mathieu-Costello, O. (1990) Effects of hypoxia on capillary orientation in anterior tibialis muscle of highly active mice. *Respir. Physiol.* **82**, 1–10.

Porter, M.M., Vandervoort, A.A. and Lexell, J. (1995) Aging of the human muscle: structure, function and adaptability. *Scan. J. Med. Sci. Sports.* **5**, 127–8.

Potter, R.F. and Groom, A.C. (1983) Capillary diameter and geometry in cardiac and skeletal muscle studied by means of corrosion casts. *Microvasc. Res.* **25**, 68–84.

Poulin, M.J., Cunningham, D.A., Paterson, D.H. *et al.* (1993) Ventilatory sensitivity to CO_2 in hyperoxia and hypoxia in older humans. *J. Appl. Physiol.* **75**, 2209–16.

Poulsen, T.D., Klausen, T., Richalet, J.P. *et al.* (1998) Plasma volume in acute hypoxia: comparison of a carbon monoxide rebreathing method and dye dilution with Evans' blue. *Eur. J. Appl. Physiol.* **77**, 457–61.

Povea, C., Schmitt, L., Brugniaux, J. *et al.* (2005) Effects of intermittent hypoxia on heart rate variability during rest and exercise. *High Alt. Med. Biol.* **6**, 215–25.

Powell, F.L. and Garcia, N. (2000) Physiological effects of intermittent hypoxia (Review). *High Alt. Med. Biol.* **1**, 125–36.

Prabhakar, H.R. (2000) Oxygen sensing by the carotid body chemoreceptors. *J. Appl. Physiol.* **88**, 2287–95.

Prabhakar, H.R. and Jacono, F.J. (2005) Cellular and molecular mechanisms associated with carotid body adaptations to chronic hypoxia. *High Alt. Med. Biol.* **6**, 112–120.

Prabhakar, H.R. and Overholt, J.L. (2000) Cellular mechanisms of oxygen sensign at the carotid body: haem and ion channels. *Respir. Physiol.* **122**, 209–21.

Prabhakar, H.R. and Peng, Y.J. (2004) Peripheral chemoreceptors in health and disease. *J. Appl. Physiol.* **96**, 359–66.

Pretorius, H.A. (1970) Effect of oxygen on night vision. *Aerospace Med.* **41**, 560–2.

Priban, I. (1963) An analysis of some short term patterns of breathing in man at rest. *J. Physiol. (Lond.)* **166**, 425–34.

Prisk, G.K., Elliott, A.R. and West J.B. (2000) Sustained microgravity reduces the human ventilatory response to hypoxia but not to hypercapnia. *J. Appl. Physiol.* **88**, 1421–30.

Pritchard, J.S. and Lane, D.J. (1974) Intestinal absorption studied in patients with chronic obstructive airways disease. *Thorax* **29**, 609.

Pugh, L.G.C.E. (1950) Physiological studies on HMS *Vengeance*: Royal Navy cold weather cruise 1994, *MRC Royal Naval Personnel Research Committee RNP 49/561*.

Pugh, L.G.C.E. (1955) Report on Cho Oyu 1952 and Everest 1953 expeditions. (Unpublished archival material held in the Archival Collection in High Altitude Medicine and Physiology at University of California, San Diego, USA.)

Pugh, L.G.C.E. (1957) Resting ventilation and alveolar air on Mount Everest: with remarks on the relation of barometric pressure to altitude in mountains. *J. Physiol. (Lond.)* **135**, 590–610.

Pugh, L.G.C.E. (1958) Muscular exercise on Mt. Everest. *J. Physiol. (Lond.)* **141**, 233–61.

Pugh, L.G.C.E. (1959) Carbon monoxide hazard in Antarctica. *BMJ* **1**, 192–6.

Pugh, L.G.C.E. (1962a) Physiological and medical aspects of the Himalayan Scientific and Mountaineering Expedition, 1960–61. *BMJ* **2**, 621–33.

Pugh, L.G.C.E. (1962b) Solar heat gain by man in the high Himalaya: UNESCO Symposium on Environmental Physiology and Psychology, Lucknow, India, pp. 325–9.

Pugh, L.G.C.E. (1963) Tolerance to extreme cold at altitude in a Nepalese pilgrim. *J. Appl. Physiol.* **18**, 1234–8.

Pugh, L.G.C.E. (1964a) Man at high altitude. *Scientific Basis of Medicine, Annual Review* 32–54.

Pugh, L.G.C.E. (1964b) Blood volume and haemoglobin concentration at altitudes above 18000 ft (5500 m). *J. Physiol.* **170**, 344–54.

Pugh, L.G.C.E. (1964c) Animals in high altitudes: man above 5000 m mountain exploration, in *Handbook of Physiology, Adaptation to the Environment,* section 4 (eds. D.B. Dill, E.F. Adolph and C.C. Wilber), Washington, DC, pp. 861–8.

Pugh, L.G.C.E. (1964d) Cardiac output in muscular exercise at 5800 m (19,000 ft). *J. Appl. Physiol.* **19**, 441–7.

Pugh, L.G.C.E. (1965) Altitude and athletic performance *Nature* **207**, 1397–8.

Pugh, L.G.C.E. (1966) Clothing insulation and accidental hypothermia in youth. *Nature* **209**, 1281–6.

Pugh, L.G.C.E. (1967) Cold stress and muscular exercise with special reference to accidental hypothermia. *BMJ* **2**, 333–7.

Pugh, L.G.C.E. (1969) Blood volume changes in outdoor exercise of 8–10 h duration. *J. Physiol. (Lond.),* **200**, 345–51.

Pugh, L.G.C.E. and Band, G. (1953) Appendix VI: Diet, in *The Ascent of Everest* (ed. J. Hunt), Hodder and Stoughton, London, pp. 263–9.

Pugh, L.G.C.E. and Ward, M.P. (1956) Some effects of high altitude on man. *Lancet* **2**, 1115–21.

Pugh, L.G.C.E., Gill, M.B., Lahiri, S., Milledge, J.S., Ward, M.P. and West, J.B. (1964) Muscular exercise at great altitudes. *J. Appl. Physiol.* **19**, 431–40.

Pulfery, S.M. and Jones, P.L. (1996) Energy expenditure and requirement while climbing above 6,000 m. *J. Appl. Physiol.* **81**, 1306–11.

Purkayastha, S.S., Bhaumik, G., Sharma, R.P. *et al.* (2000) Effects of mountaineering training at high altitude (4,350 m) on physical work performance of women. *Aviat. Space Environ. Med.* **71**, 685–91.

Pyne, D.B., Gleeson, M., McDonald, W.A., Clancy, R.L., Perry Jr., C. and Fricker P.A. (2000) Training strategies to maintain immunocompetence in athletes (Review). *Int. J. Sports Med.* **21**(Suppl 1), S51–60.

Radomski, M.N. and Boutelier, C. (1982) Hormone response of normal and intermittent cold pre-adapted humans to continuous cold. *J. Appl. Physiol.* **53**, 610–16.

Raff, H., Jankowski, B.M., Engeland, W.C. and Oaks, M.K. (1996) Hypoxia *in vivo* inhibits aldosterone and aldosterone synthase mRNA in rats. *J. Appl. Physiol.* **81**, 604–10.

Raff, H. and Kohandarvish, S. (1990) The effect of oxygen on aldosterone release from bovine adrenocortical cells *in vitro. Endocrinology,* **127**, 682–7.

Raguso, C.A., Guinot, S.L., Janssens, J-P., Kayser, B. and Pichard, C. (2004) Chronic hypoxia: common traits between chronic obstructive pulmonary disease and altitude. *Curr. Opin. Clin. Nutr. Metab. Care.* **7**, 411–7.

Rahn, H. and Fenn, W.O. (1955) *A Graphical Analysis of the Respiratory Gas Exchange,* American Physiological Society, Washington, DC.

Rahn, H. and Otis, A.B. (1949) Man's respiratory response during and after acclimatization to high altitude. *Am. J. Physiol.* **157**, 445–62.

Rai, R.M., Malhotra, M.S., Dimri, G.P. and Sampathkumar, T. (1975) Utilization of different quantities of fat at high altitude. *Am. J. Clin. Nutr.* **28**, 242–5.

Raichle, M.E. and Hornbein, T.F. (2001) The high-altitude brain, in *High Altitude: An Exploration of Human Adaptation* (eds. T.F. Hornbein and R.B. Schoen), Marcel Dekker, New York, pp. 377–423.

Raifman, M.A., Berant, M. and Levarsky, C. (1978) Cold weather and rhabdomyolysis. *J. Paediatr.* **93**, 970–1.

Raja, K.B., Pippard, M.J., Simpson, R.J. and Peters, T.J. (1986) Relationship between erythropoiesis and the enhanced intestinal uptake of ferric iron in hypoxia in the mouse. *Br. J. Haematol.* **64**, 587–93.

Ramirez, G., Bittle, P.A., Hammond, M. *et al.* (1988) Regulation of aldosterone secretion during hypoxemia at sea level and moderately high altitude. *J. Clin. Endocrinol. Metab.* **67**, 1162–5.

Ramirez, G., Hammon, M., Agousti, S.J. *et al.* (1992) Effects of hypoxemia at sea level and high altitude on sodium excretion and hormonal levels. *Aviat. Space Environ. Med.* **63**, 891–8.

Ramirez, G., Herrera, R., Pineda, D. *et al.* (1995) The effects of high altitude on hypothalamic–pituitary secretory dynamics in men. *Clin. Endocrinol.* **43**, 11–18.

Ramirez, G., Pineda, D., Bittle, P.A. *et al.* (1998) Partial renal resistance to arginine vasopressin as an adaptation to high altitude living. *Aviat. Space Environ. Med.* **69**, 58–65.

Ramos, D.A., Kruger, H., Muro, M. and Arias-Stella, J. (1967) Patologica del hombre nativo de las grande alturas: investigacion de las causes de muerte en 300 autopsias. *Bon. Sanit. Panam.* **62**, 497–507.

Rankinen, T., Pérusse, L., Gagnon, J. *et al.* (2000) Angiotensin-converting enzyme ID polymorphism and fitness phenotype in the HERITAGE Family Study. *J. Appl. Physiol.* **88**, 1029–35.

Rankinen, T., Wolfarth, B., Simoneau, J.-A. *et al.* (2000a) No association between the angiotensin-converting enzyme ID polymorphism and elite endurance athlete status. *J. Appl. Physiol.* **88**, 1571–5.

Rastogi, C.K., Malholtra, M.S., Srivastava, M.C. *et al.* (1977) Study of the pituitary–thyroid functions at high altitude in man. *J. Clin. Endocrinol. Metab.* **44**, 447–52.

Ratan, R.R., Siddiq, A., Aminova, L. *et al.* (2004) Translation of ischemic preconditioning to the patient: prolyl hydroxylase inhibition and hypoxia inducible factor-1 as novel targets for stroke therapy. *Stroke* **35**, 2687.

Rathat, C., Richalet, J.-P., Herry, J.-P. and Largmighat, P. (1992) Detection of high-risk subjects for high altitude diseases. *Int. J. Sports Med.* **13**, S76–8.

Rathat, C., Richalet, J.-P., Larmignat, P. and Herry, J.-P. (1993) Neck irradiation by cobalt therapy and susceptibility to acute mountain sickness. *J. Wilderness Med.* **4**, 231–2.

Ravenhill, T.H. (1913) Some experience of mountain sickness in the Andes. *J. Trop. Med. Hyg.* **16**, 313–20.

Raynaud, J., Drouet. L., Martineaud, J.P. *et al.* (1981) Time course of plasma growth hormone during exercise in humans at altitude. *J. Appl. Physiol.* **50**, 229–33.

Read, J. and Fowler, K.T. (1964) Effect of exercise on zonal distribution of pulmonary blood flow. *J. Appl. Physiol.* **19**, 672–8.

RCP (1966) *Report of Committee on Accidental Hypothermia,* Royal College of Physicians, London.

Rebuck, A.S. and Campbell, E.J.M. (1974) A clinical method for assessing the ventilatory response to hypoxia. *Am. Rev. Respir. Dis.* **109**, 345–50.

Recavarren, S. and Arias-Stella, J. (1964) Right ventricular hypertrophy in people born and living at high altitudes. *Br. Heart J.* **26**, 806–12.

Reed, D.J.C. (1967) A clinical method of assessing the ventilatory response to carbon dioxide. *Australas. Ann. Med.* **16**, 20–32.

Reeves, J.A. (2004) Is increased hematopoiesis needed at altitude? *J. Appl. Physiol.* **96**, 1579–80.

Reeves, J.T. and Grover, R.F. (1975) High-altitude pulmonary hypertension and pulmonary edema. *Prog. Cardiol.* **4**, 99–118.

Reeves, J.T. and Grover, R.F. (2005) Insights by Peruvian scientists into the pathogenesis of human chronic hypoxic pulmonary hypertension. *J. Appl. Physiol.* **98**, 384–9.

Reeves, J.T. and Weil, J.V. (2001) Chronic mountain sickness. A view from the crows nest. *Ad. Exper. Med. Biol.* **542**, 419–37.

Reeves, J.T., Moore, L.G., McCullough, R.E. *et al.* (1985) Headache at high altitude is not related to internal carotid arterial blood velocity. *J. Appl. Physiol.* **59**, 909–15.

Reeves, J.T., Groves, B.M., Sutton, J.T. *et al.* (1987) Operation Everest II: preservation of cardiac function at extreme altitude. *J. Appl. Physiol.* **63**, 531–9.

Reeves, J.T., Wagner, J., Zafren, K. *et al.* (1994) Seasonal variation in barometric pressure and temperature: effect on altitude illness, in *Hypoxia and Molecular Medicine* (eds. J.R. Sutton, C.S. Houston and G. Coates), Queen City Printers, Burlington, VT, pp. 275–81.

Regard, M., Oelz, O., Brugger, P. and Landis, T. (1989) Persistent cognitive impairment in climbers after repeated exposure to extreme altitude. *Neurology* **39**, 210–13.

Reichl, M. (1987) Neuropathy of the feet due to running on cold surfaces. *BMJ* **294**, 348–9.

Reinhart, W.H., Kayser, B., Singh, A., Waber, U., Oelz, O. and Bärtsch, P. (1991) Blood rheology and acute mountain sickness and high-altitude pulmonary edema. *J. Appl. Physiol.* **71**, 934–8.

Reitan, R.M. and Davison, L.A. (eds.) (1974) *Clinical Neuropsychology: Current Status and Applications,* Winston, Washington, DC.

Reite, M., Jackson, D., Cahoon, R.L. and Weil, J.V. (1975) Sleep physiology at high altitude. *Electroencephalogr. Clin. Neurophysiol.* **38**, 463–71.

Remillard, C.V. and Yuan, J.X. (2005) High altitude pulmonary hypertension: role of K^+ and Ca^{2+} channels. *High Alt. Med. Biol.* **6**, 133–46.

Remmers, J.E. and Mithoefer, J.C. (1969) The carbon monoxide diffusing capacity in permanent residents at high altitudes. *Respir. Physiol.* **6**, 233–44.

Ren, X. and Robbins, P.A. (1999) Ventilatory responses to hypercapnia and hypoxia after 6h passive hyperventilation in humans. *J. Physiol. (Lond.)* **514**(3), 885–94.

Rennie, D. (1973) Field studies in hypoxia and the kidney, in *Cornell Seminars in Nephrology* (ed. E.L. Becker), Wiley, New York, pp. 193–206.

Rennie, D. (1989) Will mountain trekkers have heart attacks? *JAMA* **261**, 1045–6.

Rennie, D. and Morrissey, J. (1975) Retinal changes in Himalayan climbers. *Arch. Ophthalmol.* **93**, 395–400.

Rennie, D. and Wilson, R. (1982) Who should not go high, in *Hypoxia: Man at Altitude* (eds. J.R. Sutton, N.L. Jones, and C.S. Houston), Thieme-Stratton, New York, pp. 186–90.

Rennie, D., Lozano, R., Monge, C. *et al.* (1971a). Renal oxygenation in male Peruvian natives living permanently at high altitude. *J. Appl. Physiol.* **30**, 450–6.

Rennie, D., Marticorena, E., Monge, C. and Sirotzky, L. (1971b) Urinary protein excretion in high altitude residents. *J. Appl. Physiol.* **31**, 257–9.

Rennie, D., Frayser, R., Gray, G. and Houston, C. (1972) Urine and plasma proteins in men at 5,400 m. *J. Appl. Physiol.* **32**, 369–73.

Rennie, I.D.B. and Joseph, B.L. (1970) Urinary protein excretion in climbers at high altitude. *Lancet* **1**, 1247–51.

Rennie, M.J., Babij, P., Sutton, J.R. *et al.* (1983) Effects of acute hypoxia on forearm leucine metabolism, in *Hypoxia, Exercise and Altitude* (eds. J.R. Sutton, C.S. Houston and N.L. Jones), Liss, New York, pp. 317–24.

Reshetnikova, O.S., Burton, G.J. and Milovanov, A.P. (1994) Effects of hypobaric hypoxia on the fetoplacental unit: the morphometric diffusing capacity of the villous membrane at high altitude. *Am. J. Obstet. Gynecol.* **171**, 1560–5.

Reynafarje, B. (1962) Myoglobin content and enzymatic activity of muscle and altitude adaptation. *J. Appl. Physiol.* **17**, 301–5.

Reynolds, R.D., Lickteig, J.A., Howard, M.P. and Deuster, P.A. (1998) Intake of high fat and high carbohydrate foods by humans increased with exposure to increasing altitude during an expedition to Mt. Everest. *J. Nutr.* **128**, 50–5.

Reynolds, R.D., Lickteig, J.A., Deuster, P.A. *et al.* (1999) Energy metabolism increases and regional body fat decreases while regional muscle mass is spared in humans climbing Mt. Everest. *J. Nutr.* **129**, 1307–14.

Rhodes, J. (2005) Comparative physiology of hypoxic pulmonary hypertension: historical clues from brisket disease (Review). *J. Appl. Physiol.* **98**, 1092–100.

Ricart, A., Maristany, J., Fort, N. *et al.* (2005) Effects of sildenafil on the human response to acute hypoxia and exercise. *High Alt. Med. Biol.* **6**, 43–9.

Rice, L., Ruiz, W., Driscoll, T. *et al.* (2001) Neocytolysis on descent from Altitude: a newly recognised mechanism for the control of red cell mass. *Ann. Intern. Med.* **134**, 652–6.

Richalet, J.-P. (1990) The heart and adrenergic system, in *Hypoxia: the Adaptations* (eds. J.R. Sutton, G. Coates and J.E. Remmers), Dekker, Philadelphia, pp. 231–40.

Richalet, J.-P., Keromes, A., Dersch, B. *et al.* (1988) Caractéristiques physiologiques des alpinistes de haute altitude. *Sci. Sports* **3**, 89–108.

Richalet, J.-P., Rutgers, V., Bouchet, P. *et al.* (1989) Diurnal variation of acute mountain sickness, colour vision, and plasma cortisol and ACTH at high altitude. *Aviat. Space Environ. Med.* **60**, 105–11.

Richalet, J.-P., Hornych, A., Rathat, C., Aumont, J., Lormignat, P. and Rémy, P. (1991) Plasma prostaglandins, leukotrienes and thromboxane in acute high altitude hypoxia. *Respir. Physiol.* **85**, 205–15.

Richalet, J.-P., Souberbielle, J.C., Antezana, A.M. *et al.* (1994) Control of erythropoiesis in humans during prolonged exposure to the altitude of 6542 m. *Am. J. Physiol.* **266**, R756–64.

Richalet, J.-P., Dechaux, M., Bienvenu, A. *et al.* (1995) Erythropoiesis and renal function at the altitude of 6,542 m. *Jpn. J. Mount. Med.* **15**, 135–50.

Richalet, J-P., Robach, P., Jarrot, S. *et al.* Operation Everest III (COMEX '97). (1999) Effects of prolonged and progressive hypoxia on humans during a simluated ascent to 8,848 M in a hypobaric chamber. *Adv. Exp. Med. Biol.* **474**, 297–317.

Richalet, J.-P., Vargas Donoso M., Jiménez D. *et al.* (2002) Chilean miners commuting from sea level to 4500 m: a prospective study. *High Alt. Med. Biol.* **3**, 159–66.

Richalet, J.P., Gratadour, P., Robach, P. *et al.* (2005a) Sildenafil inhibits altitude-induced hypoxemia and pulmonary hypertension. *Am. J. Respir. Crit. Care Med.* **171**, 275–81. E-pub 29 October 2004.

Richalet, J-P., Rivera, M., Bouchet, P. *et al.* (2005b) Acetazolamide: a treatment for chronic mountain sickness. *Am. J. Resp. Crit. Care Med.* **172**, 1427–33.

Richardson, R.S., Tagore, K., Haseler, L.J. *et al.* (1998) Increased $\dot{V}o_{2max}$ with right-shifted Hb–O$_2$ dissociation curve at a constant O$_2$ delivery in dog muscle in situ. *J. Appl. Physiol.* **84**, 995–1002.

Richardson, R.S., Newcomer, S.C. and Noyszewski, E.A. (2001) Skeletal muscle intracellular Po$_2$ assessed by myoglobin desaturation: response to graded exercise. *J. Appl. Physiol.* **91**, 2679–85.

Richardson, T.Q. and Guyton, A.C. (1959) Effects of polycythemia and anemia on cardiac output and other circulatory factors. *Am. J. Physiol.* **197**, 1167–79.

Riley, D.J. (1991) Vascular remodeling, in *The Lung: Scientific Foundations* (eds. R.C. Crystal and J.B. West), Raven Press, New York, pp. 1189–98.

Riley, R.L. and Houston, C.S. (1951) Composition of alveolar air and volume of pulmonary ventilation during long exposure to high altitude. *J. Appl. Physiol.* **3**, 526–34.

Riley, R.L., Shephard, R.H., Cohn, J.E., Carroll, D.G. and Armstrong, B.W. (1954) Maximal diffusing capacity of the lungs. *J. Appl. Physiol.* **6**, 573–87.

Ri-Li, G., Chase, P.J., Witkowski, S. *et al.* (2003) Obesity: associations with acute mountain sickness. *Ann. Intern. Med.* **139**, 253–7.

Rinpoche, R. (1973) *Tibetan Medicine,* Wellcome Institute of the History of Medicine, London.

Rl, Y. and Herschensohn, H.L. (1964) Changes in lung volumes of emphysema patients upon short exposures to simulated altitude of 18,000 feet. *Aerosp. Med.* **35**, 1201–3.

Roach, R. and Hackett, P.H. (1992) Hyperbaria and high altitude illness, in *Hypoxia and Mountain Medicine* (eds. J.R. Sutton, C.S. Houston and G. Coates), Queen City Printers, Burlington, VT, pp. 266–73.

Roach, R.C., Bärtsch, P., Hackett, P.H. and Oelz, O. (1993) The Lake Louise acute mountain sickness scoring system, in *Hypoxia and Mountain Medicine* (eds. J.R. Sutton, C.S. Houston and G. Coates), Queen City Printers, Burlington, VT, pp. 272–4.

Roach, R.C., Houston, C.S., Hogigman, B. *et al.* (1995) How do older persons tolerate moderate altitude? *West. J. Med.* **162**, 32–6.

Roach, R.C., Loeppky, J.A. and Icenogle, M.V. (1996) Acute mountain sickness: Increased severity during simulated altitude compared with normobaric hypoxia. *J. Appl. Physiol.* **81**, 1908–10.

Roach, R.C., Greene, E.R., Schoene, R.B. and Hackett, P.H. (1998) Arterial oxygen saturation for prediction of acute mountain sickness. *Aviat. Space Environ. Med* **69**, 1182–5.

Roach, R.C., Maes, D., Sandoval, D. *et al.* (2000) Exercise exacerbates acute mountain sickness at simulated high altitude. *J. Appl. Physiol.* **88**, 581–5.

Robach, P., Déchaux, M., Jarrot, S. *et al.* (2000) Operation Everest III: role of plasma volume expansion on VO$_2$max during prolonged high-altitude exposure. *J. Appl. Physiol.* **89**, 29–37.

Robarch, P., Lafforque, E., Olsen, N.V. *et al.* (2002) Recovery of plasma volume after 1 week of exposure at 4,350 m. *Eur. J. Physiol.* **444**, 821–8.

Robach, P., Schmitt, L., Brugniaux, J.V. *et al.* (2006) 'Living high–training low': Effect on erythropoiesis and aerobic performance in highly-trained swimmers. *Eur. J. Appl. Physiol.* **96**, 423–33. E-pub 3 December 2005.

Roberovsky, V. (1896) The Central Asian Expedition of Capt. Roberovsky and Lt. Kozloff. *Geogr. J.* **8**, 161.

Roberts, A.C., Butterfield, G.E., Cymerman, A., Reeves, J.T., Wolfel, E.E. and Brooks, G.A. (1996) Acclimatization to 4,300 m altitude decreases reliance on fat as a substrate. *J. Appl. Physiol.* **81**, 1762–71.

Roberts, A.D., Clark, S.A., Townsend, N.E. *et al.* (2003) Changes in performance, maximal oxygen uptake and maximal accumulated oxygen deficit after 5, 10 and 15 days of live high:train low altitude exposure. *Eur. J. Appl. Physiol.* **88**, 390–5. E-pub 7 November 2002.

Roberts, D., Smith, D.J., Donnelly, S. and Simard, S. (2000) Plasma-volume contraction and exercise-induced hypoxiaemia modulate erythropoietin production in healthy humans. *Clin. Sci.* **98**, 39–45.

Robertson, J.A. and Shlim, D.R. (1991) Treatment of moderate acute mountain sickness with pressurization in a portable hyperbaric (Gamow) bag. *J. Wilderness Med.* **2**, 268–73.

Robin, E.D. and Gardner, F.H. (1953) Cerebral metabolism and hemodynamics in pernicious anemia. *J. Clin. Invest.* **32**, 598.

Roca, J.M., Hogan, M.C., Storey, D. *et al.* (1989) Evidence for tissue limitation of $\dot{V}o_{2max}$ in normal man. *J. Appl. Physiol.* **67**, 291–9.

Rock, P.B., Johnson, T.S., Larsen, R.F. *et al.* (1989) Dexamethasone prophylaxis for acute mountain sickness. Effect of dose level. *Chest* **95**, 568–73.

Rogers, T.A. (1971) The clinical course of survival in the Arctic. *Hawaii Med. J.* **30**, 31–4.

Röggla, G., Röggla, M., Podolsky, A. *et al.* (1996) How can acute mountain sickness be quantified at moderate altitude? *J. R. Soc. Med.* **89**, 141–3.

Röggla, G., Röggla, M., Wagner, A. *et al.* (1994) Effect of low dose sedation with diazepam on ventilatory response at moderate altitude. *Wien Klin. Woch.* **106**, 649–51.

Röggla, G., Moser, B. and Röggla, M. (2000) Effect of temazepam on ventilatory response at moderate altitude (letter). *BMJ* **320**, 56.

Roi, G.S., Giacometti, M. and Von Duvillard, S.P. (1999) Marathons in altitude. *Med. Sci. Sports Exerc.* **31**, 723–8.

Roncin, J.P., Schwartz, F. and D'Arbigny, P. (1996) EGb 761 in control of acute mountain sickness and vascular reactivity to cold exposure. *Aviat. Space Environ. Med.* **67**, 445–52.

Rose, D.M., Fleck, B., Thews, O. and Kamin, W.E. (2000) Blood gas-analyses in patients with cystic fibrosis to estimate hypoxemia during exposure to high altitude. *Eur. J. Med. Res.* **26**, 9–12.

Rose, M.S., Houston, C.S., Fulco, C.S. *et al.* (1988) Operation Everest II: nutrition and body composition. *J. Appl. Physiol.* **65**, 2545–51.

Roskamm, F., Londry, F.K., Samek, L.L., Schlager, M., Weidermann, H. and Reindelch, H. (1969) Effects of standardised ergometer training produced at three different altitudes. *J. Appl. Physiol.* **27**, 840–7.

Ross, J.H. and Attwood, E.C. (1984) Severe repetitive exercise and haematological status. *Postgrad. Med. J.* **60**, 454–7.

Ross, R.T. (1985) The random nature of cerebral mountain sickness (letter) *Lancet* **1**, 990–1.

Rossis, C.G., Yiacoumettis, A.M. and Elemenoglou, J. (1982) Squamous cell carcinoma of the heel developing at site of previous frostbite. *J. R. Soc. Med.* **75**, 715–18.

Rothwell, N.J. and Stock, M.J. (1983) Luxuskonsumption. Diet-induced thermogenesis and brown fat: the case in favour. *Clin. Sci.* **64**, 19–23.

Rotta, A., Canepa, A., Hurtado, A., Velásquez, T. and Chávez, R. (1956) Pulmonary circulation at sea level and at high altitudes. *J. Appl. Physiol.* **9**, 328–36.

Roughton, F.J. (1945) Average time spent by blood in human lung capillary and its relation to the rates of CO uptake and elimination in man. *Am. J. Physiol.* **143**, 621–33.

Roughton, F.J.W. (1964) Transport of oxygen and carbon dioxide, in *Handbook of Physiology*, Section 3, *Respiration*, Vol. 1 (eds. W.O. Fenn and H. Rahn), American Physiological Society, Washington, DC, pp. 767–825.

Roughton, F.J.W. and Forster, R.E. (1957) Relative importance of diffusion and chemical reaction rates in determining rate of exchange of gases in the human lung, with special reference to true diffusing capacity of pulmonary membrane and volume of blood in the lung capillaries. *J. Appl. Physiol.* **11**, 291–302.

Roussel, B., Dittmar, A., Delhomm, C. *et al.* (1982) Normal and pathological aspects of skin blood flow measurements by thermal clearance method, in *Biomedical Thermology* (eds. M. Guthrie, E. Albert and R. Alar), Liss, New York, pp. 421–9.

Rowell, G. (1982) High altitude pulmonary oedema during rapid ascent, in *Hypoxia: Man at High Altitude* (eds. J.R. Sutton, N.L. Jones and C.S. Houston), Thieme Stratton, New York, pp. 168–71.

Roy, S.B., Guleria, J.S., Khanna, P.K., Manchanda, S.C., Pande, J.N. and Subba, P.S. (1969) Haemodynamic studies in high altitude pulmonary oedema. *Br. Heart J.* **31**, 52–8.

Ruiz, L. and Peñaloza, D. (1977) Altitude and hypertension. *Mayo Clin. Proc.* **52**, 442–5.

Russell, E. (1975) A multiple scoring method for the assessment of complex memory functions. *J. Consult. Clin. Psychol.* **43**, 800–9.

Ruttledge, H. (1934) *Everest 1933.* Hodder and Stoughton, London, p. 78.

Ruttledge, H. (1937) *Everest: the Unfinished Adventure,* Hodder and Stoughton, London, p. 212.

Ryn, Z. (1970) Mental disorders in alpinists under conditions of stress at high altitudes, Doctoral thesis, University of Cracow, Poland.

Ryn, Z. (1971) Psychopathology in alpinism. *Acta Med. Pol.* **12**, 453–67.

Ryujin, D.T., Mannebach, S.C., Samuelson, W.M. and Marshall, B.C.(2001) Oxygen saturation in adult cystic fibrosis patients during exercise at high altitude. *Pediatr. Pulmonol.* **32**, 437–41.

Sadikali, F. and Owor, R. (1974) Hypothermia in the tropics. A review of 24 cases. *Trop. Geogr. Med.* **26**, 265–70.

Sahn, S.A., Lakshminarayan, S., Pierson, D.J. and Weil, J.V. (1974) Effect of ethanol on the ventilatory responses to oxygen and carbon dioxide in man. *Clin. Sci. Mol. Med.* **49**, 33–8.

Saito, H., Nishimura, M., Shinano, H. *et al.* (1999) Effect of mild hypoxia on airway responsiveness to methacholine in subjects with airway obstruction. *Chest* **116**, 1653–8.

Saito, S., Tobe, K., Harada, N. *et al.* (2002) Physical condition among middle altitude trekkers in an ageing society. *Am. J. Emerg. Med.* **20**, 291–4.

Sakaguchi, E. and Yurugi, R. (1983) Retinal haemorrhages at simulated high altitude. *Jpn. J. Mount. Med.* **3**, 107–8.

Saldana, M. and Arias-Stella, J. (1963a) Studies on the structure of the pulmonary trunk. I. Normal changes in the elastic configuration of the human pulmonary trunk at different ages. *Circulation* **27**, 1086–93.

Saldana, M. and Arias-Stella, J. (1963b) Studies on the structure of the pulmonary trunk. II. The evolution of the elastic configuration of the pulmonary trunk in people native to high altitudes. *Circulation* **27**, 1094–100.

Saldana, M. and Arias-Stella, J. (1963c) Studies on the structure of the pulmonary trunk. III. The thickness of the media of the pulmonary trunk and ascending aorta in high altitude natives. *Circulation* **27**, 1101–4.

Saldana, M.J., Salem, L.E. and Travezan, R. (1973) High altitude hypoxia and chemodectoma. *Hum. Pathol.* **4**, 251–63.

Saldeen, T. (1976) The microembolism syndrome. *Microvasc. Res.* **11**, 187–259.

Salimi, Z. (1985) Assessment of tissue viability by scintigraphy. *Postgrad. Med.* **17**, 133–4.

Saltin, B. (1967) Aerobic and anaerobic work capacity at 2300 m. *Med. Thorac.* **24**, 205–10.

Saltin, B. and Gollnick, P.D. (1983) Skeletal muscle adaptability: significance for metabolism and performance, in *Handbook of Physiology*, Section 10 (ed. L.D. Peachey), American Physiological Society, Bethesda, MD, pp. 555–631.

Salvaggio, A., Insalaco, G., Marrone, O. *et al.* (1998) Effects of high-altitude periodic breathing on sleep and arterial oxyhaemoglobin saturation. *Eur. Respir. J.* **12**, 408–13.

Samaja, M., Veicsteinas, A. and Cerretelli, P. (1979) Oxygen affinity of blood in altitude Sherpas. *J. Appl. Physiol.* **47**, 337–41.

Samaja, M., Mariani, C., Prestini, A. and Cerretelli, P. (1997) Acid–base balance and O_2 transport at high altitude. *Acta Physiol. Scand.* **159**, 249–56.

Samaja, M., Crespi, T., Guazzi, M. and Vandergriff, K.D. (2003) Oxygen transport in blood at high altitude: role of the hemoglobin–oxygen affinity and impact of the phenomena related to hemoglobin allosterism and red cell function. *Eur. J. Appl. Physiol.* **90**, 351–9.

Sampson, J.B., Cymerman, A., Burse, R.J. *et al.* (1983) Procedures for the measurement of acute mountain sickness. *Aviat. Space Environ. Med.* **54**, 1063–73.

Sanchez, C., Merino, C. and Figallo, M. (1970) Simultaneous measurement of plasma volume and cell mass in polycythemia of high altitude. *J. Appl. Physiol.* **30**, 775–8.

Sandoval, D. (1997) Women, exercise, and high acute mountain sickness, in *Women at Altitude* (eds. C.S. Houston and G. Coates), Queen City Printers, Inc., Burlington, VT, pp. 42–52.

San Miguel, J.L., Spielvogel, H., Berger, J. *et al.* (2002) Effect of high altitude on protein metabolism in Bolivian Children. *High Alt. Med. Biol.* **3**, 377–86.

Santolaya, R.B., Lahiri, S., Alfaro, R.T. and Schoene, R.B. (1989) Respiratory adaptation in the highest inhabitants and highest Sherpa mountaineers. *Respir. Physiol.* **77**, 253–62.

Santos, J.L., Perez-Bravo, F., Carrasco, E., Calvillan, M. and Albala, C. (2001) Low prevalence of type 2 diabetes despite a high average body mass index in the Aymara natives from Chile. *Nutrition* **17**, 305–9.

Sarnquist, F.H., Schoene, R.B., Hackett, P.H. and Townes, B.D. (1986) Hemodilution of polycythemic mountaineers: effect on exercise and mental function. *Aviat. Space Environ. Med.* **57**, 313–17.

Sartori, C., Allemann, Y., Trueb, L. *et al.* (1999a) Augmented vaso-reactivity in adult life associated with perinatal vascular insult. *Lancet* **353**, 2205–7.

Sartori, C., Vollenweider, L., Löffler, B-M. *et al.* (1999b) Exaggerated endothelin release in high-altitude pulmonary edema. *Circulation* **99**, 2665–8.

Sartori, C., Allemann, Y., Duplain, H. *et al.* (2002) Salmeterol for the prevention of high-altitude pulmonary edema. *N. Engl. J. Med.* **346**, 1631–6.

Sartori, C., Duplain, H., Lepori, M. *et al.* (2004) High altitude impairs nasal transepithelial sodium transport in HAPE-prone subjects. *Eur. Respir. J.* **23**, 916–20.

Sato, M., Severinghaus, J.W., Powel, F.L. *et al.*(1992) Augmented hypoxic ventilatory response in men at altitude. *J. Appl. Physiol.* **73**, 101–7.

Sato, M., Severinghaus, J.W. and Bickler, P. (1994) Time course of augmentation and depression of hypoxic ventilatory response at altitude. *J. Appl. Physiol.* **77**, 313–16.

Saunders, P.U., Telford, R.D., Pyne, D.B. *et al.* (2004) Improved running economy in elite runners after 20 days of simulated moderate-altitude exposure. *J. Appl. Physiol.* **96**, 931–7. E-pub 7 November 2003.

Saunders, R. (1789) Some account of the vegetable and mineral productions of Boutan and Tibet. *Philos. Trans. R. Soc.* **79**, 79–111.

Savard, G.K., Cooper, K.E., Veal, W.L. and Malkinson, T.J. (1985) Peripheral blood flow during rewarming from mild hypothermia in humans. *J. Appl. Physiol.* **58**, 4–13.

Savonitto, S., Cardellino, G., Doveri, G. *et al.* (1992) Effects of acute exposure to altitude (3460 m) on blood pressure response to dynamic and isometric exercise in men with systemic hypertension. *Am. J. Cardiol.* **70**, 1493–7.

Savourey, G., Moirant, C., Eterradossi, J. and Bittel, J. (1995) Acute mountain sickness relates to sea-level partial pressure of oxygen. *Eur. J. Appl. Physiol.* **70**, 469–76.

Savourey, G., Garcia, N., Caravel, C. *et al.* (1998) Pre-adaptation, adaptation and de-adaptation to high altitude in humans: hormonal and biochemical changes at sea level. *Eur. J. Appl. Physiol.* **77**, 37–43.

Savourey, B., Launay, J.-C., Besnard, Y., Guinet, S. and Travers, S. (2003) Normo- and hypobaric hypoxia: are there any physiological differences? *Eur. J. Appl. Physiol.* **89**, 122–6.

Sawhney, R.C. and Malhotra, A.S. (1991) Thyroid function in sojourners and acclimatized low landers at high altitude in man. *Horm. Metab. Res.* **23**, 81–4.

Sawhney, R.C., Chabra, P.C., Malhotra, A.S. *et al.* (1985) Hormone profiles at high altitude in man. *Andrologia* **17**, 178–84.

Sawhney, R.C., Malhotra, A.S., Singh, T. *et al.* (1986) Insulin secretion at high altitude in man. *Int. J. Biometeorol.* **30**, 23–8.

Saxena, S., Kumar, R., Madan, T. *et al.* (2005) Association of polymorphisms in pulmonary surfactant protein A1 and A2 genes with high-altitude pulmonary edema. *Chest* **128**, 1611–9.

Schaefer, O., Eaton, R.D.P., Timmermans, F.J.W. and Hildes, J.A. (1980) Respiratory function impairment and cardiopulmonary consequences in long term residents of the Canadian Arctic. *Can. Med. Assoc. J.* **119**, 997–1004.

Scherrer, U., Vollenweider, L., Delabays, A. *et al.* (1996) Inhaled nitric oxide for high-altitude pulmonary edema. *N. Engl. J. Med.* **334**, 624–9.

Schirlo, C., Pavlicek, V., Jacomet, A. *et al.* (2002) Characteristics of the ventilatory response in subjects susceptible to high altitude pulmonary edema during acute and prolonged hypoxia. *High Alt. Med. Biol.* **3**, 267–76.

Schmid, J.P., Noveanu, M., Gaillet, R., Hellige, G., Wahl, A. and Saner, H. (2006) Safety and exercise tolerance of acute high altitude exposure (3454 m) among patients with coronary artery disease. *Heart* **92**, 921–5.

Schmid-Schonbein, H. and Neumann, F.J. (1985) Pathophysiology of cutaneous frost injury: disturbed microcirculation as a consequence of abnormal flow behaviour of the blood. Application of new concepts of blood rheology, in *High Altitude Deterioration* (eds. J. Rivolier, P. Cerretelli, J. Foray and P. Segantini), Karger, Basel, pp. 20–38.

Schmidt, W. (2002) Effects of intermittent exposure to high altitude on blood volume and erythropoietic activity. *High Alt. Med. Biol.* **3**, 167–76.

Schmidt, W., Brabant, C., Kröger, C. *et al.* (1990) Atrial natriuretic peptide during and after maximal and submaximal exercise under normoxic and hypoxic conditions. *Eur. J. Appl. Phsyiol.* **61**, 398–407.

Schmidt, W., Eckhart, K.U., Hilgendorf, A., Strauch, S. and Bauer, C. (1991) Effects of maximal and submaximal exercise under normoxic and hypoxic condition on serum erythropoietin level. *Int. J. Sports Med.* **12**, 457–61.

Schmidt, W., Heinicke, K., Rojas, J. *et al.* (2002) Blood volume and hemoglobin mass in endurance athletes from moderate altitude. *Med. Sci. Sports Exerc.* **34**, 1934–40.

Schneider, M., Bernasch, D., Weymann, J., Holle, R. and Bartsch, P. (2002) Acute mountain sickness: influence of susceptibility, preexposure, and ascent rate. *Med. Sci. Sports Exerc.* **34**, 1886–91.

Schoch, H.J., Fischer, S. and Marti, H.H. (2002) Hypoxia-induced vascular endothelial growth factor expression causes vascular leakage in the brain. *Brain* **125**, 2549–57. (brain.oupjournals.org).

Schoeller, D.A. and Van Santen, E. (1982) Measurement of energy expenditure in humans by doubly labelled water method. *J. Appl. Physiol.* **53**, 955–9.

Schoene, R.B. (1982) Control of ventilation in climbers to extreme altitude. *J. Appl. Physiol.* **43**, 886–90.

Schoene, R.B. (2001) Limits of human lung function at high altitude. *J. Exp. Biol.* **204**, 3121–7.

Schoene, R.B., Lahiri, S., Hackett, P.H. *et al.* (1984) Relationship of hypoxic ventilatory response to exercise performance on Mount Everest. *J. Appl. Physiol.* **56**, 1478–83.

Schoene, R.B., Roach, R.C., Hackett, P.H. *et al.* (1985) High altitude pulmonary edema and exercise at 4400 m on Mount McKinley. Effect of expiratory positive airway pressure. *Chest* **87**, 330–3.

Schoene, R.B., Hackett, P.H., Henderson, W.R. *et al.* (1986) High altitude pulmonary edema. Characteristics of lung lavage fluid. *JAMA* **256**, 63–9.

Schoene, R.B., Hackett, P.H. and Roach, R.C. (1987) Blunted hypoxic chemosensitivity at altitude and sea level in an elite high altitude climber, in *Hypoxia and Cold* (eds. J.R. Sutton, C.S. Houston and G. Coates), Praeger, New York, p. 532 (abstract).

Schoene, R.B., Swenson, E.R., Pizzo, C.J. *et al.* (1988) The lung at high altitude: bronchoalveolar lavage in acute mountain sickness and pulmonary edema. *J. Appl. Physiol.* **64**, 2605–13.

Scholander, P. (1960) Oxygen transport through hemoglobin solution. *Science* **131**, 585–90.

Schultze-Werninghaus, G. (2006) Should asthma management include sojourns at high altitude? *Chem. Immunol. Allergy* **91**, 16–29.

Schwandt, H-J., Heyduck, B., Gunga, H-C. and Röcker, L. (1991) Influence of prolonged physical exercise on the erythrpoietin concentration in blood. *Eur. J Appl. Physiol.* **63**, 463–6.

Scoggin, C.H., Hyers, T.M., Reeves, J.T. and Grover, R.F. (1977) High-altitude pulmonary edema in the children and young adults of Leadville, Colorado. *N. Engl. J. Med.* **297**, 1269–72.

Seccombe, L.M., Kelly, P.T., Wong, C.K. *et al.* (2004) Effect of simulated commercial flight on oxygenation in patients with interstitial lung disease and chronic obstructive pulmonary disease. *Thorax* **59**, 966–70.

Sediame, S., Zerah-Lancner, F., d'Ortho, M.P., Adnot, S. and Harf, A. (1999) Accuracy of the i-STAT bedside gas analyzer. *Eur. Respir. J.* **14**, 214–7.

Selkon, J. and Gould, J.C. (1966) Bacteriology, in *Report on IBP Expedition to North Bhutan* (eds. F.S. Jackson, R.W.D. Turner and M.P. Ward), Royal Society, London, pp. 88–98.

Selland, M.A., Stelzner, T.J., Stevens, T. *et al.* (1993) Pulmonary function and hypoxic ventilatory response in subjects susceptible to high altitude pulmonary edema. *Chest* **103**, 111–16.

Sellassie, S.H. (1972) *Ancient and Medieval Ethiopian History to 1270,* United Printers, Addis Ababa, Ethiopia.

Semenza, G.L. (2000) Surviving ischemia: adaptive responses mediated by hypoxia-inducible factor 1. *J. Clin. Invest.* **106**, 809–12.

Semenza, G.L., Agani, F., Iyer, N. *et al.* (1998) Hypoxia-inducible factor-1: from molecular biology to cardiopulmonary physiology. *Chest* **114**, 40S–45S.

Semple, P. d'A. (1986) The clinical endocrinology of hypoxia, in *Aspects of Hypoxia* (ed. D. Heath), Liverpool University Press, Liverpool, pp. 147–61.

Serebrovskaya, T.V. and Ivashkevich, A.A. (1992) Effects of a 1-yr stay at altitude on ventilation, metabolism and work capacity. *J. Appl. Physiol.* **73**, 1749–55.

Serebrovskaya, T.V., Karaban, I.N., Kolesnikova, T.M. *et al.* (1999) Human hypoxic ventilatory response with blood dopamine content under intermittent hypoxic training. *Can. J. Physiol. Pharmcol. Rev.* **77**, 967–73.

Serebrovskaya, T.V., Karaban, I.N., Kolesnikova, E.E. *et al.* (2000) Geriatric men at altitude: hypoxic sensitivity and blood dopamine changes. *Respiration* **67**, 253–60.

Severinghaus, J.W. (1977) Pulmonary vascular function. *Am. Rev. Respir. Dis.* **115** (Suppl.), 149–58.

Severinghaus, J.W. (1995) Hypothetical roles of angiogenesis, osmotic swelling, and ischemia in high-altitude cerebral edema. *J. Appl. Physiol.* **79**, 375–9.

Severinghaus, J.W. and Carcelen, A. (1964) Cerebrospinal fluid in man native to high altitude. *J. Appl. Physiol.* **19**, 319–21.

Severinghaus, J.W., Mitchell, R.A., Richardson, B.W. and Singer, M.M. (1963) Respiratory control at high altitude suggesting active transport regulation of CSF pH. *J. Appl. Physiol.* **18**, 1155–66.

Severinghaus, J.W., Bainton, C.K. and Carcelen, A. (1966a) Respiratory insensitivity to hypoxia in chronically hypoxic man. *Respir. Physiol.* **1**, 308–34.

Severinghaus, J.W., Chiodi, H., Eger, E.I. *et al.* (1966b) Cerebral blood flow in man at high altitude. *Circ. Res.* **19**, 274–302.

Shapiro, C.M., Goll, C.C., Cohen, G.R. and Oswald, I. (1984) Heat production during sleep. *J. Appl. Physiol.* **56**, 671–7.

Sharma, A., Sharma, P.D., Malhotra, H.S. *et al.* (1990) Hemiplegia as a manifestation of acute mountain sickness. *J. Assoc. Physicians India* **38**, 662–4.

Sharma, S.C. (1980) Platelet count on acute induction to high altitude. *Thromb. Haemost.* **43**, 24.

Sharma, S.C. (1981) Platelet adhesiveness in temporary residents of high altitude. *Thromb. Res.* **21**, 685–7.

Sharma, S.C. (1982) Platelet count and adhesiveness on induction to high altitude by air and road. *Int. J. Biometeorol.* **26**, 219–24.

Sharma, V.M. and Malhotra, M.S. (1976) Ethnic variations in psychological performance under altitude stress. *Aviat. Space Environ. Med.* **47**, 248–51.

Sharma, V.M., Malhotra, M.S. and Baskaran, A.S. (1975) Variations in psychomotor efficiency during prolonged stay at high altitude. *Ergonomics* **18**, 511–16.

Sharma, S.C., Balasubramanian, V. and Chadha, K.S. (1980) Platelet adhesiveness in permanent residents of high altitude. *Thromb. Haemost.* **42**, 1508–12.

Sharp, C.R. (1978) Hypoxia and hyperventilation, in *Aviation Medicine Physiology and Human Factors* (ed. J. Ernsting), Tir-Med Books, London, p. 78.

Sharp, F.R., Bergeron, M. and Bernaudin, M. (2001) Hypoxia-inducible factor in brain. *Adv. Exp. Med. Biol.* **502**, 273–91.

Shepard, R.H., Varnauskas, E., Martin, H.B. *et al.* (1958) Relationship between cardiac output and apparent diffusing capacity of the lung in normal men during treadmill exercise. *J. Appl. Physiol.* **13**, 205–10.

Shephard, R.J. (1985) Adaptation to exercise in the cold. *Sports Med.* **2**, 59–71.

Shi, Z.Y., Ning, X.H., Huang, P.G. *et al.* (1979) Comparison of physiological responses to hypoxia at high altitudes between highlanders and lowlanders. *Sci. Sin.* **22**, 1446–69.

Shigeoka, J.W., Colice, G.L. and Ramirez, G. (1985) Effect of normoxemic and hypoxemic exercise on renin and aldosterone. *J. Appl. Physiol.* **59**, 142–8.

Shih, W.J., Riley, C., Magoun, S. and Ryo, U.Y. (1988) Intense bone imaging agent uptake in the soft tissues of the lower legs and feet relating to ischemia and cold exposure. *Eur. J. Nucl. Med.* **14**, 419–21.

Shipton, E. (1938) *Blank on the Map,* Hodder and Stoughton, London, p. 265.

Shipton, E. (1943) *Upon That Mountain,* Hodder and Stoughton, London, pp. 129–30.

Shlim, D.R. and Houston, R. (1989) Helicopter rescues and deaths among trekkers in Nepal. *JAMA* **261**, 1017–19.

Shlim, D.R., Nepal, K. and Meijer, H.J. (1991) Suddenly sypmtomatic brain tumors at altitude. *Ann. Emerg. Med.* **20**, 315–6.

Shlim, D.R., Hackett, P., Houston, C., Steel, P., Nelson, D. and Hultgren, N. (1995) Diplopia at high altitude. *Wild. Environ. Med.* **6**, 341.

Shukitt-Hale, B., Banderet, L.E. and Lieberman, H.R. (1991) Relationships between symptoms, moods, performance, and acute mountain sickness at 4700 meters. *Aviat. Space Environ. Med.* **62**, 865–9.

Shukla, V., Singh, S.N., Vats, P. *et al.* (2005) Ghrelin and leptin levels of sojourners and acclimatized lowlanders at high altitude. *Nutr. Neurosci.* **8**, 161–5.

Siebkhe, H., Breivik, H., Rod, T. and Lind, B. (1975) Survival after 40 minutes' submersion without cerebral sequelae. *Lancet* **1**, 1275–9.

Siesjo, B.K. (1992a) Pathophysiology and treatment of focal cerebral ischemia. Part I. Pathophysiology. *J. Neurosurg.* **77**, 169–84.

Siesjo, B.K. (1992b) Pathophysiology and treatment of focal cerebral ischemia. Part II. Mechanisms of damage and treatment. *J. Neurosurg.* **77**, 337–54.

Siesjo, B.K. and Kjallquist, A. (1969) A new theory for the regulation of extra-cellular pH in the brain. *Scand. J. Clin. Lab. Invest.* **24**, 1–9.

Sime, F., Peñaloza, D., Ruiz, L. *et al.* (1974) Hypoxemia, pulmonary hypertension, and low cardiac output in newcomers at low altitude. *J. Appl. Physiol.* **36**, 561–65.

Simon, H.U., Grotzer, M., Nikolaizik, W.H., Blaser, K. and Schoni, MH. (1994) High altitude climate therapy reduces peripheral blood T lymphocyte activation, eosinophilia, and bronchial obstruction in children with house-dust mite allergic asthma. *Pediatr. Pulmonol.* **17**, 304–11.

Simon-Schnass, I. and Korniszewski, L. (1990) The influence of vitamin E on rheological parameters in high altitude mountaineers. *Int. J. Vitam. Nutr. Res.* **60**, 26–34.

Singh, I. and Chohan, I.S. (1972a) Abnormalities of blood coagulation at high altitude. *Int. J. Biometerol.* **16**, 283.

Singh, I. and Chohan, I.S. (1972b) Blood coagulation at high altitude predisposing to pulmonary hypertension. *Br. Heart J.* **34**, 611–17.

Singh, I., Kapila, C.C., Khanna, P.K., Nanda, R.B. and Rao, B.D.P. (1965) High-altitude pulmonary oedema. *Lancet* **1**, 229–34.

Singh, I., Chohan, I.S. and Mathew, N.T. (1969) Fibrinolytic activity in high altitude pulmonary oedema. *Ind. J. Med. Res.* **57**, 210–17.

Singh, I., Malhotra, M.S., Khanna, P.K. *et al.* (1974) Changes in plasma cortisol, blood antidiuretic hormone and urinary catecholamine in high altitude pulmonary oedema. *Int. J. Biometeorol.* **18**, 211–21.

Singh, I., Chohan, J.S., Lal, M. *et al.* (1977) Effects of high altitude stay on the incidence of common diseases in man. *Int. J. Biometeorol.* **21**, 93–122.

Singh, M.V., Rawal, S.B. and Tyagi, A.K. (1990) Body fluid status on induction, reinduction and prolonged stay at high altitude on human volunteers. *Int. J. Biometeorol.* **34**, 93–7.

Sirén, A.-L., Fratelli, M., Brines, M. *et al.* (2001) Erythropoietin prevents neuronal apoptosis after cerebral ischemia and metabolic stress. *Proc. Natl Acad. Sci. USA* **98**, 4044–9.

Siri, W.E., Van Dyke, D.C., Winchell, H.S. *et al.* (1966) Early erythropoietin, blood, and physiological responses to severe hypoxia in man. *J. Appl. Physiol.* **21**, 73–80.

Siri, W.E., Cleveland, A.S. and Blanche, P. (1969) Adrenal gland activity in Mount Everest climbers. *Fed. Proc.* **28**, 1251–6.

Slater, J.D.H., Tuffley, R.E., Williams, E.S. *et al.* (1969) Control of aldosterone secretion during acclimatization to hypoxia in man. *Clin. Sci.* **37**, 327–41.

Slutsky, A.S. and Strohl, K.P. (1980) Quantification of oxygen saturation during episodic hypoxemia. *Am. Rev. Respir. Dis.* **121**, 893–5.

Smith, C. (1999) Blood pressures of Sherpa men in modernizing Nepal. *Am. J. Hum. Biol.* **11**, 469–79.

Smith, C.A., Bisgard, G.E., Nielsen, A.M. *et al.* (1986) Carotid bodies are required for ventilatory acclimatization to chronic hypoxia. *J. Appl. Physiol.* **60**, 1003–10.

Smith, C.A., Dempsey, J.A. and Hornbein, T.F. (2001) Control of breathing at high altitude, in *High Altitude* (eds. T.F. Hornbein and R.B. Schoene), Lung Biology in Health and Disease, vol 161, Marcel Dekker, New York, pp. 140–8.

Smyth, R. (1988) Alpine runners racing danger. *Observer* (London), 7 August.

Snellgrove, D. (1961) *Himalayan Pilgrimage,* Cassirer, Oxford.

Snodgrass, A.M. (1993) The early history of the Alps. *Alpine J.* **98**, 213–22.

Snyder, L.R.G., Born, S. and Lechner, A.L. (1982) Blood oxygen affinity in high- and low-altitude populations of the deer mouse. *Respir. Physiol.* **48**, 89–105.

Sobrevilla, L.A., Romero, L., Moncloa, F. *et al.* (1967) Endocrine studies of high altitude. III. Urinary gonadotrophins in subjects native to and living at 14000 feet and during acute exposure of men living at sea level to high altitude. *Acta Endocrinol.* **56**, 369–75.

Somers, V.K., Anderson, J.V., Conway, J. *et al.* (1986) Atrial natriuretic peptide is released by dynamic exercise in man. *Horm. Metab. Res.* **18**, 871–2.

Somervell, T.H. (1925) Note on the composition of alveolar air at extreme heights. *J. Physiol. (Lond.)* **60**, 282–5.

Somervell, T.H. (1936) *After Everest,* Hodder and Stoughton, London, p. 132.

Son, Y.A. (1979) Quantitative estimation of haemoglobin and its fractions in permanent mountain dwellers in the Tyan'-Shan' and Pamir. *Hum. Physiol.* **5**, 208–10.

Song, S.Y., Asaji, T., Tanizaki, Y. *et al.* (1986) Cerebral thrombosis at altitude. Its pathogenesis and the problems of prevention and treatment. *Aviat. Space Environ. Med.* **57**, 71–6.

Sorensen, S.C. (1970) Ventilatory acclimatization to hypoxia in rabbits after denervation of peripheral chemoreceptors. *J. Appl. Physiol.* **28**, 836–9.

Sorensen, S.C. and Milledge, J.S. (1971) Cerebrospinal fluid acid–base composition at high altitude. *J. Appl. Physiol.* **31**, 28–30.

Sorensen, S.C. and Mines, A.H. (1970) Ventilatory responses to acute and chronic hypoxia in goats after sinus nerve section. *J. Appl. Physiol.* **28**, 832–4.

Sorensen, S.C. and Severinghaus, J.W. (1968) Respiratory sensitivity to acute hypoxia in man at sea level and at high altitude. *J. Appl. Physiol.* **24**, 211–16.

Specht, H. and Fruhmann, G. (1972) Incidence of periodic breathing in 2000 subjects without pulmonary or neurological disease. *Bull. Physio-Pathol. Respir.* **98**, 1075–83.

Speechley-Dick, M.E., Rimmer, S.J. and Hodson, M.E. (1992) Exacerbation's of cystic fibrosis after holidays at high altitude – a cautionary tale. *Respir. Med.* **86**, 55–6.

Spicuzza, L., Casiraghi, N., Gamboa, A. *et al.* (2004) Sleep-related hypoxaemia and excessive erythrocytosis in Andean high-altitude natives. *Eur. Resp. J.* **23**, 41–6.

Spriet, L.L., Cledhill, N., Froese, A.B. and Wilkes, D.L. (1986) Effect of graded erythrocythemia on cardiovascular and metabolic responses to exercise. *J. Appl. Physiol.* **61**, 1942–8.

Stathokostas, L., Jacob-Johnson, S., Petrella, R.J. and Paterson, D.H. (2004) Longitudinal changes in aerobic power in older men and women. *J. Appl. Physiol.* **97**, 781–9.

Staub, N.C. (1986) The hemodynamics of pulmonary edema. *Clin. Respir. Physiol.* **22**, 319–22.

Steele, P. (1971) Medicine on Mount Everest. *Lancet* **ii**, 32–9.

Stein, R.A. (1972) *Tibetan Civilization,* Faber, London, pp. 26–37.

Steinacker, J.M., Liu, Y., Boning, D. *et al.* (1996) Lung diffusion capacity, oxygen uptake, cardiac output and oxygen transport during exercise before and after a Himalayan expedition. *Eur. J. Appl. Physiol. Occup. Physiol.* **74**, 187–93.

Steinacker, J.M., Tobias, P., Menold, E. *et al.* (1998) Lung diffusing capacity and exercise in subjects with previous high altitude pulmonary edema. *Eur. Respir. J.* **11**, 643–50.

Steinbrook, R.A., Donovan, J.C., Gabel, R.A. *et al.* (1983) Acclimatization to high altitude in goats with ablated carotid bodies. *J. Appl. Physiol.* **44**, 16–21.

Stelzner, T.J., O'Brien, R.F., Sato, K. and Weil, J.V. (1988) Hypoxia-induced increases in pulmonary transvascular protein escape in rats. Modulation by glucocorticoids. *J. Clin. Invest.* **82**, 1840–7.

Stephens, D.H. (1982) Sleeping snugly in damp bedrooms. *J. R. Soc. Health* **6**, 272–5.

Stewart, A.G., Bardsley, P.A., Baudouin, S.V. *et al.* (1991a) Changes in atrial natriuretic peptide concentrations during intravenous saline infusion in hypoxic cor pulmonale. *Thorax* **46**, 829–34.

Stewart, A.G., Thompson, J.S., Rogers, T.K. and Morice, A.H. (1991b) Atrial natriuretic peptide-induced relaxation of pre-constricted isolated rat perfused lungs: a comparison in control and hypoxia-adapted animals. *Clin. Sci.* **81**, 201–8.

Stock, M.J., Norgan, N.G., Ferro-Luzzi, A. and Evans, E. (1978a) Effect of altitude on dietary-induced thermogenesis at rest and during light exercise in man. *J. Appl. Physiol. Respir. Environ. Exerc. Physiol.* **45**, 345–9.

Stock, M.J., Chapman, C., Stirling, J.L. and Campbell, I.T. (1978b) Effects of exercise, altitude, and food on blood hormone and metabolite levels. *J. Appl. Physiol: Respir. Environ. Exerc. Physiol.* **45**, 350–4.

Stokes, W. (1854) *The Diseases of the Heart and Aorta,* Hodges and Smith, Dublin, p. 320.

Stoneham, M.D. (1995) Anaesthesia and resuscitation at altitude. *Eur. J. Anaesthesiol.* **12**, 249–57.

Strauss, R.H., McFadden, E.R., Ingram, R.H. *et al.* (1978) Influence of heat and humidity on the airway obstruction induced by exercise in asthma. *J. Clin. Invest.* **61**, 433–40.

Stray-Gundersen, J., Chapman, R.F. and Levine, B.D. (2001) 'Living high–training low' altitude training improves sea level performance in male and female elite runners. *J. Appl. Physiol.* **91**, 1113–20.

Strong, L.H., Gin, G.K. and Goldman, R.F. (1985) Metabolic and vasomotor insulative responses occurring on immersion in cold water. *J. Appl. Physiol.* **58**, 964–77.

Suarez, J., Alexander, J.K. and Houston, C.S. (1987) Enhanced left ventricular systolic performance at high altitude during Operation Everest II. *Am. J. Cardiol.* **60**, 137–42.

Sui, G.J., Lui, Y.H., Cheng, X.S. *et al.* (1988) Subacute infantile mountain sickness. *J. Pathol.* **155**, 161–70.

Sumner, D.S., Boswick, J.A. and Doolittle, W.H. (1971) Prediction of tissue loss in human frostbite with xenon-133. *Surgery* **69**, 899–903.

Sumner, D.S., Criblez, T. and Doolittle, W. (1974) Host factors in human frostbite. *Mil. Med.* **139**, 454–61.

Sun, J.H., Lin, Z.P. and Hu, X.L. (1985) An observation on the development of normal children age between 7–17 years at three elevations (abstract), 2nd High Altitude Symposium, Qinghai, China (unpublished proceedings).

Sun, S., Oliver-Pickett, C., Ping, Y. *et al.* (1996) Breathing and brain blood flow during sleep in patients with chronic mountain sickness. *J. Appl. Physiol.* **81**, 611–18.

Sun, S.F. (1985) Epidemiology of hypertension on the Tibetan plateau (abstract), 2nd High Altitude Symposium, Qinghai, China (unpublished proceedings).

Sun, S.F., Droma, T.S., Zhang, J.G. *et al.* (1990) Greater maximal O_2 uptake and vital capacities in Tibetan than Han residents of Lhasa. *Respir. Physiol.* **79**, 151–62.

Suri, M.L., Vijayan, G.P., Puri, H.C. *et al.* (1978) Neurological manifestations of frostbite. *Indian J. Med. Res.* **67**, 292–9.

Surks, M.I. (1966) Elevated PBI, free thyroxine, and plasma protein concentration in man at high altitude. *J. Appl. Physiol.* **21**, 1185–90.

Suslov, F.P. (1994) Basic principles of training at high altitude. *New Studies in Athletes IAAF Quart. Mag.* **2**, 45–9.

Sutton, J.R. (1977) Effect of acute hypoxia on the hormonal response to exercise. *J. Appl. Physiol. Respir. Environ. Exerc. Physiol.* **42**, 587–92.

Sutton, J.R. (1987) Energy substrates and hypoglycaemia, in *Hypoxia and Cold* (eds. J.R. Sutton, C.S. Houston and G. Coates), Prager, New York, pp. 487–92.

Sutton, J.R., Bryan, A.C., Gray, G.W. *et al.* (1976) Pulmonary gas exchange in acute mountain sickness. *Aviat. Space Environ. Med.* **47**, 1032–7.

Sutton, J.R., Viol, G.W., Gray, G.W. *et al.* (1977) Renin, aldosterone, electrolyte, and cortisol responses to hypoxic decompression. *J. Appl. Physiol. Respir. Environ. Exerc. Physiol.* **43**, 421–4.

Sutton, J.R., Houston, C.S., Mansell, A.L. *et al.* (1979) Effect of acetazolamide on hypoxemia during sleep at high altitude. *N. Engl. J. Med.* **301**, 1329–31.

Sutton, J.R., Houston, C.S. and Jones, N.L. (1983) *Hypoxia, Exercise, and Altitude,* Liss, New York.

Sutton, J.R., Houston, C.S. and Coates, G. (1987) *Hypoxia: the Tolerable Limits,* Benchmark Press, Indianapolis.

Sutton, J.R., Reeves, J.T., Wagner, P.D. *et al.* (1988) Operation Everest II: oxygen transport during exercise at extreme simulated altitude. *J. Appl. Physiol.* **64**, 1309–21.

Svedenhag, J., Henriksson, J. and Sylven, C. (1983) Dissociation of training effects on skeletal muscle mitochondrial enzymes and myoglobin in man. *Acta Physiol. Scand.* **117**, 213–18.

Swenson, E.R. (2006) Carbonic anhydrase inhibitors and hypoxic pulmonary vasoconstriction. *Respir. Physiol. Neurobiol.* **151**, 209–16.

Swenson, E.R. and Hughes, J.M.B. (1993) Effects of acute and chronic acetazolamide on resting ventilation and ventilatory responses in men. *J. Appl. Physiol.* **74**, 230–7.

Swenson, E.R., Leatham, K.L., Roach, R.C. *et al.* (1991) Renal carbonic anhydrase inhibition reduces high altitude sleep periodic breathing. *Respir. Physiol.* **86**, 333–43.

Swenson, E.R., Duncan, T.B., Goldberg, S.V. *et al.* (1995) Diuretic effect of acute hypoxia in humans: relationship to hypoxic ventilatory responsiveness and renal hormones. *J. Appl. Physiol.* **78**, 377–83.

Swenson, E.R., MacDonald, A., Vatheuer, M. *et al.* (1997) Acute mountain sickness is not altered by a high carbohydrate diet nor associated with elevated circulating cytokines. *Aviat. Space Environ. Med.* **68**, 499–503.

Swenson, E.R., Mongovin, S., Gibbs, S. *et al.* (2000) Stress failure in high altitude pulmonary edema (HAPE). *Am. J. Respir. Crit. Care Med.* **161**, A418.

Swenson, E.R., Maggiorini, M., Mongovin, S. *et al.* (2002) Pathogenesis of high-altitude pulmonary edema: inflammation is not an etiologic factor. *JAMA* **287**, 2228–35.

Taber, R. (1994) A child in the pressure bag: a case. *ISMM Newsletter* **4**(1), 4–5.

Takeno, Y., Kamijo, Y.I. and Nose, H. (2001) Thermoregulatory and aerobic changes after endurance training in a hypobaric hypoxic and warm environment. *J. Appl. Physiol.* **91**, 1520–8.

Talbott, J.H. and Dill, D.B. (1936) Clinical observations at high altitude. *Am. J. Med. Sci.* **192**, 626–39.

Tansey, W.A. (1973) Medical aspects of cold water immersion: a review. *US Navy Submarine Medical Research Laboratory Report* NSMRL, 763, NTIS Document AD-775–687.

Tansley, J.G., Fatmian, M., Howard, L.S.G.E. *et al.* (1998) Changes in respiratory control during and after 48 h of isocapnic and poikilocapnic hypoxia in humans. *J. Appl. Physiol.* **85**, 2125–34.

Tappan, D.V. and Reynafarje, B.D. (1957) Tissue pigment manifestation of adaptation to high altitude. *Am. J. Physiol.* **190**, 99–103.

Tasker, J. (1981) *Everest the Cruel Way*, Eyre Methuen, London.

Tatsumi, K., Pickett, C.K. and Weil, J.V. (1991) Attenuated carotid body hypoxic sensitivity after prolonged hypoxic exposure. *J. Appl. Physiol.* **70**, 748–55.

Taylor, M.S. (1999) Lumbar sympathectomy for frostbite injuries of the foot. *Mil. Med.* **164**, 566–7.

Tek, D. and Mackey, S. (1993) Non-freezing cold injury in a marine infantry battalion. *J. Wild. Med.* **4**, 353–7.

Tenney, S.M. and Ou, L.C. (1970) Physiological evidence for increased tissue capillarity in rats acclimatized to high altitude. *Respir. Physiol.* **8**, 137–50.

Tenney, S.M. and Ou, L.C. (1977) Ventilatory response of decorticate and decerebrate cats to hypoxia and CO_2. *Respir. Physiol.* **29**, 81–2.

Tewari, S.C., Jayaswal, R., Kasturi, A.S. *et al.* (1991) Excessive polycythaemia of high altitude. Pulmonary function studies including carbon monoxide diffusion capacity. *J. Assoc. Physicians India* **39**, 453–5.

The Times (1999) Queen Victoria's Gurkha was a trailblazer extraordinary, 8 July, p. 50.

Theis, M.K., Honigman, B., Yip, R., McBride, D., Houston, C.S. and Moore, L.G. (1993) Acute mountain sickness in children at 2835 metres. *Am. J. Dis. Child.* **147**, 143–5.

Thews, O., Fleck, B., Kamin, W.E.S. and Rose, D.-M. (2004) Respiratory function and blood gas variables in cystic fibrosis patients during reduced environmental pressure. *Europ. J. Appl. Physiol.* **92**, 493–7.

Thomas, D.J., Marshall, J., Ross Russell, R.W. *et al.* (1977) Cerebral blood-flow in polycythaemia. *Lancet* **2**, 161–3.

Thomas, P.K., King, R.H.M., Feng, S.F. *et al.* (2000) Neurological manifestations in chronic mountain sickness: the burning feet-burning hands syndrome. *J. Neurol. Neruosurg. Psychiatry* **69**, 447–52.

Thomas, P.W. (1894) Rocky Mountain sickness. *Alpine J.* **17**, 140–9.

Thompson, D.G., Richelson, E. and Malagelada, J.R. (1983) A perturbation of upper gastro-intestinal function by cold stress. *Gut* **24**, 277–83.

Thompson, R.L. and Hayward, J.S. (1996) Wet cold exposure and hypothermia: thermal and metabolic responses to prolonged exercise in rain. *J. Appl. Physiol.* **81**, 1128–37.

Thompson, W.O., Thompson, P.K. and Dailey, M.M. (1928) The effect of posture on the composition and volume of the blood in man. *J. Clin. Invest.* **5**, 573–604.

Tierman, C.J. (1999) Splenic crisis at high altitude in two white men with sickle cell trait. *Ann. Emerg. Med.* **33**, 230–3.

Tikusis, P., Ducharme, M.B., Moroz, D. and Jacobs, I. (1999) Physiological responses on exercise fatigued individuals exposed to wet cold conditions. *J. Appl. Physiol.* **86**, 1319–25.

Tilman, H.W. (1948) *Mount Everest 1938,* Cambridge University Press, Cambridge, pp. 93–4.

Tilman, H.W. (1952) *Nepal Himalaya*, Cambridge University Press, Cambridge.

Tilman, H.W. (1975) Practical problems of nutrition, in *Mountain Medicine and Physiology* (eds. C. Clarke, M. Ward and E. Williams), Alpine Club, London, pp. 62–6.

Timmons, B.A., Ararujo, J. and Thomas, T.R. (1985) Fat utilization in a cold environment. *Med. Sci. Sports Exerc.* **17**, 673–8.

Ting, S. (1984) Cold induced urticaria in infancy. *Pediatrics* **73**, 105–6.

Tiollier, E., Schmitt, L., Burnat, P. *et al.* (2005) Living high–training low altitude training: effects on mucosal immunity. *Eur. J. Appl. Physiol.* **94**, 298–304.

Tissandier, G. (1875) Le voyage à grande hauteur du ballon 'Le Zenith'. *La Nature Paris* **3**, 337–44.

Tissot van Patot, M., Grill, A., Chapman, P. *et al.* (2003) Remodelling of uteroplacental arteries is decreased in high altitude placentae. *Placenta* **24**, 326–30.

Tissot van Patot, M.C., Leadbetter, G., Keyes, L.E. *et al.* (2005) Greater free plasma VEGF and lower soluble VEGF receptor-1 in acute mountain sickness. *J. Appl. Physiol.* **98**, 1626–9. E-pub 13 January 2005.

Tolman, K.G. and Cohen, A. (1970) Accidental hypothermia. *Can. Med. Assoc. J.* **103**, 1357–61.

Tomashefski, J.F., Feeley, D.R. and Shillito, F.H. (1966) Effects of altitude on emphysematous blebs and bullae. *Aerosp. Med.* **37**, 1158–62.

Tomiyama, Y., Brian Jr., J.E. and Tod, M.M. (2000) Plasma viscosity and cerebral blood flow. *Am. J. Physiol. Heart Circ. Physiol.* **279**, H1949–54.

Torgovicky, R., Azaria, B., Grossman, A. *et al.* (2005). Sinus vein thrombosis following exposure to simulated high altitude. *Aviat. Space Environ. Med.* **76**, 144–6.

Townes, B.D., Hornbein, T.F., Schoene, R.B., Sarnquist, F.H. and Grant, I. (1984) Human cerebral function at extreme altitude, in *High Altitude and Man* (eds. J.B. West and S. Lahiri), American Physiological Society, Bethesda, MD, pp. 32–6.

Townsend, N.E., Gore, C.J., Hahn, A.G. *et al.* (2002) Living high–training low: increased hypoxic ventilatory response of well-trained endurance athletes. *J. Appl. Physiol.* **93**, 1498–505.

Townsend, N.E., Gore, C.J., Hahn, A.G. *et al.* (2004) Hypoxic ventilatory response is correlated with increased submaximal exercise ventilation after live high, train low. *Europ. J. Appl. Physiol.* **94**, 207–15.

Tozzi, C.A., Poiani, G.J., Harangozo, A.M., Boyd, C.D. and Riley, D.J. (1989) Pressure-induced connective tissue synthesis in pulmonary artery segments is dependent on intact endothelium. *J. Clin. Invest.* **84**, 1005–12.

Travis, S.P.L. and Menzies, I.S. (1992) Intestinal permeability: functional assessment and significance. *Clin. Sci.* **82**, 471–88.

Travis, S.P.L., A'Court, C., Menzies, I.S. *et al.* (1993) Intestinal function at altitudes above 5000 m (abstract). *Gut* **34**, T165.

Treating accidental hypothermia (editorial). (1978) *BMJ* **2**, 1383–4.

Treatment of Hypothermia (eds. R.S. Pozos and L.E. Wittmers), Croom Helm, London/University of Minnesota Press, Minneapolis, pp. 143–51.

Tripathy, V. and Gupta, R. (2005) Birth weight among Tibetans at different altitudes in India: are Tibetans better protected from IUGR? *Am. J. Hum. Biol.* **17**, 442–50.

Truijens, M.J., Toussaint, H.M., Dow, J. and Levine, B.D. (2003) Effect of high-intensity hypoxic training on sea-level swimming performances. *J. Appl. Physiol.* **94**, 733–43. E-pub 11 October 2002.

Tschop, M., Strasburger, C.J., Hartmann, G. *et al.* (1998) Raised leptin concentration at high altitude associated with loss of appetite (letter). *Lancet* **352**, 1119–20.

Tsianos, G., Eleftheriou, K.I., Hawe, E. *et al.* (2005) Performance at altitude and angiotensin I-converting enzyme genotype. *Eur. J. Appl. Physiol.* **93**, 630–5.

Tsukimoto, K., Mathieu-Costello, O., Prediletto, R., Elliott, A.E. and West, J.B. (1991) Ultrastructural appearances of pulmonary capillaries at high transmural pressures. *J. Appl. Physiol.* **71**, 573–82.

Tsukimoto, K., Yoshimura, N., Ichioka, M. *et al.* (1994) Protein, cell, and leukotriene B4 concentrations of lung edema fluid produced by high capillary transmural pressures in rabbit. *J. Appl. Physiol.* **76**, 321–67.

Tucker, A. and Rhodes, J. (2001) Role of vascular smooth muscle in the development of high altitude pulmonary hypertension: an interspecies evaluation. *High Alt. Med. Biol.* **2**, 349–60.

Tuffley, R.E., Rubenstein, D., Slater, J.D.H. and Williams, E.S. (1970) Serum renin activity during exposure to hypoxia. *J. Endocrinol.* **48**, 497–510.

Turek, Z., Kreuzer, F. and Hoofd, L.J.C. (1973) Advantage or disadvantage of a decrease of blood oxygen affinity for tissue oxygen supply at hypoxia; a theoretical study comparing man and rat. *Pflügers Arch.* **342**, 185–97.

Turek, Z., Kreuzer, F. and Ringnalda, B.E.M. (1978) Blood gases at several levels of oxygenation in rats with a left shifted blood oxygen dissociation curve. *Pflügers Arch.* **376**, 7–13.

Turino, C.M., Bergofsky, E.H., Goldring, R.M. and Fishman, A.P. (1963) Effect of exercise on pulmonary diffusing capacity. *J. Appl. Physiol.* **18**, 447–56.

Unger, C., Weiser, J.K., McCullough, R.E. *et al.* (1988) Altitude, low birth weight, and infant mortality in Colorado. *JAMA* **259**, 3427–32.

Ungley, G.G., Channell, G.D. and Richards, R.L. (1945) The immersion foot syndrome. *Br. J. Surg.* **33**, 17–31.

Utiger, D., Bernasch, D., Eichenberger, U. and Bärtsch, P. (1999) Transient improvement in high altitude headache by sumatriptan in a placebo controlled trial (abstract), in *Hypoxia: Into the Next Millennium* (eds. R.C. Roach, P.D. Wagner and P.H. Hackett), Plenum/Kluwer, New York, p. 435.

Vachiery, J.L., McDonald, T., Moraine, J.J. *et al.* (1995) Doppler assessment of hypoxic pulmonary vasoconstriction and susceptibility to high altitude pulmonary oedema. *Thorax* **50**, 22–7.

Valdivia, E. (1958) Total capillary bed in striated muscle of guinea pigs native to the Peruvian mountains. *Am. J. Physiol.* **194**, 585–9.

Valencia-Flores, M., Rebollar, V., Santiago, V. *et al.* (2004) Prevalence of pulmonary hypertension and its association with respiratory disturbances in obese patients living at moderately high altitude. *Int. J. Obes. Relat. Metab. Disord.* **28**, 1174–80.

Valletta, E.A., Piacentini, G.L., Del Col, G. and Boner, A.L. (1997) FEF25-75 as a marker of airway obstruction in asthmatic children during reduced mite exposure at high altitude. *J. Asthma.* **34**, 127–31.

van den Elshout, X.X., van Herwaarden, C.L. and Folgering H.T. (1991) Effects of hypercapnia and hypocapnia on respiratory resistance in normal and asthmatic subjects. *Thorax* **46**, 28–32.

Van Osta, A., Moraine, J.J., Melot, C., *et al.* (2005) Effects of high altitude exposure on cerebral hemodynamics in normal subjects. *Stroke* **36**, 557–60. E-pub 3 February 2005.

Van Ruiten, H.J.A. and Daanen, H.A.M. (1999) Cold induced vasodilatation at altitude (abstract), in *Hypoxia: Into the Next Millennium* (eds. R.C. Roach, P.D. Wagner and P.H. Hackett), Plenum/Kluwer, New York, p. 436.

van Velzen, E., van den Bos, J.W., Benckhuijsen, J.A., van Essel, T., de Bruijn, R. and Aalbers, R. (1996) Effect of allergen avoidance at high altitude on direct and indirect bronchial hyperresponsiveness and markers of inflammation in children with allergic asthma. *Thorax* **51**, 582–4.

Vardy, J., Vardy, J. and Judge, K. (2005) Can knowledge protect against acute mountain sickness? *J. Public Health (Oxford).* **27**, 366–70. E-pub 18 October 2005.

Vargas, M., León-Velarde, F., Monge, C.C. *et al.* (1998) Similar hypoxic ventilatory response in sea-level natives and Andean natives living at sea level. *J. Appl. Physiol.* **84**, 1024–9.

Vasquez, R. and Villena, M. (2001) Normal hematological values for healthy persons living at 4000 meters in Bolivia. *High Alt. Med .Biol.* **2**, 361–7.

Vats, P., Singh, S.N., Shyam, R. *et al.* (2004) Leptin may not be responsible for high altitude anorexia. *High Alt. Med. Biol.* **5**, 90–2.

Vaughan, B.E. and Pace, N. (1956) Changes in myoglobin content of the high altitude acclimatized rat. *Am. J. Physiol.* **185**, 549–56.

Vaughn, P.B. (1942) Local cold injury – menace to military operations. A review. *Mil. Med.* **145**, 305–11.

Velásquez, M.T. (1956) *Maximal Diffusing Capacity of the Lungs at High Altitudes.* Report 56–108, USAF School of Aviation Medicine, Randolph Air Force Base, TX.

Velasquez, T. (1976) Pulmonary function and oxygen transport, in *Man in the Andes: a Multidisciplinary Study of High-altitude Quechua* (eds. P.T. Baker and M.A. Little), Dowden, Hutchinson & Ross, Stroudsburg PA, pp. 237–60.

Vella, M.A., Jenner, C., Betteridge, D.J. and Jowett, N.I. (1988) Hypothermia induced thrombocytopenia. *J. R. Soc. Med.* **81**, 228–9.

Ventura, N., Hoppeler, H., Seiler, R., Binggeli, A., Mullis, P. and Vogt, M. (2003) The response of trained athletes to six weeks of endurance training in hypoxia or normoxia. *Int. J. Sports Med.* **24**, 166–72.

Viault, F. (1890) Sur l'augmentation considerable de nombre des globules rouges dans le sang chez les habitants des haut plateaux de l'Amérique du Sud. *Comptes Rendus, Hebdomaire Des Seances de l'Academie Des Sciences (Paris)*, **III**, 917–18. English translation (1981) in *High Altitude Physiology* (ed. J.B. West), Hutchinson Ross, Stroudsburg PA, 1981, pp. 333–4.

Viault, F. (1891) Sur la quantité d'oxygène contenue dans le sang des animaux des hauts plateaux de l'Amérique du Sud. *C. R. Acad. Sci. (Paris)* **112**, 295–8.

Villafuerte, F.C., Cardenas, R., and Monge-C.C. (2004) Optimal hemoglobin concentration and high altitude: a theoretical approach for Andean men at rest. *J. Appl. Physiol.* **96**, 1579–8.

Virmani, S.K. and Swamy, A.S. (1993) Cranial nerve palsy at high altitude. *J. Assoc. Physicians India* **41**, 460.

Virokannas, H. and Anttonen, H. (1993) Risk of frostbite in vibration-induced finger cases. *Arctic Med. Res.* **52**, 69–72.

Viswanathan, R., Subramanian, S. and Radha, T.C. (1979) Effect of hypoxia on regional lung perfusion, by scanning. *Respiration* **37**, 142–7.

Vitzthum, V.J. (2001) The home team advantage: reproduction in women indigenous to high altitude (Review). *J. Exp. Biol.* **204(Pt 18)**, 3141–50.

Vitzthum, V.J. and Wiley, A.S. (2003) The proximate determinants of fertility in populations exposed to chronic hypoxia (Review). *High Alt. Med. Biol.* **4**, 125–39.

Vitzthum, V.J., Ellison, P.T., Sukalich, S., Caceres, E. and Spielvogel, H. (2000a) Does hypoxia impair ovarian function in Bolivian women indigenous to high altitude? *High Alt. Med. Biol.* **1**, 39–49.

Vitzthum, V.J., Spielvogel, H., Caceres, E. and Gaines, J. (2000b) Menstrual patterns and fecundity among non-lactating and lactating cycling women in rural highland Bolivia: implications for contraceptive choice. *Contraception* **62**, 181–7.

Vitzthum, V.J., Bentley, G.R., Spielvogel, H. *et al.* (2002) Salivary progesterone levels and rate of ovulation are significantly lower in poorer than in better-off urban-dwelling Bolivian women. *Hum. Reprod.* **17**, 1906–13.

Vivona, M.L., Matthay, M., Chabaud, M.B., Friedlander, G. and Clerici, C. (2001) Hypoxia reduces alveolar epithelial sodium and fluid transport in rats: reversal by beta-adrenergic agonist treatment. *Am. J. Respir. Cell. Mol. Biol.* **25**, 554–61.

Vizek, M., Picket, C.K. and Weil, J.V. (1987) Increased carotid body sensitivity during acclimatization to hypobaric hypoxia. *J. Appl. Physiol.* **63**, 2403–10.

Vock, P., Fretz, C., Franciolli, M. and Bartsch, P. (1989) High-altitude pulmonary edema: findings at high-altitude chest radiography and physical examination. *Radiology* **170**, 661–6.

Vock, P., Brutsche, M.H., Nanzer, A. and Bartsch, P. (1991) Variable radiomorphologic data of high altitude pulmonary edema. Features from 60 patients. *Chest* **100**, 1306–11.

Voelkel, N.F., Hegstrand, L., Reeves, J.T., McMurty, I.F. and Molinoff, P.B. (1981) Effects of hypoxia on density of β-adrenergic receptors. *J. Appl. Physiol.* **50**, 363–6.

Vogel, J.A. and Harris, C.W. (1967) Cardiopulmonary responses of resting man during early exposure to high altitude. *J. Appl. Physiol.* **22**, 1124–8.

Vogel, J.A., Hansen, J.E. and Harris, C.W. (1967) Cardiovascular responses in man during exhaustive work at sea level and high altitude. *J. Appl. Physiol.* **23**, 531–9.

Vogel, J.A., Hartley, L.H. and Cruz, J.C. (1974) Cardiac output during exercise in altitude natives at sea level and high altitude. *J. Appl. Physiol.* **36**, 173–6.

Vogt, M., Puntschart, A., Geiser, J., Zuleger, C., Billeter, R. and Hoppeler, H. (2001) Molecular adaptations in human skeletal muscle to endurance training under simulated hypoxic conditions. *J. Appl. Physiol.* **91**, 173–82.

Von Euler, U.S. and Liljestrand, G. (1946) Observations on the pulmonary arterial blood pressure in the cat. *Acta Physiol.* **22**, 1115–23.

Vonmoos, S., Nussberger, J., Waeber, J. *et al.* (1990) Effect of metoclopramide on angiotensin, aldosterone and atrial peptide during hypoxia. *J. Appl. Physiol.* **69**, 2072–9.

Vorstrup, S., Henriksen, L. and Paulson, O.B. (1984) Effect of acetazolamide on cerebral blood flow and cerebral metabolic rate for oxygen. *J. Clin. Invest.* **74**, 1634–9.

Vovk, A., Smith, W.D.F., Paterson, N.D., Cunningham, D.A. and Patterson, D.H. (2004) Peripheral chemoreceptor control of ventilation following sustained hypoxia in young and older adult humans. *Exp. Physiol.* **86**, 647–56.

Vuolteenaho, O., Koistinen, P., Martikkala, V. *et al.* (1992) Effect of physical exercise in hypobaric conditions on atrial natriuretic peptide secretion. *Am. J. Physiol.* **263**, R647–52.

Waddell, L.A. (1899) *Among the Himalayas,* Constable, London, pp. 261–2.

Wagenvoort, C.A. and Wagenvoort, N. (1973) Hypoxic pulmonary vascular lesions in man at high altitude and in patients with chronic respiratory disease. *Pathol. Microbiol.* **39**, 276–82.

Wagenvoort, C.A. and Wagenvoort, N. (1976) Pulmonary venous changes in chronic hypoxia. *Virchows Arch. [A]* **372**, 51–6.

Waggener, T.B., Brusil, P.J., Kronauer, R.E. *et al.* (1984) Strength and cycle time of high-altitude ventilatory patterns in unacclimatized humans. *J. Appl. Physiol.* **56**, 576–81.

Wagner, P.D. (1988) An integrated view of the determinants of maximum oxygen uptake, in *Oxygen Transfer from Atmosphere to Tissues,* vol. 227 (eds. N.C. Gonzalez and M.R. Fedde), Plenum, New York, pp. 246–56.

Wagner, P.D. (1996) A theoretical analysis of factors determining $\dot{V}_{O_{2max}}$ at sea level and altitude. *Respir. Physiol.* **106**, 329–43.

Wagner, P.D. and West, J.B. (1972) Effects of diffusion impairment of O_2 and CO_2 time courses in pulmonary capillaries. *J. Appl. Physiol.* **33**, 62–71.

Wagner, P.D., Saltzman, H.A. and West, J.B. (1974) Measurement of continuous distributions of ventilation–perfusion ratios: theory. *J. Appl. Physiol.* **36**, 588–99.

Wagner, P.D., Sutton, J.R., Reeves, J.T., Cymerman, A., Groves, B.M. and Malconian, M.K. (1987) Operation Everest II. Pulmonary gas exchange during a simulated ascent of Mt. Everest. *J. Appl. Physiol.* **63**, 2348–59.

Wagner, P.D., Hedenstierna, G. and Rodriguez-Roisin, R. (1996) Gas exchange, expiratory flow obstruction and the clinical spectrum of asthma. *Eur. Respir. J.* **9**, 1278–82.

Wagner, P.D., Araoz, M., Boushel, R. *et al.* (2002) Pulmonary gas exchange and acid-base status at 5,260 m in high-altitude Bolivians and acclimatized lowlanders. *J. Appl. Physiol.* **92**, 1393–400.

Walker, J.T. (1885) Four years journeyings through great Tibet by one of the trans-Himalayan explorers of the Survey of India. *Proc. R. Geogr. Soc.* **7**, 65–92.

Waller, D. (1990) *The Pundits: British Exploration of Tibet and Central Asia,* University Press of Kentucky, Lexington, KY.

Walter, R., Maggiorini, M., Scherrer, U., Contesse, J. and Reinhart, W.H. (2001) Effects of high-altitude exposure on vascular endothelial growth factor levels in man. *Eur. J. Appl. Physiol.* **85**, 113–17.

Wanderer, A.A. (1979) An 'allergy' to cold. *Hosp. Pract.* **14**, 136–7.

Wang, L.C.H. (1978) Factors limiting maximum cold induced heat production. *Life Sci.* **23**, 2089–98.

Ward, M.P. (1954) High altitude deterioration, in: A discussion on the physiology of man at high altitude. *Proc. R. Soc., Series B, London* **143**, 40–2.

Ward, M.P. (1968) Diseases occurring at altitudes exceeding 17500 ft. MD thesis, University of Cambridge, pp. 66–9.

Ward, M.P. (1973) Periodic respiration. *Am. R. Coll. Surg. Engl.* **52**, 330–4.

Ward, M.P. (1974) Frostbite. *BMJ* **1**, 67–70.

Ward, M.P. (1975) *Mountain Medicine, a Clinical Study of Cold and High Altitude,* Crosby Lockwood Staples, London.

Ward, M.P. (1987) Cold, hypoxia and dehydration, in *Hypoxia and Cold* (eds. J.R. Sutton, C.S. Houston and G. Coates), Prager, New York, pp. 475–86.

Ward, M.P. (1990) Tibet: human and medical geography. *J. Wilderness Med.* **1**, 36–46.

Ward, M.P. (1991) Medicine in Tibet. *J. Wilderness Med.* **2**, 198–205.

Ward, M.P. (1993) The first ascent of Mount Everest, 1953: the solution of the problem of the 'last thousand feet'. *J. Wilderness Med.* **4**, 312–18.

Ward, M.P. and Jackson, F.S. (1965) Medicine in Bhutan. *Lancet* **1**, 811–13.

Warren, C.B.M. (1939) Alveolar air on Mount Everest. *J. Physiol. (Lond.)* **96**, 34–5.

Washburn, B. (1962) Frostbite. What it is – and how to prevent it – emergency treatment. *N. Engl. J. Med.* **266**, 974–89.

Webb, P. (1951) Air temperature in respiratory tracts of resting subjects in cold. *J. Appl. Physiol.* **4**, 378–82.

Webb, P. (1986) After drop of body temperature during re-warming – an alternative explanation. *J. Appl. Physiol.* **60**, 385–90.

Wedin, B., Vanggaard, L. and Hirvonen, J. (1979) 'Paradoxical undressing' in fatal hypothermia. *J. Forensic Sci.* **24**, 543–53.

Wedzicha, J.A., Cotes, P.M., Empey, D.W. *et al.* (1985) Serum immunoreactive erythropoietin in hypoxic lung disease with and without polycythaemia. *Clin. Sci.* **69**, 413–22.

Weeke, J. and Gundersen, H.J.G. (1983) The effect of heating and cold cooling on serum T.S.H., G.H. and norepinephrine in resting normal man. *Acta Physiol. Scand.* **47**, 33–9.

Wehrlin, J.P. and Marti, B. (2006) Live high–train low associated with increased haemoglobin mass as preparation for the 2003 World Championships in two native European world class runners. *Br. J. Sports Med.* **40**, e3; discussion e3.

Wehrlin, J.P., Zuest, P., Hallen, J. and Marti, B. (2006) Live high - train low for 24 days increases hemoglobin mass and red cell volume in elite endurance athletes. *J. Appl. Physiol.* **100**, 1938–45.

Weibel, E.R. (1970) Morphometric estimation of pulmonary diffusion capacity. *Respir. Physiol.* **11**, 54–75.

Weil, J.V. (1986) Ventilatory control at high altitude, in *Handbook of Physiology,* Sec. 3, vol. II (eds. N.S. Cherniack and J.G. Widdicome), American Physiological Society, Bethesda, MD, pp. 703–27.

Weil, J.V. (2004) Sleep at high altitude. *High Alt. Med. Biol.* **5**, 180–9.

Weil, J.V. and White, D.P. (2001) Sleep, in *High Altitude* (eds. T.F. Hornbein and R.B. Schoene), Marcel Dekker, New York, pp. 707–76.

Weil, J.V., Byrne-Quinn, E., Sodal, I.E. *et al.* (1970) Hypoxic ventilatory drive in normal man. *J. Clin. Invest.* **49**, 1061–72.

Weil, J.V., Byrne-Quinn, E., Ingvar, E. *et al.* (1971) Acquired attenuation of chemoreceptor function in chronically hypoxic man at high altitude. *J. Clin. Invest.* **50**, 186–95.

Weil, J.V., Kryger, M.H. and Scoggin, C.H. (1978) Sleep and breathing at high altitude, in *Sleep Apnea Syndromes* (eds. C. Guilleminault and W. Dement), Liss, New York, pp. 119–36.

Weiss, E.A. (1991) Environmental heat illness, in *Proceedings of the First World Congress on Wilderness Medicine,* Wilderness Medical Society, Point Reyes Station, CA, pp. 347–57.

Weisse, A.B., Moschos, C.B., Frank, M.L. *et al.* (1975) Haemodynamic effects of staged haematocrit reduction in patients with stable cor pulmonale and severely elevated haematocrit. *Am. J. Med.* **58**, 92–8.

Weitz, C.A. and Garruto, R.M. (2004) Growth of Han migrants at high altitude in central Asia. *Am. J. Hum. Biol.* **16**, 405–19.

Weller, A.S., Millard, C.E., Stroud, M.A. *et al.* (1997) Physiological responses to a cold, wet and windy environment during prolonged intermittent walking. *Am. J. Physiol.* **272** (*Regulatory Integrative Comp. Physiol.* **41**) R226–33.

Welsh, C.H., Wagner, P.D., Reeves, J.T. *et al.* (1993) Operation Everest II: spirometric and radiographic changes in acclimatized humans at simulated high altitudes. *Am. Rev. Respir. Dis.* **147**, 1239–44.

Wen, T.C., Sadamoto, Y., Tanaka, J. *et al.* (2002) Erythropoietin protects neurons against chemical hypoxia and cerebral ischemic injury by up-regulating Bcl-xL expression. *J. Neurosci. Res.* **67**, 795–803.

West, J.B. (1962a) Diffusing capacity of the lung for carbon monoxide at high altitude. *J. Appl. Physiol.* **17**, 421–6.

West, J.B. (1962b) Regional differences in gas exchange in the lung of erect man. *J. Appl. Physiol.* **17**, 893–8.

West, J.B. (1981) *High Altitude Physiology: Benchmark Papers in Physiology,* vol. 15, Hutchinson Ross, Stroudsburg, PA, p. 328.

West, J.B. (1982) Diffusion at high altitude. *Fed. Proc.* **41**, 2128–30.

West, J.B. (1983) Climbing Mt. Everest without oxygen: an analysis of maximal exercise during extreme hypoxia. *Respir. Physiol.* **52**, 265–79.

West, J.P. (1985a) *Everest – the Testing Place.* McGraw-Hill, New York.

West, J.B. (ed.) (1985b) *Best and Taylor's Physiological Basis of Medical Practice,* 11th edn, Williams and Wilkins, Baltimore, MD.

West, J.B. (1986a) Highest inhabitants in the world. *Nature* **324**, 517.

West, J.B. (1986b) Lactate during exercise at extreme altitude. *Fed. Proc.* **45**, 2953–7.

West, J.B. (1986c) *Ventilation/blood Flow and Gas Exchange*, 5th edn, Blackwell Scientific Publications, Oxford.

West, J.B. (1988a) Rate of ventilatory acclimatization to extreme altitude. *Respir. Physiol.* **74**, 323–33.

West, J.B. (1988b) Tolerable limits to hypoxia on high mountains, in *Hypoxia: the Tolerable Limits* (eds. J.R. Sutton, C.S. Houston and G. Coates), Benchmark Press, Indianapolis, pp. 353–62.

West, J.B. (1988c) *High Life: A History of High-altitude Physiology and Medicine*. Oxford University Press, Oxford, pp. 358–63.

West, J.B. (1990) *Ventilation/Blood flow and Gas Exchange*, 5th edn, Blackwell Scientific, Oxford.

West, J.B. (1993a) Acclimatization and tolerance to extreme altitude. *J. Wilderness Med.* **4**, 17–26.

West, J.B. (1993b) The Silver Hut expedition, high-altitude field expeditions, and low-pressure chamber simulations, in *Hypoxia and Molecular Medicine* (eds. J.R. Sutton, C.S. Houston and G. Coates), Queen City Printers, Burlington, VT, pp. 190–202.

West, J.B. (1995) Oxygen enrichment of room air to relieve the hypoxia of high altitude. *Respir. Physiol.* **99**, 225–32.

West, J.B. (1996a) Prediction of barometric pressures at high altitudes with the use of model atmospheres. *J. Appl. Physiol.* **81**, 1850–4.

West, J.B. (1996b) T.H. Ravenhill and his contributions to mountain sickness. *J. Appl. Physiol.* **80**, 715–24.

West, J.B. (1997) Fire hazard in oxygen-enriched atmospheres at low barometric pressures. *Aviat. Space Envir. Med.* **68**, 159–62.

West, J.B. (1998) *High Life: a History of High-Altitude Physiology and Medicine*, Oxford University Press, New York.

West, J.B. (1999a) Barometric pressures on Mt. Everest: new data and physiological significance. *J. Appl. Physiol.* **86**, 1062–6.

West, J.B. (1999b) The original presentation of Boyle's law. *J. Appl. Physiol.* **87**, 1543–5.

West J.B. (2001) Safe Upper Limits for Oxygen Enrichment of Room Air at High Altitude. *High Alt Med Biol* **2**: 47–51.

West, J.B. (2002a) Highest permanent human habitation. *High Alt. Med. Biol.* **3**, 401–7.

West, J.B. (2002b) Potential use of oxygen enrichment of room air in mountain resorts. *High Alt. Med. Biol.* **3**, 59–64.

West, J.B. (2004a) Gulmuf–Lhasa rail link: an enormous challenge in high altitude medicine. *High Alt. Med. Biol.* **5**, 3.

West, J.B. (2004b) The physiologic basis of high-altitude disease. *Ann. Intern. Med.* **141**, 789–800.

West, J.B. (2005a) *Respiratory Physiology – The Essentials,* 7th edn, Williams & Wilkins, Baltimore, MD.

West J.B. (2005b) Robert-Boyle's landmark book of 1660 with the first experiments on rarified air. *J. Appl. Physiol.* **98**, 31–9.

West, J.B. and Mathieu-Costello, O. (1992a) High altitude pulmonary edema is caused by stress failure of pulmonary capillaries. *Intl. J. Sports Med.* **13**(Suppl 1), S54–8.

West, J.B. and Mathieu-Costello, O. (1992b) Strength of the pulmonary blood–gas barrier. *Respir. Physiol.* **88**, 141–8.

West, J.B. and Mathieu-Costello, O. (1992c) Stress failure of pulmonary capillaries: role in lung and heart disease. *Lancet,* **340**, 762–7.

West, J.B. and Readhead, A. (2004) Working at high altitude: medical problems, misconceptions, and solutions. *Observatory* **124**, 1–14.

West, J.B. and Wagner, P.D. (1977) Pulmonary gas exchange, in *Bioengineering Aspects of the Lung* (ed. J.B. West), Dekker, New York, pp. 361–457.

West, J.B. and Wagner, P.D. (1980) Predicted gas exchange on the summit of Mt Everest. *Respir. Physiol.* **42**, 1–16.

West, J.B., Lahiri, S., Gill, M.B. *et al.* (1962) Arterial oxygen saturation during exercise at high altitude. *J. Appl. Physiol.* **17**, 617–21.

West, J.B., Lahiri, S., Maret, K.H., Peters, R.M. Jr and Pizzo, C.J. (1983a) Barometric pressures at extreme altitudes on Mt. Everest: physiological significance. *J. Appl. Physiol.* **54**, 1188–94.

West, J.B., Hackett, P.H., Maret, K.H. *et al.* (1983b) Pulmonary gas exchange on the summit of Mount Everest. *J. Appl. Physiol.* **55**, 678–87.

West, J.B., Boyer, S.J., Graber, D.J. *et al.* (1983c) Maximal exercise at extreme altitudes on Mount Everest. *J. Appl. Physiol.* **55**, 688–98.

West, J.B., Peters, R.M., Aksnes, G., Maret, K.H., Milledge, J.S. and Schoene, R.B. (1986) Nocturnal periodic breathing at altitudes of 6300 and 8050 m. *J. Appl. Physiol.* **61**, 280–7.

West, J.B., Tsukimoto, K., Mathieu-Costello, O. and Prediletto, R. (1991) Stress failure in pulmonary capillaries. *J. Appl. Physiol.* **70**, 1731–42.

West, J.B., Mathieu-Costello, O., Jones, J.H. *et al.* (1993) Stress failure of pulmonary capillaries in racehorses with exercise-induced pulmonary hemorrhage. *J. Appl. Physiol.* **75**, 1097–109.

West, J.B., Colice, G.L., Lee, Y.-J. *et al.* (1995) Pathogenesis of high-altitude pulmonary edema: direct evidence of stress failure of pulmonary capillaries. *Eur. Respir. J.* **8**, 523–9.

Westendorp, R.G.J., Frölich, M. and Meinders, A.E. (1993) What to tell steroid substituted patients about the effects of high altitude? *Lancet* **342**, 310–11.

Westendorp, R.G., Blauw, G.J., Frolich, M. and Simons, R. (1997) Hypoxic syncope. *Aviat. Space Environ. Med.* **68**, 410–4.

Westerterp, K.R. (2001) Limits to sustainable human metabolic rate. *J. Exper. Biol.* **204**, 3183–7.

Westerterp, K.R., Kayser, B., Brouns, F. *et al.* (1992) Energy expenditure climbing Mt. Everest. *J. Appl. Physiol.* **73**, 1815–19.

Westerterp, K.R., Kayser, B., Wouters, L., Le Trong, J.-L. and J.-P. Richalet (1994) Energy balance at high altitude of 6,542 m. *J. Appl. Physiol.* **77**, 862–6.

Westerterp, K.R., Robach, P., Wouters, L. and Richalet, J.-P. (1996) Water balance and acute mountain sickness before and after arrival at high-altitude of 4,350 m. *J. Appl. Physiol.* **80**, 1968–72.

Westerterp, K.R., Meijer, E.P., Rubbens, M., Robarch, P. and Richalet, J.P. (2000) Operation Everest III: energy and water balance. *Eur. J. Physiol.* **439**, 483–8.

Westerterp-Plantegna, M.S., Westerterp, K.R., Rubbens, M., Verwegen, C.R., Richalet, J.-P. and Gordette, B. (1999) Appetite at high altitude [(Operation Everest III Comex-97)]: A simulated ascent of Mount Everest. *J. Appl. Physiol.* **87**, 391–9.

Weston, A.R., Karamizrak, O., Smith, A. *et. al* (1999) African runners who lived at sea level exhibited greater fatigue resistance, lower lactate accumulation and higher oxidative activity. *J. Appl. Physiol.* **86**, 915–23.

Wetter, T.J., Harms, C.A., Nelson, W.B., Pegelow, D.F. and Dempsey, J.A. (1999) Influence of respiratory muscle work on $\dot{V}O_2$ and leg blood flow during submaximal exercise. *J. Appl. Physiol.* **87**, 643–51.

Whayne, T.F. and Severinghaus, J.W. (1968) Experimental hypoxic pulmonary edema in the rat. *J. Appl. Physiol.* **25**, 729–32.

White, M.M., McCullough, R.E., Dyckes, R., Robertson, A.D. and Moore, L.G. (2000) Chronic hypoxia, pregnancy and endothelium-mediated relaxation in guinea pig uterine and thoracic arteries. *Am. J. Physiol.* **278**, H2069–75.

Whittaker, S.R.F. and Winton, F.R. (1933) The apparent viscosity of blood flowing in the isolated hind limb of the dog and its variation with corpuscular concentration. *J. Physiol.* **78**, 339–69.

Whittembury, J., Lozano, R. and Monge, C.C. (1968) Influence of cell concentration in the electrometric determination of blood pH. *Acta Physiol. Lat. Am.* **18**, 263–5.

Whymper, E. (1891–1892) *Travels among the Great Andes of the Equator.* John Murray, London.

Wickramasinghe, H. and Anholm, J.D. (1999) Sleep and breating at high altitude. *Sleep Breath.* **3**, 89–102.

Wickwire, J. (1982) Pulmonary embolus and/or pneumonia on K2, in *Hypoxia, Man at Altitude* (eds. J.R. Sutton, N.L. Jones and C.S. Houston), Thieme Stratton, New York, pp. 173–6.

Wiedman, M. and Tabin, G.C. (1999) High-altitude retinopathy and altitude illness. *Ophthalmology* **106**, 1924–6.

Wielicki, K. (1985) Broad peak climbed in one day. *Alpine J.* **90**, 61–3.

Wilber, R.L., Holm, P.L., Morris, D.M., Dallam, G.M. and Callan, S.D. (2003) Effect of F(I)O(2) on physiological responses and cycling performance at moderate altitude. *Med. Sci. Sports Exerc.* **35**, 1153–9.

Wiles, P.G., Grant, P.J., Jones, R.G. *et al.* (1986) Lowered skin blood flow at exhaustion. *Lancet* **2**, 295.

Wilkerson, J.A., Bangs, C.C. and Hayward, J.S. (1986) *Hypothermia, Frostbite and Other Cold Injuries,* The Mountaineers, Seattle, p. 45.

Wilkins, D.C. (1973) Acclimation to heat in the Antarctic, in *Polar Human Biology* (eds. O.G. Edholm and E.K.E. Gunderson), Heinemann Medical, London, pp. 171–81.

Wilkinson, R., Milledge, J.S. and Landon, M.J. (1993) Microalbuminuria in chronic obstructive lung disease. *BMJ* **307**, 239–40.

Will, D.H., McMurty, I.F., Reeves, T.J. *et al.* (1978) Cold-induced pulmonary hypertension in cattle. *J. Appl. Physiol.* **45**, 469–73.

Williams, E.S. (1961) Salivary electrolyte composition at high altitude. *Clin. Sci.* **21**, 37–42.

Williams, E.S. (1975) Mountaineering and the endocrine system, in *Mountain Medicine and Physiology* (eds. C. Clarke, M. Ward and E. Williams), Proceedings of a

Symposium for Mountaineers, Expedition Doctors and Physiologists, Alpine Club, London, pp. 38–44.

Williams, E.S., Ward, M.P., Milledge, J.S., Withey, W.R., Older, M.W.J. and Forsling, M.L. (1979) Effect of the exercise of seven consecutive days hill-walking on fluid homeostasis. *Clin. Sci.* **56**, 305–16.

Willison, J.R., Thomas, D.J., DuBoulay, G.H. *et al.* (1980) Effects of high haematocrit on alertness. *Lancet* **1**, 846–8.

Wilson, D.F., Roy, A. and Lahiri, S. (2005) Immediate and long-term responses of the carotid body to high altitude (Review). *High Alt. Med. Biol.* **6**, 97–111.

Winearls, C.G., Oliver, D.O., Pippard, M.J. *et al.* (1986) Effect of human erythropoietin derived from recombinant DNA on the anaemia of patients maintained by chronic haemodialysis. *Lancet* **2**, 1175–7.

Winkle, R.K., Mader, T.H., Parmley, V.C., White, L.J. and Polse, K.A. (1998) The etiology of refractive changes at high altitude following radial keratotomy: hypoxia versus hypobaria. *Ophthalmology* **105**, 282–6.

Winslow, R.M. and Monge, C.C. (1987) *Hypoxia, Polycythemia, and Chronic Mountain Sickness*, Johns Hopkins University Press, Baltimore, MD. (a) pp. 182–4, (b) pp. 64–74.

Winslow, R.M., Monge, C.C., Statham, N.J. *et al.* (1981) Variability of oxygen affinity of blood: human subjects native to high altitude. *J. Appl. Physiol.* **51**, 1411–16.

Winslow, R.M., Samaja, M. and West, J.B. (1984) Red cell function at extreme altitude on Mount Everest. *J. Appl. Physiol.* **56**, 109–16.

Winslow, R.M., Monge, C.C., Brown, E.G. *et al.* (1985) Effects of hemodilution on O_2 transport in high-altitude polycythemia. *J. Appl. Physiol.* **59**, 1495–502.

Winslow, R.M., Chapman, K.W., Gibson, C.C. *et al.* (1989) Different haematologic response to hypoxia in Sherpas and Quechua Indians. *J. Appl. Physiol.* **66**, 1561–9.

Winter, R.J.D., Melaegros, L., Pervez, S. *et al.* (1987a) Plasma atrial natriuretic factor and ultrastructure of atrial specific granules following chronic hypoxia in rats. *Clin. Sci.* **72**, 26P.

Winter, R.J.D., Davidson, A.C., Treacher, D.F. *et al.* (1987b) Plasma atrial natriuretic factor in chronically hypoxaemic patients with pulmonary hypertension. *Clin. Sci.* **73**, 51P.

Winter, R.J.D., Meleagros, L., Pervez, S. *et al.* (1989) Atrial natriuretic peptide levels in plasma and in cardiac

tissues after chronic hypoxia in rats. *Clin. Sci.* **76**, 95–101.

Winterborn, M., Bradwell, A.R., Chesner, I. and Jones, G. (1986) Mechanisms of proteinuria at high altitude. *Clin. Sci.* **70**, 58P.

Winterstein, H. (1911) Die Regulierung der Atmung durch das Blut. *Pflügers Arch. Ges. Physiol.* **138**, 167–84.

Winterstein, H. (1915) Neue Untersuchungen über die physikalisch-chemische Regulierung der Atmung. *Biochem. Z.* **70**, 45–73.

Withey, W.R., Milledge, J.S., Williams, E.S. *et al.* (1983) Fluid and electrolyte homeostasis during prolonged exercise at altitude. *J. Appl. Physiol.* **55**, 409–12.

Wittenberg, J.B. (1959) Oxygen transport: a new function proposed for myoglobin. *Biol. Bull.* **117**, 402–3.

Wohns, R.N. (1986) Tranisient ischemic attacks at high altitude. *Crit. Care Med.* **14**, 517–8.

Wohns, R.N.W. (1987) Transient ischemic attacks at high altitude, in *Hypoxia and Cold* (eds. J.R. Sutton, C.S. Houston and G. Coates), Praeger, New York, p. 536.

Wolde-Gebriel, Z., Demeke, T., West, C.E. and Van der Haar, F. (1993) Goitre in Ethiopia. *Br. J. Nutr.* **69**, 257–68.

Wolfel, E.E., Groves, B.M., Brooks, G.A. *et al.* (1991) Oxygen transport during steady state submaximal exercise in chronic hypoxia. *J. Appl. Physiol.* **70**, 1129–36.

Wolfel, E.E., Selland, M.A., Mazzeo, R.S. and Reeves, J.T. (1994) Systemic hypertension at 4,300 m is related to sympathoadrenal activity. *J. Appl. Physiol.* **76**, 1643–50.

Wolff, C.B. (1980) Normal ventilation in chronic hypoxia. *J. Physiol.* **308**, 118–19P.

Wolff, C.B. (2000) Cerebral blood flow and oxygen delivery at high altitude. *High Alt. Med. Biol.* **1**, 33–8.

Wood, S., Norboo, T., Lilly, M., Yoneda, K. and Eldridge, M. (2003) Cardiopulmonary function in high altitude residents of Ladakh. *High Alt. Med. Biol.* **4**, 445–54.

Woods, D., Hickman, M., Jamshidi ,Y. *et al.* (2001) Elite swimmers and the D allele of the ACE I/D polymorphism. *Hum. Genet.* **108**, 230–2.

Woods, D.R. and Montgomery, H.E. (2001) Angiotensin-converting enzyme and genetics at high altitude. *High Alt. Med. Biol.* **2**, 201–10.

Woods, D.R., Brull, D. and Montgomery, H.E. (2000) Endurance and the ACE gene. *Sci. Prog.* **83**, 317–36.

Woods, D.R., Pollard, A.J., Collier, D.J. *et al.* (2002) Insertion/deletion polymorphism of the angiotensin

I-converting enzyme gene and arterial oxygen saturation at high altitude. *Am. J. Respir. Crit. Care Med.* **166**, 362–6.

Woolcott, O.O., Castillo, O.A., Torres, J., Damas, L. and Florentini, E. (2002) Serum leptin levels in dwellers from high altitude lands. *High Alt. Med. Biol.* **3**, 245–6.

Wren, A.M., Seal, L.J., Cohen, M.A. *et al.* (2001) Ghrelin enhances appetite and increases food intake in humans *J. Clin. Endocrinol. Metabol.* **86**, 5992–5.

Wright, A.D., Imray, C.H., Morrissey, M.S., Marchbanks, R.J. and Bradwell, A.R. (1995) Intracranial pressure at high altitude and acute mountain sickness. *Clin. Sci.* **89**, 201–4.

Wu, T.Y. (1994a) Low prevalence of systemic hypertension in Tibetan native highlanders. *ISMM Newsletter* **4**(1), 5–7.

Wu, T. (1994b) Children on the Tibetan plateau. *ISMM Newsletter* **4**(3), 5–6.

Wu, T.Y. (2000) Take note of altitude gastrointestinal bleeding. *ISMM Newsletter* **10**(2), 9–10.

Wu, T.Y. (2005) Chronic mountain sickness on the Qinghai–Tibetan plateau. *Chin. Med. J.* **118**, 161–8.

Wu, T-Y. and Liu, Y.R. (1995) High altitude heart disease. *Chin. J. Pediatr.* **6**, 348–50.

Wu, T-Y., Zhang, Q., Jin, B. *et al.* (1992) Chronic mountain sickness (Monge's disease): an observation in Quinghai–Tibet plateau, in *High Altitude Medicine* (eds. G. Ueda, J.T. Reeves and M. Sekiguchi), Sinshu University Press, Matsumoto, pp. 314–24.

Wu, T., Wang, X., Wei, C. *et al.* (2005) Hemoglobin levels in Qinghai-Tibet: different effects of gender for Tibetans versus Han. *J. Appl. Physiol.* **98**, 598–604. E-pub 16 July 2004.

Xie, Y., Zhu, W.Z., Zhu, Y., Chen, L., Zhou, Z.N. and Yang, H.T. (2004) Intermittent high altitude hypoxia protects the heart against lethal Ca^{2+} overload injury. *Life Sci.* **76**, 559–72.

Xu, F. and Severinghaus, J.W. (1998) Rat brain VEGF expression in alveolar hypoxia: possible role in high-altitude cerebral edema. *J. Appl. Physiol.* **85**, 53–7.

Xu, K. and Lamanna, J.C. (2006) Chronic hypoxia and the cerebral circulation. *J. Appl. Physiol.* **100**, 725–30.

Yagi, H., Yamada, H., Kobayashi, T. and Sekiguchi, M. (1990) Doppler assessment of pulmonary hypertension induced by hypoxic breathing in subjects susceptible to high altitude pulmonary edema. *Am. Rev. Respir. Dis.* **142**, 796–801.

Yamaguchi, S., Matsuzawa, S., Yoshikawa, S. *et al.* (1991) Effect of acclimatization and deacclimatization on hypoxic ventilatory response. *Jpn. J. Mount. Med.* **11**, 77–84.

Yamamoto, W.S. and Edwards, M.W. (1960) Homeostasis of carbon dioxide during intra-venous infusion of carbon dioxide. *J. Appl. Physiol.* **15**, 807–18.

Yanagidaira, Y., Sakai, A., Kashimura, O. *et al.* (1994) The effects of prolonged exposure to cold on hypoxic pulmonary hypertension in rats. *J. Wilderness Med.* **5**, 11–19.

Yanda, R.L. and Herschensohn, H.L. (1964) Changes in lung volumes of emphysema patients upon short exposures to simulated altitude of 18,000 feet. *Aerosp. Med.* **35**, 1201–3.

Yang, S.P., Bergo, G.W., Krasney, E. and Krasney, J.A. (1994) Cerebral pressure-flow and metabolic responses to sustained hypoxia: effect of CO2. *J. Appl. Physiol.* **76**, 303–13.

Yarnell, P.R., Heit, J. and Hackett, P.H. (2000) High-altitude cerebral edema (HACE): the Denver/Front Range experience. *Semin. Neurol.* **20**, 209–17.

Yaron, M., Waldman, N., Niermeyer, S. *et al.* (1998) The diagnosis of acute mountain sickness in preverbal children. *Arch. Pediatr. Adolesc. Med.* **152**, 683–7.

Yaron, M., Niermeyer, S., Lindgren, K.N. and Honigman, B. (2002) Evaluation of diagnostic criteria and incidence of acute mountain sickness in preverbal children. *Wild. Environ. Med.* **13**, 21–6.

Yaron, M., Niermeyer, S., Lindgren, K.N., Honigman, B., Strain, J.D. and Cairns, C.B. (2003) Physiologic response to moderate altitude exposure among infants and young children. *High Alt. Med. Biol.* **4**, 53–9.

Yaron, M., Lindgren, K.N., Halbower, A.C., Weisberg, M., Reite, M. and Niermeyer, S. (2004) *High Alt. Med. Biol.* **5**, 314–20.

Yoneda, I. and Watanabe, Y. (1997) Comparison of altitude tolerance and hypoxia symptoms between non-smokers and habitual smokers. *Aviat. Space Environ. Med.* **68**, 807–11.

Young, A.J., Muza, S.R., Sawka, M.N. *et al.* (1986) Human thermo-regulatory responses to cold air are altered by repeated cold water immersion. *J. Appl. Physiol.* **60**, 1542–8.

Young, P.M., Rose, M.S., Sutton, J.R. *et al.* (1989) Operation Everest II: plasma lipid and hormonal responses during a simulated ascent of Mt Everest. *J. Appl. Physiol.* **66**, 1430–5.

Young, A.J., Sawka, M.N., Muza, S.R. *et al.* (1996) Effects of erythrocyte infusion on V_{o2max} at high altitude. *J. Appl. Physiol.* **81**, 252–9.

Young, A.J., Castellani, J.W., O'Brian, C. *et al.* (1998) Exertional fatigue, sleeplessness and negative energy balance increases susceptibility to hypothermia. *J. Appl. Physiol.* **85**, 1210–17.

Zacarian, S.A. (1985) Cryogenics: the cryolesions and the pathogenesis of cryonecrosis, in *Cryosurgery for Skin and Cutaneous Diseases,* Mosby, St Louis, MO.

Zaccaria, M., Rocco, S., Noventa, D. *et al.* (1998) Sodium regulating hormones at high altitude: basal and post-exercise levels. *J. Clin. Endocrinol. Metab.* **83**, 570–4.

Zaccaria, M., Ermolao, A., Bonvicini, P., Travain, G. and Varnier, M. (2004) Decreased serum leptin levels during prolonged high altitude exposure. *Eur. J. Appl. Physiol.* **92**, 249–53.

Zafren, K. (1998) Hyponatremia in a cold environment. *Wild. Environ. Med.* **9**, 54–5.

Zafren, K., Reeves, J.T. and Schoene, R. (1996) Treatment of high-altitude pulmonary edema by bed rest and supplemental oxygen. *Wild. Environ. Med.* **7**, 127–32.

Zamudio, S .(1997) Ovarian Hormone Influences on Fluid Volume Regulation at High Altitude, in *Women at Altitude* (eds. C.S. Houston and G. Coates), Queen City Printers, Inc., Burlington, VT, pp. 35–41.

Zamudio, S. (2003) The placenta at high altitude (Review). *High Alt. Med. Biol.* **4**, 171–91.

Zamudio, S., Baumann, M.U. and Illsley, N.P. (2006) Effects of chronic hypoxia in vivo on the expression of human placental glucose transporters. *Placenta* **27**, 49–55.

Zhang, E.G., Burton, G.J., Smith, S.K., Charnock-Jones, D.S. (2002) Placental vessel adaptation during gestation and to high altitude: changes in diameter and perivascular cell coverage. *Placenta* **23**, 751–62.

Zhang, Y.B. (1985) *An Introduction to Medical Research in Qinghai*, High Altitude Medical Research Institute, Qinghai, China.

Zhao, L., Mason, N.A., Morrell, N.W. *et al.* (2001) Sildenafil inhibits hypoxia-induced pulmonary hypertension. *Circulation* **104**, 424–8.

Zhongyuan, S., Xuehan, N., Shoucheng, Z. *et al.* (1980) Electrocardiogram made on ascending the mount Qomolangma from 50 m A.S.L. *Sci. Sin.* **23**, 1316–25.

Zhongyuan, S., Deming, Z., Changming, L. and Miaoshen, Q. (1983) Changes of electroencephalogram under acute hypoxia and relationship between tolerant ability to hypoxia and adaptation ability to high altitudes. *Sci. Sin.* **26**, 58–69.

Zhu, W.Z., Xie, Y., Chen, L., Yang, H.T. and Zhou, Z.N. (2006) Intermittent high altitude hypoxia inhibits opening of mitochondrial permeability transition pores against reperfusion injury. *J. Mol. Cell. Cardiol.* **40**, 96–106. E-pub 8 November2005.

Zhuang, J., Droma, T., Sun, S. *et al.* (1993) Hypoxic ventilatory responsiveness in Tibetan compared with Han residents of 3,658 m. *J. Appl. Physiol.* **74**, 303–11.

Zieliński J., Koziej, M., Mańkowski, M. *et al.* (2000) The quality of sleep and periodic breathing in healthy subjects at an altitude of 3200 metres: sleep at high altitude. *High Alt. Med. Biol.* **1**, 331–6.

Zimmerman, G.A. and Crapo, R.O. (1980) Adult respiratory distress syndrome secondary to high altitude pulmonary edema. *West. J. Med.* **133**, 335–7.

Zuntz, N., Loewy, A., Müller, F. and Caspari, W. (1906) *Höhenklima und Bergwanderungen in ihrer Wirkung auf den Menschen,* Bong, Berlin. An English translation of the relevant passages can be found in *High Altitude Physiology* (ed. J.B. West), Hutchinson Ross, Stroudsburg, PA, 1981.

Index